The Financial Management of Hospitals

Fourth Edition

The Financial Management of Hospitals

Fourth Edition

by
Howard J. Berman
and
Lewis E. Weeks

Health Administration Press
Ann Arbor, MI
1979

Printing History

First Edition
First Printing—November 1971
Second Printing—January 1973
Third Printing—July 1973

Second Edition
First Printing—March 1974
Second Printing—November 1974
Third Printing—July 1975
Fourth Printing—June 1976

Third Edition
First Printing—August 1976
Second Printing—November 1977
Third Printing—November 1978

Fourth Edition
First Printing—September 1979

Library of Congress Cataloging in Publication Data

Berman, Howard J
  The financial management of hospitals.

  Bibliography: p.
  Includes index.
  I. Hospitals—Business management. 2. Hospitals—
Finance. I. Weeks, Lewis E., joint author.
II. Title.
RA971.3.B48 1979   658.1'5932   79-16947
ISBN 0-914904-33-7

To Marilyn and Frances, our wives, for their patience and understanding about the demands of time this manuscript has taken.

Foreword

When my good friends and colleagues, Howard Berman and Lew Weeks, advised me that they were in the process of completing still another edition of *The Financial Management of Hospitals* my reaction was one of some incredulity. After all, it was only yesterday or thereabouts that the last edition appeared (actually it was 1976). And when they subsequently did me the honor of asking that I provide a foreword to the new edition, as with the previous three, I concluded that I might be regarded as somewhat of a talisman in view of the enormously successful reception of the predecessors!

But it is with considerable vicarious pride and satisfaction that these comments are made: pride in that the field-at-large has so well recognized the merits of the publication in its various versions and satisfaction in that at long last a critical need is being addressed, i.e., the emergence of solid material specific to hospital financial management, which this publication so well typifies.

The Financial Management of Hospitals in all of its editions has kept foremost the needs of two audiences, the respective worlds of practice and academia. The authors have succeeded admirably in serving both.

Obviously a further edition suggests both new material and the updating of old, and such is amply evident in this latest version. And again this fact well reflects the dynamics of the era as applied to hospital financial management and the book's considerable value to practitioner, teacher, and student alike in this context.

The term "classic" is sometimes rather loosely applied in the literature of all fields, but such an encomium seems appropriate to the volume that is now in your hands. The 1971 First Edition appeared when there was an appalling paucity of relevant literature. Fortunately that circumstance has substantially changed in less than a decade, but *The Financial Management of Hospitals* continues in its reincarnations as an invaluable resource.

Andrew Pattullo
Senior Vice President
W. K. Kellogg Foundation
Battle Creek, Michigan
April 3, 1979

Preface

The authors have been gratified by the reception and recognition which the previous editions of this work have received. We hope that this, the fourth edition, warrants the continued acceptance by both our colleagues and our students. It has been prepared with careful regard to their comments, criticisms, and quality standards.

In writing the edition, we have attempted to revise and update the third edition both to reflect the changing health care financial environment and to make it a more complete reference and teaching document. Each chapter has been reviewed and material has been added or modified as necessary. Statistical data has also been updated to reflect current performance and facts. In particular, Part II has been revised adding material on legislated rate review as well as a new section on Medicaid. The chapter on the "future" has been revised to reflect the implications of recent social and economic developments and changes in public attitudes. Also, the Bibliography has been changed and enlarged to capture the growing body of literature.

As was the case with the previous editions, the responsibility for any errors or oversights must lie with the authors. The credit for any contributions which this work might make, however, must still accrue to our colleagues who have advised us and to our students who have taught us.

Particular appreciation should also be expressed to all those who helped with the previous editions and to Maureen Dillon, Louise Kurylo, Arthur Leyland, and Joan Miller for their help and advice in preparing this edition.

Howard J. Berman
Lewis E. Weeks

HOWARD J. BERMAN was Assistant Professor of Hospital Administration, the Program in Hospital Administration, the University of Michigan, when the first edition of this book was originally written. He presently is a Vice President of the American Hospital Association. He received his bachelor's degree from the University of Illinois in finance and his master's in hospital administration from the University of Michigan. He has contibuted articles on hospital finance and management to various journals in the health field and has lectured to both hospital and financial managers. He has served as a member of the Task Force on Financial Management of the Association of University Programs in Health Administration. Currently he serves on the Advisory Board of the Cooperative Information Center and the Editorial Boards of *Inquiry* and *Topics in Health Care Financing*. Additionally, he holds a faculty appointment at the University of Chicago.

LEWIS E. WEEKS until recently was editor of *Abstracts of Hospital Management Studies* and of the Cooperative Information Center for Hospital Management Studies at the University of Michigan. He was the founding editor of the Health Administration Press. Presently he is the editor of INQUIRY. He received his master's degree in history from the University of Michigan and his doctorate in communication arts from Michigan State University. He has written articles for health profession journals and a monograph on Progressive Patient Care. He was coeditor with John R. Griffith of *Progressive Patient Care: An Anthology* and coauthor with John R. Griffith and James H. Sullivan of *The McPherson Experiment*. With John R. Griffith and Robert A. DeVries he was coauthor of the Research Report, *A Reappraisal of the McPherson Experiment in Progressive Patient Care*. He was editor of *Education of a Hospital Trustee*. He was coeditor with Howard J. Berman of *Economics in Health Care* and coeditor with Howard J. Berman and Gerald E. Bisbee, Jr. of *The Financing of Health Care*.

Contents

Part I
Introduction

"Management progress begins with an understanding of why, and proceeds based on a knowledge of how."—Seth

Chapter 1

Financial Management

The notion that competent financial management is necessary for efficient and effective hospital operations is accepted as a truism by most administrators. Why, however, is competent financial management necessary? What is financial management's usefulness or value in hospital operations and how can this usefulness be maximized?

Usually and erroneously, financial management is associated with the complex and often confusing world of accounting and seemingly esoteric tools (cash flow analysis, statements of sources and uses of funds, and budgets) which accompany the practice of accounting. It has been viewed historically as a specialized area of management; separate and apart from the general management of operations. This has been due primarily to the fact that:

1. Financial management personnel have *failed to communicate* with operational management; they have not directed their efforts and reports to the needs of other managers and the hospital in total.
2. Operational management has been focusing its attention on individual functions rather than concentrating and coordinating all aspects of the operation toward achievement of a common objective.

Thus, financial management traditionally has not been a part of the mainstream of operational management.

This traditional role and position, however, is changing and financial management is rapidly becoming an integral component of total operational management. What is the operational benefit of this change? In order to answer not only this question but also

1

those set out above, it is first necessary to define the objective of management.

Objective of Management

In the case of the commercial enterprise the objective of management is not difficult to identify. It is basically that of maximizing owner's wealth. Quite simply, management must administer the assets of the enterprise in order to obtain the greatest wealth for the owners; i.e., management must maximize the value $E/R = W$, where "E" is the earning or profits from the assets, "R" is the capitalization rate or the subjective estimate of the likelihood of receiving the projected profits from the assets, and "W" is the value of the firm or the owner's wealth.

Given that management's objective is to maximize owner's wealth, the usefulness of financial management becomes clear. However, as indicated above, owner's wealth (W) is a function of the earnings (E) of the firm and the risk associated with the actual receipt of those earnings (R). Therefore, management's goal is to find that combination of E and R which will yield the highest possible value of W. In order to do this, management must not only use its general managerial skills, i.e., planning, organizing, coordinating, motivating, and controlling to maximize E, but also its financial management skills to evaluate and select earnings streams and minimize R. Thus, if management is to maximize W, it must either be lucky or use financial tools and techniques.

In the case of a nonprofit enterprise, such as a voluntary hospital, where the guidelines of return on investment and profitability are either not available or not meaningful, the objective of management is somewhat more difficult to define. If one assumes that a hospital is needed, i.e., the community is not overbedded, then intuitively one could suggest that the long run objective of hospital management is to perpetuate the continued operation of the hospital by ensuring that total revenues at least equal total costs or expenses. However, this objective, while obviously realistic and pragmatic, is limited in scope and overly simplistic, for it focuses on only one aspect of management's responsibilities. It ignores not only the basic health care function and purpose of the hospital, but also management's obligation to the community which a hospital serves. Therefore, it is unacceptable and must be expanded and modified.

Hospitals are vital and necessary community resources. As such, they should be managed for the benefit of the community. Therefore, in the case of a hospital, the objective of management should be to provide the community with the services which it needs, at an acceptable level of quality, and at the least possible cost. This objective not only implicitly includes the foregoing revenue cost equality goal, for the hospital must continue in existence if it is to provide service to the community, but also goes beyond it. It both establishes management's responsibility to the community and provides a general set of operating criteria.

It should be noted that other objective functions have been suggested for hospital management. These alternatives range from the simple, but realistic, objective of employment security to profit maximization. Between these extremes are management goals such as, recovery of cost, output maximization, quality maximization, output and quality maximization, and cash flow maximization. While these various goals have been hypothesized, none has been subjected to vigorous empirical testing. Moreover, they all lack pragmatic insight into either the social/societal role of the hospital, the realities of hospital financing, or the intrinsically dynamic nature of a hospital's operating requirements. Nevertheless, they can be useful analytical devices; while not substituting for the strategic and planning value of the foregoing statement of management's objective, they do provide an added dimension for understanding operational behavior.

Value of Financial Management

Given this objective, the value of financial management can be readily seen. Primarily, financial management tools and techniques can aid management in providing the community with quality services at least cost by furnishing the data which are necessary for making intelligent capital investment decisions, by guiding the operations of certain hospital subsystems, and by providing the systems and data needed to monitor and control operations.

Financial management techniques, such as present value (discounted flow) analysis and internal rate of return analysis, can be used to determine the cost implications of the various capital investment opportunities available to a hospital. These techniques provide management with the quantitative data which are needed not only to develop capital budgets knowledgeably, but also to take advantage of investment opportunities which will reduce the cost of care.

Admittedly, cost is not the only factor which should be considered in hospital investment decisions. The needs of the com-

Figure 1-1

Operational Value and Usefulness of Financial Management

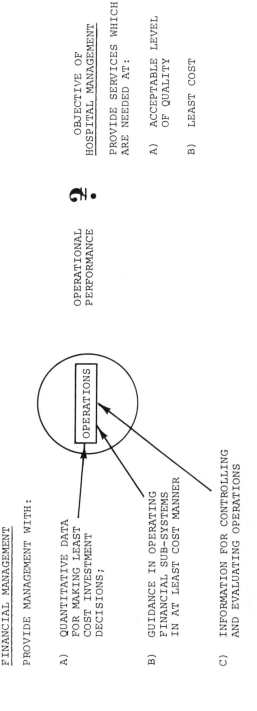

FINANCIAL MANAGEMENT

PROVIDE MANAGEMENT WITH:

A) QUANTITATIVE DATA FOR MAKING LEAST COST INVESTMENT DECISIONS;

B) GUIDANCE IN OPERATING FINANCIAL SUB-SYSTEMS IN AT LEAST COST MANNER

C) INFORMATION FOR CONTROLLING AND EVALUATING OPERATIONS

OPERATIONS

OPERATIONAL PERFORMANCE

OBJECTIVE OF HOSPITAL MANAGEMENT

PROVIDE SERVICES WHICH ARE NEEDED AT:

A) ACCEPTABLE LEVEL OF QUALITY

B) LEAST COST

FINANCIAL MANAGEMENT PROVIDES DATA AND MANAGEMENT TECHNIQUES WHICH CAN ASSIST MANAGEMENT IN GUIDING OPERATIONAL PERFORMANCE IN ORDER TO MEET THE HOSPITAL'S OBJECTIVE.

munity, the level of quality, and the capacity of the organization to achieve the various alternatives must also be weighed in the decision process. At times, these noneconomic factors may transcend cost implications and management may select other than the least cost alternative. However, if management is to make this decision wisely, it must be aware of the cost implications of the various alternative opportunities. This awareness can only be obtained through the use of the above financial management techniques.

Financial management tools and techniques also can aid management in a more direct way than just providing quantitative information for capital investment decision making. A hospital can be viewed as a complex system composed of a number of simple subsystems. Some of these subsystems, such as accounts payable and receivable management, cash and short-term investment management and inventory management, are basically financial activities and can be operated at least cost through the use of such financial practices and techniques as: accounts receivable factoring, economic order quantity models, cash forecasting, internal control procedures, etc.

Additionally, financial management tools can help management to meet its objectives in a third way. Cost finding reports, expense and revenue budgets, and position and operating statements provide management with the information necessary to control internal operations.

Cost finding provides data on actual operational performance by cost center. This information can be compared to budgeted performance expectations in order to identify problem areas which require attention and to obtain an index of operational performance. These data, along with information provided via the position and operating statements, will also give management the material needed to evaluate and control the hospital's capital structure, i.e., evaluate and control the proportion of capital obtained from various sources.

Cost finding is also of value to management in another way. If, over the long run, revenues are to at least equal expenses or costs, then management must, as accurately as possible, determine the costs of each revenue producing area. Cost finding is the best available technique for accomplishing this. The data obtained through cost finding furnish not only the information necessary for negotiating equitable reimbursement rates with third party payers but also, when combined with a schedule of charges and a revenue budget, the information necessary for establishing an adequate charge structure. Obviously, both of these functions must be carried out successfully if management is to ensure a revenue-expense equality and the continued existence of the hospital.

Thus, financial management can play a critical role in assisting management to achieve its operational objective (see Figure 1-1). Its usefulness, though mainly in the areas of cost control and reduction, is not limited to these factors. As has been indicated, financial management techniques are of help in assuring a revenue-expense equality. However, this and other uses of financial management tools are basically by-products, flowing almost automatically from its primary cost and operational control values.

A Word of Clarification

A pause should be made at this time in order to clarify a point. The discussion so far in the book has focused on financial management and its importance in operating any type of enterprise. It should be made clear that throughout the chapter financial management rather than accounting was emphasized and that the importance of the financial manager and not that of the accountant was being stressed. The distinction being drawn may appear subtle and perhaps even unimportant. However, it is critical and deserves this moment of clarification in order to minimize future misunderstandings.

Financial management, as previously mentioned, is usually associated with the practice of accounting. However, though the two may be associated, they are not synonymous. Accounting can be described as the art of collecting, summarizing, analyzing, reporting, and interpreting in monetary terms, information about the enterprise. This is an important function, but is is not financial management.

Financial management can be described as the art both of obtaining the funds which the enterprise needs in the most economic manner and of making the optimal use of those funds once obtained. Financial management can then be viewed as a decision process. Like all decision processes it needs information and facts if it is to function accurately, and certain techniques and tools if it is to function efficiently. Financial management techniques and tools provide the means for efficiency. The accounting system and the accountant provide the data needed for accuracy.

The two functions then are linked, with financial management building on accounting. Financial management utilizes accounting, and the information it produces, to determine how to more effectively operate the enterprise. The difference between the two can be viewed as one of scope, for financial management both includes and goes beyond accounting.

This difference in scope makes it important that we expand our horizon and not talk or think in terms of accounting only, but rather in terms of financial management and the financial manager. An accountant with an enlarged scope and perspective of operation can be a financial manager. However, accounting, by definition, cannot be financial management, for its goal is informational—not operational.

Financial management is accounting—plus. It is the use of the data generated by the accounting system for improved operations. In view of today's political climate and management environment, improved operations, and hence financial management, are necessities.

Organization of the Text

The answers to the questions posed at the outset of this discussion should now be obvious. Competent financial management is a necessity for efficient hospital management, for it provides the information and tools necessary for controlling operations and reducing costs. The objective of this text is to acquaint the health services manager with both the potential which exists for improved operations through the use of the foregoing financial management tools, and the mechanics of these tools.

It is neither expected nor hoped that an administrator will develop a sufficient facility with the tools and mechanics which will be discussed to perform personally the financial management function in his hospital. However, it is hoped that he will develop a sufficient familiarity and understanding of financial management to be cognizant of the need for competent financial management, to be aware of the tools and techniques which should be utilized, and to be able to evaluate the performance of his financial manager. It is to this end that the following text is designed.

Part I—Introduction—is intended to provide the reader with the background material and an initial understanding of the financial environment in which a hospital exists. Chapter 2 sets out the accounting principles and conventions which apply to hospitals, and Chapter 3 discusses the internal organization which is necessary for effective financial management. Part II—Sources of Operating Revenue—can also be considered to be background material, though of a somewhat different nature.

It is unusual to include a section on sources of operating revenue in a financial management text. However, hospitals maintain a unique operating relationship with their sources of revenue, i.e., with third party purchasers of care. Hospitals, while treating many individual patients, are paid for services which they provide to these individuals by relatively few sources. These sources, because of their economic power, are able to affect substantially the financial status of an individual hospital by the method or procedure which they use to pay that hospital. Therefore, if one is to understand the financial parameters within which a hospital operates and within which financial management in general and working capital management in particular must function, it is necessary first to understand how hospitals are paid and what can be the effect of this payment mechanism.

Part II discusses in detail the nature of the hospital-third party relationship, the philosophies and payment guidelines of various third party cost based reimbursement agreements, and the mechanics of determining hospital costs. Additionally, in order to fully cover the subject areas, the mechanics of rate setting are also examined in this part.

Working Capital Management—Part III—builds on the foundation set out in Part II. It examines the operation of the financial subsystems of the hospital and the application and usefulness of financial management techniques in operating these systems in a least cost manner. The emphasis of this section is both on defining the nature, sources, and costs of working capital and on discussing how financial management techniques can be used not only to minimize a hospital's investment in working capital but also to maximize the return which can be obtained from those assets which must be so invested. Each component of working capital is examined and the techniques for determining the optimal level of investment in each asset are explored. Also included in this section is a discussion of the management reports which are needed to effectively evaluate, control, and guide working capital operations.

Part IV is a section of four chapters on the budget: its value in financial management; its preparation; its effect on staff participation and accountability; and its need for a reporting system.

Part V is a brief section which focuses on the future trends in hospital financing and on the nature of the operational environment which can be expected. Like all projections it is a bit speculative. Nevertheless, it serves to bring into an interesting focus a variety of critical issues.

The organization of the text has been designed first to build a knowledge of the financial environment of the hospital and then,

based upon this knowledge, to examine specific financial management tools and their application and utilization in hospital management. Thus, there is a pyramiding and increasing sophistication of the subject matter, culminating in an understanding of
financial reports and the knowledge necessary to both evaluate the
operations of the financial subsystems of a hospital and determine
the nature of needed changes and improvements.

Suggested Readings*

General

American Institute of Certified Public Accountants. *Hospital Audit
Guide.*
Berman, Howard J. "Financial Management: Necessity or Nicety?" *Hos-
pital Administration*, Summer 1970.
Cleverly, William O. *Financial Management of Health Care Facilities*,
Selections.
Davis, Karen, "Economic Theories of Behavior in Nonprofit, Private Hos-
pitals." *Economic and Business Bulletin*, Winter 1972.
Lindsay, Robert, Jr. and Sametz, Arnold W. *Financial Management, An
Analytical Approach*, Chapter 2.
Silvers, J.B. "Identity Crisis: Financial Management in Health." *Health
Care Management Review*, Fall 1976.
Symonds, Curtis W. *Basic Financial Management*, Chapter 1.
Warren, David G. *Problems in Hospital Law, Third Edition*, Chapters 14
and 15.

Budgeting

American Hospital Association. *Budgeting Procedures for Hospitals.*
Bartizal, John R. *Budget Principles and Procedures.*
Durbin, Richard L. and Springall, W. Herbert. *Organization and Admin-
istration of Health Care*, Chapter 8.

Cost Control

American Hospital Association. *Cost Finding and Rate Setting for Hospitals.*
Bulloch, James. "Responsibility Accounting—A Results Oriented Appraisal System." *Management of Personnel Quarterly*, Winter 1964, pp.
25–31.

---

*Full publishing details for works cited in Suggested Readings will be found in
Bibliography A or B at the end of this volume.

Foyle, William R. "Evaluations of Methods of Cost Analysis."

Hiett, Tee H., Jr. "Fiscal Controls for Hospital Departments." *Proceedings Eighteenth Annual Institute of American Institute of Industrial Engineers,* pp. 158–163.

Capital Investment Decisions

American Hospital Association. *Capital Financing for Hospitals.*

Griffith, John R. *Quantitative Techniques for Hospital Planning and Control.*

Quirin, G. David. *The Capital Expenditure Decision.*

Van Horne, James C. *Financial Management and Policy, Part II.*

Appendix 1-A Corporate Tax Statutes of Hospitals

As has been indicated, the objective of this text is to acquaint the administrator of a nonprofit hospital with both the potential which exists for improved operations through the use of financial management tools and the mechanics of such tools. However, before going on, it should be made clear what is meant by "nonprofit." Perhaps the best technique for clarifying the meaning of "nonprofit" is to review the Internal Revenue Code, for "nonprofit" is a term which primarily relates to the hospital's tax status.

Summary of the Internal Revenue Code[1]

Corporate Taxation—Section 11

    A. A tax is hereby imposed for each taxable year on the taxable income of every corporation.

    B. The tax is to be progressive in nature ranging from 17 to 46 percent of taxable income.[2]

Exemption from Corporate Taxation—Section 501-C-3

    A. Corporations operated exclusively for religious, charitable, safety or educational purposes are exempt from corporate

---

[1]Internal Revenue Code of 1954 as amended to date.

[2]

Taxable Income	Rate
$0–$25,000	17%
$25,001–$50,000	20%
$50,001–$75,000	30%
$75,001–$100,000	40%
Over $100,000	46%

taxes if no part of their net earnings goes to the benefit of any private individual.

B. In order to qualify for exemption, hospitals must meet the following requirements:[3]
   1) be organized as a nonprofit, charitable organization whose purpose is caring for the sick;
   2) not restrict the use of its facilities to a particular group of physicians or surgeons.

Maintenance of Exemption—Section 503

A. A hospital, in order to maintain its tax exemption, must refrain from engaging in any prohibited transactions.

B. Prohibited transactions are defined as any transaction in which a Section 501-C-3 corporation:
   1) lends any part of its income without receiving adequate security or interest;
   2) pays any compensation in excess of reasonable salary levels;
   3) makes any investments for more than adequate consideration;
   4) sells any assets for less than adequate consideration;
   5) subverts in any other manner substantial portions of its income or assets.

C. If a hospital engages in any of these acts with an individual who is either an owner or an employee of the hospital, then it is engaging in a prohibited transaction and cannot maintain its tax exemption.

Thus, "nonprofit" does not mean that the hospital cannot earn a profit. Rather, it simply means that no part of the hospital's net earnings (profit) can inure to the benefit of any private individual. It is in this sense that the term will be used in this text.

Appendix 1-B Revenue Ruling 69-545[4]

Advice has been requested whether the two nonprofit hospitals described below qualify for exemption from Federal income tax

---

[3]It should be noted that in the original Code, a third requirement was also included; "operate to the extent of its financial ability, for the benefit of those not able to pay for services."

[4]Also released as Technical Information Release 1022, dated Oct. 8, 1969.

under section 501(c)(3) of the Internal Revenue Code of 1954. The articles of organization of both hospitals meet the organizational requirements of section 1.501(c)(3)-1(b) of the Income Tax Regulations, including the limitation of the organizations' purposes to those described in section 501(c)(3) of the Code and the dedication of their assets to such purposes.

Situation 1. Hospital A is a 250-bed community hospital. Its board of trustees is composed of prominent citizens in the community. Medical staff privileges in the hospital are available to all qualified physicians in the area, consistent with the size and nature of its facilities. The hospital has 150 doctors on its active staff and 200 doctors on its courtesy staff. It also owns a medical office building on its premises with space for sixty doctors. Any member of its active medical staff has the privilege of leasing available office space. Rents are set at the rates comparable to those of other commercial buildings in the area.

The hospital operates a full time emergency room and no one requiring emergency care is denied treatment. The hospital otherwise ordinarily limits admissions to those who can pay the cost of their hospitalization, either themselves, or through private health insurance, or with the aid of public programs such as Medicare. Patients who cannot meet the financial requirements for admission are ordinarily referred to another hospital in the community that does serve indigent patients.

The hospital usually ends each year with an excess of operating receipts over operating disbursements from its hospital operations. Excess funds are generally applied to expansion and replacement of existing facilities and equipment, amortization of indebtedness, improvement in patient care, and medical training, education, and research.

Situation 2. Hospital B is a 60-bed general hospital which was originally owned by five doctors. The owners formed a nonprofit organization and sold their interests in the hospital to the organization at fair market value. The board of trustees of the organization consists of the five doctors, their accountant, and their lawyer. The five doctors also comprise the hospital's medical committee and thereby control the selection and the admission of other doctors to the medical staff. During its first five years of operations, only four other doctors have been granted staff privileges at the hospital. The applications of a number of qualified doctors in the community have been rejected.

Hospital admission is restricted to patients of doctors holding staff privileges. Patients of the five original physicians have accounted for a large majority of all hospital admissions over the years. The hospital maintains an emergency room, but on a relatively inactive basis, and primarily for the convenience of the patients of the staff doctors. The local ambulance services have been instructed by the hospital to take emergency cases to other hospitals in the area. The hospital follows the policy of ordinarily limiting admissions to those who can pay the cost of the services rendered. The five doctors comprising the original medical staff have continued to maintain their offices in the hospital since its sale to the nonprofit organization. The rental paid is less than that of comparable office space in the vicinity. No office space is available for any of the other staff members.

Section 501(c)(3) of the Code provides for exemption from Federal income tax of organizations organized and operated exclusively for charitable, scientific, or educational purposes, no part of the net earnings of which inures to the benefit of any private shareholder or individual.

Section 1.501(c)(3)-1(d)(2) of the regulations provides that an organization is not organized or operated exclusively for any purpose set forth in section 501(c)(3) of the Code unless it serves a public rather than a private interest.

Section 1.501(c)(3)-1(d)(2) of the regulations states that the term "charitable" is used in section 501(c)(3) of the Code in its generally acceptable legal sense.

To qualify for exemption from Federal income tax under section 501(c)(3) of the Code, a nonprofit hospital must be organized and operated exclusively in furtherance of some purpose considered "charitable" in the generally accepted legal sense of that term, and the hospital may not be operated, directly or indirectly, for the benefit of private interests.

In the general law of charity, the promotion of health is considered to be a charitable purpose. "Restatement (Second), Trusts," sec. 368 and sec. 372; "IV Scott on Trusts" (3rd ed. 1967), sec. 368 and sec. 372. A nonprofit organization whose purpose and activity are providing hospital care is promoting health and may, therefore, qualify as organized and operated in furtherance of a charitable purpose. If it meets the other requirements of section 501(c)(3) of the Code, it will qualify for exemption from Federal income tax under section 501(a).

Since the purpose and activity of Hospital A, apart from its related educational and research activities and purposes, are providing hospital care on a nonprofit basis for members of its community, it is organized and operated in furtherance of a purpose considered "charitable" in the generally accepted legal sense of that term. The promotion of health, like the relief of poverty and the advancement of education and religion, is one of the purposes in the general law of charity that is deemed beneficial to the community as a whole even though the class of beneficiaries eligible to receive a direct benefit from its activities does not include all members of the community, such as indigent members of the community, provided that the class is not so small that its relief is not of benefit to the community. "Restatement (Second), Trust," sec. 368, comment (b) and sec. 372, comments (b) and (c); "IV Scott on Trusts" (3rd ed. 1967), sec. 368 and sec. 372.2. By operating an emergency room open to all persons and by providing hospital care to all those persons in the community able to pay the cost thereof either directly or through third party reimbursement, Hospital A is promoting the health of a class of persons that is broad enough to benefit the community.

The fact that Hospital A operates at an annual surplus of receipts over disbursements does not preclude its exemption. By using its surplus funds to improve the quality of patient care, expand its facilities, and advance its medical training, education, and research programs, the hospital is operating in furtherance of its exempt purposes.

Furthermore, Hospital A is operated to serve a public rather than a private interest. Control of the hospital rests with its board of trustees, which is composed of independent civic leaders. The hospital maintains an open medical staff, with privileges available to all qualified physicians. Members of its active medical staff have the privilege of leasing available space in its medical building. (For more information see Revenue Ruling 69-464). It operates an active and generally accessible emergency room. These factors indicate that the use and control of Hospital A are for the benefit of the public and that no part of the income of the organization is inuring to the benefit of any private individual nor is any private interest being served.

Accordingly, it is held that Hospital A is exempt from Federal income tax under section 501(c)(3) of the Code.

Hospital B is also providing hospital care. However, in order to qualify under section 501(c)(3) of the Code, an organization must be organized and operated *exclusively* for one or more of the purposes set forth in that section. Hospital B was initially established as a proprietary institution operated for the benefit of its owners. Although its ownership has been transferred to a nonprofit organization, the hospital has continued to operate for the private benefit of its original owners who exercise control over the hospital through the board of trustees and the medical committee. They have used their control to restrict the number of doctors admitted to the medical staff, to enter into favorable rental agreements with the hospital, and to limit emergency room care and hospital admission substantially to their own patients. These facts indicate that the hospital is operated for the private benefit of its original owners, rather than for the exclusive benefit of the public. See "Sonora Community Hospital v. Commissioner," 46 T.C. 519 (1966), aff'd 397 F.2d 814 (1968).

Accordingly, it is held that Hospital B does not qualify for exemption from Federal income tax under section 501(c)(3) of the Code. In considering whether a nonprofit hospital claiming such exemption is operated to serve a private benefit, the Service will weigh all of the relevant facts and circumstances in each case. The absence of particular factors set forth above or the presence of other factors will not necessarily be determinative.

Even though an organization considers itself within the scope of Situation 1 of the Revenue Ruling, it must file an application on Form 1023, Exemption Application, in order to be recognized by the Service as exempt under section 501(c)(3) of the Code. The application should be filed with the District Director of Internal Revenue for the district in which is located the principal place of business or principal office of the organization. See section 1.501.(a)-1 of the regulations.

Revenue Ruling 56-185, O.B. 1956-1, 202, sets forth requirements for exemption of hospitals under section 501(c)(3) more restrictive than those contained in this Revenue Ruling with respect to caring for patients without charge or at rates below cost. In addition, the fourth requirement of Revenue Ruling 56-185 is ambiguous in that it can be read as implying that the possibility of "shareholders" or "members" sharing the assets of a hospital upon its dissolution will not preclude exemption of the hospital as a charity described in section 501(c)(3) of the Code. Section 1.501(c)(3)-1(b)(4) of the regulations promulgated subsequent to Revenue Ruling 56-185 makes it clear, however, that an absolute dedication of assets to charity is a precondition to exemption under section 501(c)(3) of the Code.

Revenue Ruling 56-185 is hereby modified to remove therefrom the requirements relating to caring for patients without charge or, at rates below cost. Furthermore, requirement four has been modified by section 1.501(c)(3)-1(b)(4) of the regulations.

It is interesting to note that, though Revenue Ruling 69-545 eliminated the requirement relating to caring for patients without charge from the exemption qualification criteria, the gap has, at least, been partially filled by revisions to Title 42 of the Public Health Act. The thrust of the revisions to Part 53 (Grants, Loans and Loan Guarantees for Construction and Modernization of Hospitals and Medical Facilities) Subpart L (Community Service; Services for Persons Unable to Pay; Nondiscrimination) can be summarized as requiring that institutions receiving—or having received—Hill-Burton assistance are obligated to make available a reasonable volume of services to persons unable to pay.[5] Compliance to this requirement is presumed if the institution:

●either budgets for the support of, and makes available on request, uncompensated services at a level not less than the lesser of 3 percent of operating costs or 10 percent of all Federal assistance provided under the Act; or

●certifies that it will not exclude any person from admission on the ground that such person is unable to pay.

---

[5]*Federal Register*, Vol. 37, No. 142, July 22, 1972 and *Federal Register*, Vol. 40, No. 194, October 6, 1975.

Chapter 2

Accounting Principles for Hospitals

It is somewhat unusual to begin a text on financial management with a discussion of accounting principles, and one may ask "Why do so here?" The answer, quite simply, is that if hospital managers are to understand the value of financial management for improved hospital operations and feel comfortable in its use, they must have a full understanding of the financial workings of the hospital. The best way to obtain such an understanding is to begin with a review of accounting principles.

An understanding of these principles is critical to the knowledgeable use of financial data, for they determine the nature and character of the financial information which the manager receives. Therefore, if a manager is to be able to understand and properly evaluate and utilize financial data, he must first understand the principles which guide the collection and presentation of these data.

The purpose of this chapter is thus twofold. First, it is to review and point out the differences and similarities between commercial and hospital accounting practices. Some of the material which will be discussed should be familiar. Therefore, little attention will be devoted to the mechanical workings or applications of these principles, for they should already be understood. However, those readers with questions as to mechanics or applications should consult any familiar beginning or intermediate accounting text.

The second objective of this chapter is to provide some familiarity with, and orientation to, the financial environment of the hospital. Thus, attention will be devoted to the unique features of hospital accounting.

Basic Accounting Concepts

Accounting practices have developed over a long period of years. During this time, several basic concepts have been accepted and adopted by accountants as fundamental guides which define the manner in which accounts should be kept. The need for such guides should be quite easily understood.

Without general rules or guides for the recording of business transactions and the preparation of accounts, it would be impossible for accounting information to be understandable and useful to various parties. This would be the case, for there would be no common basis for recording transactions. Similar transactions, if accounting records are to be understood, must yield, at least in terms of the accounting records, similar results. If this end is to be attained, certain basic concepts must be used in preparing accounting records. Thus, over the years accountants have adopted a basic body of theory which is used as a guide for preparing all accounting records. In this way uniformity is obtained and accounting records are understandable and useful to all persons who need them.

Presented below are six basic accounting principles or concepts with which managers should be familiar and which they should understand if they are to be able to use accounting data and reports. It should be pointed out that accounting is not a static art. Some of these principles are continually being questioned and reviewed and, in time, will be modified. However, they are currently the accepted guide, and while the reader may question the propriety of some, he should, at this point, accept and attempt to understand these principles so that he will be able to utilize accounting data and financial reports knowledgeably.

Entity Concept. For accounting purposes the hospital or, for that matter, any other business is personified and viewed as an entity capable of taking economic actions. Thus, the accountant considers the hospital as an entity which is separate and distinct from its employees, contributors and governing board. Accounts are kept for the business entity—not for the persons associated with the entity—and reflect the events which affect the business.

As a corollary to the entity concept, accountants have also assumed that the entity will be one of continuing activity—it will be a going concern with an almost indefinite life. The persons associated with the entity may come and go, but the entity will remain. Thus, in preparing statements and reports, the accountants's method and valuations should reflect the continuity assumption instead of the assumption that the entity will be liquidated and that its assets and liabilities should be valued at their current worth or liquidation price.

Transactions Concept. Given that a hospital is an accounting entity, the results of all transactions affecting that entity must be included in the accounting records and reports. The value and need for this general rule should be quite clear. If accounting data and reports are to be dependable and valid, all transactions of the entity must be included. If this is not done, then the accounting records can be manipulated to describe any operational picture which is desired. Therefore, complete recording and disclosure of all transactions is necessary if an accurate presentation of financial condition is to be had.

However, the necessity of reporting all transactions does not necessarily mean that all transactions must be reported on an individual basis. Individualized reporting would result in financial reports being too cumbersome to be useful management tools. Therefore, it is acceptable reporting practice to summarize transactions—as long as the effect of every transaction is reported and a "fair" statement of financial condition is presented.

Cost Valuation Concept. The previous statement sets forth as a general rule that all transactions must be included in the accounting record. The question which can be raised at this point is: At what value should these transactions be recorded? This is perhaps one of the most difficult questions facing accountants, for a number of values exist for any given asset or liability: sale price, replacement cost, purchase price, to name a few. Faced with this dilemma, accountants and others have found that cost, or the price paid to acquire an item, is generally the most useful basis of valuation for purposes of the permanent accounting record.

Admittedly, the use of this cost as the basis for valuation has some drawbacks. Over time, especially during periods of fluctuating prices, the value of an item can vary substantially. In this situation, the accounting value of an item will only accurately reflect the value of an item as of the time it is acquired and will not show its current worth. Also, cost valuation requires that something of value be given up for an item in order for that item to be recorded in the account. This means, therefore, that the intangible assets of an enterprise, such as the skill of management, reputation, and special expertise, are generally not included in accounting records.[1]

Recognizing these weaknesses of cost valuation, some have argued that a different basis should be used—a basis which shows at all times the current value of the operation. However, there are several compelling reasons for the continued use of a cost basis of valuation.

Cost has the important advantage over all other bases of valuation in that it is determinable, definite, objective, and verifiable. Cost is the only basis of valuation which is definite and not a matter of conjecture or opinion. If sale or replacement cost were used as the basis for valuation of any item not only would value be subject to varying opinions and judgments, but also the necessity of determining a value for each item at the end of the accounting period would be a costly and laborious task with questionable benefits in view of the costs involved. Thus, if accounting reports are to provide consistent and factual figures, cost should be used as the basis of valuation.

In addition to the permanent accounting reports based on cost, management may feel that it is desirable to prepare supplementary reports designed to reflect price level change. This approach to the asset valuation problem not only allows for the benefits of cost valuation to be retained, but also allows for the effects of price level changes to be reflected in the accounting reports. In this way, the advantages of cost valuation and the potential advantages of price level adjustments to cost are both available.

Double Entry Concept. The accounting records should not only reflect, on a cost basis, all transactions of the entity, but also be constructed in such a manner as to reflect the two aspects of each transaction, i.e., the change in asset forms or the change in assets, and the change in the source of financing—liabilities. For example, if a hospital purchases an automobile for cash, not only must the cash account be adjusted, but also an entry must be made

---

[1] It should be noted that tangible assets may, from time to time, be obtained as contributions or donations. In such cases, in order to avoid understating the worth of the enterprise, these assets should be recorded in the accounts even though, in the usual sense, nothing of value has been given up to obtain the assets. In instances of this nature, accountants have assumed that the basis of valuation or cost is equal to the fair market value of the assets as of the time they are received. Intangible assets are also occasionally valued in the accounting records by means of a "goodwill" entry which is equal to the difference between the accounting value and the price paid for an asset. This entry, however, is generally not found in hospital accounting records.

to show the acquisition of a fixed asset. If the hospital had borrowed funds in order to finance the car, two entries would still have to be made. One entry would have to be made to show the acquisition of the fixed asset and another entry would have to be made to reflect the source of financing, i.e., the liability which was incurred. Thus, if the accounting records are to reflect fully the effect of any given transaction, two entries must be made.

Accounting records, therefore, are constructed on the basis of a double entry system, with every transaction affecting at least two items. This is a concept with which all should be familiar, for it is really no more than just requiring that the debit entries balance the credit entries.

Accrual Concept. Just as the cost valuation concept provides the guide for recording assets and liabilities, the accrual concept provides the guide for accounting for revenues and expenses. The accrual concept can be more easily understood if it is viewed not as a theoretical concept, but rather as a system of accounting—a system which requires that revenue, and for that matter losses, be recorded in the accounts when realized and that expenses be recorded in the period in which they contribute to operations.

The desirability of handling revenues and expenses in this manner should be clear. As was discussed earlier, accounting records and reports should accurately reflect the effects of all transactions. However, in any given accounting period, net income represents the results of all transactions or operations within that period. Thus, the accounting records should also accurately reflect net income. In order to do this, the records must include only those revenues and expenses which apply to the given period and exclude all revenues and expenses which result from transactions of other accounting periods.

This matter of properly allocating income and expenses to the appropriate fiscal period is often a difficult problem to accountants. Faced with this problem, accountants have developed two rules to aid them in allocating revenues and expenses. Simply stated, these rules are: (1) revenues and losses should be recorded in the period in which they are realized; and (2) expenses should be recorded in the period in which they contribute to operations.

These two guides provide objective tests for determining when revenues and expenses should be recorded. Realization of a revenue, or loss, means that the gain or loss must be definitely established and the amount must be determined before an accounting entry is made. Thus, for example, securities must be sold before the gain or loss from holding the securities is entered into the accounting record.

In allocating expenses, a somewhat different guide is used. As has been stated above, expenses are recognized in the period during which they contribute to operations. This notion can be illustrated by assuming that employees are paid in January for work performed in December. Using the contribution test, the expense should be allocated to December, the month in which the contribution to operations was made, not to January. Thus, the expense should be recognized and recorded in the accounts not when the wages are paid but rather when the work is done.

The use of these two rules allows accountants to allocate revenues and expenses to the proper accounting period. In this way, the accounting reports accurately present the operating results of the period.

Matching Concept. The use of the realization and contribution rules allows accounting to bring together related income and expenses in an accurate manner in the same accounting period. However, if the results of a particular operation are to be described objectively, not only must income and expenses of the same accounting period be brought together, but also associated revenues and expense items must be matched in order to properly determine net income.

If it were not necessary to match related items of revenue and expense, then it would be possible to manipulate income from different types of activities in order to produce whatever type of operating picture is desired. Thus, the necessity of matching is similar to the necessity for including the results of all transactions in the accounts. Only by matching expenses against related revenues can the results of a particular operating activity be accurately and objectively presented.

Accounting Conventions

The foregoing concepts should not be regarded as infallible rules to be followed in every situation. Instances may arise wherein it would be desirable to make certain exceptions in the application of these concepts. Additionally, in practice, the above concepts are modified by certain conventions, the most important of which are: materiality, consistency, conservatism, and industry practices.

Materiality

Accounting is not intended to be an abstract academic exercise. Rather, it should be a useful tool for management's evaluation and control of operations. Thus, the accounting report should not attempt to reflect a great number of events which are so insignificant that the work and cost of recording them are not justified by the benefit received. For example, the matching principle requires that expenses be matched against related revenue. However, in a large operation, such as a hospital, an insignificant amount of revenue may be obtained from the selling of scrap material. Strict adherence to theory would require that the expenses involved in collecting and selling such scrap material be offset against the revenues obtained. However, unless the revenues from the sale or the expenses related to those revenues are of real importance, it is neither particularly helpful nor necessary to adhere strictly to theory. The point involved here is one of materiality.

Materiality, however is counterbalanced by the notion of full disclosure. This notion requires that significant data be accurately and completely reflected in the accounting reports. Thus, it is difficult to give any firm guidelines as to what is material or immaterial. Materiality varies with the relative amount and relative importance of the transactions being considered. One's decisions should be based upon common sense and a judgment of the importance of the transaction to the total operation.

Consistency

If the full benefits of accounting reports are to be obtained, one must be able to compare the reports of any given year with those of prior years. In order to obtain such comparability, the reports must be prepared on a consistent basis. Without such consistency, the value and usefulness of accounting reports are severely limited. Thus, accountants place considerable emphasis on consistency, and changes in the methods of keeping accounts should not be made without careful consideration.

Conservatism

In accounting, the doctrine of conservatism means, when the proper valuation of an asset is in doubt, the asset should be recorded in the accounts in a manner which will be least likely to overstate its value. It should be noted, however, that there is nothing inherent in this doctrine requiring an understatement of asset values. Unfortunately, few practices in accounting are more misunderstood than that of conservatism. Conservatism just provides accountants with a guide for valuing assets in questionable situations. If the value of an asset is in doubt, it is more prudent to understate than overstate the value. If there is no doubt as to the value of an asset, then there is no need to apply this doctrine.

Industry Practices

In addition to the above conventions, various industries also may have unique accounting practices which affect the way accounting records are kept and reports are presented. The hospital industry is one such industry. The remainder of this chapter will be devoted to discussing the particular accounting conventions of the hospital industry.

Hospital Accounting

The foregoing concepts and conventions have been developed primarily for use by profit-making enterprises. These guidelines, however, are also equally applicable to hospitals and hospital accounting. Hospitals, though differing in orientation from commercial enterprises, are still a form of business. Therefore, the principles of sound business management, such as the above accounting guides or rules, are just as applicable to hospitals as they are to General Electric, Ford Motor Company, Consolidated Edison or any other commercial enterprise. The nonprofit operating philosophy of most hospitals should neither constitute an excuse nor be used as a justification for irresponsible management or accounting practices. Hospital accounting practices should thus be based upon the above rules and conventions.

In addition to the above guides, the American Hospital Association has recommended that hospitals adopt two other accounting conventions. It has suggested that in order to more clearly report the effects of all hospital transactions that a fund accounting system be used. Also, the American Hospital Association has suggested that in order to provide for consistency between hospitals that a uniform chart of accounts be adopted by all hospitals. These two conventions are discussed in some detail below.

Fund Accounting

Fund accounting is an approach to the organization of accounting records which hospitals have adopted as the means of meeting a need which arose early in their development as community institutions. Quite simply, fund accounting requires that a hospital maintain a separate set of accounting records for each distinct phase of financial activity, function, or responsibility. This means that a single hospital may have four or five sets of records or books, as opposed to the one set which is generally used by a commercial enterprise.

One way to conceptualize what is involved in fund accounting is to view the hospital as an operating company with several divisions. Each division operates as an entity with its own accounts and profit objective and deals with the other divisions, in the same manner, as if they were completely separate operations.

Similarly, in fund accounting each distinct phase of financial activity is handled as if it were a separate accounting entity with its own particular objective and purpose. The accounts within each fund are self-balancing, i.e., debits equal credits and can be used to produce balance sheets and income statements. Interfund transactions, though in reality being within the same total entity, are handled in principle as though they involved entirely separate enterprises. Thus, fund accounting is a technique for establishing, within a single hospital, separate accounting subentities, each representing a distinct phase of financial operations or managerial responsibility.

The American Hospital Association has recommended that hospitals establish at least the following funds or accounting subentities:[2]

Operating Fund	fund used to account for the resources, obligations, and capital of the regular day-to-day operations of the hospital;
Endowment Fund	fund used to account for donor restricted assets given to the hospital, the principal amount of which is to be maintained intact and only the income from which is expendable;
Plant Fund	fund used to account for the hospital's investment in buildings, land, equipment, and reserves to replace these assets, as well as related long-term debts;

---

[2]*Chart of Accounts for Hospitals:* American Hospital Association, Chapter 2.

Specific Purpose Fund   fund used to account for cash or
                                   other current assets restricted to the
                                   financing of specific activities;

Construction Fund   fund used to account for transac-
                                   tions related to the acquisition or
                                   construction of new plant assets.

Though the American Hospital Association recommends the above major funds, its guidelines are flexible. A particular hospital may never need to use the Specific Purpose Fund and may only periodically need the Construction Fund. Conversely, some hospitals may need additional funds in order to properly account for certain actions of their governing board. Therefore, a hospital's fund accounting system can and should be custom tailored to meet its own unique needs and should not be unduly bound by the above guidelines.

Given this background, the reader may question the necessity of using a fund accounting system. Many hospital accounting authorities also question the need for fund accounting.[3] As has been indicated, fund accounting was adopted by hospitals as a response to a need which arose early in their development as community institutions. Hospitals, because of their objective of service to the community, are often the recipients of large gifts and endowments which are given as trusts to be used for specific purposes. Acceptance of such gifts places a hospital in a fiduciary position wherein it is legally obligated to conform to the restrictions placed upon the use of the donated funds. In order to carry out this obligation, it was felt that there was a need for a separate accounting for those assets whose use was to be limited to particular activities or functions. Fund accounting was developed in order to provide for this accounting need.

In addition to the need for separate accounts or funds to account for restricted donations, hospitals were also faced with another situation which mediated toward the development of fund accounting. Prior to World War II, the responsibility for the mainte-

---

[3]The American Institute of Certified Public Accountants (AICPA) has also raised the question of the necessity of fund accounting. The AICPA has noted that reporting on a fund accounting basis may be helpful where needed to achieve a proper segregation and presentation of unrestricted resources from those resources over which the board has little, if any, discretion because of externally imposed restrictions. If an organization has restricted resources and elects not to report on a fund accounting basis, disclosure of all material restrictions should be made.

nance, supervision, and construction of the physical plant was often the responsibility of the governing board. As such, it was a completely separate sphere of activity from the responsibility for day-to-day general operations. In this kind of situation, it is not difficult to understand how an accounting system using subentities developed. The accounting system just reflected the actual operating situation, i.e., responsibility for the different phases of operation was separated and, therefore, the accounting system for these activities should also be separated.

Today, however, there is no longer this dichotomy of function. A hospital manager is responsible for both the maintenance and supervision of the physical plant and the day-to-day general operations of the hospital. Given that this dichotomy no longer exists, there is no reason to use an accounting technique which misrepresents the actual operating situation. Rather, a system which reflects the single sphere of responsibility should be used. Therefore, the plant and general fund should be merged. In this way, not only can the accounting and reporting process be simplified, but also the distorted picture of managerial responsibility depicted by the use of a separate plant fund can be corrected. Figure 2-1 illustrates the differences between a fund accounting balance sheet and a merged balance sheet.

Some may argue that the Endowment and Specific Purpose Funds, as well as the Construction Fund, can be merged with the Operating Fund if full disclosure is provided. It is questionable, though, if such a merger is administratively desirable or legally possible. A discussion of the legal implications of Endowment Fund management and accounting is beyond the scope of this book. Therefore, it will be left as a moot point which must be determined individually for a particular hospital after discussion with its legal counsel.

The critical factors for the hospital manager to realize and understand, however, are the following:

a. that fund accounting is the most commonly used hospital accounting system;
b. that fund accounting requires the creation of a separate accounting entity for each distinct financial activity or responsibility of the hospital;
c. that a hospital's fund accounting system should be designed to meet its own unique situation, i.e., if the organization structure is appropriate, funds should be merged—such as the operating and plant funds—or, if necessary, additional funds should be created.

Figure 2-1
Caryn County General Hospital
Balance Sheet
As of 12/31/73 (000)

I-Fund Accounting Balance Sheet

Assets		*Liabilities and Capital*	
General Fund		General Fund	
Cash	$ 7	Accounts Payable	$ 15
Marketable Securities	5	Salaries Payable	5
Accounts Receivable	125	Total General Fund	
Inventories	15	Liabilities	20
		General Fund Capital	132
Total	$152	Total	$152
Specific Purpose Fund		Specific Purpose Fund	
Cash	$ 5	Specific Purpose Fund	
Marketable Securities	15	Capital	$ 20
Total	$ 20	Total	$ 20
Plant Fund		Plant Fund	
Land	$ 20	Mortgage	$ 80
Buildings		Plant Fund Capital	123
(net of dep.)	100		
Fixed Equipment			
(net of dep.)	50		
Major Movable Equip-			
ment (net of dep.)	30		
Cash	3		
Total	$203	Total	$203
Total Assets	$375	Total Liabilities and	$375
		Capital	

II-Merged Balance Sheet

Assets		*Liabilities and Capital*	
Current Assets		Current Liabilities	
Cash	$ 15	Accounts Payable	$ 15
Marketable Securities	20	Salaries Payable	5
Accounts Receivable	125		
Inventories	15		
Total	$175	Total	$ 20
Fixed Assets		Long-Term Liabilities	
Land	$ 20	Mortgage	$ 80
Building			
(net of dep.)	100		
Fixed Equipment		Capital	$275
(net of dep.)	50		
Major Movable Equip-			
ment (net of dep.)	30		
Total	$200	Total	$355
		Total Liabilities and	
Total Assets:	$375	Capital	$375

The mechanics of fund accounting will be left to the accountants and hospital accounting texts. Readers with questions as to mechanics should consult any hospital accounting text such as *Introduction to Hospital Accounting* by Seawell (see Suggested Readings).

In addition to fund accounting, the American Hospital Association has also recommended that a hospital adopt a uniform chart of accounts, i.e., a uniform account classification system. A chart of accounts is actually nothing more than a listing of the account titles, with numerical symbols, for all the asset, liability, capital, revenue, and expense accounts of a hospital.

The notion of what a chart of accounts is can be understood most easily by examining a sample chart of accounts. Table 2-1 is an excerpt from the chart of accounts of a particular hospital. As can be seen in the right-hand column, all the journal account titles which the hospital has for each category of assets are listed. The left-hand column lists the numerical classification code for each account. A complete chart of accounts would contain a listing, each with its corresponding account number, of all the journal accounts of the hospital.

Table 2-2 is a summary of the overall numbering system suggested by the American Hospital Association. As can be seen from the table, the three numbers at the left of the decimal point indicate the control or primary account classification, and the two digits to the right indicate the secondary account classification. For example, account number 111.20 from Table 2-1 can be translated as follows:

$$\underbrace{111}.\underbrace{20}$$

Primary Classification	Secondary Classification
First Digit = Asset (nature of Acct.)	Fourth Digit = ⎫ Bank Savings account refinement of the
Second Digit = Operating Fund (fund group)	account classi-
	Fifth Digit = ⎭ fication
Third Digit = Investment (account classification)	

Thus, the account numbers indicate, to the experienced reader, that the account is not only an asset account in the Operating Fund, but also that the asset is a temporary investment. The fourth and fifth digits just further specify the identity of the account, i.e., indicate that it is a bank savings.

Table 2-1

Sample Chart of Acounts

Assets:
Operating Fund

110.00–110.49	*Cash*
110.00	Cash on Deposit—General Fund
110.00	Cash on Deposit—Payroll
110.20	Cash on Deposit—Supplies and Expense
110.50–110.99	*Cash Imprest Funds*
110.50	Cashiers Change Fund
110.51	Cafeteria Change Fund
110.52	Nightbox
110.53	X-Ray Change Fund
110.60	Brink's Revolving Change Fund
110.70	Laboratory Machine Fund
110.80	U.S. Post Office—Stamp Fund
111.00–111.99	*Investments*
111.20	Savings R. and M. Friedman Bank
112.00–112.09	*Accounts and Notes Receivable*
112.00	Accounts Receivable—Inpatients
112.01	Accounts Receivable—Outpatients
112.10–112.19	*Allowance for Uncollectable Receivables*
112.10	Reserve for Doubtful Accounts
112.11	Reserve for Blue Cross
112.12	Reserve for Medicare Adjustments
112.20–112.29	*Recoveries of Accounts Written Off*
112.20	Other Accounts Receivable—Suspense
112.21	Reserve for Bad Debts—Suspense
112.30–112.39	*Other Receivables*
112.30	Tuition Receivable
112.31	Taxes Receivable—Current
112.32	Accounts Receivable—X-Ray Room Rent
112.33	Accounts Receivable—Clearance

Table 2-2
Summary—Numerical Coding System—Primary Classification

110–196 Assets	110–114	Operating Fund
	120–122	Specific Purpose Fund
	130–132	Endowment Fund
	140–146	Plant Fund
	150–155	Construction Fund
	160–196	Other Funds
217–298 Liabilities	217	Operating Fund
	227	Specific Purpose Fund
	237–238	Endowment Fund
	247–248	Plant Fund
	257–258	Construction Fund
	267–298	Other Funds
219–299 Capital Accounts		Operating Fund
	219	Specific Purpose Fund
	229	Endowment Fund
	239	Plant Fund
	249	Construction Fund
	259	Other Funds
	269–299	
310–599 Revenue Accounts	310–499	Patient Service Revenue
	500–529	Deductions from Revenue
	530–599	Other Revenue
600–999 Expense Accounts	600–699	Nursing Service
	700–799	Other Professional Services
	800–899	General Services
	900–949	Fiscal Services
	950–979	Administration Services
	980–999	Unassigned Expenses

Summary—Logic of Coding System

Asset, Liability, and Capital Accounts	Revenue Accounts	Expense Accounts

Primary Classification

First digit	Nature of account, e.g., asset, liability, capital	Nature of revenue and expense accounts—classified by unit; e.g.
Second digit	Fund Group	402—Laboratory-Clinical
		435—Anesthesiology
Third digit	Account classification; e.g., cash, inventory, revenue by nursing unit, etc.	601—Nursing Service-Administration
		735—Anesthesiology

Table 2-2 (Continued)

Secondary Classification

Fourth Digit ⎧ Additionally, classification codes available for use
            ⎨ as needed, to provide for refinement of the
Fifth Digit ⎩ primary classification.

The internal operational value of a chart of accounts is twofold. First, a chart of accounts, through the use of numerical account titles, facilitates the performance of the entire accounting process, from the collection of data to the presentation of reports, not only by saving clerical time and effort, but also by reducing the number of errors. Also, the chart of accounts, by requiring the systematic organization of accounts, provides the basis for management control of operations through responsibility accounting and management by objectives. Thus, a chart of accounts is a basic and necessary element in any accounting system and should be utilized by all hospitals.

In addition to the above internal operational benefits, other benefits can be obtained through the use of a common or uniform chart of accounts by all hospitals. Adoption of the uniform chart of accounts recommended by the American Hospital Association provides individual hospitals with the opinions of experts as to the most effective and efficient ways of recording, classifying, and summarizing financial information. Uniformity also allows for an improved exchange of information among hospitals and between hospitals and the various large purchasers of hospital care.[4] Lastly, the adoption of a uniform chart of accounts assists national and state hospital and other health care organizations in the gathering of financial data. The knowledge derived from the analysis of this information can provide tremendous benefits to the entire hospital industry. Thus, in order to obtain the full benefits available from the use of a chart of accounts, it is recommended that hospitals not only use a chart of accounts, but also that they adopt the system recommended by the American Hospital Association.

Admittedly, no two hospitals are exactly alike. It follows, therefore, that no two hospitals will have exactly the same charts of accounts. In designing its chart of accounts, the American Hospital Association was well aware of this problem and designed a system

---

[4]It should be noted that one must exercise caution in making interhospital comparisons. Admittedly, uniformity does facilitate interhospital comparisons. However, uniformity of reporting should not be interpreted as either meaning or implying exact comparability of operations.

which is flexible enough to meet the specific requirements of all hospitals while still maintaining a basic uniformity for the recording and reporting of financial data. The recommended chart of accounts provides the basis for operational accountability, comparability, and control while at the same time being sufficiently general to be a useful guideline for all hospitals.

There is little value at this point, in discussing the recommended chart of accounts in more detail. Those readers who desire additional information should refer to the American Hospital Association's publication entitled *Chart of Accounts for Hospitals*. For the moment, the hospital manager should just be aware of and understand the internal operational values of a chart of accounts and the additional benefits which can be obtained by adopting a uniform chart of accounts.

Suggested Readings

American Hospital Association. *Chart of Accounts for Hospitals,* Chapters 2,3.

American Institute of CPA. "Hospital Audit Guide."

Foyle, William R. "Merge the Plant and General Funds, Why Not?" *Hospital Accounting,* June 1965, pp. 2–5.

Moyer, C.A. and Mautz, R.K. *Intermediate Accounting,* Chapter 2.

Seawell, L. Vann. *Hospital Accounting and Financial Management,* Chapters 1,3.

Seawell, L. Vann. *Introduction to Hospital Accounting.*

Chapter 3

Financial Organization: The Hospital

A well managed hospital operation is generally not the result of individual genius or effort. Rather, it is the product of the efforts and intellects of a group of individuals organized to function in concert. Organization provides the mechanism for allocating responsibilities and channeling efforts so that not only will all necessary tasks be performed, but also that all work will be coordinated and controlled in order to achieve the objectives of the hospital in the most efficient and effective manner. Sound organization in all areas is thus one of the critical elements necessary for effective management. (See Appendix 3, this chapter.)

Sound organization can take many forms. There is no single "right" or "proper" organizational structure which can be recommended for all hospitals. The type of organization plan best suited for any given hospital depends on the size and characteristics of the operation, the probabilities and nature of any future expansion, and the personality and style of the hospital's management group. However, certain patterns of organization have been found to be practicable, and certain guiding principles can be applied with uniformity in almost all situations.

The purpose of this chapter is to examine these principles and practices as they relate to the financial organization structure of a hospital. Admittedly, they will not be ideally applicable in all situations. However, they do provide the basis for the financial organization of a hospital and should be understood if the reader is to obtain a working knowledge of hospital financial management.

Organization Structure

The governing board of a voluntary hospital is vested by law with the ultimate authority and responsibility for managing all of a hospital's business. Therefore, the governing board is responsible for all phases of hospital operations, including financial operations. Thus, as is indicated in Figure 3-1, the financial organization structure of a hospital begins with the governing board.

The governing board itself, however, does not personally manage a hospital's financial operations. Rather, it generally utilizes the same basic staff/line combination approach which it employs to carry out many of its other responsibilities. That is, not only does it delegate line responsibility for the actual management of financial operations to certain hospital employees, but also it generally delegates the responsibility for ensuring that financial operations are properly managed to a committee of trustees which acts in a staff capacity to the board. Thus, line responsibility for financial operations is delegated to administration (the chief executive officer) and also a finance committee is usually appointed to ensure that financial operations are performed appropriately.

The finance committee acts as the control or "check" in a hospital's system of financial checks and balances. It is responsible for overseeing the financial operations and position of the hospital, ensuring that adequate working and long-term capital are available, and for advising the board on all fiscal and investment matters.[1]

In addition to the finance committee, the board also usually appoints or elects one of its members to serve as the hospital's treasurer. In a commercial enterprise the treasurer is generally a full-time employee of the firm whose function is primarily custodial. He is responsible for safeguarding the assets of the firm, supervising the receipt and disbursement of cash, and ensuring that the operation is adequately financed. As the custodian of the firm's assets, he counterbalances the chief financial officer, who controls the process by which assets are handled, in order to provide an adequate system of financial checks and balances.

The financial structure of the hospital, due to legal and philosophical constraints, has not developed in the same manner as that of the commercial corporation. The treasurer, as a member of the

---

[1]Some hospitals may have a separate budget committee to review the budget and examine any deviation and also a building fund committee to raise certain long-term capital. However, these functions can, if desired, be performed by the finance committee.

Figure 3-1

Financial Organization Structure—Voluntary General Hospital

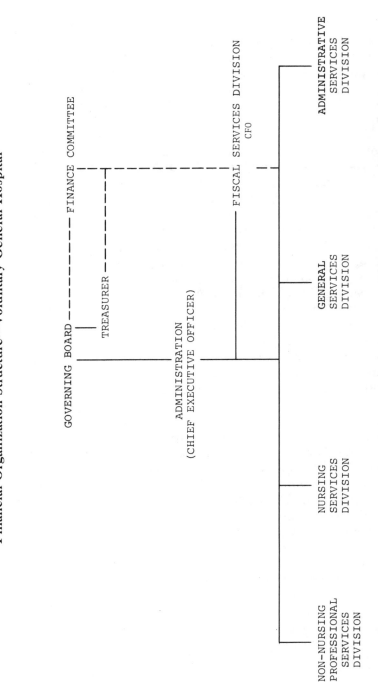

governing board, is usually not an employee of the hospital and does not devote his full time to the day-to-day management of the hospital's financial operations. Also, the duties traditionally assigned to the treasurer in a commercial corporation are delegated, in a hospital corporation, to adminstration, the chief financial officer, and the finance committee. The hospital treasurer serves as the chairman of the finance committee and through this mechanism carries out his custodial duties and provides the means for a system of financial checks and balances.

This approach to financial organization, though commonly used, obviously can be questioned. It may be argued that it is difficult, if not impossible, to obtain an adequate system of checks and balances, if the treasurer is not an employee of the hospital devoting his full attention to financial operations. Additionally, the case can be made that as the size of the hospital increases, both the custodial and cash management functions not only increase, but also become more critical. Thus a full-time employee-treasurer is needed in order to adequately carry out these functions. Whether these arguments are valid or not is a moot point, for, as has been indicated, there is no single "right" or "proper" organization structure. There is nothing inherent in the foregoing plan to summarily preclude its usefulness or effectiveness. It does seem reasonable, though, to expect that at some size level the employment of a treasurer becomes advantageous. At what point this size level is reached, however, will differ from hospital to hospital and must be determined individually by each institution, based on the costs and potential benefits.

Line Responsibility

The Joint Commission on Accreditation of Hospitals, in its standards for accrediting of hospitals, has established as a basic standard or requirement that:

> The governing body, through its chief executive officer, shall provide for the control and use of the physical and financial resources of the hospital.

It further goes on and interprets this standard as meaning that:

> Responsibility for implementing the policies of the governing body relative to the control and the effective utilization of the physical and financial resources of the hospital should be given to the chief executive officer.

Thus, the line responsibility or the responsibility for actually managing the day-to-day financial operation lies with the hospital's administrator or chief executive officer.[2]

It is impossible, however, for the chief executive officer or administrator to exercise personal supervision over all aspects of the hospital's operations. The demands, both internal and external, which require the administrator's personal attention and expertise, and the technical nature of operations, have increased to the point where the administrator must delegate the personal supervision and management of many tasks to members of his staff. Thus, the direct supervision of financial operations is delegated to the chief financial officer.[3]

The fact that the administrator delegates the day-to-day responsibility for financial management does not mean that he can or should ignore this phase of operations. He should actively involve himself in all financial policy, capital investment and capital acquisition decisions. However, the day-to-day supervision and management of financial operations should be left to the chief financial officer (CFO), with the administrator just satisfying himself, through various reporting and control mechanisms, that the CFO is properly carrying out his responsibilities.

As the party with the direct responsibility for financial management, the CFO, regardless of his actual title, is the hospital's chief financial officer and occupies the most critical position in the financial organization structure. Historically, the role and managerial value of the controller has been inappropriately defined, focusing on bookkeeping and business office management instead of management accounting and financial management. Thus, the managerial value and usefulness of both the CFO and financial management have been de-emphasized. Often, neither the administrator nor the governing board realized the value of financial planning and data or the significance of the controller's potential contribution. Consequently, the caliber of financial management generally found in hospitals has been, at best, inadequate and at times nonexistent.

However, the pendulum is now swinging in the other direction. Pressures from third party payers, government agencies, and the

---

[2]*Standards for Accreditation of Hospitals:* Joint Commission on Accreditation of Hospitals, page 7.

[3]The title of the Chief Financial Officer will vary from hospital to hospital. In some institutions, the position may be identified as the Controller. In others, it may be the Vice President of Fiscal Services. As a rule of thumb, the function should carry a title which is generally similar to that of other line managers.

public, regarding both hospital costs and the efficacy of hospital management, have caused both administrators and trustees to realize the need and value of quality financial management and the necessity of having a qualified controller as an executive officer at the policy-making level. Thus, it is reasonable to expect that the management role and function of the CFO will become increasingly important in the future.

What, though, is the function and role of the CFO? If an administrator is to be able to satisfy himself that the controller is properly carrying out his financial management responsibilities, he must first be familiar with and understand the CFO's function. Therefore, a discussion of the specific functions of the CFO is germane at this point.

Chief Financial Officer's Functions

The Committee on Ethics and Eligibility Standards of the Financial Executives Institute has defined the CFO's function as follows:

1. To establish, coordinate and maintain, through authorized management, an integrated plan for the control of operations. Such a plan would provide, to the extent required in the business, cost standards, expense budgets, sale forecasts, profit planning, and programs for capital investment and financing, together with the necessary procedures to effectuate the plan.

2. To measure performance against approved operating plans and standards, and to report and interpret the results of operations to all levels of management. This function includes the design, installation and maintenance of accounting and cost systems and records, the determination of accounting policy and the compilation of statistical records as required.

3. To measure and report on the validity of the objectives of the business and on the effectiveness of its policies, organization structure and procedures in attaining those objectives. This includes consulting with all segments of management responsible for policy or action concerning any phase of the operation of the business as it relates to the performance of this function.

4. To report to government agencies, as required, and to supervise all matters relating to taxes.

5. To interpret and report on the effect of external influences on the attainment of the objectives of the business. This

function includes the continuous appraisal of economic and social forces and of government influences as they affect the operations of the business.

6. To provide protection for the assets of the business. This function includes establishing and maintaining adequate internal control and auditing, and assuring proper insurance coverage.

The Committee's definition is designed primarily for the controller of a commercial firm. However, the generic problems of management do not vary significantly between industries. Admittedly, hospitals differ in some respects for their commerical counterparts, but the basic problems of planning and organizing operations, obtaining adequate financing, controlling costs, measuring and reporting performance, etc. are the same in all instances. Thus, the above definition is sufficiently broad in concept to be applicable to the hospital CFO.

In order to simplify discussion of the controller's function it may be advisable to recast the above definition into a more functionally oriented listing. Although there is some overlap between categories, the controller's primary or basic functions and activities can be set out as follows:

The Planning Function. The development and maintenance of an integrated budget or plan of operations is often felt to be the major and most critical function of the CFO. The objective of a hospital can generally be stated as that of providing its community with the services which it needs at both an acceptable level of quality, and at the least possible cost. This is a complex goal which cannot be achieved unless the efforts of all departments are carefully coordinated and planned. Planning is, thus, a necessity for effective operations. However, it should be understood at the outset that the plan is the hospital's plan, not the CFO's, and that all members of management must participate in its development and support its objective.

The CFO's role in planning should be one of educating management to the need for a plan, coordinating the preparation of the plan, examining and testing the plan for adequacy and accuracy, and translating the final plan into financial terms. The CFO is only a counselor and coordinator. The responsibility for planning for each separate operational function must lie with the appropriate department head and administrator.

The Recording Function. The systematic recording of financial transactions is commonly viewed as, and traditionally has been, the principal function of the hospital CFO. Pressures for improved financial management, though, are forcing the CFO to delegate the actual performance of this function to the accounting specialist members of his staff, and to devote his own time and energies to more comprehensive financial problems. Nevertheless, the CFO is still responsible for ensuring that all financial transactions are accounted for and that accurate records are maintained. Thus, although he may delegate actual performance of this activity, he should carefully supervise its accomplishment.

The various specific aspects or components of the recording function are discussed further in the following section.

The Measuring Function. Management needs to have information available from the measurement and evaluation of the actual operational performance so that the hospital's objectives can be met and its plan of operations carried out. This function can perhaps be understood most easily if it is viewed as the feedback loop and monitor for the planning function. The planning function sets the standards for operations and the measuring function ascertains and analyzes the level of actual performance. The results of these two functions can be compared in order to determine the extent of any deviation between planned and actual performance, and the nature of any necessary corrective action. Together, these functions—along with the reporting function—provide the basis for management control of operations.

It should be noted that the CFO does not personally enforce control of operations. Rather, his role is one of assisting functional management—just as it is in planning—by providing the information needed to control operations and to achieve the desired objectives and level of performance. In order to perform this role properly, not only should the CFO provide measures of actual performance, but also he should assist in evaluating performance and review the mechanism by which data are gathered. Thus he can assure that sufficient data are available and that they are being provided on a timely basis.

The Reporting Function. Viewed from an internal management standpoint, the reporting function is closely related to the planning and measuring functions. Without reporting, planning operations and measuring of actual performance are just exercises in futility. Reporting is the mechanism by which information is communicated, and planning and measuring are brought together in order to provide the basis for controlling operations. Effective control is impossible without an appropriate and efficient reporting system.

The CFO's reporting responsibilities, however, go beyond just the preparation and presentation of figures, charts and other reports. To be effective, the CFO must also interpret the presented information so that its meaning and implications are understandable to all members of management. This aspect of the reporting function is critical, for without interpretation the managerial usefulness of reports is, at best, limited. Thus, if management is to obtain the information necessary to direct and control operations, the CFO must not only provide information, but also analyze or interpret the data so that its managerial usefulness is clear.

In addition to the above internal responsibilities, the reporting function also carries with it external reporting obligations, e.g., cost reports for third party payers, informational returns for the Internal Revenue Service, financial reports for lenders, trustees, and the public. These reports, though of marginal internal management value, are important for the overall well-being and operation of a hospital. The CFO, therefore, to adequately fulfill his reporting function, must carry out both its internal and external aspects.

The Advising Function. The advisory function of the CFO is closely linked to the reporting function and actually can be considered as a component of that function. However, because of the significance of the contribution which the CFO can make through the proper exercise of this function, it is specifically set out in order to emphasize its importance.

Through measuring and reporting on the validity of the institution's objectives and the effectiveness of its policies, and its organization and procedures in achieving those objectives, the CFO can not only force management to evaluate the hospital's current operational status, but also aid in the establishment of future operating policies. Additionally, the CFO, by analyzing the impact of external political-economic factors, can advise management as to what actions must be taken in order to achieve the desired operational goals. Thus, the CFO occupies a unique position, as a counselor to management, responsible both for ensuring that total operational achievements are periodically evaluated and for aiding in the establishment of future operational guidelines.

The Recording Function: Further Discussion

As has been indicated, the recording function has in the past been the principal activity of the hospital CFO. The major items included in this function have been (1) the development and operation of the hospital's general accounting system, (2) the design and custody of all of the books, records, and forms needed to record financial transactions, and (3) the development and installation of an adequate system of internal control. The first two items are of a technical accounting nature and as such are not really appropriate to this text. Readers wishing detailed information in these areas should consult any basic accounting text such as, *Hospital Financial Accounting: Theory and Practice* by L. Vann Seawell. The third item, however, is basic to sound financial management and merits further discussion.

Internal control has been defined by the Committee on Auditing Procedures of the American Institute of Certified Public Accountants as:

> the plan of organization and all of the coordinate methods and measures adopted within a business to safeguard its assets, check the accuracy and reliability of its accounting data, promote operational efficiency, and encourage adherence to prescribed managerial policies.

Thus, internal control involves not only the control or safeguarding of assets, but also the plan of organization and all the methods and procedures that relate to operational efficiency. In a broad sense, therefore, internal control can be viewed as including two basic types or areas of controls—accounting controls and administrative controls.

Accounting controls are concerned mainly with safeguarding the assets of the hospital and assuring the reliability of the financial records. Administrative controls are concerned mainly with operational efficiency and adherence to managerial policies. It should be noted, though, for purposes of internal management, that the two areas are interrelated and both are needed if control is to be achieved.

The Committee on Auditing Procedures specifies four items which are necessary for a satisfactory control system:[4]

1. A plan of organization that provides an appropriate segregation of functional responsibilities;
2. A system of authorization and record procedures adequate to provide accounting control over assets, liabilities, revenues and expenses;

---

[4]Committee on Auditing Procedures, *Auditing Standards and Procedures*, "Statement on Auditing Procedures, No. 33" (1963), page 27.

3. Sound practices to be followed in performance of the duties and functions of each of the organizational departments;
4. A degree of quality of personnel commensurate with responsibilities.

Organization Plan. As has been discussed earlier, there is no single "right" or "proper" organizational structure for all hospitals. However, regardless of the specific organization plan adopted, certain basic principles of organization are applicable in all cases. Specifically, the organizational structure should establish clear lines of authority and responsibility, create independence of operation, demark custodial and record-keeping responsibilities, ensure that an individual is not responsible to more than one person, and provide for proper spans of control. These organizational features are essential not only for internal control, but also for effective operational management.

Accounting Procedures. A formal system of authorization and record procedures is as critical for internal control as is a sound organization plan. Procedures provide the prescribed manner by which all types of transactions should be handled, including the records, forms, and accounts to be used and the authorization or approvals which are needed. Authorizations are of particular importance, for they provide not only the checks and balances needed to control any given procedure but also, when combined with the proper forms, the documentation necessary for both the accounting records and external audits. Thus, in essence, procedures and authorizations are complementary. That is, procedures specify a given process, and authorizations provide the mechanism for ensuring that the process or procedures are properly carried out. Together, they provide the basis for accounting control.

Operating Practices. In addition to formal accounting procedures, a sound system of operational practices and authorizations is also requisite for effective internal control. Just as accounting procedures provide the mechanism for ensuring that transactions are documented and that accounting records are adequate, operating procedures provide the means for ensuring that transactions proceed efficiently and that proper checks and balances exist.

Fundamental to sound operating procedures are such practices as:

—obtaining competitive bids from suppliers;
—matching packing slips against purchase orders and suppliers' invoices;

—prenumbering all forms and checks,
—maintaining individual records of all capital assets;
—separating custody and record-keeping responsibilities;
—requiring dual signatures on checks;
—reconciling general and subsidiary ledgers.

A complete listing of all of the practices which should be employed in order to assure proper internal controls of operations is beyond the scope of this text. Readers desiring additional information in this area should consult the American Hospital Association's manual, *Internal Control and Internal Auditing for Hospitals.*

Quality Personnel. The final, and perhaps the most important factor necessary for internal control, is an adequate number of qualified personnel who are capable of carrying out established procedures and practices in an efficient manner. Organization plans and procedural manuals are inanimate. They cannot, in themselves, perform the various tasks which they prescribe; only people can vitalize procedures. Therefore, if procedures are to be carried out properly and if internal control is to be more than just charts and manuals, the employees of the hospital must be of the quality and possess the skills necessary to carry out their tasks in the prescribed manner. Without adequate personnel, it is impossible to operate an effective system of internal control.

It should be noted, however, that though qualified personnel are necessary in all areas, the internal auditor is the key employee in any internal control system. The internal auditor is responsible for not only protecting the hospital's assets against fraud, error, and loss, but his functions also include:

—reviewing and appraising the soundness, adequacy and application of accounting, financial, and operating controls;
—ascertaining the extent of compliance with established policies, plans, and procedures;
—ascertaining the reliability of accounting and other data developed within the organization;
—appraising the quality of performance in carrying out assigned responsibilities.[5]

He is, in effect, the man who monitors the internal control system, assuring both that it is functioning and that it is functioning properly.

---

[5]"Statement of the Responsibilities of the Internal Auditor," Institute of Internal Auditors, New York, 1967.

In order to perform this task, he should occupy a staff position and report directly to the controller. In this way he will have the organizational independence necessary to avoid conflicts of interest and the freedom to appraise operations objectively.

Checklist. In addition to the above basic characteristics, the American Hospital Association also suggests that the following checklist can be used to appraise the adequacy of an internal control system.[6]

1. Does the hospital have a current organization chart?
2. Are the accounting and treasury functions satisfactorily defined and segregated?
3. To whom does the chief accounting officer report?
4. Does the hospital have an internal auditor? To whom does he report? Outline briefly the scope of the internal audit work.
5. Is a chart of accounts used?
6. Is a current accounting manual being used?
7. Are monthly statements to management prepared and furnished, along with supporting analyses and explanatory comments?
8. Are the monthly statments—relative to material variances from standards, budgets or prior periods—discussed with the board of directors, executive committee, treasurer, department heads, etc.?
9. Are costs and expenses under budgetary control?
10. Has the general policy concerning insurance coverage been defined by the board of directors? Is the insurance coverage periodically reviewed by a responsible officer or employee?
11. Are journal entries (a) adequately explained and supported and (b) approved by a reponsible employee?
12. Are all employees required to take annual vacations? Have provisions been made for the temporary reassignment of duties in the absence of an employee on vacation, etc.?
13. Does a responsible employee maintain a calendar or follow-up file on such matters as the due dates of tax returns and special reports, the expiration dates of the period of limitations on tax refund claims, etc.?
14. What is the hospital's policy concerning its key employees (such as purchasing agents, departmental or division man-

---

[6]*Internal Control and Internal Auditing for Hospitals*, American Hospital Association, pp. 10–11.

agers, etc.) having any direct or indirect ownership or profit participation in outside business enterprises with which the hospital does business? What procedures are followed to determine that such a policy is being complied with?

Readers desiring a detailed discussion of policies and procedures relative to any of the above items should refer to the previously mentioned American Hospital Association manual.

Independent Auditors

In addition to an internal auditor, prudent management requires that an external independent auditor be utilized by the hospital. An independent auditor differs from an internal auditor in that:

—he is not an employee of the hospital;
—his primary concern is not the needs of internal management, but rather the needs of external agencies and organizations;
—his review of operations is limited to basically financial matters;
—he is only incidently concerned with the detection and prevention of fraud; and
—his examination of the hospital is periodic as opposed to continuous.

The value and usefulness of an independent auditor lies as much in business convention as it does in operational control.

The opinion of an independent auditor, concerning the financial statements of a hospital, is the best possible indication of whether persons who are not associated with the hospital may justifiably rely upon those statements in making financial decisions.[7] The assumed need for such an opinion is derived from an implicit value judgment concerning the self-interest and character of internal management.

Whether this value judgment is valid is a moot point. Audited financial statements, bearing an independent opinion, have come to be commonly accepted both as being credible and as containing data which can be freely relied upon by the external agencies and organizations. This position and philosophy is recognized by the Federal government under the Medicare program, by Blue Cross plans, and by state governments under their rate review and public disclosure programs.

---

[7]Howard F. Stettler, *Systems Based Independent Audits*, Prentice-Hall, p. 1. See also American Institute of CPA, "Hospital Audit Guide," 1972.

Figure 3-2
Organization Chart
Fiscal Services Division

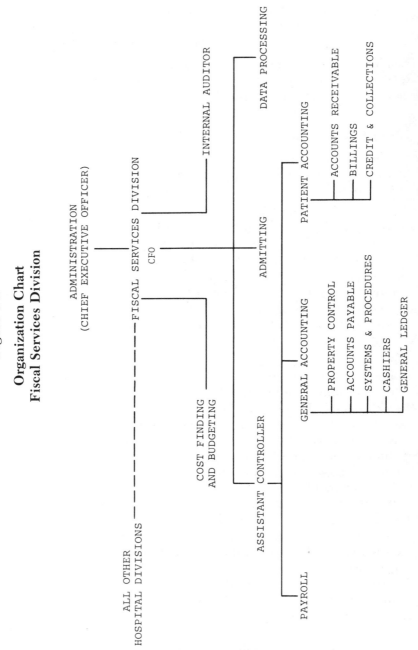

An independent auditor is also of value in terms of operational control. Due to his financial and attitudinal independence from the hospital, he is not an employee of the hospital and his code of ethics requires independent thought and action—he provides a check and balance, at least in regard to financial matters, on both the internal auditor and the entire concern. The value of this "fail-safe" mechanism is obvious and in itself justifies the use of an independent auditor.

In selecting an auditor, careful consideration should be given to his technical competence and independence. At a minimum, the auditor should be a certified public accountant. Admittedly, certification does not guarantee technical competence. However, it is evidence that, at least at one point in time, he has demonstrated his qualifications to render competent service. Hence, certification should be considered a basic requisite for selection.

The matter of the auditor's independence must also be weighed in the selection process. The auditor must be financially independent of his client in that "Any direct financial interest or material indirect financial interest is prohibited as is any relationship to the client, such as . . . voting trustee, director, officer, or key employee."[8] He also must be independent in terms of his fee not being contingent upon his findings or results of the service. Lastly, the auditor's independence must not be compromised by his being selected by the very persons whose work he would be reviewing. In operational terms this means that the governing board, or one of its committees—such as the Finance Committee, as opposed to the chief executive officer or the controller, should select the auditor.

List of Functions

Given the foregoing material, one should have a general understanding of the functional responsibilities of the CFO. This understanding can be clarified further by examining the organization chart pictured in Figure 3-2.

Figure 3-2 illustrates the broad scope and importance of the CFO's responsibilities. If a CFO is to carry out these responsibilities properly, he must possess not only a knowledge of accounting principles and procedures, but also the ability to interpret and analyze accounting and statistical data, communicate with and

---

[8]Article 101, American Institute of Certified Public Accountants', "Code of Ethics."

motivate employees and other managers, and utilize accounting data not as an end in itself, but rather as the means to both effective financial and hospital management. The CFO, thus, must be more than just an accountant. He must have both the imagination to convert static accounting data into management information and the technical skill to employ such information as an aid in managing not only the financial operations of the hospital, but also total operations.

Conclusion

The CFO obviously occupies a key position in the organizational structure of the hospital. The demands upon a chief executive officer's time and the specialized technical complexities of financial operations prohibit an administrator from personally supervising day-to-day financial operations. Therefore, in order to properly fulfill his fiscal responsibilities, an administrator must obtain the services of a competent CFO and ensure that the CFO adequately carries out functions of his position. The remainder of this text is devoted to providing an administrator with the background and knowledge necessary to aid him in evaluating both a CFO's performance and the financial condition of a hospital.

Suggested Readings

American Hospital Association. *Internal Control and Internal Auditing for Hospitals.*

American Institute of Certified Public Accountants. *Hospitals Audit Guide.*

Bower, James B. and Schlosser, Robert E. "Internal Control—Its True Nature." *The Accounting Review*, April 1965, pp. 338–344.

Caruana, Russell A. *A Guide to Organizing The Hospital's Fiscal Services Division.*

Heckert, Josiah B. and Willson, James D. *Controllership*, Chapters 1, 2, and 6.

Murphy, Thomas. "The Hospital Treasurer and Controller: Duties and Responsibilities." *Hospital Financial Management*, April 1970, pp. 11–14.

Shelton, Robert M. "The Hospital Financial Manager Today." *Hospital Financial Managment*, April 1970, pp. 4, 5, 6, 40, 41.

Taylor, Philip J. and Nelson, Benjamin O. *Management Accounting for Hospitals*, Chapters 1 and 12.

Tonkin, G. W. "The Controller's Role on the Management Team." *Hospital Financial Management*, April 1970, pp. 7–9.

Appendix 3 Illustrative Hospital Organization Charts

Figure 3-1 depicts a representative hospital organization structure. However, as discussed, there is no single "right" or "proper" organizational structure. To illustrate this point, several alternative organization structures are presented below.

Alternative 1—Smaller Hospitals*

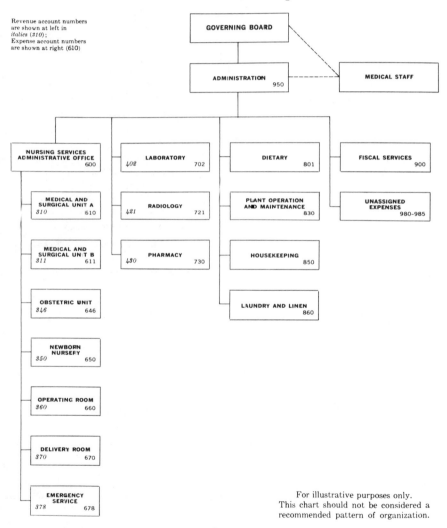

For illustrative purposes only.
This chart should not be considered a
recommended pattern of organization.

*Reprinted with permission from *Chart of Accounts for Hospitals*, published by the American Hospital Association, 1966, p. 130.

Alternative 2*

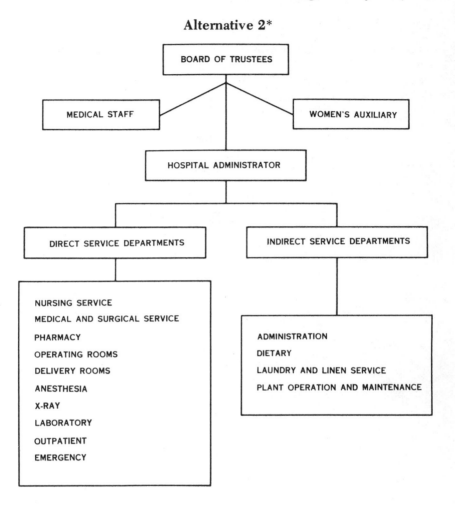

*L. Vann Seawell, *Principles of Hospital Accounting,* Physicians' Record Co., page 329. Reprinted with permission.

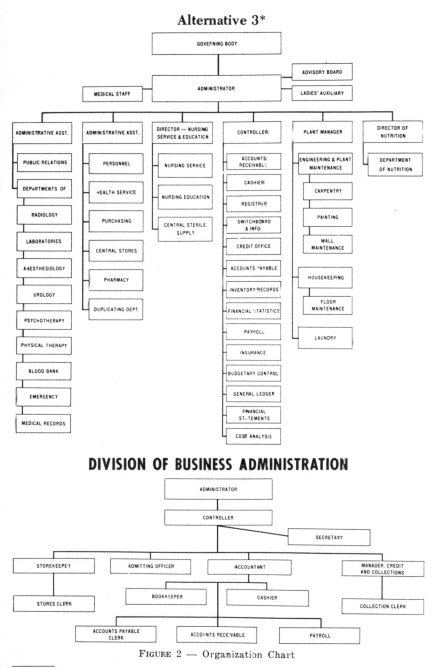

FIGURE 2 — Organization Chart

*L. Vann Seawell, *Hospital Accounting and Financial Management*, Physicians' Record Co., page 14. Reprinted with permission.

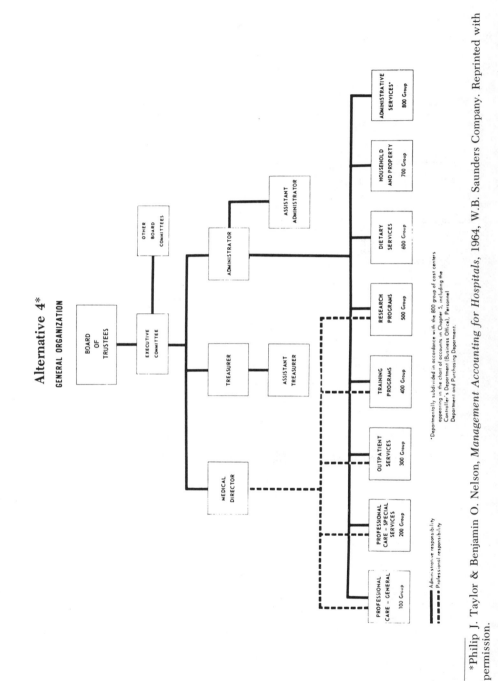

Alternative 4*

GENERAL ORGANIZATION

*Philip J. Taylor & Benjamin O. Nelson, *Management Accounting for Hospitals*, 1964, W.B. Saunders Company. Reprinted with permission.

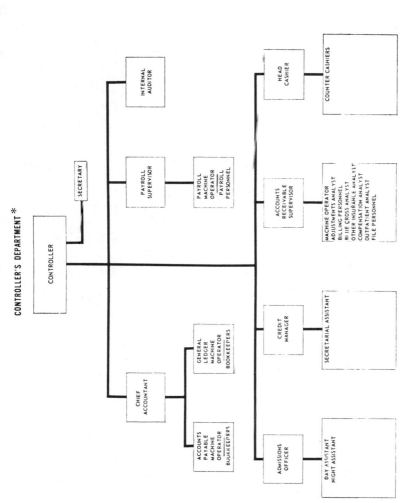

CONTROLLER'S DEPARTMENT *

CONTROLLER

SECRETARY

INTERNAL AUDITOR

PAYROLL SUPERVISOR

PAYROLL MACHINE OPERATOR
PAYROLL PERSONNEL

CHIEF ACCOUNTANT

ACCOUNTS PAYABLE MACHINE OPERATOR
BOOKKEEPERS

GENERAL LEDGER MACHINE OPERATOR
BOOKKEEPERS

ADMISSIONS OFFICER

DAY ASSISTANT
NIGHT ASSISTANT

CREDIT MANAGER

SECRETARIAL ASSISTANT

ACCOUNTS RECEIVABLE SUPERVISOR

MACHINE OPERATOR
ADJUSTMENTS ANALYST
BILLING PERSONNEL
BLUE CROSS ANALYST
OTHER INSURANCE ANALYST
COMPENSATION ANALYST
OUTPATIENT ANALYST
FILE PERSONNEL

HEAD CASHIER

COUNTER CASHIERS

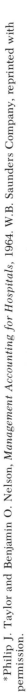

*Philip J. Taylor and Benjamin O. Nelson, *Management Accounting for Hospitals*, 1964. W.B. Saunders Company, reprinted with permission.

Alternative 5—Manufacturing Corporation*

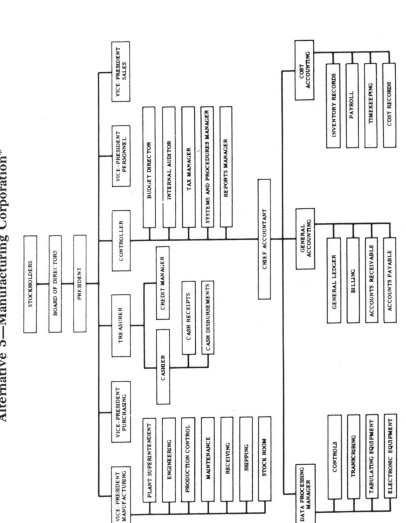

*Howard F. Stettler, *Systems Based Independent Audits* © 1967. Reprinted by permission of Prentice-Hall, Inc., Englewood Cliffs, N.J.

Alternative 6—Manufacturing Corporation*

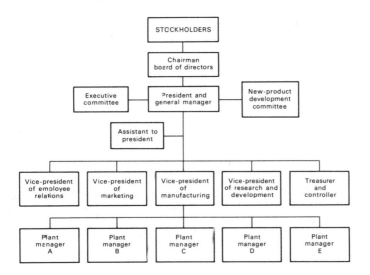

Alternative 7—Manufacturing Corporation*

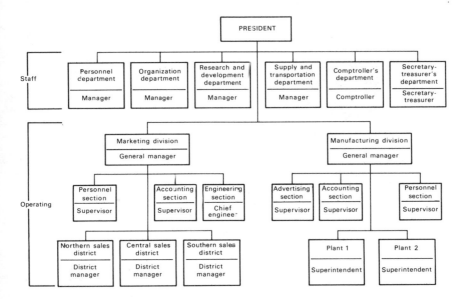

---

*From *Management Theory and Practice* by Ernest Dale, Copyright, 1965. Used with the permission of McGraw-Hill Book Company.

Part II

Sources of
Operating Revenues

It is somewhat unorthodox to include in a text on financial management a discussion of the sources of operating revenue available to a firm. However, in the case of hospital financial management, if a complete understanding of the hospital's financial environment is to be obtained, this approach may be the best way to start, for a unique relationship exists between hospitals and the actual payers for care.

Hospitals, though treating many individual patients, are paid for the services which they provide by a relatively few sources. These sources, because of their relative economic power, are able to affect the financial status of an individual hospital substantially by their payment methods or procedures. Therefore, it seems advisable, before examining the application of financial management tools and techniques to hospital management, first to consider how hospitals are paid.

The Past is Prologue

By way of introduction, it is instructive to begin by first looking backward. Like many complex phenomena, the beginnings of the current patterns of hospital payment are difficult to trace. The history of the present financing system reflects both an overlapping of ideas—as different people in different geographic areas were attempting to solve the same problems at the same time—and a rediscovery—under new circumstances—of previously tried mechanisms. However, out of this image, a thread of logic, which portrays a reasonable systematic development process, can be deciphered.

Prior to the turn of the century, most hospitals billed and were paid on, what would be now called, an all inclusive rate. That is, hospitals charged all patients the same daily rate. This single rate covered all services which the hospital provided.

By today's standards, this sort of "flat" rate approach is admittedly simplistic. However, when viewed in the context of times—wherein hospitals provided only limited services and had an undifferentiated product—the approach not only provided for equity but also represented an administratively sound way to operate.

The flat rate approach served as a workable mechanism until hospitals began to provide more complex as well as differentiated products. The development of specific techniques in surgery, the increased use of anesthesia, and the discovery of the Roentgen ray enabled the hospital product to improve and different products to be provided to different patients. As a result, hospitals established a system of special services charges; patients who used particular services paid separately for them. The intent of the special services charge system was simply to maintain equity between patients who used particular services and those who did not.

Special services and special service charges grew in variety and amount with the introduction of laboratory services, physical therapy, drugs, and so forth. By the 1920s, it was not unusual for a patient's total amount of special service charges to exceed the regular daily service charges.

The growth in special service charges, combined with a general increase in hospital charges, resulted in adverse public reaction to both hospital costs and the *a la carte* approach to billing. As a result of this reaction, the hospital industry began to reconsider—as a means of spreading costs among patients—the practicability of an all inclusive rate financing system.

The early use of the inclusive rate system in the 1920s applied only to certain special services such as laboratory examinations. A few years later the principle was applied to certain admissions by diagnosis such as tonsillectomies and maternity service. In the early 1930s, all inclusive rates were established by some hospitals for all inpatients. These rates varied only as to the length of stay of the patient and the type of accommodations occupied.

While the industry, in general, was moving back to an all inclusive rate payment mechanism, a complementary—and perhaps, more important—innovation was being introduced in Ohio. In 1919, the State of Ohio introduced, for purposes of workmen's compensation payment, the concept of an all inclusive rate based on audited costs. The significance of this concept should not be lost for it provided half the foundation for over 40 years of hospital payment systems. With the introduction of "audited costs," the basis of payment to hospitals not only shifted in terms of decision loci but also, in terms of reliance on objective quantifiable data— cost.

In the early 1920s, the State of Pennsylvania implemented a variation of the Ohio mechanism by paying hospitals on the bais of the estimated cost per day. In the 1930s, the Federal government first became involved, through the Children's Bureau, in hospital care reimbursement. Like Ohio, the Federal government also added an innovation. In this instance, the concept was that of "reimbursable cost." That is, as opposed to full hospital costs, the Children's Bureau only paid the costs per day which were applicable to patient care, excluding costs which were not for direct patient care, i.e., administrative and benefits.

With the introduction of the notion of reimbursable costs, the other half of the payment system foundation was in place. Throughout the next four decades, with the exception of the period in the 1930s when Blue Cross Plans were getting started and a flat rate system was used, a variety of retrospective, prospective, incentive and disincentive systems have been used to pay hospitals. Similarly, the methods of calculating costs and obtaining increased uniformity of calculation among hospitals evolved. While each of these systems and methods built upon and differed from the other, central to each—as well as to the current system—has been and is the notion of audited reimbursable cost.

It is upon this foundation which the following chapters should be considered.

Chapter 4

Sources of Revenue

Introduction

Hospitals are big business. In fact, hospitals are one of the biggest industries in the country. The operation and management of a hospital, however, is in many ways unlike that of other businesses. The distinction between the operation of hospitals and commercial enterprises is particularly apparent in regard to the sources of the revenues which are obtained to support the institution.

With most businesses the source of revenue is the sale of goods or services. The nonhospital business buys or manufactures goods and/or provides services at a certain price and sells those products in a competitive or quasicompetitive market at prices which hopefully will return a profit. Most businesses are run for profit, which tends to challenge management and to force it to produce efficiently and competitively in order to return a profit to the owners.

At one time hospitals were maintained basically to care for the critically or chronically ill and depended on benefactors and philanthropists to finance any deficits. Today, due to increased utilization of hospitals and greater costs of operation, the benefactor alone cannot subsidize hospital operations. He may furnish capital funds at some time in his life to erect a hospital building to bear his name, but taxes have eaten into his income to such a degree that he no longer stands ready at each year-end to make up the hospital's operating losses.

Most of today's hospitals are not managed as profit-making, competitive institutions and, as stated, they generally do not have philanthropists who will make up their deficits. Today, voluntary hospitals depend on "third parties" as their major source of revenue.

Who is a third party? The third party (besides the hospital and patient who are the first two parties) is Blue Cross, the commercial insurance company, Medicare, Medicaid, Workmen's Compensation, or any agent other than the patient who contracts to pay all or part of a patient's hospital bill. A third party is the major source of revenue for the hospital, is a sure source of revenue, and is a party that can be depended upon to pay its bill within a certain payment system and within a reasonably constant time period. Therefore, the third party is a highly important factor in the operation of a hospital.

The share of total hospital expenses paid by the third party will vary from area to area and from hospital to hospital. On average, however, one can think of hospital revenues (collections, not charges) as coming, in rounded figures from:

Blue Cross payments	30%
Government agencies	30%
Commercial and independent insurance	30%
Self-pay	10%

One might infer from these figures that there was a distribution of payments at the same rate or price among the various payers. This is far from true, for there is a double standard of payment which many think is unfair and unjust.

The major purchasers of hospital care today, Blue Cross and the Federal government (principally Medicare and Medicaid), usually pay on a "cost" or "cost-plus" basis because they say they are wholesale buyers of care. The remainder of the purchasers of hospital care pay at rates higher than the "cost" or "cost-plus" reimbursement formulas. Some of these higher charges are partially covered by commercial insurance policies which pay certain indemnities for specified services. Any balance beyond the stated indemnities would be charged directly to the patient. The same is true for "deductibles" and services beyond those allowed under a third party policy, such as the amount disallowed for certain outpatient services or the difference between the rate for a two-bed room allowed under the policy and the rate for the private room which was used.

On the face of it, this method of charges and payments seems plausible and quite fair. As indicated earlier, most voluntary community hospitals are not operated for profit. In fact, they are classified as "not-for-profit." Under this not-for-profit arrangement, the major portion of Blue Cross contracts calls for "cost-plus" reimbursements, Medicare pays "costs," the insurance companies pay the benefits allowed under the insurance contract, and the self-pay patient pays the balance, which might seem his just share.

Unfortunately, there are two factors which place Mr. Self-Pay Patient in a very uncomfortable position where he is unable to do much to protect himself against the uncontrolled explosion in the price of hospital care. First, there is no incentive for the not-for-profit hospital to contain costs as long as costs are "reasonable" and will be allowed by Blue Cross and the government. There is no real price competition in the market place between hospitals which would establish a base for reasonable prices. What competition there is, is status competition which will be discussed later.

The second tragic factor for Mr. Self-Pay is that he purchases services at retail in a system where all the other major payers for care purchase service at "cost" or very slightly above "cost." However, the problem is not that the third party puchasers pay "cost," but rather that cost as defined by the purchasers is neither total accounting cost nor economic cost. Thus, what is not allowed as "cost" by third party payers must be paid by someone else and that "someone else" is the only one left, Mr. Self-Pay, who must pay the highest rate of all.

This last point is critical and deserves further clarification. In accounting terms, cost can be defined as any release of value. That is, a cost is incurred any time something of value—usually money—is given up in order to obtain something else. Thus, costs are equal to the money given up to obtain labor and capital necessary to operate the hospital and treat patients. This definition of costs would probably be accepted in theory by both hospitals and third parties. However, third parties do not feel that this approach represents an equitable basis for paying hospitals. Instead, they suggest there are two types of costs: the full costs defined above (the total costs incurred in operating the hospital); and reimbursable costs, which differ from full costs in that they do not include all the costs involved in operating the hospital. Every hospital has many legitimate costs which might not be evident to one unfamiliar with the administration of a hospital.

A hospital is a complex organization with problems peculiar to its field. It develops expenses in its operation, some of which may seem only tangential to the care of patients, yet which can be pointed to as part of the total process of medical and nursing care. The legitimacy of some of these costs has been rejected by the large third party purchasers of care who feel the costs are not directly related to the care their clients are receiving, that they are not directly related to any of the nursing, medical or paramedical services they are purchasing.

Over the years, the justification for allowing the so-called tangential or peripheral costs under the reimbursement formulas has been debated by the hospitals, Blue Cross, and the government. Some of the costs have been allowed, others have been disallowed or are still under discussion. In the meantime, the costs being debated are still being incurred by hospitals and are still being paid by Mr. Self-Pay.[1]

It has been mentioned, but bears repeating, that all of the expenses a hospital incurs are not considered allowable costs and consequently Mr. Self-Pay, from whom ten to twelve percent of the hospital's revenue comes, must pay the disallowed costs if the hospital can find no other source of payment.

Debated Areas of Hospital Costs

A discussion of the debated areas of hospital costs should illustrate and clarify the problem.

Depreciation of Buildings and Equipment

Depreciation could be said to be merely a recognition that things wear out and need to be replaced. If allowance is made for this depreciation and the money value is set aside, with price levels constant, then the buildings and equipment can be replaced as they wear out. This is simplified language.

Unfortunately, depreciation cannot be discussed with such simplified language. Depreciation is an expense of doing business, whether in a supermarket or in a community hospital. There is no question in the mind of the supermarket operator that depreciation of buildings and moveable equipment is a real cost of doing business, but the hospital has often in the past had to "debate" whether depreciation should be an allowable cost under third party reimbursement formulas.

For the most part, third parties now accept and recognize depreciation as a legitimate operating expense and allow its inclusion in the reimbursement formula. This acceptance, however, has not ended the controversy surrounding depreciation, for hospitals and

---

[1]The commercial firms are operating under another set of rules which allow them to offer protection on a defined benefit basis or on a wide coverage basis, such as the major medical policy, with a deductible factor—both conditions under rates based on actuarial figures.

third parties now have shifted the debate from whether depreciation should be considered as a legitimate operating expense to what the conditions should be for accepting it as an expense. The conditions or debatable points are likely to be: whether the amount to be depreciated should be the historical (original) cost or the replacement cost of the buildings and equipment; what the estimated life of the items should be; and what the method of computing depreciation should be. Historical cost generally is and should be used in calculating depreciation in reimbursement formulas; estimated life of buildings and equipment is determined by past practice and by rulings of the Internal Revenue Service; and the actual depreciation is computed by a method agreeable to both parties.[2,3]

Three of the common methods of computing depreciation are: straight line; sum-of-the-years in digits, and double declining balance. The last two methods are often referred to as accelerated depreciation. In the first two methods the sum to be depreciated would be the historical cost less the estimated salvage value, and would be computed over the "lifetime" by an agreed upon method. The third method depreciates the *total* historical cost leaving a balance at the end of the period which would be an amount similar to the salvage value allowed under the other methods.

The straight line method of calculating depreciation is to divide

---

[2]The argument for the use of historical cost rather than replacement cost for computing depreciation can be based on the definition of depreciation. The historical cost method is correct if depreciation is considered as a means of allocating previously incurred costs to the proper time periods during which the facilities are used up. Replacement of worn-out facilities should be a separate problem. Replacement can be financed from the depreciation fund without being related to the method of computing depreciation.

[3]Though historical cost has been the traditional standard for reporting asset values and computing depreciation, the Securities and Exchange Commission (SEC) in 1976, adopted regulations that would require certain companies to disclose replacement cost information in financial statements filed with the Commission. The SEC's ruling initially applies only to public corporations that have inventories and gross property, plant, and equipment which aggregate more than $100 million and which comprise more than 10 percent of assets.

Such companies are required to disclose the estimated current replacement cost of inventories and productive capacity at the end of each fiscal year for which a balance sheet is required and the approximate amount of cost of sales and depreciation based on replacement cost for the two most recent full fiscal years.

The SEC's initial efforts, though appropriately flexible—and allowing for imprecision, are an attempt to assure that financial reports reflect current business economics. More importantly, the SEC's initiative sets a new precedent, which if extended can not only radically change financial reporting and corporate management behavior—but also, if extended to the full health industry, can have profound implications on health planning, hospital payment, etc.

Table 4-1
Depreciation by Three Methods

Historical Cost $60,000
Salvage Value $5,000
Net Cost to be Depreciated $55,000

Historical Cost To be Depreciated $60,000

STRAIGHT LINE			SUM-OF-YEARS DIGIT					DOUBLE DECLINING BALANCE		
Deprec. year	Depreciation Amt. this yr.	Deprec. to date		Deprec. year	Est. life	Depreciation Amt. this yr.	Deprec. to date	Deprec. year	Depreciation Amt. this yr.	Deprec. to date
1	$5,500	$ 5,500		1	10	$10,000	$10,000	1	$12,000	$12,000
2	$5,500	$11,000		2	9	$ 9,000	$19,000	2	$ 9,600	$21,600
3	$5,500	$16,500		3	8	$ 8,000	$27,000	3	$ 7,680	$29,280
4	$5,500	$22,000		4	7	$ 7,000	$34,000	4	$ 6,144	$35,424
5	$5,500	$27,500		5	6	$ 6,000	$40,000	5	$ 4,915	$40,339
6	$5,500	$33,000		6	5	$ 5,000	$45,000	6	$ 3,932	$44,271
7	$5,500	$38,500		7	4	$ 4,000	$49,000	7	$ 3,146	$47,417
8	$5,500	$44,000		8	3	$ 3,000	$52,000	8	$ 2,517	$49,934
9	$5,500	$49,500		9	2	$ 2,000	$54,000	9	$ 2,013	$51,947
10	$5,500	$55,000		10	1	$ 1,000	$55,000	10	$ 1,611	$53,558

the cost of the item to be depreciated less the salvage value by the number of years of estimated life. For example, a $60,000 item with a salvage value of $5,000 would leave a balance of $55,000 for depreciation. If the estimated life was ten years, the depreciation allowed each year would be 1/10 of the balance after subtracting the salvage value, or $5,500.

Under the sum-of-the-years digit method, the amount to be depreciated is multiplied by a fraction made up of a numerator which equals the number of years of estimated life remaining and of a denominator equal to the sum of the total years of life. To use the same set of figures as in the first example, depreciation by the sum-of-years method would be computed as follows: the first year,

$$\$55,000 \times \frac{10 \text{ (Years of estimated life remaining)}}{55 \text{ (sum of total years } 10 + 9 + 8 + 7}_{+6 +5 +4 +3 +2 +1 = 55)} = \$10,000;$$

the second year, $\$55,000 \times \frac{9}{55} = \$9,000$; the third year the fraction

would be $\frac{8}{55}$, and so on.

With the double declining method, depreciation is figured by dividing the total historical cost by half the number of estimated years of life the first year; thereafter, each year divide the remaining balance by half of the total years of life. In the example used before, figuring by the double declining balance method, the depreciation the first year is computed by dividing $60,000 by 5 (half the estimated life years), or $12,000, leaving a balance of $48,000. The second year the $48,000 is divided by 5 to give a depreciation of $9,600, leaving a balance of $38,400, and so on.

The method of depreciation which a hospital can use under the "cost" and "cost-plus" formulas of reimbursement must be negotiated in many cases because there are differences in the depreciation rates by the accelerated methods (the sum-of-the-years digit method and the declining balance method) from the straight line method, particularly in the first five years. Table 4-1 illustrates the differences and the management implications of the accelerated methods.

During times of rising price levels, it is important to recover capital costs through depreciation as quickly as possible so that the hospital's capital funds can be re-invested in order to protect against the lower purchasing power caused by inflation and rising price levels. The usefulness of accelerated depreciation to gain this protection becomes apparent when one realizes that depreciation funds can be invested or used immediately for capital purposes in dollars which reflect current value. If it is necessary to wait a few years longer to receive depreciation funds, and prices rise, the funds obtained through depreciation will buy less. Therefore, during periods of rising prices it is important for the hospital to depreciate its buildings and equipment at accelerated rates in order to have depreciation funds with the greatest possible purchasing power for replacement purposes.

Debt Principal as an Allowable Cost

Hospitals, as do individuals, often buy buildings, land and major equipment on deferred payments. The purchase is usually financed under a plan providing for payments on the principal, plus an interest charge on the unpaid balance, much as an individual finances the purchase of a home. The individual certainly thinks of the monthly payment on his home as an expense for which he must budget and plan. The hospital must also make provisions to meet the principal and interest payments on its debt. However, considering the hospital's payment as an allowable expense in the cost reimbursement formulas raises an interesting question which reasonably can be asked: Should payments on debt be an allowed cost under reimbursement formulas for hospital care?

In the previous section depreciation was shown as a method of recovering the historical cost, less salvage value, of buildings and equipment over the estimated lifetime of the items. Thus, depreciation compensates the hospital for the expense of purchasing buildings and equipment. If the payments on the principal of the debt were allowed as an expense, and if an expense item were also allowed for depreciation on buildings and equipment, then there would be two allowances (double allowance) for the cost of buildings and equipment. If depreciation is the route used to allow for the cost of buildings and equipment, as it should be, then there is an orderly method to recover the cost of buildings and equipment over the estimated lifetime of those items, no matter how they were acquired: by cash, deferred payments, or by gifts. Thus, there is no need for additional funds to amortize debt because funds for this purpose are provided through depreciation expense payments.

Debt principal payments are not recognized as allowable cost by either Blue Cross, or the Federal government. Accelerated depreciation, with depreciation funded, should be the method of accounting for the cost of buildings and equipment. It would seem that anyone arguing for double allowance is in a very untenable position.

The special problem of how to cover the need for extra capital for facilities, for added services or for the acquisition of additional land is discussed in item 8, "Plus Factor as an Allowable Cost."

Education as an Allowable Cost

Education is an expense item in hospitals which varies greatly with the size of the hospital and the services it offers. Some small hospitals spend little or nothing in this area. At the other extreme, the large university teaching hospital has training expenses for medical students, residents, and nurses in addition to medical faculty costs, paramedical training courses, continuing education, and other hospital in-service activities. For purposes of the reimbursement formulas, reasonable net costs are allowed for approved patient-related educational purposes. The net cost is the balance after grants, scholarships, and other monies paid in support of the educational program have been deducted from the total expense incurred. This approach to paying educational costs is quite reasonable. The only debatable point here is the relation of the cost to the patient. The administrator should consider educational programs necessary to the operation of his hospital as patient-related, for the prime purpose of the institution is to give the best possible care to the patient.

Research as an Allowable Cost

Research has the same criteria for acceptance as an allowable cost under reimbursement formulas as educational costs: the research expense should be net expense after deduction of grants, gifts for research, and other monies designated for research; and the research must be patient-related. Patient relationship is sometimes more difficult to interpret with research than with education because research, by nature, might seem to be more "pure" than "applied." If the hospital determines that the research it approves is pragamatic, the administrator should insist that it is patient-related and that the net expense be allowed as a reimbursable cost. Research is a necessary ingredient of a dynamic process such as the provision of health care, and should be allowed in total as a reimbursable expense.

Bad Debts as Allowable Cost

Blue Cross and Medicare (as well as other government programs) buy and pay for hospital service according to an arrangement agreed upon by the buyer and provider of the services. The agencies buying services pay for all they buy at an agreed rate so, at least in theory, there are no bad debts in this contractual relationship. Although bad debts may not arise directly from the hospital-third party relationship, there are at least two attitudes about the third party's responsibilities for bad debts. One attitude might be: if the hospital has bad debts resulting from services furnished to self-pay patients, it cannot expect Blue Cross or Medicare to consider the bad debts as an allowable cost in their reimbursement formulas. However, there is a possible exception in which bad debts occur in third party relationships. If Blue Cross or Medicare deducts certain amounts from the benefits of patients (according to contract or agreement), the hospital must bill the patient directly for the deducted amounts. These deducted amounts are difficult and costly to collect and often become bad debts. There is some justification for the allowance of this kind of bad debt as an expense item under the payment formula.

A second attitude might be that a hospital must be financially viable in order to furnish Blue Cross subscribers and Medicare clients with services on a "cost" basis. Furthermore, the hospital cannot remain in a viable state if all its real costs are not met. Therefore, aside from overcharging the self-pay patient and/or depending on fund drives or benefactors to pay off bad debts and some of the other real costs which have been disallowed in reimbursement formulas, the hospitals are going to have to insist that the third party purchasers of care pay their fair shares of all the real operating costs.

Interest Expense as an Allowable Cost

Interest expense is generally recognized as a legitimate claim. However, the term "net interest" is used in reimbursement negotiations to mean the interest expense a hospital incurs less any interest the hospital receives on investments. For accounting purists, this is an abhorrent practice to combine the two in this manner. Nevertheless, there is no disagreement that interest paid is an expense, and that interest earned generally should be credited against operating expenses by proper accounting methods. However, the two are discrete and different items and deserve to be so treated.

Interest paid by the hospital for purposes agreed on as legitimate by the hospital and the third party should be allowed as an expense. Interest earned by the hospital should be considered separately from interest paid—not as a bookkeeping item only—

but on the characteristics of each transaction of business producing interest or dividends. For example, under the present Medicare reimbursement formula, interest earned on investments of
funds from the depreciation account can be added to that account
without deducting any part of the earnings from the allowance
(under the reimbursement formula) for the interest the hospital
pays on its obligations. In the same manner, interest or dividends
earned on investments from other special purpose funds should be
credited to those funds.

Interest paid by the hospital is an expense. Interest earned by
the hospital can be revenue or it can be money paid into an account for a special purpose. Special purpose funds, in the final
analysis, are eventually used to support the hospital's health care
delivery system and furnish needed dollars which will not be
requested from the Blue Cross, Medicare or the public. There are
several ways the interest-earned dollars flow through the system,
but ultimately the patient benefits. "Net interest" is a fiction and
as such should be dropped from discussions of the very real problems faced in providing quality hospital care.

Free Service, Allowances, or Discounts as Allowable Costs

These items are considered under the heading of revenue rather
than cost by Blue Cross and the government, even though the
hospital would prefer to include them as expenses. A service being furnished at a discount (or free) is a service being furnished at
a rate agreed upon by the hospital and the other party, whether
the party be an employee, a staff physician, a student or an indigent patient. The hospital would like to include all discounts and
allowances as costs recoverable from Blue Cross and the government, as well as from the private patient.

It would seem fair to consider discounts and allowances as deductions from the prices charged patients or other purchasers.
Therefore, the revenue is reduced, not an expense incurred, when
services or goods are sold at reduced prices.

Free service, whether it be charity or an unpaid bill which must
be charged off, represents a cost. Someone must pay for that cost
which is inescapable in operating a general hospital. Since it is a
kind of cost which is always present, it would seem fair to spread
the payment of this cost to all who use the hospital. Presently, the
self-pay patient pays the costs no one else wants to assume or
which cannot be met by contributions or other nonoperating
sources of revenue.

Plus Factor as an Allowable Cost

A better term should be coined than "plus factor" for a necessary cost element now to be discussed so it will not be confused with the "cost-plus" allowed under certain Blue Cross contracts for certain unforeseen costs or contingencies. Besides "cost-plus" there is also need for another plus factor, a certain small percentage of the capital invested in the hospital plant which would be allowed each year for growth, for increases in the cost of replacement of existing facilities and equipment, and to keep abreast of the state of the art. This in no way implies that the plus factor should be sufficient for large building programs or for added services, but merely to ensure that the hospital does not fall behind with its present facilities. This plus factor is not acceptable to the third parties, but it is an economic cost and a reality of need which will not disappear and which should be viewed as a reasonable and necessary cost of operation.

The Position of the American Hospital Association

The AHA has issued three documents in the past fifteen years which have had a direct bearing on the question of hospital revenues. The first publication was *Principles of Payment for Hospital Care* revised in 1963; the second was *Statement on the Financial Requirements of Health Care Institutions and Services* in 1969; the third was the *Financial Requirements of Health Care Institutions and Services* in 1977.

In *Principles,* the Association addressed itself to several of the questionable items of expense for which hospitals request allowance as cost in the Blue Cross and government reimbursement formulas. By 1969, the evolution in the thinking of AHA was evident. Although the same questions of allowable costs were included, the descriptive words were different. In 1969, the AHA was now looking at the relationship of the health care institution and the wholesale purchaser of services from a wider perspective—even a more philosophic frame of reference. The 1977 policy document reaffirms and updates the 1969 *Statement of Financial Requirements of Health Care Institutions and Services,* emphasizing that all purchasers of health care must recognize and share fully in the total financial requirements of institutions providing care. It also highlights the concept of the institution needing, as a capital requirement, adequate reserves.

The Association was talking about "the health care institution" instead of the "hospital," was recommending areawide planning, and was speaking of the purchaser meeting "the full financial requirements of the providers." Many of the words were changed in 1969 from those of the 1963 "Principles" which might have had bad connotations for the major purchasers. The new view was wider, more prospective, and was an attempt to consider the hospital financial system as an entity rather than the sum of several diverse pieces.

The three documents will be discussed in detail because they deal with problem areas which affect the solvency of almost all hospitals.

Principles of Payment for Hospital Care—1963

The American Hospital Association, in this document, discussed the problems its member hospitals faced in being reimbursed for hospital care given to Blue Cross subscribers or to patients whose care was paid for by a government agency. The summary of the major recommendations given below indicates both a need for change in the hospital-third party contracts—and a change in the attitudes on several of the debatable issues already discussed in this chapter.

The recommendations included:

(1) The amount and method of payment to hospitals should ensure fair and adequate payment for the provider of service; that essential services be maintained; and that encouragement be given to develop higher standards of service. (This was a good general statement to serve as a preamble).

(2) Agencies purchasing hospital services should pay the costs incurred in providing the services, and total payments should not exceed total hospital charges for those services during the accounting period. (Again, a generalization that costs incurred in providing services should be paid, but that payments should not exceed regular hospital charges.)

(3) There should be a uniform reimbursement rate for similar services for all third party agencies.

(4) Third parties should not be expected to pay for a portion of the cost of a specific case which has been or will be paid from other revenues. (As an example, the care of a traffic accident victim might be totally or partially paid for as an automobile insurance benefit. This is accepted practice.)

(5) Charges to self-pay patients should be based upon and reasonably related to costs. (Strangely enough, in a commentary on this point, it was stated that charges to self-pay patients should not

be less than composite cost. In practice, the self-pay patient usually pays more than the "cost" allowed under the reimbursement formulas.)

(6) Hospitals furnishing services to beneficiaries of third party purchasers should make essential facilities and high quality service available with "due regard to economy and efficiency." (This is a necessary point for a document of this kind, even if it is self-evident.)

(7) "Rates of payment should reflect current hospital costs" thus making it necessary that providers and buyers of hospital service have a workable method of compensating for changing costs. (A formula is necessary to compensate for changing costs because in some instances the periods for reconciling accounts under the reimbursement formulas can be several months or a year apart. If costs should change rapidly, as they often do, a hospital could be caught with a rate of payment well below actual cost.)

(8) Payments to different hospitals for the same service may differ because of variation of costs reflecting occupancy rate, hospital design and equipment, medical staff, employee's salaries, services offered, location of hospital (urban, rural, suburban), and other details. (This difference of conditions in hospitals, which may vary the cost of providing the same service, is understood and accepted.)

(9) "The determination of reimbursable cost requires acceptance and use of uniform definitions, accounting, statistics and reporting"—preferably using A.H.A. financial publications as guides. (If there is to be a uniform method of computing reimbursable cost, there certainly should be uniformity in accounting and record-keeping.)

(10) The principle of average cost per inpatient day should be applied in reimbursement cost formulas when the patients for whom a third party contracting agency is responsible are average for the hospital. This makes it necessary to take into consideration accommodations (private, semiprivate, ward), type of unit or service (obstetrics, medical, surgical, chronic care), and other special conditions. (This is another reasonable recommendation pointed toward all parties being treated alike in charges for service whether the patient's care is being paid under Blue Cross, Medicare, or self-pay plans.)

(11) Expenditures for medical research, "over and beyond the usual care of patients," should not be included in reimbursable cost. (This would seem to necessitate definition of allowable net

expense for medical research, including what medical research is related to patient care and what is not. This might be a problem difficult to negotiate in some instances.)

(12) The net cost of medical, nursing, and other related education should be an allowable cost. (This was discussed earlier in the chapter where net cost was determined by subtracting grants, tuition allowances, and other monies designated for education from the total cost of education.)

(13) Bad debts, unpaid costs of the indigent and medically indigent, and courtesy allowances should not be included in reimbursable cost but should be considered as deductions from earned income. (The authors have taken a view different from A.H.A. on this point. Earlier in the chapter bad debts and other unpaid costs were called costs which should be allowed in the reimbursement formulas; discounts were considered reductions in revenue, but not an allowable cost.)

(14) Ordinary remodeling should be charged against maintenance repairs as an expense item; remodeling which enhances capital value should be capitalized and, therefore, not included in reimbursable costs. (This should not be controversial.)

(15) Net interest (as explained earlier in the chapter) at a reasonable rate incurred on capital or other indebtedness should be allowed in determining reimbursable costs. (This, too, is generally acceptable.)

(16) Expenses incurred by hospitals providing services of sisters or other members of religious orders should be allowed as operating expenses at rates no greater than those paid employees for similar work. (This is common practice.)

(17) Income received from government agencies, foundations and others to support projects or pay salaries of special employees who ordinarily would not be employed by the hospital should be deducted from expenses in determining reimbursable cost. (Hospitals should not oppose this reasonable recommendation.)

(18) A separate cost for the nursery care of newborns should be allowed. (This recommendation of a separate cost center for nursery care of newborns was prompted by special instances where nursery care is a substantial unit of care and the special costs involved might influence the average cost of care of the whole hospital. By separating costs of the nursery, other patient costs could be figured more fairly.)

(19) Depreciation of buildings and equipment should be allowed (and be used for capital purposes) in accordance with the

recommendations of A.H.A.'s *Uniform Chart of Accounts and Definitions for Hospitals.* (The A.H.A. believes its rates of depreciation have become standard, and this is probably true.)

(20) Expenses for inpatient and outpatient services should be segregated. (This is necessary because of the difference in Blue Cross reimbursement rates for inpatients and outpatients, and because cost factors and conditions in the two sectors are different, thus affecting any cost analysis.)

(21) Hospitals should not be required to use funds from endowment funds or restricted gifts to reduce third party payments. (This is a reiteration of the principle that third parties who purchase hospital service on a cost-based formula should pay the total costs of providing that service, thus obviating a need for the hospital to supplement the third party payment from any source.)

(22) Income from endowment funds or gifts designated for the care of specific groups of third party beneficiaries should be used to reduce third party payments for persons in such groups. (This is a fair proposal.)

(23) "Hospitals should not be required to use net income from nonpatient service to reduce third party payments." (Net income from rental of office space or from sharing of facilities with other organizations might be considered a revenue different from interest received on investments. However, a question might arise as to whether net income from nonpatient services should not indirectly reduce the charges to all classes of purchasers, certainly not to third party payers alone.)

(24) The A.H.A. "Principles" also include the obligations of the parties, as applicable: to keep and make available adequate records; to furnish satisfactory service and payment; to make reports in the form and at the time agreed upon; to make studies of factors of the services provided in order to promote quality of care and economy of cost; and for the hospitals to act in association in order to develop more uniform standards and practices.

All the points noted in the A.H.A. "Principles" are pertinent and deserve consideration and study by all parties concerned on a continuing basis, for the administration of a hospital and the care of its patients is a fluid, ever-changing process.

Statement on the Financial Requirements of Health Care Institutions and Services—1969

The "Statement" proposes a program which would provide proper financing of the health care system and calls for the system to accept "the community's right to insist on proper planning within that system." The "Statement" is labeled as a set of general guidelines and is couched in rather euphemistic terms to sweeten the words previously used to describe some of the debated elements of reimbursement formulas.

It is important for the reader to note how the A.H.A. stresses the responsibility of all purchasers of care to bear their proportionate shares of the operating and capital costs of the health care institutions, and how the community and the area planning agencies are considered participating partners along with the providers and purchasers of health care.

Briefly summarized, the "Statement" made the following points:

1. *The purchasers of care collectively should pay the total financial requirements of the health care institutions* (both current operating requirements and capital needs) which are listed below.

   (a) Salaries, wages, employee's fringe benefits, services, supplies, normal maintenance, minor building modifications, and applicable taxes. (These expenses are normal, regular and noncontroversial with the possible exception of the interpretation of "minor building modifications.")

   (b) Interest on funds borrowed for capital needs and operating cash purposes. Interest on external loans for plant capital purposes would be reduced by income earned on investments of operating funds, endowments, gifts, and grants when such income was not assigned for specific purposes. The above offset would not apply to income on funds borrowed for current operating cash needs if the amount and application of the funds were "consistent with prudent fiscal management." (This is the net interest concept again, but with the added consideration of the interest earned on investment of borrowed current operating funds not being used to offset interest paid on borrowed funds. The A.H.A. may find difficulty in obtaining agreement on this exemption from the offset. This could be a bargaining point which could be disallowed in exchange for some other advantage.)

   (c) Financial needs for approved educational programs above amounts covered by tuition, grants, scholarships, and other sources. (This is the "net educational cost" discussed earlier.)

   (d) Financial needs for approved research projects related to patient care above amounts covered by grants and other contributions. (This is the "net research cost" discussed earlier.)

(e) All purchasers of care should be responsible for their appropriate share of the bad debts. (This is a little ambiguous as to what the "appropriate share" is, yet it is an important point the A.H.A. is making: that *all* purchasers should be responsible for a share of the bad debt. In the past, bad debts have not usually been considered an allowable cost.)

(f) The cost of care of patients unable to pay—the medically indigent—should be appropriately shared by all purchasers of care. (The situation is directly parallel to the bad debts provision in the paragraph above—and is as important as that point.)

(g) Capital needs are discussed generally under the headings:

(1.) Plant capital needs for preservation and replacement of plant and equipment; improvement of plant; expansion of plant; and amortization of plant capital indebtedness.

(2.) Operating cash needs to meet the fluctuating day-to-day obligations.

(3.) Return on investment for proprietary (for-profit) health care institutions. (The A.H.A. "Statement" avoids the use of the words "depreciation" and "plus factor" and seems to be suggesting that a capital fund be established into which would be paid depreciation of buildings and equipment, gifts, grants and appropriations and some payment from patient services. From this seemingly suggested fund could be paid sums for: acquisition of land; replacement and major modernization of buildings; expansion of plant, equipment and services; and for amortization of capital indebtedness. Also, the need for operating funds demands a method for raising such monies. The purpose of A.H.A. seems to be to establish this need for capital funds and operating funds and for the advisability of all purchasers of care paying their proportionate shares of these needs. Apparently it is assumed that these financial requirements could be negotiated by the large purchasers and the health care institution under suggested formulas. One point lightly touched upon was a recommendation that health care institutions being run for profit be allowed a fair return on their investment. If this is allowed, then it would seem that not-for-profit hospitals could rightfully ask for a "plus factor" for growth and to hedge against inflation in lieu of the return on investment.)

2. *The role and responsibilities of the health care institution*

(a) According to the "Statement," the health care institution should maintain high quality of care, promote effective utilization of its patient care services, and inform and educate the community to the proper use of health care facilities. The institution should investigate the opportunities of sharing services, such as purchasing, laundry and computers, with other facilities. Ongoing planning, both short- and long-term, should be the rule. Financial data should be available to the contracting parties and, when indicated, to the public.

(b) The contracting parties should strive to offer benefits as liberal as possible, and should advise the public members covered by prepayment plans to contract for as wide a coverage as possible. The contracting parties should strive to improve the efficiency of their administration of the health care dollar while making retroactive appeal methods available for adjustment of charges. The parties should disclose information to the public on the utilization and financing of services.

(c) Areawide planning councils for health care should cooperate and assist both health care institutions and contracting parties and also liaison with general community planning agencies. The councils should aid the community with respect to the "appropriateness, adequacy, priority and location of health care services and facilities." The A.H.A. would have the areawide planning council be an approving agency for new buildings and expansion plans as well as for puchase of major equipment. The capital spending fund the A.H.A. would establish would be operative for new major spending under the advice of the area planning council.

(d) The community is expected to support its health care institution with cash contributions and moral reinforcement.

American Hospital Association Policy, 1977

The 1977 American Hospital Association policy is fundamentally a reaffirmation of the 1969 Statement. It does, however, differ from its predecessor in that it more firmly addresses the concept of operating margin, emphasizing that institutions must include in their financial requirements a factor which will enable them to assure that adequate resources will be available to finance necessary changes, i.e., new technology, expansion, working capital requirements, and so forth. The 1977 Statement also emphasizes that all purchasers must recognize and share fully in the institutions' total financial requirements. In this regard, the point is made that "Any apportionment that permits a purchaser to assume a lesser responsibility is not appropriate and does not alter the total financial requirements of the health care institution. Rather, it requires other purchasers to make up the deficiency."

The 1977 policy statement is presented below:

Financial Requirements of Health Care Institutions and Services

Introduction

The delivery of health services requires a vast array of professional services, institutions, allied health organizations and educational programs, research activities, and community health projects. A high-quality health care delivery system is dependent upon the commitment of sufficient resources and their effective management. The system must ensure that necessary services are provided to the public in an effective, efficient, and economic manner. Coordination of the components of the health care delivery system and self-discipline of all participants within the system are necessary to meet this end. Three interrelated functions whereby such coordination and self-discipline can be achieved are effective planning, effective utilization, and effective management. These functions share the ultimate purpose of maintaining the highest standards of quality in the delivery of health care.

The health care delivery system has and should continue to have multiple sources of financing that must meet total financial requirements. These sources of financing should recognize that health care institutions must be financed at a level that supports the health objectives of the community, including uncompensated care costs as defined herein. The health care delivery system and its financing should be sufficiently flexible to change as needs of the community change and as new and effective technologies are developed so that the total financial requirements can continue to be met.

Elements of Financial Requirements

Institutional financial stability requires that there be a realistic appraisal of the two major financial components: (1) current operating requirements and (2) operating margin.

Meeting these financial requirements will enable the institutions to maintain and improve current programs and facilities and to initiate new programs and facilities consistent with community needs and advances in medical science.

Health care institutions differ in size, scope, and types of ownership and services, and therefore their operating and capital requirements differ. However, all elements of financial requirements must be reflected in the payments to health care institutions to provide adequately for demonstrated financial needs. The elements of financial requirements are described below.

Current Operating Requirements

Current operating requirements include the following costs:

1. Patient care
    These costs include, but are not limited to, salaries and wages, employee benefits, purchased services, interest expense, supplies, insurance, maintenance, minor building modification, leases, applicable taxes, depreciation, and the monetary value assigned to services provided by members of religious orders and other organized religious groups.

2. Patients who do not pay
    It must be recognized that a portion of the total financial requirements will not be met by certain patients who:
    a. Fail to fully meet their incurred obligation for services rendered,
    b. Are relieved wholly or in part of their responsibilities because of their inability to pay for services rendered. Therefore, these unrecovered financial requirements must be included as a current operating requirement for those who pay.

3. Education
    Where financial needs for educational programs having appropriate approval have not been met through tuition, schol-

arships, grants, or other sources, all purchasers of care must assume their appropriate share of the financial requirements to meet these needs.

4. Research
    Appropriate health care services and patient-related clinical research programs are an element of the total financial requirements of an institution. The cost of these programs should be met primarily from endowment income, gifts, grants, or other sources.

Operating Margin

In order to meet the total financial requirements of an institution, a margin of net patient care revenues in excess of current operating requirements must be maintained. This difference will provide necessary funds for working capital requirements, capital requirements, and return on equity.

1. Working capital requirements
Financial stability is dependent on having sufficient cash to meet current fiscal obligations as they come due.

2. Capital requirements
Health care institutions are expected to meet demands resulting from such factors as population shifts, discontinuance of other existing services, and changes in the public's demand for types of services delivered. In order to be in a position to respond to such changing community needs, health care institutions must anticipate and include such capital needs in their financial requirements. There must be assurances that adequate resources will be available to finance recognized necessary changes.

The capital requirements of a health care institution must be evaluated and approved by its governing authority in the context of the institution's role and mission in the community's health care delivery system. Coordination among the health care institution's governing authority, administration, and medical staff and the cooperation among health organizations and the appropriate areawide health planning agency are essential to this evaluation.

a. Major renovations and repairs
    Funds must be provided for necessary major repairs of plant and equipment to ensure compliance with changing regulatory standards and codes and to finance planned and approved renovation projects.

b. Replacement of plant and equipment
Because of deterioration and obsolescence, assets must be replaced and modernized based on community needs for health care services. Funds that reflect the changes in general price levels must be available for the replacement and modernization of plant and equipment.

c. Expansion
Sufficient funds must be available for the acquisition of additional property, plant, and equipment when consonant with community needs.

d. New technology
Advances in medical science and advances in technology of delivering health services often require additional expenditures. Sufficient financial resources must be available for continued additional investment in the improvement of plant and equipment, consonant with community needs, so that health care institutions can keep pace with changes in the health care delivery system.

3. Return on equity
Investor-owned institutions should receive a reasonable return on their owners' equity.

Responsibilities of Purchasers for
Meeting Financial Requirements

Each institution's total financial requirements should be apportioned among all purchasers of care in accordance with each purchaser's use of the institution and measurable impact on the operations of the institution. Any apportionment that permits a purchaser to assume a lesser responsibility is not appropriate and does not alter the total financial requirements of the health care institution. Rather, it requires other purchasers to make up the deficiency.

Responsibilities of Providers

Health care institutions have an obligation to disclose to the public evidence that their funds are being effectively utilized in accordance with their stated purpose of operation. Institutions also have a responsibility not only to purchasers of care but also to their community to provide effective management. An institution's goals and the methods that it uses to achieve (sic) those goals should be consonant with community planning and the resources in that community.

Authors' Plan of Study of Problems in Part II

The authors have taken what may appear to be an unusual approach to discussing hospital financial management by electing to discuss the subject of hospital revenues. In the preceding pages, it has been implied that the problems related to the sources of revenue are vital to the operation of a solvent hospital. It has been shown that third parties, or "contracting parties" as A.H.A. states it, buy at wholesale rates on a "cost" or "cost-plus" basis where cost is not uniform due to the differing interpretations of cost. Furthermore, the self-pay patient has been pictured as one who pays a higher rate than Blue Cross or the government because his bill must absorb costs disallowed by the big purchasers.

The administrator and his financial advisers are thus faced with the problem of generating enough revenue to meet the actual dollar costs of day-to-day operation, to make major repairs and replacements of buildings and equipment, to finance expansion of land, plant, equipment, and added services as the demand justifies.

So we can say as a gross financial problem revenue is critical. If this is the case, then it follows that more must be known about the costs to justify the rates and charges to produce the revenue. Beyond that, more must be known about the contracting parties who buy hospital services under special reimbursement formulas. Finally, consideration must be given to the changes that may take place in the coming years.

With the above needs in mind, cost analysis will be described in the next chapter. Methods of allotting costs to centers of the hospital which produce revenue will be outlined. The methods will entail apportioning the salaries, supplies and overhead expenses of the service departments which do not produce revenue to the departments which do. The total expense of the revenue departments (determined by adding the costs apportioned from the non-revenue departments) then can be used as a basis for determining reimbursable "costs" and for setting rates and charges.

The chapter on cost analysis will be followed by one on Blue Cross and one on Medicare. In both of these chapters the philosophies of providing care of these two large purchasers will be examined, along with their methods of payment.

A later chapter will examine the relation of costs to charges and some methods of setting rates based upon that relationship.

Suggested Readings

American Hospital Association. "Equity in Financing" from *Report of the Task Force on the Principles of Payment for Hospital Care*, pp. 27–44.

American Hospital Association. "Principles of Payment for Hospital Care."

American Hospital Association. *Statement on the Financial Requirements of Health Care Institutions and Services.*

Bowers, James B.; Connors, Edward J.; Mosier, John E.; Rowley, Clyde S. *Hospital Income Flow.*

Foyle, William R. "Debatable Elements of Hospital Cost" in McNerney, Walter et al. *Hospital and Medical Economics,* pp. 935–956.

Mannix, John R. "Blue Cross Reimbursement of Hospitals."

Appendix 4-A

Blue Cross System's Policy Statement on Payment to Health Care Institutions*

The adoption, by the American Hospital Association in 1969 of the *Statement On The Financial Requirements of Health Care Institutions and Services*, as well as the pursuant adoption of the *Policy on the Implementation of the Statement on the Financial Requirements of Health Care Institutions and Services* and the *Guidelines for Review and Approval of Rates for Health Care Institutions and Services by a State Commission*, has raised several public policy issues which have long been a concern of Blue Cross. The debate over national health insurance has undoubtedly sharpened the issues. Three issues fundamental to the financing of health care are addressed below:

—what elements should be considered in calculating rates of payment;
—what should be the method of payment; and
—what should be the locus of the rate determination decision.

Rates of Payment

The elements of cost which should be evaluated in calculating rates of payment for health care institutions have been delineated in the American Hospital Association's *Statement on the Financial Requirements of Health Care Institutions and Services*. This *Statement* identifies the community obligations of health care institutions and presents a reasonable model for structuring adequate rates of payment to institutions which meet the requisite obligations. As such, it should be supported by Blue Cross as a reasonable guide to Plan/provider negotiations.

In implementing the *Statement*, it should be recognized that the proposed method of rate calculation neither demands nor presupposes a single rate of payment for all purchasers. Rather, the method requires only that contracting agencies pay their "appro-

---

*Adopted by The Blue Cross Association November 14, 1972.

priate share" of an institution's financial requirements, i.e., each class of purchaser pays its unique economic cost.*

Research by the American Hospital Association, in regard to nursing care for the aged, has demonstrated that economic cost can differ significantly by class of purchaser. Similar research by Massachusetts Blue Cross has not only demonstrated the same result, but also shown that the potential magnitude of cost differential between classes of purchasers can, in some instances, be as much as twelve percent.

If the *Statement's* principle of "appropriate share" is to be achieved and if equity is to be obtained—both between payer and provider and among payers—rates must be calculated to reflect not only elements of cost, but also each class of purchaser's impact on a provider's incurrence of any particular element of cost. In operational terms, this means, for example, that:

—cost elements such as working capital financing, credit and collection expenses, nursing care expenses, which vary due to the business practices or characteristics of a class of purchaser, should be reflected in payment rates on the basis of actual cost incurrence—not on the basis of a uniform distribution;

—approved plant capital costs should be reflected in payment rates on a proportionate basis, with historical cost providing the payment ceiling and with negotiated capital advances acting as credits against future capital obligations;

—the financing of free services (patients unable to pay) should be reflected in payment rates on a negotiated basis. The economic cost concept demands that government and other programs which have traditionally paid less than their share should close the gap as rapidly as possible;**

---

*Economic cost per class of purchaser can be defined as the sum of the present tangible and present and future intangible costs which an institution incurs in the process of providing care to a particular class of purchaser, such as Blue Cross members. It basically consists of the cost elements outlined in the *Statement*, adjusted to reflect actual cost incurrence. Relative to other classes of purchasers Blue Cross generates smaller amounts of some of the costs mentioned. For example, lower costs are due to Blue Cross contractual agreements with providers which reduce business risks, to prompt payment practices, and, in some cases, to the provision of working capital advances. Other factors, such as increased claims preparation time, can increase Blue Cross cost. All the factors should be reflected in determining Blue Cross' economic cost.

**In calculating Blue Cross' obligation, its open enrollment practices, extensive conversion and transfer privileges, and service benefits must be taken into account. These factors not only set Blue Cross apart from other carriers, but also reduce the amount of both free services and reductions of income by making coverage available to persons who otherwise might not be able to obtain it. This economic fact should be recognized in determining Blue Cross' economic cost.

—costs of community services, such as research and education, should be borne primarily by the community with participation by purchasers occurring only on a negotiated basis;

—reductions of income, due to items such as bad debts, should be reflected in payment rates on the basis of actual experience and performance—not on a proportionate basis;

—payment rates should reflect measures of cost per unit of services that the provider, payer, and community agree are appropriate responsibilities of the payer.

In essence, rates must be established on the basis of each class of purchaser's economic costs and should vary, if economically justified and only to the extent of such justification, to reflect differences in cost. It is essential that all participants in the delivery system recognize this principle, for it is only by determining rates for all purchasers on the basis of economic reality that an adequately and equitably financed health care system can be achieved. The technology necessary to implement this principle exists; its application is now needed.

Further, it is vital, if the public is to be well served, that health care institutions and purchasers meet the obligations and responsibilities set out in Chapter V of the *Statement,* both separately and jointly. A major dimension of economic cost must be community as well as individual institutional need.

A concern for adequate payment must be joined by concerns for short range and long range planning, effective utilization, broader benefits, public disclosure and responsible administration. It is only by combining sound financing with a responsiveness to community needs that long-run equity can be achieved.

Method of Payment

Ideally, the payment method not only should aid in improving the operation of the entire health care system through controls and incentives, but also should assure that each class of purchaser's payment equals its share of total economic cost. The selection of effective payment methods is critical to the proper functioning of the total delivery system.

No one payment method has emerged that combines the strengths and eliminates the weakness of all others. Of the several prospective and retrospective methods of payment that are currently in use, or being considered for use, none empirically has proved itself to be the "best" method. Much rhetorical interest and support has been generated for particular concepts, such as controlled charges (Indiana), budget negotiations (Rhode Island), prospective projection (New York), performance review (Maryland), etc., but objective evidence for decision making is limited.

Compounding the matter is the uncertainty surrounding the basic policy issue of whether a single, uniform method or a pluralistic approach will produce the best long-term results. Theoretically, the use by all purchasers of care of a single method of paying providers and monitoring performance should enable both providers and purchasers to obtain operating economies. These economies should result from the elimination of procedural duplication and the simplification of administrative processing.

On the other hand, a pluralistic approach also can result, theoretically, in operating economies. Multiple payment methods, each in contrast to the other, either at a given point in time or over time, can yield total system economies, due to each method's attempt to demonstrate the best total result. The magnitude of these economies—as a result of concentrating on total expenses as opposed to focusing on a particular system, e.g., administrative expenses—potentially can exceed the economies which could be obtained through the administrative reforms of a single payment methodology. Also, we should keep in mind that any given method of payment cannot be judged in the abstract; its ultimate validation is only against contrasting approaches.

Existing payment methods should be evaluated and further experimentation should be conducted. Blue Cross fully recognizes this need and the import of its outcome, and encourages health care institutions to join with it in a series of projects to investigate both areas.

Rate Determination Decision

The matter of the locus and design of the rate determination decision, i.e., who should participate in the rate-setting function and in what manner, is fundamental to both the operation of the financing mechanism and the larger question of the basic management character of the health care system.

Essentially, the issue centers on the relative merits of government regulation of carrier rates and contracts, in conjunction with rigorous negotiation between carriers and providers, versus government regulation of both carrier rates and contracts and provider rates. Several variations on each theme are possible.

Limited experience to date reveals problems with various approaches. This experience needs to be extended and systematized, and innovations need to be added.*

Providers have been frustrated not only by inadequate payment, but also by line-by-line review of budgets, tantamount to external management of the institution. Some negotiations, in given areas, have been exemplary. Others have been marked by unproductive strife. The essential elements of success need to be distilled before any given pattern is uncritically advocated.

Implications

The fact of continuously rising health care costs and the potential of national health insurance have combined with several other factors to create a climate which demands improvements in the present system of financing health care. Blue Cross recognizes not only the need for reform, but also the equally critical need to establish operative models for guiding future decisions. However, if system-wide reform is to be accomplished effectively, it should be grounded in solutions whose efficacy has been demonstrated.

Blue Cross both supports and offers to join health care institutions in demonstration projects designed to identify approaches and mechanisms for improving the financing system.

As a matter of policy, Blue Cross is committed to establishing a financing system which both adequately meets the needs of responsibly managed health care institutions and is equitable to all classes of purchasers.

Appendix 4-B

Blue Cross Association Policy Statement on Payment to Health Care Institutions**

The Blue Cross Organization has the responsibility to provide for the public a community financing mechanism for quality health care at reasonable cost. Blue Cross Plans have committed to achieve that objective by membership standards and programs

---

*For example, a prior notice mechanism may represent a workable approach to providing procedural safeguards.

**Adopted by the Board of Governors January 14, 1978. The 1978 Policy Statement is both an affirmation and extension of the policy statement adopted by the Board of Governors in 1972.

which are designed to influence the efficient and effective delivery of health care. An important part of that commitment is the responsibility of each Plan to explore alternative means of reimbursement to participating hospitals and to insure that they are reimbursed on a basis consistent with the public interest. Four issues fundamental to the reimbursement of health care institutions are addressed below:

—what should be considered in calculating rates of payment;
—what should be the method of payment;
—what should be the locus of the rate determination decision; and
—what should be the critical elements in rate setting design.

Rates of Payment*

Elements of cost which should be considered in calculating rates for payment for health care institutions have been delineated in the American Hospital Association's *Statement on the Financial Requirements of Health Care Institutions and Services* as adopted by the AHA House of Delegates, August 1977. This *Statement* is a reasonable initial point of discussion in Plan/provider negotiations.

In negotiations, it should be recognized that:

(1) the amounts claimed for each element should be related to the community need for all resources of each facility in the community, and
(2) the proposed method of rate calculation neither demands nor presupposes a single rate of payment for all purchasers.

Community Need

Each community needs sufficient health care institutional resources to provide care of the population to be served in that community. Payment should reflect only those costs attributable to needed levels of service capacity and utilization. Efforts to identify and develop appropriate capacity for the community can be successful only if payment policies and planning programs are mutually reinforcing. Further, programs intended to encourage appropriate utilization should not be offset by payment for elements that would distribute the same total costs over a smaller unit base.

---

*Rates of Payment, as used throughout this paper, are defined as rates determined under a cost reimbursement formula or hospital billed charges.

Class of Purchaser

Within the limits determined by community need, each class of purchaser (both contracting and non-contracting payors) should pay its "appropriate" share of an institution's cost elements. This share can differ significantly by class of purchaser; the actual costs generated by each class of purchaser will vary because of different average complexity of cases, capital requirements, cash flow, unrecovered costs, and other cost elements. The extent of the difference is not likely to be uniform among institutions, or across the country; these differences are already recognized in a number of payment programs and by HEW regulations affecting Medicare payments.

If equity is to be achieved—both between payor and provider and among payors—rates of payment must reflect each class of purchaser's impact on a provider's incurrence of any particular element of cost. In operational terms, government and other programs which have traditionally paid less than their appropriate share should close the gap as rapidly as possible. This means, for example, that:

—cost elements, such as working capital financing, credit and collection expenses, and nursing care expenses, which vary due to the business practices or characteristics of a class of purchaser, should be reflected in payment rates on the basis of actual cost incurrence—not on the basis of uniform distribution;

—approved plant capital costs should be reflected in payment rates on a proportionate basis, with historical cost providing the payment ceiling and with negotiated capital advances acting as credits against future capital obligations;

—the financing of free services (patients unable to pay) should be reflected in payment rates only after negotiation;

—reductions of income, due to items such as bad debts, should be reflected in payment rates on the basis of actual experience and performance—not on a proportionate basis;

—the cost of community services, such as research and education, should be borne primarily by the community with participation by purchasers occuring only after negotiation; and

—payment rates should reflect measures of cost for such units of services that the provider, payor, and community agree are appropriate responsibilities of the payor.

Blue Cross Plan subscribers, for instance, generate, relative to other classes of purchasers, significantly smaller amounts of certain of these costs, due, for example, to the Plan's contractual agreements with providers which reduce business risk and its prompt payment practices and, in some cases, provision of working capital advances. Other factors, such as increased claims preparation time, can increase Blue Cross Plan cost to the institution. These factors should be reflected in determining Blue Cross Plan subscribers' contribution to the elements of costs generated by the institution.

Other payor characteristics can also affect the elements of costs of an institution. An insurance carrier's open enrollment practices, extensive conversion and transfer privileges, and service benefits should be taken into account. These factors not only set Blue Cross Plans apart from other carriers, but also reduce the amount of free services and other reductions of income by making coverage available to persons who otherwise might not be able to obtain it. This economic fact should be recognized in determining a Blue Cross Plan's payments.

In essence, rates must be established on the basis of the elements of cost generated by each class of purchaser. Rates should vary only to the extent they can be economically justified. It is essential that all participants in the delivery system recognize this principle. It is only by determining rates for each purchaser on the basis of economic reality that an adequately and equitably financed health care system can be achieved. This principle is recognized by the AHA *Statement of Financial Requirements*, revised August 1977, which says: "Each institution's total financial requirements should be apportioned among all purchasers of care in accordance with each purchaser's *use* of the institution and *measurable impact on the operations of the institution*" (emphasis added).

A concern for adequate payment must be joined by concerns for sound community and institutional health care program planning, effective utilization review, broader benefit programs, public disclosure and responsible administration. It is only by combining sound financing with a recognition of, and responsiveness to, community needs and resource constraints, that long-run equity and cost effectiveness can be achieved.

Method of Payment

Ideally, the payment should aid in improving—through controls and incentives—the operation of the entire health care delivery system. It should assure that each class of purchaser's payment equals its appropriate share of necessary elements of costs. Thus, the selection of effective payment methods is critical to the proper functioning of the total delivery system.

No one payment method has emerged that combines the strengths and eliminates the weaknesses of all others. Of the several prospective and retrospective methods of payment that are currently in use, or being considered for use, none has empirically proven itself to be the "best" method. Experiments are currently being conducted and evaluated and others are being proposed. Support exists for particular concepts, but neither enough time nor enough information exists to permit a definitive evaluation of success for any one method in any particular environment.

Moreover, there is reason to doubt whether a single, uniform method, universally applied, will produce the best long-term results. Although a single method of paying providers and monitoring performance has the appeal of uniformity and perhaps simplicity, a single method is not likely to be the most effective and efficient method for particular circumstances.

On the other hand, different payment methods can be tailored to a particular community circumstance. Providers in each community can help the Plan develop a payment arrangement that best fits the community needs. Within that total community approach, each method is appropriate for its setting and can thereby contribute to the availability of quality health care services in an efficient and effective manner. Any given method of payment cannot be judged in the abstract; its ultimate validation is in its superiority to a contrasting approach in a particular circumstance.

In this framework, any method of payment selected should include: (1) payment systems that support or encourage capital planning and utilization review decisions consistent with community and medical needs; (2) payment limits as may be set forth by prospective budgets or community-wide determinations, by the community or other organizational entities; (3) voluntarily organized, rigorous negotiations between provider and payors; and (4) disclosure of critical institutional management and cost data for specific services and diagnoses.

Existing payment methods should be evaluated and further experimentation should be conducted. The Blue Cross organization recognizes this need and the import of its outcome, and encourages health care institutions to join with it in a series of projects to investigate all reasonable methods.

Design of Rate Determination System

The locus of the decision and the design of the rate determination process—who should participate in the rate setting function and what are to be included in that design—are fundamental to both the operation of the financing mechanism and the larger question of the basic management character of the health care system.

Locus of the Decision

A major issue is whether government regulation of carrier rates and carrier contracts with providers should be within the framework of rigorous negotiations or by a regulated system of provider rate setting for all payors. Again, no one arrangement has been demonstrated to meet all desirable objectives. Negotiated rates between providers and payors permit greater flexibility to adapt to specific circumstances without the rigidities introduced by government regulation of rate specifies. Negotiated rates also permit a greater range of experimental arrangements. Experience to date suggests the need for more experimentation and innovation; state mandated review systems have not demonstrated their efficacy.

The essential elements of success need to be distilled before any given pattern is uncritically advocated. The locus of the decision should best be kept where the negotiating parties can retain and exercise the greatest flexibility to adapt to local circumstances and where programs in support of planning, utilization, and cost containment controls can be introduced and evaluated more effectively.

Wherever voluntary programs in local circumstances do not result in controlling costs and achieving equity among providers and payors, consideration would need to be given to implementing specific state regulatory programs. Implementation of such programs, however, should be restricted to the particular problems encountered in the local situations rather than total state regulation of the program.

Critical Elements in Rate Setting Design

Any well designed rate determination system should have several elements combined in whatever emphasis is appropriate for each local situation: Necessary elements in the design would include:

—*Disclosure* of corporate structure, officer affiliations, and financial and operating data similar to that required of other segments of the economy. Public interest oriented organizations should have the same obligation to report these data as those operating in the for-profit system. Such information would increase effectiveness of rate bargaining between providers and payors, help identify where costs are significantly different among providers for similar services and diagnoses, and encourage appropriate utilization and capital decision making.

—*Linkage of capital planning decisions with payment.* Based on community approved capital budgeting and certificate of need approvals, negotiated payment arrangements could exclude, for example, payments for depreciation, interest, rate of return, and direct operating costs associated with capital expenditures determined to be unneeded in the community.

—*Limits on payment* based on prospective budgets. Prospective budgets may be derived from national guidelines for the rate of increase in hospital receipts or expenditures, from area-wide agreements, or from rigorous bargaining between payors and hospitals.

—*Incentive arrangements* to encourage improved performance. Arrangements could include sharing of savings in excess of goals established by limits.

—*Technical assistance programs* to help those institutions which have remediable cost escalation situations.

—*Negotiated rates* based on intensive bargaining with providers on an area-wide basis, using maximum data available in accordance with a public policy of disclosure of critical operating and financial data.

These elements should provide the basis for an effective payment program for the Blue Cross organization. Still, there may be unusual circumstances in which the parties in a voluntary effort cannot obtain necessary data to negotiate successfully on matters of payment. A mutually developed arbitration process should help resolve unnegotiated issues.

Conclusion

The fact of continuously rising health care costs and the potential of national health insurance have combined with several other factors to create a climate which demands improvements in the present system of financing health care. The Blue Cross organization recognizes not only the need for reform, but also the equally critical need to establish operative models for guiding future decision. If system-wide reform is to be effectively accomplished, however, it should be grounded in solutions whose efficacy have been demonstrated.

The elements of a well designed payment program can be combined into different arrangements, and each of them can be carefully evaluated for structure and effectiveness. The Blue Cross organization both supports and offers to join health care institutions in demonstration projects designed to identify approaches and mechanisms for improving the financing system.

As a matter of policy, the Blue Cross organization is committed to establishing a financing system which serves the public and adequately meets the needs of responsibly managed, community needed, health care institutions, and is equitable to all classes of purchasers.

Chapter 5
Cost Analysis

In Chapter 4 the importance of the sources of revenue to the financial status and position of hospitals was emphasized. It was pointed out that the great majority of the hospital's revenue comes from Blue Cross and Medicare, which base their reimbursements on "costs." Certain costs are considered debatable; in fact, some seemingly legitimate costs are not even allowed in the reimbursement formulas. Hence, management necessarily must put great stress on cost finding or analysis, must formulate reasonable guidelines for the definition of cost, and must establish a firm base for all cost claims through cost analysis.

Thus, cost finding has become a resource tool for financial management in hospitals, particularly in recent years. On the one hand, cost finding has become a necessary procedure in apportioning costs to the patient care areas in order to comply with the reimbursement formulas of Medicare, Medicaid, and some Blue Cross plans.

On the other hand, any successful business, hospital or other, has to have a management team which is cost informed, which plans with cost information at hand, which invests the business's capital with solid knowledge of the company's cost situation, and which sets prices and wages on the basis of "real" costs. That cost information comes from accurate cost finding.

The hospital's administrator, controller, and finance committee need accurate cost finding more than the executives of many other businesses because they operate on as little or less "net profit" than a giant supermarket or a chain of discount department stores. Also, they have less flexibility and less control of their financial environment.

100

A hospital cannot set rates and charges which are realistically related to costs unless the cost finding system accurately allocates both direct and indirect costs to the patient unit or patient service. Staffing of the nursing units, maintenance department, or an ancillary service should be done only with knowledge of the "real costs" as well as the real needs. Routine personnel problems involving financial questions (let alone union negotiations) should be approached only with sound cost information. Certainly, budgeting or any other projections of the financial future need solid grounding in the cost analysis of past performance.[1]

The hospital's purchasing department has worries of cost and inventory control, the dietary department has needs for cost controls down to the pennies per meal, laundry and housekeeping must consider their costs compared to contracted services—all these needs demand good cost information which comes with accurate cost finding methods.

Hospital administration handles millions of dollars of the community's money each year while walking a precarious path between rising costs and inadequate revenue. Hospitals cannot survive without the best possible cost information—the best possible cost finding or analysis.

It has been said, with some truth, that the need to develop cost figures for government and insurance claims has made for better financial management and administration in hospitals.

Cost finding, as it will be discussed in the following pages, will be considered the process of allocating all costs of operating the hospital to cost centers or departments which produce revenue.[2] Cost finding or cost analysis has also been defined as "the process of manipulating or rearranging the data or information in the existing accounts in order to obtain the costs of the services rendered by the hospital."[3] In other words, cost finding is a means of spreading the costs of plant maintenance, plant operations, and

---

[1] The value of cost finding in budgeting and internal control of operations in the hospital is great. The budgeting process is discussed in Part IV.

[2] "All costs" includes salaries, supplies and other expenses of doing business, including depreciation.

[3] Three terms (cost finding, cost analysis, and cost accounting) will be used frequently in this text which may cause some confusion because they have a common end product arrived at by two different techniques. *Cost finding and cost analysis* are used synonymously to refer to the technique of allocating direct and indirect hospital costs as explained in this chapter. They refer to an after-the-fact procedure in which data are taken from completed general accounting forms and then distributed to cost centers. *Cost accounting* is a procedure which is a part of the ongoing general accounting system in which the cost allocations are done as the accounting forms are being prepared.

other general service departments or cost centers in a reasonable way to nursing care, operating room, emergency room, pharmacy, and other departments or revenue centers which enter charges for services provided for patients. An equitable cost determination for filing claims with the government or Blue Cross is a necessity; likewise, rates and charges for services billed to other payers should be related to costs determined by some equitable method.

There seems to be a reasonable basis for relating charges patients are asked to pay to the costs of the hospital services they receive. The costs of the services are not only those expenses (salaries, supplies, food, medication) directly connected with the department providing the service, but also include such "overhead" items as maintenance, administration, depreciation, housekeeping, laundry, plant operation, and medical records. If the total costs of operating the hospital are to be recovered from the patients who receive service, an accurate assignment of all costs must be made to the departments providing services patients pay for.

Some rational process of analyzing costs and assigning them appropriately to the proper patient service departments is patently necessary.

Prerequisites

There are five prerequisites a cost analysis system should meet if its function is to be fulfilled and if it is to operate efficiently.

1. There should be an organization chart and a chart of accounts relating to it.
2. There should be an identification of all cost centers as either general service cost centers or as final cost centers to which all costs are ultimately assigned.
3. There should be an accurate accounting system capable of accumulating financial data by cost center.
4. There should be a comprehensive information system capable of collecting nonfinancial data by cost center and by the total hospital providing: (a) the basis for distribution of costs from general service centers to final cost centers; and (b) the basis for calculating unit cost by final cost center.
5. A methodology for cost analysis should be chosen which is most practicable for the hospital situation.

The organization chart and the related chart of accounts. These have been discussed in Part I. These two items provide the road map by which costs can be routed through cost finding to the final cost center and a framework for the distinct functions of each center.

Identification of all cost centers. In the chart of accounts, cost centers should be established for all centers of activity and responsibility in the hospital. Some of the cost centers represent patient-centered activities, while others are primarily for general services such as: providing heat, light, and food; keeping the floors and walls clean; washing the linen; shoveling the snow; and doing the many other tasks necessary to the satisfactory operation of a complex organization such as a hospital. The hospital charges the patient directly for services such as: room, board, and nursing (under a daily rate); drugs and dressings; x-ray; laboratory; physical therapy; and other therapeutic treatments and diagnostic procedures. These charges are usually itemized on his bill. However, the costs of many services (such as maintenance, housekeeping and laundry) are not entered on the bill as direct charges. Thus, the second prerequisite in a cost analysis system is to identify (a) cost centers which produce revenue (room charge, etc.) and (b) the general service cost centers which do not produce revenue (maintenance, housekeeping, laundry, etc.). This identification is necessary because all the expenses, direct or indirect, incurred by the general service centers (non-revenue-producing centers) must be allocated to the revenue-producing centers which are the final cost centers in the cost analysis process.

Accurate accounting system. After cost centers have been designated either as general service centers or as final cost centers, the accounting system must be accurate enough to accumulate and appropriately assign all financial data to the various cost centers. This is a necessary prerequisite not only if the direct costs of each cost center are to be accurately determined, but also if accurate total cost data are to be obtained.

Comprehensive information system on nonfinancial data. As suggested in the paragraph above, much of the expense is not incurred by the cost centers independently, but is expense shared by many cost centers which, therefore, must be prorated among the cost centers if accurate total cost data are to be obtained. In order to prorate equitably, it is necessary to have several kinds of nonfinancial data which can be used in dividing the cost among all centers. This nonfinancial information may include such statistics as square footage of each center, gross payrolls per center, number of employees per center, number of meals served, pounds of laundry washed, number of records processed, or number of patients cared for.

Methods of cost analysis. Several methods are commonly used in cost analysis, including:

—direct apportionment
—the step-down method
—double apportionment
—algebraic or multiple apportionment.

Direct Apportionment

Allotting the cost incurred by non-revenue-producing departments to revenue departments by direct apportionment can be done by any one of several methods. The most simple and most illogical way is for administration to determine arbitrarily the percentage of the non-revenue-connected expense each revenue center is to bear. Other yardsticks can be based on the percentage each revenue department represents of the total square footage of the hospital's buildings, or of the number of employees, payroll, pounds of laundry, patient days, or number of purchase requisitions. The reader can probably expand the list of possibilities even further. For instance, a person trained in the retail business might suggest: "Why not allot costs of the nonrevenue cost centers or departments to revenue departments in ratio to the revenue generated by each of those departments?"

Direct allocation, though administratively and clerically simple, is an inappropriate cost finding methodology, for it: (1) ignores the exchanges of services between non-revenue-producing departments; and (2) does not compensate for the different demands for services by revenue departments on nonrevenue departments. For an example of the first point, the maintenance department might be called upon to do a large amount of work for the laundry. Since both departments are nonrevenue departments, there would be no means under direct allocation of charging any of the cost of the maintenance department to the laundry. To illustrate the second point: the Intensive Care Unit may need more housekeeping service proportionately than any other nursing unit. For exchange of services between nonrevenue and revenue departments, the allocation of costs may not be in relation to the service provided. Consequently, direct allocation is neither a method of cost analysis recommended by the authors nor one accepted by most third parties.

The Step-Down Method

The step-down method is a more advanced cost finding technique than direct allocation, for it involves the distribution of the costs of nonrevenue-producing departments to other nonrevenue departments and, in turn, finally to revenue departments. The term "step-down" is used because of the format in which distributions of nonrevenue department costs are made. The costs of the nonrevenue department serving the most departments (both revenue and nonrevenue) are distributed first; the nonrevenue department serving the second largest number of departments is distributed next; the one serving the third largest number next, and so on. This technique results in a workpaper which resembles a staircase or steps. Hence, the name of the method is obtained.

To explain the step-down distribution graphically, a ten-month cost apportionment of Community Hospital (Exhibit A) is used. The order of departments for apportionment was determined as "Plant Operations, Maintenance and Repairs" across the page to "Superintendence and House Orderlies."

Column 1 lists all the departments; Column 2 gives the square footage of each department; Column 3, the Total Operating and Professional Services Expenses to be distributed. For example, the expense to be distributed for "Plant Operation" is $64,115.90.

Look across horizontal Row A to the third heading, "Plant Operation" and note beneath the heading that the basis of allocation of this expense is square footage.

Column 4 shows how the total expenses of the plant operation ($64,115.90) are distributed among the other departments, both nonrevenue and revenue, on the basis of the percentage of the total square footage of the hospital excluding that allotted for plant operation.

In Column 5 the $23,047.55 expense total of Maintenance and Repairs ($21,176.88 from Column 3 and $1,870.67 from Column 4, which was charged by Plant Operations to Maintenance and Repairs) is distributed to all remaining departments in ratio to the square footage of those departments.

The Laundry Department total of $22,311.74 shown in Column 7 was derived from the original department total of $18,287.18 in Column 3 plus $2,937.06 from Plant Operations in Column 4 and $1,087.50 from Maintenance and Repairs in Column 5. The laundry expense is prorated according to the total pounds of laundry issued as expressed in percentages in Column 6.[4]

---

[4]Besides square footage and pounds of laundry, it should be noted that other yardsticks are listed in horizontal Row B for use in cost allotment: patient days (Col. 10, 11); percentage of record-keeping (Col. 11); departmental payroll (Col. 13, 16, 17); and priced requisitions (Col. 14, 15).

Community Hospital

Exhibit A —Step-Down Method

A. Department			Plant Operations	Maintenance and Repairs
	Departmental Square Footage	Total Operating and Professional Services Expenses		
B. Basis of Allocation			Sq. Footage	Sq. Footage
(1)	(2)	(3)	(4)	(5)
Plant Operation	3,564	$ 64,115.90	$64,115.90	
Maintenance	1,349	21,176.88	1,870.67	$23,047.55
Laundry	2,118	18,287.18	2,937.06	1,087.50
Housekeeping	1,245	49,409.75	1,726.46	639.26
Purchasing and Stores	1,228	6,144.34	1,702.88	630.53
Dietary — less revenue	3,592	62,173.72	4,981.06	1,844.34
Medical Records	1,225	19,831.70	1,698.72	628.99
Administrative	1,703	100,216.17	2,361.56	874.42
Central Supply	1,007	8,684.57	1,396.42	517.05
Medical and Surgical	118	2,846.33	163.63	60.59
Nursing Service		232,808.70		
Nursing Supervision and				
House Orderlies	209		289.82	107.31
Nursing Service				
Centers:				
Intensive Care	1,380		$ 1,913.67	$ 708.57
Intermediate Care	3,744		5,191.84	1,922.38
Continuing Care	4,148		5,752.07	2,129.82
Self Care	4,919		6,821.24	2,525.69
Pediatrics	2,445		3,390.50	1,255.40
Obstetrical	3,117		4,322.37	1,600.44
Sub Totals:	19,753		$27,391.69	$10,142.30
Emergency Room	712	5,504.79	$ 987.33	365.58
Operating Room	3,903	30,213.87	5,412.33	2,004.02
Delivery Room	3,313	21,475.76	4,594.17	1,701.08
Nursery	1,325	14,008.18	1,837.39	680.33
Pharmacy	343	39,225.89	475.64	176.11
Radiology	1,384	53,093.20	1,919.20	710.63
Laboratory	603	29,417.44	836.18	309.62
Anesthesia		2,897.98		
Oxygen		4,314.22		
Physical Therapy	886	9,555.02	1,228.62	454.93
Occupational Therapy	220	4,832.93	305.07	112.96
TOTAL:	49,800	$800,234.52	$64,115.90	$23,047.55

Community Hospital

Laundry		Housekeeping	Purchasing and Stores	Dietary — less Revenue	Medical Records
	Amount				
Percentage of Total Pounds Issued		Sq. Footage	Sq. Footage	Patient Days	Estm'd Percentage of Record Keeping and Patient Days
(6)	(7)	(8)	(9)	(10)	(11)
	$22,311.74				
		$51,775.47			
		1,531.17	$10,008.92		
2.8%	624.73	4,478.79	892.18	$74,994.82	
		1,527.43	304.28		
		2,123.44	423.00		
10.5%	2,342.73	1,255.61	250.13		
		147.13	29.31		
		260.60	51.91		
5.3%	$ 1,182.52	$ 1,720.69	$ 342.76	$ 4,207.21	4.10%
14.0	3,123.65	4,668.32	929.95	16,986.33	17.72
14.9	3,324.45	5,172.06	1,020.30	19,371.16	19.22
15.0	3,346.76	6,133.41	1,221.81	18,898.69	19.12
4.3	959.40	3,048.62	607.31	7,079.51	6.17
18.5	4,127.67	3,886.52	774.22	8,451.92	8.67
72.0%	$16,064.45	$24,629.62	4,906.35	$74,994.82	75.00%
2.1%	$ 468.55	$ 887.78	176.85		5.00%
3.9	870.16	4,866.57	969.46		
		4,130.92	822.90		
		1,652.12	329.11		
		427.68	85.19		
1.0	223.12	1,725.68	343.77		
.3	66.93	751.87	149.77		15.00
					5.00
7.4	1,651.07	1,104.74	220.07		
		274.32	54.64		
100.0%	$22,311.74	$51,775.47	$10,008.92	$74,994.82	100.0%

Community Hospital

Exhibit A (con't.)

A. Department	Medical Records	Administrative, less Telephone	Central Supply	Medical and Surgical
B. Basic of Allocation	Amount	Departmental Payroll	Priced Requisitions	Priced Requisitions
(1)	(12)	(13)	(14)	(15)
Plant Operation				
Maintenance				
Laundry				
Housekeeping				
Purchasing and Stores				
Dietary — less revenue				
Medical Records	$23,991.12			
Administrative		$105,998.59		
Central Supply		2,840.76	$17,287.27	
Medical and Surgical				$3,246.99
Nursing Service				
Nursing Supervision and House Orderlies				
Nursing Service Centers:				
Intensive Care	$ 1,009.43	$ 11,055.65	$ 1,822.08	$ 586.73
Intermediate Care	4,075.49	16,005.79	2,160.91	695.18
Continuing Care	4,647.68	19,291.75	1,777.13	571.79
Self Care	4,534.32	12,825.83	2,207.59	710.44
Pediatrics	1,698.57	6,815.71	565.29	181.84
Obstetrical	2,027.85	3,953.75	1,557.59	501.01
Sub Totals:	7,993.34	$ 69,948.48	$10,090.59	$3,246.99
Emergency Room	$ 1,199.56	$ 1,187.18	$ 409.71	
Operating Room		7,123.11		
Delivery Room		4,568.54		
Nursery		4,685.14	4,254.39	
Pharmacy		2,437.97	2,359.71	
Radiology		3,285.96	172.87	
Laboratory	3,598.66	4,971.33		
Anesthesia	1,199.56			
Oxygen				
Physical Therapy		3,370.75		
Occupational Therapy	———	1,579.37	———	———
TOTAL:	$23,991.12	$105,998.59	$17,287.27	$3,246.99

Community Hospital

Nursing Service	Superintendence and House Orderlies				
		Total Nursing Cost	Patient Days	Nursing Costs Per Pat. Day	Total Expense of Revenue Producing Departments
Departmental Payroll	Departmental Payroll				
(16)	(17)	(18)	(19)	(20)	(21)
$232,808.70					
$44,279.43	$44,989.07				
$ 29,806.47	$ 7,112.77	61,468.55	1,230	$49.97	
43,135.50	10,293.50	109,188.84	4,971	21.97	
51,996.38	12,407.99	127,472.58	5,670	22.48	
34,557.42	8,246.50	102,029.70	5,531	18.45	
18,381.60	4,386.43	48,370.18	2,072	23.34	
10,651.90	2,541.88	44,397.12	2,473	17.95	
$188,529.27	$44,989.07	$492,926.97	21,947	$22.46	
					$ 11,187.33
					51,459.52
					41,547.76
					25,551.98
					43,001.35
					61,301.56
					40,101.80
					4,097.54
					4,314.22
					17,585.20
					7,159.29
$232,808.70	$44,989.07				$307,307.55

Figure 5-1

Cost Finding

Double Distribution Method

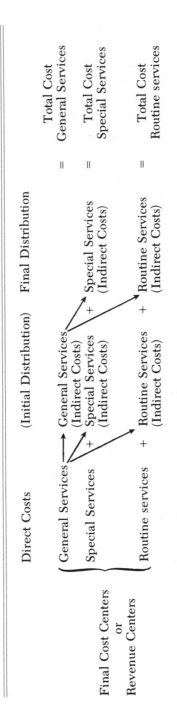

The step-down process is continued through Column 18 until the six nursing care units have absorbed their proportionate share of costs of the nonrevenue service departments plus their own operating costs which are totaled in Column 18. Finally, in Column 21, the revenue departments other than nursing are shown as having absorbed their allotted shares of the costs of nonrevenue departments of the hospital. The sum of nursing costs in Column 19 ($492,926.97) and the total expense of the other revenue-producing departments ($307,307.55 in Column 21) equal the total operating and professional service expenses of the hospital ($800,234.52 as shown in Column 3). This completes the distribution of all expenses to revenue-producing departments.

It should be noted that the step-down method has been criticized as not allowing fully for interdepartmental charges between the different nonrevenue departments. As an example, the Housekeeping Department was the fourth nonrevenue department to have its cost distributed in Exhibit A of the step-down method. None of the housekeeping costs could be distributed to Plant Operation, Maintenance, or Laundry because those departments had already been closed out. Likewise, laundry charges could not be charged to plant operation or maintenance because both of those departments were closed out before laundry. The step-down method does finally allot all charges to the cost centers represented by the various revenue-producing departments. At the present, step-down is a method approved by A.H.A. and by many of the third parties. However, some accountants, due to the inaccuracies inherent in the "step-down" process, advocate different methods. Among the other methods is the double apportionment method which uses two rounds of distribution in charging the nonrevenue costs to the revenue departments. An explanation of this method follows.

The Double Apportionment Method[5]

Double apportionment, or double distribution, was designed to correct one of the major weaknesses of the step-down method. This weakness was shown above to be the failure to allow fully for interdepartmental charges between non-revenue-producing departments. In double apportionment, two separate cost distribu-

---

[5]One weakness of double distribution is that it doesn't charge a department for its own services. Note in Exhibit B, Column 4, that Plant Operations expense ($64,115.90) is distributed to every department but its own.

tions are used (see Figure 5-1). In the first distribution all direct
and indirect costs of all departments are distributed to the various
cost centers according to the agreed upon basis of allocation. For
example, costs of plant operation, maintenance, housekeeping,
and purchasing are allotted to all departments (revenue and nonrevenue) in ratio to the square footage of the departments. Laundry costs are allocated to the departments served according to
pounds of laundry each used, inpatient dietary costs are distributed to units served according to the patient days formula, and so
on down the list of department costs to be distributed.[6] *After the
first distribution is completed, the costs which have been allocated to the nonrevenue departments are then redistributed to
the revenue-producing departments using the same bases of allocations as before (square footage, etc.).*

In the double distribution method there is a more equitable
allowance for exchange of services between nonrevenue departments than in the step-down method.

The following pages contain an explanation of the double apportionment method with an illustration in Exhibits B and C.

The first distribution. By using Exhibit A, the step-down cost
analysis sheet of Community Hospital, and Exhibit B for double
apportionment, the differences and similarities in step-down and
double apportionment can be shown. Basically, double apportionment is two distributions of costs to reflect as accurately as possible the interchange of services between nonrevenue departments
before costs are finally allotted to the revenue-producing departments. The information in Column 3 which shows the Total Operating and Professional Services Expenses is the same in both
methods. Column 4 is the same in both methods with the total
expense for Plant Operations distributed among all other departments on a square footage basis. The difference between the two
methods begins in Column 5. Under double apportionment the
total expenses under Maintenance and Repair would be the figure
shown in Exhibit B, Column 3 ($21,176.88). This amount would
be distributed in Column 5 to all departments for which square
footage is shown. Note that the expenses were not accumulated (it
was *not* $21,176.88 plus $1,870.67 to make $23,047.55) but was the
original expense total in Column 3, or $21,176.88. Throughout the
first distribution under the double apportionment method the
original expense total in Column 3 is used for each department.

---

[6]Other dietary costs (employees' cafeteria, for example) should be allocated to
cost centers according to utilization.

The distribution of the laundry costs to users of laundry will be in the same proportion under both methods, but the amount of expense will differ because under double apportionment just the original cost (not the accumulated cost) is distributed. The Dietary Department is also a special case of distribution of the original expense of $62,173.72 (Column 3) to the nursing units according to the patient days. The original expense of Medical Records ($19,831.70) is distributed under the formula shown in both exhibits: 75 percent to nursing units on the basis of patient days; and 25 percent among Emergency Room, Radiology, and Laboratory on the basis of estimated usage.

The Administrative expense ($100,215.17) would be distributed under double apportionment to all departments other than administration in ratio to departmental payrolls. The original expense total for Central Supply (Column 14) and Medical and Surgical Supplies (Column 15) under double apportionment would be distributed to the same departments which received the accumulated allotments under the step-down method. After the Nursing Service payroll and the Superintendence and House Orderlies payroll (Columns 16 and 17) are distributed to the nursing units, the final computation of the first distribution of the double apportionment method can be undertaken. In Column 22 (not used in Exhibit A), totals of the expenses allocated to the various departments are made horizontally across the page. Column 22 will then contain the totals of all the allocated expenses of all nonrevenue departments, reflecting the interrelations of services provided by one department for another. A second distribution will now be needed to allot the nonrevenue expenses to the revenue departments. (See Exhibit C).

The second distribution. When the horizontal totals (Column 22) have been determined for all of the nonrevenue departments, the second distribution, that of nonrevenue expenses to revenue departments, can be made. For example, the total for Plant Operations in Column 22, Exhibit B, is distributed to all the nursing units and other revenue-producing departments according to the ratio of the square footage of each revenue department to the total square footage of all revenue departments (see Exhibit C). The same bases of allocation are used in the second distribution as were used in step-down and in the first distribution of the double apportionment: square footage is used for Plant Operations, Maintenance and Repairs, Housekeeping, and Purchase and Stores; laundry usage ratio of the revenue departments would be used to

Community Hospital

Exhibit B.—First Distribution Double Apportionment Method

A. Department			Plant Operations	Maintenance and Repairs
	Departmental Sq. Footage	Total Operating and Professional Services Expenses		
B. Basis of Allocation				Sq. Footage
(1)	(2)	(3)	(4)	(5)
Plant Operation	3,564	$ 64,115.90	($64,115.90)	$ 1,557.74
Maintenance	1,349	21,176.88	1,807.67	($21,176.88)
Laundry	2,118	18,287.18	2,937.06	925.74
Housekeeping	1,245	49,409.75	1,726.46	544.16
Purchasing and Stores	1,228	6,144.34	1,702.88	536.74
Dietary — less revenue	3,592	62,173.72	4,981.06	1,569.98
Medical Records	1,225	19,831.70	1,698.72	535.42
Administrative	1,703	100,216.17	2,361.56	744.34
Central Supply	1,007	8,684.57	1,396.42	440.14
Medical and Surgical	118	2,846.33	163.63	51.58
Nursing Supervision	209	44,279.43	289.82	91.35
Nursing Service		188,529.27		
Nursing Centers				
Intensive Care	1,380		1,913.67	603.16
Intermediate Care	3,744		5,191.84	1,636.43
Continuing Care	4,148		5,752.07	1,813.00
Self Care	4,919		6,821.24	2,149.98
Pediatrics	2,445		3,390.50	1,068.66
Obstetrical	3,117		4,322.37	1,362.38
Sub Totals:	19,753		$27,391.69	$ 8,633.60
Emergency Room	712	$ 5,504.79	$ 987.33	$ 311.20
Operating Room	3,903	30,213.87	5,475.33	1,705.90
Delivery Room	3,313	21,475.76	4,594.17	1,448.04
Nursery	1,325	14,008.18	1,837.39	579.12
Pharmacy	343	39,225.89	475.64	149.92
Radiology	1,384	53,093.20	1,919.20	604.92
Laboratory	603	29,417.44	836.18	263.56
Anesthesia		2,897.98		
Oxygen		4,314.22		
Physical Therapy	886	9,555.02	1,228.62	387.26
Occupational Therapy	220	4,832.93	305.07	9616
TOTAL:	49,800	$800,234.52	$64,115.90	$21,176.88

Community Hospital

Laundry		Housekeeping	Purchasing and Stores	Dietary — less Revenue	Medical Records	
	Amount					Amount
Percentage of Total Pounds Issued		Sq. Footage	Sq. Footage	Patient Days	Estimated Percentage of Record Keeping and Patient Days	
(6)	(7)	(8)	(9)	(10)	(11)	(12)
		$ 3,625.74	$ 450.84			
		1,372.75	170.65			
	($18,287.18)	2,155.29	267.93			
		($49,409.75)	157.50			
		1,249.52	($6,144.34)			
2.8%	512.05	3,652.94	454.38	($62.173.72)		
		1,246.47	154.97			($19,831.70)
		1,732.84	215.43			
10.5%	1,920.16	1,024.65	127.39			
		120.07	14.93			
		212.67	26.44			
5.3%	969.22	1,402.18	174.57	3,484.47	4.10%	813.10
14.0%	2,560.21	3,808.60	473.60	14,082.36	17.72%	3,514.14
14.9%	2,724.79	4,220.68	524.70	16,062.55	19.22%	3,811.66
15.0%	2,743.08	5,000.19	622.25	15,668.79	19.12%	3,791.83
4.3%	786.35	2,487.84	309.30	5,869.78	6.17%	1,223.62
18.5%	3,383.13	3,171.62	394.20	7,005.77	8.67%	1,719.41
72.0%	$13,166.78	$20,091.11	$2,498.73	$62,173.72	75.00%	$14,873.76
2.1%	384.03	724.48	90.07		5.00%	991.59
3.9%	713.20	3,988.73	493.70			
		3,371.05	419.10			
		1,348.22	167.62			
		349.01	43.39			
1.0%	182.87	1,406.25	175.08		15.00%	2,974.76
.3%	54.83	613.57	76.28		5.00%	991.59
7.4%	1,353.26	900.53	112.08			
		223.86	27.83			
100.0%	$18,287.18	$49,409.75	$6,144.34	$62,173.72	100%	$19,831.70

Community Hospital

First Distribution Double Apportionment Method

Exhibit B. (con't.)

A. Department	Administrative -less Telephone	Central Supply	Medical and Surgical	Nursing Service
B. Basis of Allocation	Departmental Payroll	Priced Requisitions	Priced Requisitions	Departmental Payroll
	(13)	(14)	(15)	(16)
Plant Operation	2,004.32			
Maintenance	2,004.32			
Laundry	2,004.32			
Housekeeping	7,516.20			
Purchasing and Stores	501.08			
Dietary — less revenue	7,516.20			
Medical Records	2,004.33			
Administrative	($100,216.17)			
Central Supply	1,002.17	($8,684.57)		
Medical and Surgical			($2,846.33)	
Nursing Supervision	6,012.97			($44,279.43)
Nursing Service				
Nursing Centers				
Intensive Care	5,010.80	694.77	227.70	4,427.93
Intermediate Care	24,051.86	3,473.80	1,138.53	21,254.17
Continuing Care	11,023.77	1,563.21	512.34	9,741.46
Self Care	2,505.41	347.39	113.86	2,213.97
Pediatrics	5,010.81	694.77	227.70	4,427.93
Obstetrical	2,505.40	347.39	113.86	2,213.97
Sub Totals	$50,108.05	$7,121.33	2,333.99	
Emergency Room	5,010.81	434.23	142.32	
Operating Room	4,008.65	694.77	227.70	
Delivery Room	2,004.33	260.54	85.39	
Nursery	1,002.17	173.70	56.93	
Pharmacy	2,004.33			
Radiology	1,002.17			
Laboratory	1,002.17			
Anesthesia				
Oxygen	1,002.17			
Physical Therapy	2,004.33			
Occupational Therapy	501.08			
TOTAL:	$100,216.17	$8,684.57	$2,846.33	$44,279.43

Community Hospital
First Distribution Double Apportionment Method

Superintendence & House Orderlies	Total Nursing Cost	Patient Days	Nursing Costs Per Patient Day	Total Expense of Revenue Departments	Total Expense of Non-Revenue Departments, Accumulated Horizontally
Departmental Payroll					
(17)	(18)	(19)	(20)	(21)	(22)
	stated in column 21)	(omitted for clarity)	(omitted for clarity)		(a) 7,638.64
					(b) 5,355.39
					(c) 8,290.34
					(d) 9,944.32
					(e) 3,990.22
					(f) 18,686.61
					(g) 5,639.91
					(h) 5,054.17
					(i) 5,910.93
					(j) 350.21
($188,529.27)					(k) 6,633.25
18,852.93				(l) 38,574.50	
90,494.03				(m) 171,679.57	
41,476.44				(n) 99,226.67	
9,426.47				(o) 51,404.47	
18.852.93				(p) 44,350.19	
9,426.47				(q) 35,966.07	
				(r) 14,580.85	
				(s) 47,521.85	
				(t) 33,658.38	
				(u) 19,173.33	
				(v) 42,248.18	
				(w) 61,358.45	
				(x) 33,255.62	
				(y) 2,897.98	
				(z) 5,316.39	
				(zz) 15,541.10	
				(zzz) 5,986.93	
$188,529.27				722,740.53	77,493.99

Exhibit C
Community Hospital

	ICU	Intermed	Cont. Care	Self Care	Ped	OB	ER	OR
(a) Plant Operation	$ 305.56	$ 907.10	$ 1003.07	$ 1105.85	$ 534.73	$ 763.86	$ 114.59	$ 946.20
(b) Maintenance	214.20	642.60	696.15	803.25	374.85	535.54	80.45	642.65
(c) Laundry	580.30	1243.50	1326.40	1409.30	497.40	1658.00	248.04	415.50
(d) Housekeeping	397.76	1293.28	1292.72	1491.60	696.08	994.43	99.14	1193.28
(e) Purchasing	159.60	438.72	518.70	598.50	279.30	399.02	79.98	478.80
(f) Dietary	934.34	4671.65	4671.65	4671.65	1868.66	1868.66		
(g) Med. Records	231.24	999.11	1084.01	1078.37	348.20	488.98	282.00	
(h) Admininist.	404.32	1415.12	859.35	202.16	404.32	202.16	404.32	303.24
(i) Central Supply	472.10	2367.13	1063.18	236.05	472.10	236.05	295.55	472.10
(j) Med & Surg	28.02	140.07	63.04	14.01	28.02	14.01	17.51	28.02
(k) Nurs. Superv.	663.33	3183.95	1459.32	331.66	663.33	331.66		
Dept. Totals	$4390.77	$17302.23	$14037.59	$11942.40	$6166.99	$7492.37	$1621.58	$4479.79

Second Distribution, Double Apportionment Method

Delivery	Nursery	Phcy	Radiology	Lab	Anesth	O$_2$	P.T.	O.T.	Totals
$ 763.86	$ 229.14	$ 315.56	$ 267.33	$152.70			$ 152.70	$ 76.39	$ 7638.64
535.54	160.65	214.20	187.56	107.10			107.10	53.55	5355.39
			165.80				746.10		8290.34
994.43	298.32	397.76	298.32	198.88			198.88	99.44	9944.32
399.02	119.70	159.60	159.78	79.80			79.80	39.80	3990.22
									18686.61
			846.00	282.00					5639.91
202.16	75.81	151.62	75.81	75.81		75.81	151.62	50.54	5054.17
177.41	119.26								5910.93
10.51	7.00								350.21
									6633.25
$3082.93	$1009.88	$1238.74	$2000.60	$896.29		$75.81	$1436.20	$319.82	$77493.99

distribute Laundry expense; patient days for Dietary; and so on. Once the second distribution is completed, and all of the expenses of the nonrevenue departments resulting from the first distribution have been allocated to revenue departments and totaled, the totals for each revenue department can be brought forward from Column 21 of Exhibit B and a grand total made for each department as shown in Exhibit C.

Exhibit D shows the double apportionment system is a more accurate method of distributing hospital costs than either the direct allocation or the step-down method. Even though it does entail more clerical work, it is the most desirable of the manual systems discussed.

Community Hospital

Exhibit D—Comparison of Cost Distribution Methods

Unit	Step-Down Method	Double Apportionment Method
Intensive Care	$ 61,468.55	$ 42,965.27
Intermediate Care	109,188.84	188,981.80
Continuing Care	127,472.58	113,264.26
Self Care	102,029.70	63,346.87
Pediatrics	48,370.18	50,517.18
Obstetrical	44,397.12	43,458.44
Emergency Room	11,187.33	16,202,43
Operating Room	51,459.52	52,001.64
Delivery Room	41,547.76	36,741.31
Nursery	25,551.98	20,183.21
Pharmacy	43,001.35	43,486.92
Radiology	61,301.56	63,359.05
Laboratory	40,101.80	34,151.91
Anesthesia	4,097.54	2,897.98
Oxygen	4,314.22	5,392.20
Physical Therapy	17,585.20	16,977.30
Occupational Therapy	7,159.29	6,306.75
	$800,234.52	$800,234.52

Multiple Apportionments (the Algebraic Methods)

Some accountants have developed methods of multiple distributions of costs which are sometimes referred to as algebraic methods. Conceivably, these distributions could be done manually, but from a practical standpoint double distribution remains the most feasible manual method.

Algebraic multiple distributions are made of expenses between nonrevenue departments and then, finally, to revenue departments in an attempt to refine the cost analysis to the greatest possible degree of exactness. Although 10 or 12 distributions are made in some methods, it is most generally agreed that after four distributions there is little change in the ultimate cost figures.

To use multiple distributions to best advantage, a computer should be used. In fact, a method of distributing interrelated costs has been devised in which simultaneous equations are programmed on a computer to take into consideration all cost interrelations between departments: nonrevenue departments to nonrevenue departments to revenue departments. The resulting cost analysis system is the most exact method yet devised, but it is beyond the capabilities of the average hospital accountant. The cost of programming and computer service time makes this type of cost analysis most practicable only when performed by a central service.[7]

How the Systems Compare

At one time, William R. Foyle, a C.P.A. interested in hospital cost analysis, made a comparison of cost apportionment for three hospitals under each of the first four methods described in this direct allocation; step-down; double apportionment; and algebraic (multiple apportionment). Mr. Foyle's thesis was that the algebraic method using multiple apportionment would not only give a more accurate reckoning of the costs of the interchange of services between nonrevenue departments but would also give a more accurate distribution of costs to general care departments in relation to ancillary services. The proper distribution of costs to general care departments is particularly important where the patient mix (high Medicare admission rate, for example) especially stresses the demand for general care over that of laboratory, radiology, and other ancillary departments. Mr. Foyle could demonstrate the difference in apportionment by the various methods of cost analysis, but concluded that the mathematical method was not the only factor to be considered in cost distribution. Certain management

---

[7]One method widely used was devised by the MICAH Corporation, Ann Arbor, Michigan. The Hospital Administrative Services of the American Hospital Association also offers computerized cost analysis in their Cost Allocation Program (CAP). Dr. David Penn developed an algebra-equivalent method for Laventhol Krekstein Horwath & Horwath called a "successive iteration" method for practical use by accounting staffs.

decisions made in the beginning such as the basis of allocation (square footage, payroll allocation, accumulated costs, pounds of laundry, etc.) might widen differences more than mathematical methodologies.[8]

Conclusions

The most accurate method of cost analysis in terms of apportioning all allowable hospital costs to revenue-producing departments is a form of multiple apportionment.

In order to adjust for interdepartmental services, the simultaneous equation method programmed for a computer is the most exact. The double apportionment method is the most accurate of the feasible manual methods. Step-down, although acceptable to most third party payers, is less accurate because of the "closing" of a department for receipt of charges from other departments once its original and accumulated charges have been distributed.

A study of three hospitals showed a one or two percent variation by departments between the algebraic method (multiple apportionment) and the step-down with double apportionment coming somewhere between. Consequently, on the basis of accuracy alone, the order of preference is: (1) algebraic (multiple apportionment); (2) double apportionment; (3) step-down; and (4) direct apportionment. From a practical standpoint of time and cost of the analysis, however it would be better to consider the selection of manual methods as: (1) double apportionment; and (2) step-down.

Suggested Readings

American Hospital Association. *Cost Finding and Rate Setting for Hospitals.*

Cleverly, William O. "An Input-Output Model for Hospital Costing."

Micah Corporation. *The Micah System for Hospital Cost Analysis.*

Pearlman, Adams, Wolfe, Shuman. "Methods of Distributing the Costs on Nonrevenue Producing Centers."

Seawell, L. Vann. *Hospital Financial Accounting: Theory and Practice.*

---

[8]Foyle, William R., "Evaluation of Methods of Cost Analysis", an unpublished paper, c.1964.

Chapter 6

Blue Cross

History and Philosophy

The story of Blue Cross is said to have begun in 1929 when Dr. Justin Ford Kimball, the new Executive Vice President of Baylor University, found that the University Hospital in Dallas, Texas was in serious financial trouble because of the large amount of outstanding accounts receivable. The problem struck home to Dr. Kimball as an educator because many school teachers were prominent along the delinquent debtors.

The solution that was found for the problem in Dallas proved to be a prototype followed by many other communities. A prepayment plan for hospital care was developed under which teachers who joined the plan could pay six dollars a year and be assured of up to 21 days of hospital care in a semiprivate room at Baylor University Hospital. The prepayment plan worked: it solved the cash shortage dilemma facing the hospital and at the same time relieved the pressure of hospital bills for the teachers. By the end of 1929 1,000 teachers were enrolled. This represented about 75 percent of the total. After a time, other groups in the community joined the teachers in the prepayment plan.

The Baylor prepayment idea caught on in other parts of the country where hospitals were faced with the problems of collecting unpaid bills and where workers worried about how to pay for unexpected hospitalization during times of increasing unemployment and decreasing wages. The workers liked the security of knowing that there was a definite period of care in a definite type of accommodation paid for in advance, if they needed it. The hospital liked having the payment for the hospital care of a whole group of persons assured—and insured.

Shortly afterward other groups made contracts with hospitals in the Dallas area, but the contracts were between a certain group and a certain hospital. Multihospital prepayment contracts came later.

By 1932 plans were being developed in several communities of the country with contractual relations between each plan and more than one hospital.

In 1933, C. Rufus Rorem, Ph.D., a medical economist, joined the small staff of the American Hospital Association as Associate Director and brought with him a $100,000 grant from the Julius Rosenwald Fund for the development of group hospitalization plans. Under Rorem's guidance the Association developed criteria for acceptable group hospitalization plans. Among the features the Association recommended were:

1. The plan should be founded as a public service not-for-profit agency.
2. The coverage should be for hospital care, not for physicians' services.
3. The plan should operate with the advice of physicians, hospital trustees, and others interested in public service.
4. There should be a free choice of hospital.
5. All recognized hospitals should participate in offering services under the plan.
6. The hospitals should be responsible for providing satisfactory care.
7. The plan should be financially sound.

In practice at least, the role of the American Hospital Association grew to that of being an accrediting agent of Blue Cross plans. The group plan idea began appearing in other states: New Jersey, and Minnesota, among the first. (E.A. van Steenwyk of the Minnesota plan was the originator of the Blue Cross name and symbol.) In the various states the legislatures addressed themselves to the problems of the mushrooming hospital care plans and passed enabling acts which allowed the groups to solicit members without having financial reserves as large as required of commercial insurance firms. The enabling acts provided for state regulation of subscription rates (premiums) charged by the plans, usually by the office of the state insurance commissioner.

The question is often asked: Does Blue Cross represent the hospital or the patient? This question cannot be answered simply, for the role of Blue Cross has been changing since the founding of the first plan. As has been indicated, Blue Cross was founded to save hospitals from financial ruin by reducing outstanding accounts receivable through a plan of prepayment of hospital care. The subscribers to the prepayment plan benefited by being relieved of hospital expenses which they probably would not have been prepared to pay. Originally the prepayment plan was fostered by hospitals with the American Hospital Association in the forefront as adviser. The public was included in a minority role on Blue Cross advisory boards. To this point, Blue Cross has been hospital- as opposed to patient-oriented.

However, as Blue Cross became more widespread, as hospital costs rose, and as premium rates rose in consequence, the public became more interested in the operation of the plans. The states which set Blue Cross premium rates resisted the requests for higher rates and demanded cost containment where possible. Blue Cross was forced by circumstances to begin controls by demanding better accounting methods in hospitals, by taking a firmer attitude on certain debatable costs, by fostering utilization review, and by experimenting with various methods of rate setting.[1]

At the time when Blue Cross became more conscious of the need for hospital cost containment, and began to invite more public members to advisory boards, it can be said that Blue Cross became more subscriber-related. (See the section on trends at the end of this chapter.)

It is difficult to generalize about Blue Cross, about: its philosophy; its role; its benefits; its contracts; its membership; its reimbursement methods; or the direction in which it is going. It is difficult, if for no other reason than that there were in 1978 69 separate plans in the United States, five in Canada, one in Puerto Rico, and one in Jamaica.

But people do generalize about Blue Cross in spite of the 76 separate corporations. Some persons say Blue Cross is social insurance. Without enumerating the pros and cons for Blue Cross as social insurance, it can be safely said that the Blue Cross concept calls for nongovernmental prepayment plans for hospital expenses—and there is a social overtone, to say the least. Blue

---

[1]The most common method for setting premium rates is to have a general rate, a "community rate," for members of groups above a certain minimum size based on the utilization among groups. Rate setting formulas based on the "experience" or utilization of the different groups have also been tried. In the third quarter of 1978 among Blue Cross regular group members the ratio of those under experience-rated contracts to those under community-rated was about 3½:1.

Cross moves in the direction of one aspect of social insurance (comprehensive hospital care) in the "first day, first dollar" ideal goal of covering the whole hospital stay from the first day of admission and the first dollar of expense. Commercial insurance usually has a different base. It generally pays definite dollar indemnities for certain accommodations and for certain services.

Some of the Blue Cross contracts throughout the country limit benefits, or list hospital benefits with certain dollar or percentage deductions. Although it cannot be said that Blue Cross covers 100 percent of the hospital charges of its subscribers, the percentage of coverage is high. It might be easy to speculate that practically 100 percent of the bills would be paid by Blue Cross, except for special accommodations or extraordinary services some patients needed or demanded.

Membership

The growth of Blue Cross in number of plans and in number of members was particularly rapid from the 1930s up to 1958. In 1937 there were 37 plans with one million members; 10 years later (1947) the total membership had grown to 27 million, or 19 percent of the U.S. population. The growth spurted on until 1958 when 79 U.S. plans had 52 million members, equivalent to 30 percent of the U.S. population. Then, for the first time in over 20 years, Blue Cross membership did not increase. Unemployment in the automobile industry directly affected one of the largest groups of members.

After this period, increase in membership began again, both in gross numbers and in percentage of the U.S. population. By the end of 1973 the membership in the 74 U.S. Blue Cross plans[2] had reached a total of over 80 million or 37.7 percent of the population of the areas served. This figure included nearly 5.4 million federal employees and dependents enrolled under the Federal Employees Health Benefits Program (FEP).

The implementation of Medicare on July 1, 1966 was responsible for Blue Cross designing coverage for subscribers over 65. Subscribers thus were removed from regular membership and en-

---

[2]The number of U.S. Blue Cross plans had been reduced from 79 to 69 through mergers by the third quarter of 1978. In addition to the 69 U.S. plans, there was one in Puerto Rico and there were five in Canada, and one in Jamaica, as previously mentioned. Canadian enrollment totaled about five million in 1978; the Canadian coverage was supplemental to that furnished under the various provincial health care plans.

rolled for complementary coverage. In 1973, 7.3 million Blue Cross members had complementary coverage to Medicare. This Blue Cross coverage in effect was designed to pay for the deductibles which the individual was expected to pay under Medicare provisions.[3]

In the third quarter of 1978 the U.S. Blue Cross plans (excepting Puerto Rico) had 73,718,604 regular members enrolled.[4] This number did not include the more than eight million persons over 65 who had coverage supplemental to Medicare. See Tables 6-1 and 6-4.

Generally, groups as small as four or five members are eligible for group Blue Cross rates if 100 percent of the group enrolls. When the group is larger (15 or more), the required percentage is about 70 percent. Arrangements are made to transfer from group to group with change of employment or to a conversion policy when a subscriber leaves a group, but does not join another covered under Blue Cross. Also in the conversion, the subscriber may be charged a higher rate and receive fewer benefits.

Other fractionations in membership besides the group, nongroup division are the regular and complementary membership classifications, which in turn are subdivided into individual and family enrollment.

With group enrollments there usually is not withholding of benefits for a period of time because of pre-existing conditions (pregnancy being the most likely exception), but with nongroup enrollments there may be a waiting period for some pre-existing conditions.

Enrollments can be for an individual or for a family. Under the family contract, dependent children are usually covered up to 19 years of age, unless married before that time. In some instances a totally disabled child will be covered after the age of 19.

Administration

One should always bear in mind when speaking of "Blue Cross" that there are 76 autonomous plans in the United States, Puerto Rico, Canada, and Jamaica. However, there is a national organization, the Blue Cross Association, which is often the spokesman for the collective whole and which also acts as a clearinghouse of

---

[3]See Chapter 7.

[4]See Table 6-1 for a distribution of Blue Cross memberships by kinds of contract and group coverage.

Table 6-1

Percentage Distribution of U.S. Blue Cross Enrollment, Fourth Quarter 1978*

Type of Contract		Type of Membership	
All Contracts		*Total Membership*	
Group	77.05	Group	85.7
Nongroup	22.95	Nongroup	14.3
Total all contracts	100.0	Total membership	100.00
Regular Contracts		*Regular Membership*	
Group	69.6	Group	81.9
Nongroup	8.6	Nongroup	7.5
Subtotal	78.2	Subtotal	89.4
Complementary Coverage		*Complementary Membership*	
Group	7.4	Group	3.8
Nongroup	14.4	Nongroup	6.8
Subtotal	21.8	Subtotal	10.6
Total all contracts	100.00	Total membership	100.00

*Membership of Puerto Rico plan not included.
Source: Blue Cross Association.

research information, a coordinator of national Blue Cross contracts, and is a fiscal agent for a majority of the Medicare claims.[5]

There is no standard Blue Cross-subscriber contract for the 69 U.S. plans although there may be a slow movement in this direction because nationwide corporations, or large industrial unions, want uniform benefits for all the employees enrolled. In many instances the contracts negotiated by widespread companies call for benefits superior to those offered in some of the plans. Consequently, it has become necessary for BCA to form a subsidiary corporation to handle claims made under national contracts[6]. The largest of the national contracts, the Federal Employees Health Benefit Program, has over 5.5 million members, as already noted.

The administrative officers of the plans are paid employees, but the governing boards are composed of voluntary members representing hospitals, medicine and the public. Originally, the average ratio of the hospital members of the boards was over half and the public members about one-third. The trend has been for the hospital percentage to decrease and the public percentage to increase so that hospital members are no longer predominant in numbers[7].

The cost of administration of the plans has been impressively modest. Usually the plans report administrative costs of 5 to 6 per cent. The low cost can be accounted for partially because: Blue Cross plans do their own "selling" through salaried employees rather than through agents working on commission; they process their own claims; and they are not profit-oriented.

Contracts

There is no standard Blue Cross-hospital contract, for contracts will vary from plan to plan. However, it is evident that there is a

---

[5]There were two national Blue Cross organizations until they merged in 1960: the Blue Cross Association and the Blue Cross Commission (a child of the American Hospital Association). The purposes of the current Blue Cross Association are broadly: to coordinate the activities of the separate plans; to represent and speak for the plans on a national basis; to act as a clearinghouse for claims to be paid under contracts which covered employees of organizations which were spread over the territories of more than one plan, or for claims of members who were treated outside their own plan district. Since the merger, the national association has grown stronger. The association was strengthened again when it became the claims agent for Medicare for much of the country.

[6]Health Service Inc., a stock insurance company wholly owned by Blue Cross Association.

[7]A proposal has been made to the state legislature that Michigan Blue Cross-Blue Shield should reduce its board to 28 members with 20 of them being "subscriber representatives" which may indicate some change from the usual term "public representatives."

close relationship between any Blue Cross plan and its participating hospitals. This should not cause amazement, if one bears in mind that Blue Cross was organized originally by hospitals to save themselves from financial disaster and to take financial pressure off the patient.

A fairly typical contract might make the Plan the participating hospital's agent to sell prepayment of hospital care and to collect the fees for this coverage. In turn the plan would pay the hospital bills of its members under the benefit schedule outlined in the subscriber's contract. (This service is carried at a relatively low cost, as already noted.)

The Plan would act for participating hospitals in making reciprocal agreements with other Blue Cross plans so that subscribers of other plans could receive benefits while in the area of the Plan, and vice versa.

Many of the characteristics of Plan-hospital relationships which might be outlined in a contract are discussed in the Blue Cross profile which follows.

A Blue Cross Profile

The Blue Cross plans are not uniform in benefits, payment methods, monitoring or contract negotiation agencies, depreciation methods or allowable costs, to name a few. The circumstances are in flux so that it is difficult to present a model outside of certain "standard" or basic benefits and a few other common characteristics. In former editions, the authors used the Michigan plan contract and hospital statement of reimbursable costs as fairly common examples of those instruments, for some general understanding of Blue Cross contracts. At the present time, even Michigan Blue Cross-Blue Shield is attempting to restructure its hospital relations.

In recent years, one of the most graphic profiles of Blue Cross to emerge has been the American Hospital Association's "Resurvey of Hospital-Blue Cross Contract Provisions," issued January 1977 and based on data collected as of June 30, 1976.

One of the most dramatic questions addressed was whether payments to hospitals were based on charges or costs. The AHA survey for 1976 showed reimbursement was based as follows:

- Charge-based   50 percent
- Cost-based   50 percent

(It should be recognized that in most charge-based programs charges are based on costs, and costs are examined in much the same way they are in cost-based programs.)

Figures compiled in 1973 by the Blue Cross Association showed the ratio as cost-based 69.2 percent and charge-based 30.8 percent. See Table 6-5 for the 1976 distribution.

Compilation of Cost

Those plans operating with cost-based contracts used varied methods for computing costs. For example:

•22 plans used Average Per Diem
•5 plans used Combination Method (CRCC)
•9 plans used Departmental Method (DRCC)

Carve Out. With the implementation of Medicare and Medicaid in the mid-1960s, the patient mix in most hospitals changes and became skewed. Changes in patient mix, in costs and in length of stay led, in many instances, to the requirement that Medicare and/ or Medicaid patient data be excluded before costs be computed for Blue Cross reimbursement. The expression "carve out" was coined to connote this exclusion of Medicare/Medicaid data. AHA found that 14 Blue Cross plans in 1973 carved Medicare data, and four plans carved out Medicaid.

Allowable Costs

In cost-based or negotiated contracts allowable costs varied somewhat. Some of the so-called debatable costs are discussed below.

Depreciation. In the survey, 33 plans reported straight line depreciation, while nine plans recognized accelerated depreciation. Historical cost as a basis for computing depreciation was required by 27 plans, "price level" was the basis required by six plans. Seventeen plans required the funding of depreciation.

Interest Payments. Interest on capital indebtedness was allowed by 39 plans; interest on other than capital indebtedness was allowed by a total of 39 plans. Twenty-three plans required that total interest payments be reduced by any interest income.

Bad Debts. This item was recognized as an element of cost, regardless of source, by 30 plans, while seven plans recognized as bad debts only those incurred by Blue Cross beneficiaries.

Charity (Free Care). This was accepted as a cost item, regardless of source, by 27 plans, while two plans accepted it only for Blue Cross beneficiaries.

Debt Amortization. Payments for this purpose were allowable costs with 14 plans.

Working Capital Needs. Several methods have been used to assist hospitals with cash flow. There always has been a problem for hospital administration to meet its payroll, pay its debtors, and meet its financial obligations, while waiting for third party processing and paying of hospital claims. Six plans provided for a permanent working capital advance to member hospitals; six plans provided for periodic interim payments; two provided for sight drafts; and 13 assisted in other ways.

Contract Negotiations

These were carried on between individual hospitals and Blue Cross plans in 28 of the 66 cases for which data were reported in the 1976 survey. A summary of those data follows. Blue Cross contracts were negotiated for hospitals by:

• Individual hospitals   under 28 plans
• State hospital associations   under 25 plans
• Metropolitan hospital associations   under 5 plans
• Other   under 8 plans

Contract Standards and Requirements. Blue Cross-hospital contract standards and requirements under several of the plans are shown in Table 6-6. It should be understood that a mere listing of the number of plans having certain characteristics cannot show the combinations of characteristics as has been attempted in the table.

Contract Approval. The approval of the Blue Cross contract by the state insurance commissioner is required with 37 plans.

Benefits and Utilization. These subjects are discussed more fully later in the chapter than appeared in the AHA resurvey.

Benefits

Blue Cross benefits to subscribers vary among the contracts offered by the 76 U.S. plans as well as among group, nongroup, individual, family, and complementary coverage contracts within the individual plans.

In order to put the range of variation of benefits into perspective, the abstracts of 85 regional and national Blue Cross contracts serviced by Michigan Blue Cross in 1969 were studied. The following descriptive material emerging from that study is not exhaustive by any means, but it does serve to give a general profile of Blue Cross benefits.

An alphabetic list of services and supplies, which are included in all the contracts studied as Blue Cross benefits in participating hospitals and which might be considered standard benefits, is printed below.[8] Following the list of standard benefits is a discussion of varying benefits for other services, and for coverage of conditions requiring hospitalization.

"Standard" Blue Cross "Full" Benefits[9]
(hospital inpatient care)

Anesthesia and	Hydrotherapy
Administration	I.V. Solutions
Basal Metabolism	Laboratory
Tests (BMR)	Operating Room
Biologicals	Oxygen and
Casts	Administration
Delivery Room	Physical Therapy
Dressings	Splints
Drugs	Treatment Rooms
Electroencephalograms (EEG)	

Ambulance service generally was not included as a benefit. However, there were a few instances among the 85 contracts where $15 per trip or $25 per admission, or $40 a disability was allowed. In two contracts full coverage was given.

The blood and blood plasma supplied were usually not covered in Blue Cross contracts, although the administration of the blood and plasma generally were.

Cobalt therapy was not covered by Blue Cross although in some instances it was a Blue Shield benefit.

Conditions requiring hospitalization:
1. General acute care. There was a wide variation in the number of days of hospitalization covered in the contracts studied. The segments of care represented were 30, 70, 120, 180, 365, and 730 days. The largest number of the 85 contracts in any benefit classification was 40 in the 365 day segment, followed by 26 in the 120 day segment. In nearly every instance, a new benefit period

---

[8]Benefits for care in nonparticipating hospitals are limited in most Blue Cross subscriber contracts. They are usually limited to a certain indemnity payment per day or per service and are much lower than the benefits paid in a participating hospital.

[9]Standard and full benefits in the 85 Blue Cross contracts studied.

could begin 90 days after the first segment of benefit days was used up. The 730-day benefit was added in a few contracts for persons employed 10 years or more.

2. Maternity care. Thirty-four contracts allowed 10 days hospitalization for maternity care. The remainder were divided almost evenly between 365 and 120-day benefits. There were a few contracts which specified maximum dollar allowances such as $80, $100, or $125. Most contracts gave maternity coverage nine months or 270 days after enrollment, although five gave immediate coverage. Most contracts required enrollment under two person or family contracts, although one covered any enrolled female.

3. Complications of pregnancy were covered under much the same conditions as maternity care as to days of hospitalization allowed, prior days of enrollment required, and type of contracts needed.

4. Tuberculosis care was a benefit allowing 30 days of hospitalization in 40 of the contracts. Twelve contracts allowed 120 days, and eight contracts allowed 70 days of hospitalization. Fifteen allowed hospitalization until the disease was diagnosed. Most contracts allowed new benefit periods after 12 months, and nearly as many set the period at 90 days.

5. Nervous and mental conditions were covered by most of the Blue Cross contracts with 34 allowing 30 days of care. The remainder of the contract benefits were scattered between 31, 45, 70, 120, 365 and 730 days of care, except for 12 which paid only until the nervous or mental condition was diagnosed. New benefit periods were given after 12 months in most cases, although a 90-day period was a part of 12 contracts.

6. Alcoholism and drug addiction were conditions for which hospitalization was allowed in less than half the contracts. Care until the condition was diagnosed was allowed in 23 of the contracts. Where hospitalization was a benefit for alcoholism and drug addiciton, 12 months wait after using up benefit days was usually required before a new benefit period could start.

Dental care benefits were included in some Blue Cross contracts; often these benefits were limited to extractions or care of impactions.

Diagnostic service "toward definite disease or injury" was listed as a benefit in 20 of the 85 contract abstracts examined.

Electrocardiograms were usually a Blue Shield benefit rather than Blue Cross.

Isotopes (diagnostic and therapeutic) were not a Blue Cross benefit, although they were allowed under some Blue Shield contracts.

Miscellaneous benefits. There were a few isolated benefits which appeared in one or two instances and were scattered through the 85 contracts studied. Among those exceptional items were: audio therapy, extended care, external pacemaker, hemodialysis, intensive care, nursery, physical rehabilitation, prosthetics, visiting nurse, and weight reduction. Undoubtedly, some of the miscellaneous services might have been covered in some other contracts without being specifically itemized.

Outpatient benefits in most of the contract abstracts examined included emergency treatment of accidental injuries within 24, 48, or 72 hours. The benefits usually were: "services same as inpatient hospital benefits;" diagnostic x-ray (Blue Shield benefit); electrocardiogram (Blue Shield); and electroencephalogram (also Blue Shield). Other benefits occasionally included were: diagnostic laboratory, BMR, radiation therapy (Blue Shield), x-ray therapy (Blue Shield), radium therapy (Blue Shield), physical therapy, and minor required therapy.

Radium and x-ray therapy were listed as Blue Shield benefits in a majority of the contracts examined, although in some contracts the member was named as the payer.

Room and board was a benefit under Blue Cross contracts with the coverage usually for ward or semiprivate accommodations. In a few instances there were daily dollar limits, but this was the exception rather than the rule. The patient was billed for expenses beyond the fee for semiprivate rooms or beyond any dollar limit.

X-ray diagnostic service was usually a Blue Shield benefit. X-ray therapy benefits were listed above under "radium therapy."

Benefits: 1978 Profile

A 1978 statement about the general scope of benefits offered by Blue Cross plans which appeared in *The Blue Cross and Blue Shield Fact Book* may offer a useful summary of a rather complex national benefit picture:

> In their basic contracts, Blue Cross Plans generally offer service benefits rather than cash indemnities regardless of the hospital's charges. Payment for care is made by the Plan to the hospital or other provider rather

than to the subscriber. Preadmission testing is covered by more than 45 Plans. Outpatient services (usually for accidental injury and minor surgery, although some Plans cover medical emergencies, diagnostic testing, physical therapy, kidney dialysis and chemotherapy treatments) are also covered in Blue Cross Plans basic certificates. Under family contracts, 58 Plans cover handicapped dependent children regardless of age as long as the physical or mental condition exists.

In addition, most Blue Cross Plans offer supplementary variable front-end deductibles and 80 percent coinsurance. Maximums vary from $5,000 to an unlimited amount of extended benefits beyond the basic certificate which may include the services of a physician, surgeon, and physiotherapist, nursing home care, care in the home after hospitalization, ambulance services, prosthetic appliances, blood transfusions, prescription drugs, rental or payment for durable equipment, therapy treatments, diagnostic x-rays and laboratory services, catastrophic illness coverage as well as coverage for private duty and licensed practical nursing care in the hospital; treatment of nervous or mental conditions, drug addiction or alcoholism usually is at 50 percent coinsurance.

Blue Cross Plan subscribers receive benefits anywhere in the country. They can transfer from one Plan area to another and may change their coverage from single to family, family to single, family member to individual, group to nongroup, or from regular to complementary, without losing continuity or fulfilling any waiting periods.

Utilization

The impact of Blue Cross on the financial situations of hospitals can perhaps be best understood if one considers the huge numbers of Blue Cross subscribers, the millions of days of hospital care the subscribers use, and the millions of visits they make to hospital ambulatory clinics. The percentage of the total utilization of hospital facilities by Blue Cross subscribers is impressively large. In turn, the payment for those Blue Cross subscriber services represents a major percentage of the hospital revenue in this country. That important hospital utilization by Blue Cross subscribers is discussed in the following pages.

Table 6-2

Blue Cross Hospital Utilization,* 1964
Through 1978, United States Plans

	Admissions		Patient Days		Average Length of Stay		Outpatient Visits	
Year	Rate†	Percent change	Rate†	Percent change	Days	Percent change	Rate†	Percent change
1964	150	—	1211	—	8.08	—	80	—
1965	149	− .7	1209	− .2	8.14	.8	85	6.2
1966	139	− 6.7	1069	−11.6	7.67	−5.8	91	7.1
1967	125	−10.1	898	− 16.0	7.19	−6.3	98	7.7
1968	123	− .8	898	.2	7.31	1.7	112	14.3
1969	122	− .8	893	− .8	7.51	− .1	120	12.2
1970	124	1.6	895	.2	7.23	−1.1	141	17.5
1971	127	2.4	902	.8	7.12	−1.5	162	14.8
1972	123	− 3.2	869	− 3.7	7.04	−1.1	176	8.6
1973	123	.0	856	− 1.5	6.96	−1.1	192	9.1
1974	121	− 1.6	823	− 3.9	6.77	−2.7	213	10.9
1975	121	.0	814	− 1.1	6.72	− .7	235	10.3
1976	120	− .8	797	− 2.1	6.64	−1.2	266	13.2
1977	117	− 2.5	764	− 4.1	6.51	−2.0	277	4.1
1978	115	− 1.7	736	− 3.7	6.38	−2.0	292	5.4

*Federal employees and their dependents enrolled in the Federal Employees Health Benefits Program (FEP) are excluded 1964–1968. Utilization data for members with complementary coverage to Medicare are not included in the 1966–1978 figures. Data for Puerto Rico are not included The data for 1969–1978 are based on October 1 to September 30 figures.

†Rate per 1,000 Blue Cross members.

Source: Blue Cross Association.

Studies have been done comparing Blue Cross subscribers' utilization of hospitals with that of members of other group plans, with persons covered by commercial insurance, and with private pay patients. Usually, the Blue Cross subscriber makes more frequent use of the hospital than most of the other persons listed. However, inpatient hospital utilization tended to go down from 1964 through 1967 with a leveling-off in 1968; outpatient facility utilization increased steadily in the period 1964–1978 as shown in Table 6-2.

Table 6-3

Ratio of Blue Cross Enrollment
and Utilization to Population, 1978*

U.S. Census Region	Approximate Percentage of U.S. Population	Percentage of U.S. Blue Cross Membership	Utilization Percentages		
			Admissions	Patient Days	Outpatient Visits
Northeast	24	37.7	33.0	33.8	48.3
North Central	26	28.2	30.0	31.9	31.1
South	32	25.6	29.1	28.0	15.8
West	18	8.5	7.9	6.3	4.8

*Utilization and enrollment data from third quarter 1978.
Source: Blue Cross Association.

Blue Cross enrollment is not uniform throughout the country in ratio to population. Concentration of enrollment in ratio to population is highest in the Northeast and North Central states as shown in Table 6-3. Note also that there are significant variations in admissions, inpatient days, and outpatient visits. /

A summary of Blue Cross membership and utilization by census region is given in Table 6-4.

Reimbursement

In the Baylor experiment in prepayment of hospital bills, the plan paid hospital charges on a flat rate per patient day. In general, this was the method of payment through the early days of Blue Cross. In some cases, hospitals were asked to discount their bills because of cash shortage in plan treasuries. Discounting was good business on the part of the hospitals because it was apparent that prepayment plans were vital to the survival of hospitals. If the plans failed, hospitals might do the same.

If some persons look askance at the close relationship between Blue Cross and hospital it might be well to remember the history of the Thirties and Forties, the mutual need the two parties had for each other, and the need the public had for good hospital care.

Lawrence A. Hill has suggested that hospitals in the early days of Blue Cross were quite ready to accept the uniform flat rates paid to all hospitals in a plan area because the payments were

Table 6-4

Blue Cross Regular Membership Enrollment
and Utilization by Census Region, 1978 *

Region	Average membership	Admissions		Patient Days		Average length of stay	Outpatient Visits	
		Number	Rate**	Number	Rate**		Number	Rate**
Northeast	27,814,532	676,698	97	4,355,883	626	6.44	2,716,197	391
North Central	20,800,688	615,690	118	4,102,526	789	6.66	1,745,524	336
South	18,830,753	598,073	127	3,599,603	765	6.02	885,034	188
West	6,272,631	162,196	103	813,401	519	5.01	270,156	172
United States Total	73,718,604	2,052,657	111	12,871,413	698	6.27	5,616,911	305

*Excluding members with complementary coverage, and the Puerto Rico plan.
**Rate per 1,000 members per year.
Source: Blue Cross Association.

certain money, and because the Blue Cross subscribers did not make up a major percentage of patients served.[10]

Even during the Depression days of the 1930s, it became apparent that a flat rate was unfair to hospitals even though it was a convenient mechanism for Blue Cross in budgeting and ratesetting. Two points about flat rates were particularly unfair to hospitals. One, all hospitals did not operate with the same costs: there was a difference in services offered by hospitals, and there was a difference for certain hospitals in special overhead costs such as educational expenses. The second factor was the impact caused by the increase in percentage of Blue Cross patients on the financial condition of hospitals.[11]

It was evident some changes in reimbursement formulas had to be made. One of the first adjustments made by Michigan Blue Cross, for example, was to allow higher rates for hospitals approved by the American College of Surgeons. The adjustment charges ranged from 25 cents to $2.00 per day in addition to the usual $5.50 for ward patients and $6.00 for those in private rooms.

By July 1941, the Michigan plan was paying on a cost basis for hospital care of their patients. In 1946 a formula based on the "lesser of costs or charges" was adopted and is still being used.

By 1947 a majority of the 87 Blue Cross plans then existent had abandoned the flat rate contract. Hill's research showed:

—Thirty-three plans related payments to actual patient billings. Some imposed ceilings.
—Twelve plans paid a fixed per diem rate subject to periodic adjustment.
—Thirty-two plans retained the flat rate per diem payments with no variance among hospitals. These tended to be the smaller plans.
—Eight paid on average per diem costs.
—There were no data for two plans.

The pressure for change from flat rate to a costs or charges related formula came from the hospitals, not Blue Cross. The hospitals wanted a basic reimbursement formula which would offer protection against inflation. Hill believes an assumption existed that "cost increases sprang from causes wholly external to the hospital,

---

[10]Lawrence A. Hill, "Incentive Reimbursement—Some Explorations," an unpublished paper, 1969, is the source of much of the material on the history of Blue Cross reimbursement.

[11]By 1941 Blue Cross enrollment had risen to 7,500,000. *Modern Hospital*, Vol. 57, No. 5, November 1941, p. 106.

Table 6-5

U.S. Blue Cross Enrollment by Reimbursement Method, 1976

Reimbursement Method	Number of Plans	Percentage of Members
Cost-based	36	50.0
Charges-based (100% of charges)	24	33.4
Charges-based (99% or less of charges)	12	16.6
	72	100.0%

Source: AHA Resurvey, 1976.

and thus, hospital management was not only powerless, it was unconcerned."[12]

About 1950 cost-based reimbursement became accepted practice with Blue Cross. By 1962 cost-based reimbursement was by far the most common practice but by 1976 the ratio had changed, as shown in Table 6-5.

Cost Containment and Prospective Reimbursement

Cost containment is a phrase prominent in the consciousness of every health administrator and every third party official. The president and congress talk about putting a cap on costs in hospitals. What they are all hoping is that health care costs will not accelerate faster than the average rate of inflation in the United States. The health industry is conscious of the need to police its own house to avoid federal and state governments imposing mandatory controls. The American Hospital Association has been making a valiant effort through its Voluntary Effort (VE) program to make hospitals budget conscious and budget limiting in their operation. It was announced recently that VE saved 1.48 billion dollars during 1978 and projected 41.5 billion savings in its first five years ending in 1982. So, some success is being shown, but until hospital costs definitely can be brought in line with national economic trends, the industry will be under continuing pressure.

---

[12]An additional source on the equity in financing hospital care and particularly with methods of reimbursement is the American Hospital Association's *Report of Task Force on Principles of Payment for Hospital Care*, 1963, 61 pp.

A few years ago, incentive reimbursement was the title given for setting rates for services prospectively or projectively and allowing hospitals and other providers to benefit by sharing in any savings in costs. Now, the title most commonly used is prospective reimbursement or PR. PR is not a simple, easily defined concept except in the most general way. PR in hospitals is a method of budgeting costs for a future period and establishing a payment rate for services between the provider and the payer. The budgeting can be based on the total operation or on service departments as discrete parts of the operation, depending on the scope of the plan. The rates of payment can be based on per diem costs, per episode of illness, on length of stay, on a capitation basis, on services rendered—to name a few. Obviously, the rate of payment may have an effect on the hospital's reaction to the rate setting system. A hospital working on per diem costs might want to encourage longer stays if occupancy was below the most efficient operating level. A hospital on an episode of illness plan might make the plan more profitable by avoiding admissions of complex cases, if possible. The question of quality of care or adequacy of service is always going to be raised. If hospital stays or services are cut, are there other modes of care (nursing home, outpatient clinic, visiting nurse, or family care) which may give continuing satisfactory, if substitute, care? The whole problem of adequacy of care becomes complicated when one begins talking about quality of care, right to care, and, in fact, fair and just expectation of service on the part of the patient.

Presently (1979) there are 35 or more experiments in PR in one form or another. Many difficulties stand in the way of PR. To be successful, a plan should be acceptable and workable for all major parties: the provider, Blue Cross, Medicare, Medicaid, and the insurance companies. (As usual, the private pay patient is the endangered species.) The need for uniform accounting, budgeting, and reporting methods ultimately must be part of any statewide or regional plan.

Budgeting, of course, is the basis of rate setting. To make the budget viable, utilization review, budget control or monitoring, and other good financial management must be parts of the follow through. A provision for the renegotiation of the budget has been thought necessary by some parties to compensate or adjust for acts of God and for unforeseen events. Examples from the past used in the argument for this future renegotiation have been the unexpected rise in malpractice insurance rates in the past few years, and the unpredicted effects of legislation (the impact of Medicare and Medicaid on patient services and length of stay since 1966). It is assumed that in the future changes might occur comparable to the examples of the past.

Some of the PR experiments have revealed that a plan could not be completely designed at the onset to operate without change. In fact, PR plans might need to be experimental for several years and might need to vary from one part of the country to another. Furthermore, legal questions might arise now and then which would impede the development of a PR plan.

To this point, few, if any, plans can demonstrate that hospital inflation has been reduced to a par with U.S. inflation in general. Dr. Robert F. Allison studied a PR experiment funded by the Social Security Administration in which several Michigan hospitals worked out rate agreements with Michigan Blue Cross–Blue Shield. (This PR plan for Blue Cross subscribers affected 38 percent of the revenue of the study hospitals.) In testimony before the Michigan Insurance Bureau in July 1978, Doctor Allison said the study hospitals were currently running 3.5 percentage points over the 9.5 percent annual U.S. rate of inflation at that time. The 3.5 percentage point overage compared well with the 6.1 percentage point overage at which it had been running previously. However, the 13 percent hospital inflation rate was above the 10 percent "cost cap" Blue Cross originally wanted.

The problem is to refine the operation to lower the percentage gap while not eliminating from the budget items for services, equipment, or improvements which may reappear another year to affect that year's financial equilibrium.

It is difficult to manage a multipartite organization such as a hospital with the many centers of influence and pressure never quite synchronized. The hospital administration, the board of trustees, the medical and nursing staffs, the community, the government, Blue Cross, commercial insurance, the patients' demands for expanded services, the unionization of hospital employees, the mushrooming of paramedical personnel seeking identity, the status competition between hospitals, the lack and impotency of area planning are only a part of the discouragingly long list of factors that make cost control of patient services in a hospital an unsolved problem.

Problems also are connected with reimbursements based on charges or negotiated rates. At the present time, some persons are trying to revive the idea of a negotiated daily rate because it will save a tremendous amount of bookkeeping and will simplify billings. If this side of the picture alone were looked at, substantial savings could be demonstrated. However, to arrive at a daily rate, good cost accounting must be maintained, and frequent negotiations must be carried on to adjust the rate to current costs. Furthermore, the "new" formulas are more sophisticated and sometimes call for different daily rates according to the ordinal day of stay: the first day might be a different rate from the tenth day, as an example, because of the difference in services to be needed, traditionally, on those two days.

Reimbursement under any formula remains an administrative problem of the first magnitude.

Dr. William L. Dowling of the University of Washington, who has done much research on prospective reimbursement, in a paper titled "Prospective Reimbursement of Hospitals" published in *Inquiry* Volume XI, Number 3, encapsulated the problem when he wrote:

> In summary, hospitals can attempt to contain costs in different ways. The actions hospitals actually take under prospective reimbursement will depend largely on the payment unit used. Selection of the payment unit, therefore, depends on how one wishes to change hospital performance. Hospitals can be left free to respond to prospective reimbursement as best fits their situation, or additional external controls could be applied to influence their responses. Hospital preferences for the different payment units would depend in part on their expectations about future use. If an increase in use is expected, the output related payment units would be preferred; if a decrease is expected, the budget or capitation payment units would be preferred.

Payment of Premiums

A subtle influence on hospital utilization and on the cost of Blue Cross may be inherent in who pays the insurance premium.

In the early days of prepayment schemes for hospital care, the concern was to assure subscribers that they could have a reasonable number of days of hospital care as a benefit for monthly payments they could afford to pay. The premiums were paid to a hospital which, in consequence, was able to remain solvent during the Depression and provide needed services to the subscribers. It was a fairly simple one-to-one situation: a contract between a person and a hospital.

During the 1930s and later, complexities began to appear in the relationship between the subscriber and the provider: multihospital coverage became possible; a definition and refinement of the list of benefits developed; and the Blue Cross image emerged to make protection regional and even national in scope. Insurance coverage for hospital care became a desired goal of most American families. Linked with these changes was the development of large industrial labor unions with great power at the bargaining table. One of the fringe benefits sought by the labor unions was for the employer to share in the cost of hospital insurance as he did in the cost of social security. The trend developed for the employer to pay a share of the worker's insurance, or a share of the worker's and dependents' insurance or other combinations of payment—all moving toward the employer paying the total premium for worker and dependents.

Many thoughtful persons, while not disagreeing with payment of health insurance as a fringe benefit, have raised some questions. Is there the same prudence on the part of persons requesting services under insurance paid as a fringe benefit as compared to requests of persons who pay their own insurance premiums and know there is a direct relationship between services used and the cost of insurance? If the employers pay most or all of the premiums for health insurance, does this contribute to more frequent admission to hospital, higher costs, and higher premiums? These questions are unanswerable at present, but are worth pondering.

Dr. Grover C. Wirick, in collecting data for his recent study of Blue Cross, *Hospital Use and Characteristics of Michigan Blue Cross Subscribers*, compiled some figures on payment patterns for Blue Cross premiums from a weighted sample of Michigan subscribers. The data on employer's contributions to the premiums have not been previously published. See Figure 6-1.

Blue Cross Financial Data, Year 1977

The tremendous financial impact on the health industry of the activities of the Blue Cross plans is suggested by an examination of the assets and liabilities of the U.S. Blue Cross plans (including Puerto Rico) for the year ending December 31, 1977:

Total assets	$ 6,288,171,000
Total liabilities	4,307,748,000
Reserves	1,980,423,000
Total income	15,852,191,000
Claims expense	14,232,749,000
Administrative expense (5.9%)	915,896,000
Net income	703,546,000

Source: Blue Cross Association

Table 6-6

Profile of Standards and Requirements of Blue Cross Plans*

Number of Plans Requiring	Certificate of Need	Joint Commission on Accreditation of Hospitals	Planning Agency Approval	State Licensure	Utilization Review	Other	Not Applicable	Not Specified
2	X							
1	X	X	X					
1	X	X	X		X			
1	X	X	X		X	X		
1	X	X			X			
1	X	X			X	X		
2	X		X					
1	X		X	X				
5	X		X		X			
1	X		X		X	X		
1	X					X		
1		X						
1		X	X		X			
1		X	X		X	X		
1		X			X			
1		X			X	X		
7			X					
5			X		X			
1			X	X				
2				X				
4					X			
2						X		
13							X	
8								X

*Source: "Resurvey of Hospital-Blue Cross Contract Provisions," American Hospital Association, January 1, 1977.

Trends in Blue Cross

It is difficult to outline trends which characterize all 69 U.S. Blue Cross plans, but the following list is an attempt. Some of the trends listed may seem antithetic, and this is possible if plans try a wide spectrum of alternatives in attempting to solve the problems facing them.

1. Benefits will be more liberalized, particularly in length of stay allowed per episode of illness, and for maternity care.
2. The attitude will be more liberal toward care for mental illness, drug addiction, and tuberculosis.
3. There will be a liberalization of coverage of outpatient ambulatory care clinics and emergency rooms, since this is the growing edge for health care.
4. There will be experiments in combination with Blue Shield in major medical coverage to compete with commercial insurance.
5. There will be an examination of the Blue Cross versus the commercial insurance position to determine if Blue Cross should try to compete all-out on commercial insurance terms or should continue striving to furnish comprehensive "first day, first dollar" coverage.[13]
6. A larger public (and membership) representation will appear on the governing boards of Blue Cross plans so that management, which pays a large share of the premiums, and labor, which represents a large share of Blue Cross membership, will have voices in Blue Cross policymaking.
7. Pressure will be exerted wherever possible to keep hospital prices down through utilization control by the hospital, through more stringent accounting practices and through encouragement of regional planning and shared services.[14]
8. Blue Cross will attempt to adapt itself to the changes that take place as the United States considers possible national health insurance and/or a national health service. The experience as claims agent for Medicare, and as supplemental insuror for the over-65 Blue Cross members should serve well for whatever comes in comprehensive health protection in the next decade.

---

[13]The gravity of the situation facing Blue Cross is one of the relative numbers covered by Blue Cross and by the commercial carriers. A few years ago, the number of Blue Cross members far exceeded those covered by commercial insurance companies; now the reverse is true, Blue Cross is outnumbered.

[14]Utilization committees have been used in hospitals to prevent overstay by patients, and recertification procedures have been used to examine the need for continued stay after certain base periods. The results have not been outstanding. Uniform recordkeeping and accounting procedures to this time have been unattained goals.

Figure 6-1

Blue Cross Premium: Employers' Contributions and Subscribers' Payments

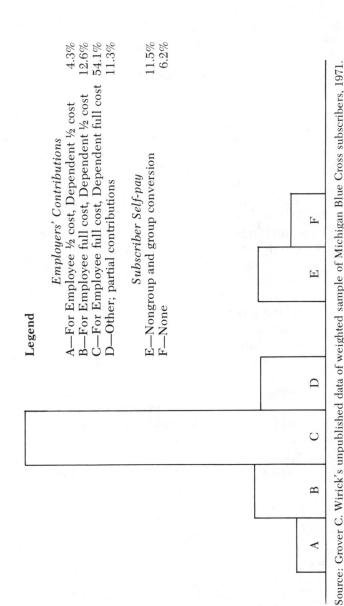

Legend

Employers' Contributions

A—For Employee ½ cost, Dependent ½ cost   4.3%
B—For Employee full cost, Dependent ½ cost   12.6%
C—For Employee full cost, Dependent full cost   54.1%
D—Other; partial contributions   11.3%

Subscriber Self-pay

E—Nongroup and group conversion   11.5%
F—None   6.2%

Source: Grover C. Wirick's unpublished data of weighted sample of Michigan Blue Cross subscribers, 1971.

9. Blue Cross will move to develop HMO style prepaid group practice coverage on a wider basis than at present so that more subscribers will have the choice of regular Blue Cross coverage vs. HMO style coverage.

In summary, it appears that in the future Blue Cross will be moving in the direction of: more comprehensive benefit coverage; wider public membership in its advisory boards; hospital cost containment; and active participation in the planning of any national health insurance.

Blue Shield

It is almost impossible to talk about Blue Cross without mentioning Blue Shield. In fact, they are often referred to collectively as "The Blues."

Blue Shield plans were organized chiefly by medical societies for prepayment of physicians' fees connected with hospital care. For most Blue Cross plans, there is a Blue Shield companion plan. Sometimes they work together and share services and billings. In other cases, there is a corporate linking such as the Michigan Blue Cross-Blue Shield. The Blues often cross over in benefits as in the cases where Blue Cross will pay for a hospital anesthetist technician, but Blue Shield will pay for an anesthesiologist.

In an earlier section of this chapter under the heading "Benefits," it can be seen that certain services and therapeutic procedures were Blue Shield, rather than Blue Cross benefits. The hospital's relationship to Blue Shield is much more limited than to Blue Cross, but it is a necessary relationship in providing health care.

The first of the plans now called Blue Shield was organized in California in 1939 by the California Medical Society under the name California Physicians Services. As the name implies, the plan offered physicians' services to members of employees groups who earned less than $3,000 a year (about an average worker's wage at that time).

In 1946, nine physician service plans formed a national association for coordination of efforts. This was called the Associated Medical Care Plans. This was the forerunner of the National Association of Blue Shield Plans which in turn became the Blue Shield Association segment of the consolidation now called the Blue Cross Association and the Blue Shield Association.

The Blue Shield symbol and name came into use in 1948 in a

Buffalo, N.Y. prepaid medical plan and was adopted by the national group that year and registered in 1951.

From a total membership in the United States of less than 10 million subscribers in 1948, the enrollment of the 70 Blue Shield plans on December 31, 1977 was equal to about one-third the population of the United States. The distribution as to coverage was:

•Group coverage	57,026,036
•Nongroup coverage	6,143,179
•Complementary Medicare	7,688,329
Total	70,857,544

More than 20 million other persons receive services from Blue Shield under fiscal arrangements with Medicare B, Medicaid, and with CHAMPUS in certain states. A stock insurance company, Medical Indemnity of America, wholly owned by Blue Shield Association, assists in enrolling and servicing national accounts.

Payment under Blue Shield is made directly to participating physicians under one of two methods. More than half the subscribers are enrolled under contracts calling for payment to physicians under the newest program, the UCR (Usual, Customary, and Reasonable) charge program. The UCR provides payments to physicians on the basis of the usual and customary fee in the locality in which they practice. The other mode of payment is the indemnity method which allows fixed dollar amounts toward payment of medical care.

The national Blue Shield Association sets rigorous standards for the local plans: they must be able to underwrite comprehensive health care benefit programs consisting of 20 broad benefit areas, must be able to offer contracts to national accounts, and must offer UCR programs.

Blue Shield plans are reaching out experimentally with new methods of payment and new areas of coverage such as: prepaid group practice, vision care, hearing care, and coverage for prolonged and catastrophic illness.

The 70 Blue Shield plans represented one of the countries large financial combinations in the report of December 31, 1977. Balances were:

•Total assets	$4,580,953,000
•Total liabilities	3,058,434,000
•Total reserves	$1,522,519,000

The income and expense totals for the U.S. Blue Shield plans (including Puerto Rico) for 1977 were:

- •Total income $11,106,501,000
- •Claims expense   9,687,157,000
- •Administrative expense (7.9%)   865,589,000
- •Net income   553,755,000

Suggested Readings

Anderson, Odin W. *Blue Cross Since 1929 Accountability and Public Trust.*

Kaitz, Edward M. *Pricing Policy and Cost Behavior in the Hospital Industry,* pp. 123–241.

Somers, H.M. and Somers, A.R. *Doctors, Patients, and Health Insurance,* pp. 257–303.

Chapter 7
Medicare and Medicaid

M Day was July 1, 1966. This was a day of great social adjustment in the United States. It was the day that health service benefits were initiated by the federal government under Medicare and Medicaid, otherwise known as Title XVIII and Title XIX of the Social Security Act.

Medicare and Medicaid together made more impact on the way we live in the United States than any other piece of social legislation since the original Social Security Act passed in the mid-Thirties during the administration of Frankin D. Roosevelt. In fact, Medicare and Medicaid have direct ties to the Roosevelt administration and every administration since then. Some kind of plan for a national health insurance or service has been conceptualized, introduced as a bill into Congress, or at least has been stated as a goal in some politician's campaign during every administration since the Thirties. President Lyndon B. Johnson chose to honor the efforts of former President Harry S. Truman to have health insurance legislation passed in Congress by flying to Independence, Missouri so that he could sign the bill which made Medicare and Medicaid into law in the presence of Mr. Truman.

Medicare and Medicaid are compromises between several divergent views of what the benefits under such plans should be, and how the plans should be financed and administered. The compromises have made administration difficult, but it is better to have compromises than no plan, or no benefits. It would seem that U.S. Representative Wilbur D. Mills (D., Ark.), Chairman of the House Ways and Means Committee in 1965 thought this way also, for he is credited with bringing about a meeting of minds through compromise. A stalemate over health legislation had been existent for years, caused by the differing positions of various Congressmen, the American Medical Association, the American Hospital Association, the Blue Cross Association, trade unions, business associations and other special interest groups.

Medicare helps pay for two kinds of service for persons 65 years of age or over: Part A (HI) is insurance for hospital care and related services; and Part B is insurance to help pay doctor's bills for service in or out of the hospital, and for other related services. This Part B insurance is also known as the Supplementary Medical Insurance Program (SMI).

Medicaid provides help in some states for the medically indigent (persons unable to pay for medical care even though they may be able to defray other ordinary living expenses). There is no age limit for Medicaid recipients; the only test is need. Many of the so-called welfare medical cases including the blind, the disabled, and crippled children come under Medicaid.

Although Medicaid has been the source of help for the medically indigent in some states since the SSA Amendments went into effect in 1966, there were other changes made under the SSA Amendments of 1972 (Public Law 92–603, H.R.I.) which further affected certain of those persons:

—Persons under 65 who have been receiving disability benefits under Social Security for at least twenty-four consecutive months are now eligible for hospital insurance under Medicare Part A and also may enroll in the medical insurance program, Part B.

—Widows, 50 or over, who were eligible for disability benefits for two years or more but did not file a disability claim because they were getting social security checks as mothers caring for young or disabled children, are eligible for Part A hospital insurance and may enroll in the Part B medical insurance program.

—Persons under 65 who need hemodialysis or renal transplantation for chronic renal disease are eligible for hospital insurance under Medicare Part A and may enroll for Part B medical insurance, if they meet certain work requirements under social security, or are receiving Social Security benefits, or are the spouses or dependent minor children of such individuals. Eligibility for coverage begins with the third month after the month in which a course of renal dialysis begins and continues through the twelfth month after the month in which an individual has a transplant or in which dialysis terminates.

Medicare (Part A) Hospital Insurance

The fact that Medicare is structured in two parts illustrates the compromise effected by Congress. Part A helps pay for hospital care, extended care, and home health service for persons 65 years of age or older who are registered under Medicare. Part A is financed by a special percentage assessment added to the Social Security payroll deduction of employees, and to the SSA contributions of the employers and the self-employed. The general fund of the federal government makes up any deficit.[1] However, there is an annual review of costs so that adjustments can be made in coinsurance ratios, if needed. The coinsurance arrangements calls for the beneficiary to pay a part of the cost and for Medicare to pay the remainder. Claims are handled through an intermediary or fiscal agent for the government. This agent usually is the local Blue Cross plan acting under a subcontract with the Blue Cross Association, or an insurance company.

The structure of Part A of Medicare satisfied the exponents of financing by payroll deduction through the Social Security Administration with supplements from the federal government when needed. Part A was also designed to meet the demands of those who favored coinsurance. The extensive claims facilities of Blue Cross and major commercial insurance companies were also needed.

The SSA Amendments, 1972, made provision for persons aged 65 and over who previously were not eligible for Medicare hospital insurance to secure such coverage on a voluntary basis by agreeing to pay a monthly hospital insurance premium and also by agreeing to enroll for Part B Medicare medical insurance. The basic premium as of July 1, 1973 for hospital insurance under this voluntary provision was $33 a month. By July 1, 1978 the basic premium for a person 65 years of age had risen to $63 a month.

Medicare (Part A) Benefits

Three kinds of facilities are the major sources of service benefits for Medicare Part A recipients: care in the hospital; care in a skilled nursing facility after a hospital stay; or services from a home health care agency to bed patients who are at home after a stay in a hospital or a skilled nursing facility[2] (See Table 7-2).

---

[1]Table 7-1 gives a profile of the increase in contributions since 1966. Both percentage of contribution rate and annual earnings base are likely to be increased in the future.

[2]Extensive changes in definition have been adopted in the use of "skilled nursing facility" to replace "extended care facility" under the SSA amendments of 1972. See section on skilled nursing facilities, page 165.

Table 7-1

Contribution Ratio for Medicare Hospital Insurance (HI) Part A

Beginning	Annual Earnings Base	Contribution Rate (%) Employee and Employer, each	Maximum Contribution each
1966	$ 6,600	0.35	23.10
1967	6,600	0.5	33.00
1968	7,800	0.6	46.80
1969	7,800	0.6	46.80
1970	7,800	0.6	46.80
1971	7,800	0.6	46.80
1972	9,000	0.6	54.00
1973	10,800	1.0	108.00
1974	12,000	1.0	120.00
1975	14,100	1.0	141.00
1976	15,300	1.0	153.00
1977	16,500	1.0	165.00
1978	17,700	1.0	177.00
1979*	22,900	1.05	240.45
1980	25,900	1.05	271.95
1981	29,700	1.30	386.10
1982	31,800	1.30	413.40
1983	33,900	1.30	440.70
1984	36,000	1.30	468.00
1985	38,100	1.35	514.35
1986	40,200	1.45	582.90
1987	42,600	1.45	617.70

*Reflects changes and estimates (years 1979–1987). Source: Social Security Administration

Benefits are governed by benefit periods. A Medicare benefit period begins the first time a person registered under Medicare enters a hospital as a bed patient and ends whenever he has not been in a hospital or in a facility offering skilled nursing care for 60 days in a row. The key to understanding the benefit period is the 60 day interval necessary between the end of one benefit period and the beginning of another.

Table 7-2

Medicare and Medicaid: Benefits, Financing, and Coinsurance

	Persons Covered	Benefits (Services)	Benefits (Length)	Methods of Financing	Coinsurance Costs
MEDICARE A	Aged 65 or older who are registered with SSA. Also exceptions for certain disabled.	Certain services from hospitals, SNFs, and home health agencies.	Hospitals: 90 days in each benefit period. SNFs: 100 days of care in each benefit period. Home health nurse or therapist: 100 visits within one year after hospital or SNF stay.	Primarily by Social Security tax of 1.05 percent of first $22,900 annual employee earnings (1979) by an employer or by self-employed.	Hospital: recipient pays first $160, and from 61st to 90th days pays $40 a day. Lifetime reserve: recipient pays $80 a day. SNF: recipient pays $20 a day from 21st through 100th day. Home health care: if recipient qualifies under Medicare A, 100 home visits, after discharge from hospital or participating SNF are fully paid by Medicare.
MEDICARE B	Aged 65 or older who are registered with SSA for Supplementary Medical Insurance.	Certain services from physicians, hospital outpatient departments and home health agencies.	Services during a calendar year.	By a monthly premium paid by the recipient and an equal amount by the federal government. Premiums can be raised as SSA benefits are raised. Premium in July 1979 was $8.70 per month per person.	Recipient pays first $60 cost of a calendar year
MEDICAID	Medically indigent, as needed.	Hospital services as inpatient or outpatient, laboratory tests, x-rays, physician's services, home health care visits.	Year	Shared federal and state program.	None

Table 7-3

Hospital Insurance (HI) Copayments for First Amounts and for 61st through 90th day of Hospitalization per Benefit Period

	Pay First	Frcm 61st to 90th Day Pay per Day	Lifetime Reserve Days Pay per Day
Prior to 1969	$ 40	$ 10	$ 20
Beginning January 1969	44	11	22
1970	52	13	26
1971	60	15	30
1972	68	17	34
1973	72	18	36
1974	84	21	42
1975	92	23	46
1976	104	26	52
1977	124	31	62
1978	144	36	72
1979	160	40	80

Source: Social Security Administration

Table 7-4

Supplementary Medical Insurance (SMI) Premiums

Before April 1, 1968	$3.00 a month
Beginning April 1, 1968	4.00
July 1, 1970	5.30
July 1, 1971	5.60
July 1, 1972	5.80
July 1, 1973	6.30
July 1, 1974	6.70
July 1, 1976	7.20
July 1, 1977	7.70
July 1, 1978	8.20
July 1, 1979	8.70*

Source: Social Security Administration
*Future increases in premiums will be possible only in percentage ratio to general increases of Social Security benefits.

Part A Hospital Coinsurance Benefits

These benefits provide for care in a semiprivate room (2–4 beds in a room) with all meals, including special diets, for up to 90 days in a benefit period. Other hospital care expenses which are included under coinsurance are:

—Drugs furnished by the hospital
—Laboratory tests
—Nursing services (regular but including special care units)[3]
—Medical supplies such as splints and casts
—Operating room and recovery room costs
—X-ray and other radiological services including radiation therapy, billed by the hospital
—Use of appliances and equipment furnished by the hospital, such as wheelchair, crutches, and braces
—Rehabilitation services, such as physical therapy, occupational therapy, and speech pathology services
—Care in a participating psychiatric hospital for not more than 190 days in a lifetime
—Blood (except for first three pints in each benefit period)

Part A Hospital Coinsurance Payment

Those in force January 1979[4] were the following: For the first 60 days in the hospital a bed patient registered under Medicare Part A pays the first $160 of the hospital bill, and for the 61st through the 90th day pays $40 a day.[5] Medicare pays all other covered charges. The initial $160 is paid only once in a benefit period, no matter if the patient is in the hospital several times.[6]

---

[3]Items not paid for under Part A coinsurance include: private duty nurses; extra charge for a private room unless patient needs it for medical reasons; telephone; radio; television; or physician's services (covered under Part B).

[4]Periodic adjustments have been necessary in the coinsurance percentages and dollar amounts because of rising costs.

[5]Besides the 90 days of hospital care allowed per benefit period, there is also a "lifetime reserve" of 60 days available to Medicare patients. If a Medicare patient needs to use more than 90 hospital days during one benefit period he may use some of his lifetime reserve days. Medicare pays all covered charges, except $80 per day for lifetime reserve days used. There is another special rule which limits benefits: a beneficiary has a lifetime limit of 190 hospital days in a psychiatric hospital.

[6]The Social Security Administration keeps a record of benefit days for the beneficiary.

Part A Skilled Nursing Facility (SNF) Coinsurance Benefits

These benefits apply to beneficiaries who become bed patients in the SNF (after leaving a hospital) for up to 100 days in each benefit period. The benefits include care in a semiprivate room (2 to 4 beds in a room) with all meals and special diets, if needed. Other expenses which are covered with coinsurance provisions include:

—Drugs furnished by the SNF
—Regular nursing service
—Physical, occupational, and speech therapy
—Medical supplies such as splints and casts
—Medical social services
—Use of appliances and equipment furnished by the SNF such as wheelchair, crutches and braces[7]

Conditions Necessary for a Patient to Qualify for Part A Extended Care Benefits

These conditions include:

—Medical needs requiring continuing nursing care
—A physician determining that a patient needs extended care and ordering such care
—The patient having been in a participating or qualified hospital for at least three days in a row before admission to SNF
—Patient being admitted to the SNF 14 days of leaving the hospital
—Patient being admitted to SNF for further treatment of condition treated in hospital.

Two new qualifying factors under the 1972 SSA Amendments affect extended care benefits: advanced approval of extended care and home health benefits; and modification of the 14-day transfer requirement for extended care benefits.

As of January 1, 1973 the Secretary of HEW was authorized to establish minimum periods during which beneficiaries would be presumed to be eligible and payment could be made for extended care or home health benefits after hospitalization. Medical conditions, length of stay, or number of visits would be the basis for the regulations. The attending physician will be required to certify

---

[7]Expenses not covered in the SNF include: private duty nursing; extra charge for a private room unless the patient needs it for a medical reason; telephone; radio; television; and physician's services (covered under Part B).

that the condition is one designated in the regulations and will furnish a plan of treatment prior to or at the time of admission or the first visit under home health service. Certifications and patient stays will be subject to review.

A waiver in the requirement that a patient is entitled to extended care benefits only if he is transferred to a SNF within 14 days of discharge from a hospital is now possible if:

—appropriate bed space is unavailable in the geographic area during the 14 day period. However, in this case, the transfer must take place within 28 days of hospital discharge.
—in cases where skilled nursing care or rehabilitative services cannot be utilized within the 14 day period due to the patient's medical condition. For example, after a fracture, physical therapy or restorative nursing might not be indicated within the regular period after hospital discharge. Therefore transfer to a SNF should be made at a time medically appropriate.

Coinsurance Provisions for Care in a Skilled Nursing Facility

These provisions call for the beneficiary to pay $20 per day for care from the 21st day through the 100th day.

Part A Home Health Coinsurance Benefits in the Patient's Home after Leaving the Hospital

These benefits can include certain services furnished by a participating home health agency.[8]

—Part-time nursing care
—Physical, occupational, and speech therapy
—Part-time services of home aides
—Medical social work
—Medical supplies furnished by the agency
—Use of medical appliances

Up to 100 visits by the nurse therapist, or other persons supplying service, are allowed within a year after the most recent discharge from a hospital or a participating SNF.

Conditions Necessary to Qualify for Part A Home Health Benefits

—Patient was in a participating (or otherwise qualified) hospital for at least three days in a row

---

[8]Medicare does not pay as a home health benefit the expenses of: full-time nursing care; drugs and biologicals; personal comfort or convenience items; or for meals delivered to the home.

—Patient is confined to his home

—Doctor determines patient needs home health care and sets up a home health plan within 14 days after discharge of patient from the hospital or a participating SNF

—The home health care plan is for further treatment of a condition for which person received services as a bed patient in the hospital or extended care facility

Medicare (Part B) Medical Insurance

Part B is the medical insurance section of Medicare designed to help pay for doctors' services, outpatient services, medical services and supplies outside the hospital coverage, and those home health services not covered in Part A (a previous stay in hospital or extended care unit is required to qualify for home health services under Part A). Part B is financed by a monthly insurance premium, $8.70 per month per person during the year beginning July 1979[9] paid by the Medicare beneficiary and a like amount contributed by the federal government.[10] The premium rate has been reviewed each year in December, and a new rate has been set to become effective in July of the following year for the years through 1972. This system was established to ensure that costs could be met by the equal contributions of the beneficiaries and the government. Under the SSA Amendments of 1972, however, beneficiary premiums for medical insurance cannot be increased unless there has been a general social security benefit increase since the current premium rate was established, and the percentage of premium increase cannot exceed the percentage of the general social security increase.

The equal contribution method of financing for Part B Medicare illustrates another of the compromises effected between differing views in health insurance proposals to the Congress. Part B also has provisions for coinsurance and for a nongovernment fiscal agent to act as the "carrier" or intermediary agent. Usually, the carrier is a Blue Shield plan or an insurance com-

---

[9] Higher rates must be paid by those beneficiaries who did not enroll within the first year of eligibility after becoming 65 years of age. After the first year the rate is about 10 percent higher, about 20 percent after the second, and about 30 percent after the third.

[10] The Part B insurnace premium is deducted from the monthly checks of those who receive Social Security benefits. Railroad Retirement benefits, or Civil Service annuities. Those who do not receive such checks, pay their premiums directly to Social Security or their premiums are paid by a state social agency (Medicaid).

pany handling claims for a state or a large area of a state. Both the coinsurance and nongovernment carrier provisions could be called compromises.

The SSA Amendments 1972 made provision to avoid levying penalties due to neglect of eligible persons to enroll in Part B (SMI) insurance. Beneficiaries receiving monthly SSA or Railroad Retirement benefits prior to age 65 are now deemed to have enrolled in SMI the month before the month they are entitled to Part A hospital insurance (HI). Those who have not previously received benefits will be deemed to enroll likewise before the HI entitlement. Disability beneficiaries will be deemed to have enrolled in the 24th consecutive month of receiving benefits. However, an individual can decline SMI, if he wishes. The requirement that beneficiaries enroll within three years of initial eligibility or re-enroll within three years of termination has been eliminated. There was no change made in the provision that only one re-enrollment is permitted after a termination, or in the approximate 10 percent increase in the basic premium for each 12 months one could have been, but was not, enrolled.

Part B Coinsurance

Part B requires the beneficiary to pay the first $60[11] in reasonable charges[12] in a calendar year. After the first $60 expense, Medicare Part B insurance will pay 80 percent of all reasonable charges for the rest of the year.

Medicare (Part B) Benefits

Benefits for Part B expenses are paid in either of two ways: (1) payment can be made to the doctor or supplier; or (2) the payment can be made directly to the beneficiary.

Under method (1) the doctor or supplier agrees to apply for the medical insurance payment at a rate not to exceed the "reasonable charge" set by the carrier. The beneficiary is responsible for any of the $60 deductible which might not have been met that year

---

[11]The provision that the first $60 Part B expense in a calendar year is deducted from benefits is modified by a special carry-over rule which covers the last three months of the year. Any Part B expenses incurred in the last three months of the calendar year which can be counted toward the $60 deductible for that year can also be counted toward the $60 annual deductible for the next calendar year.

[12]"Reasonable charges" for covered services are set by the carrier after taking into account the customary charges of the doctor or other supplier of services and after considering, as well, the customary charges made by other doctors or suppliers for that service in the community.

and for the 20 percent coinsurance of the amount above the $60 deductible.

Under method (2), after the proper forms have been signed by the doctor or supplier, the beneficiary can apply for direct payment. In turn, he can pay his doctor or supplier for services rendered.

There is a time limit for filing claims for Part B Medicare benefits which follows the rule that services received in the fourth quarter of year 1 and the services received in the first three quarters of year 2 must be filed before the end of year 3. Example: claims for services received between October 1, 1979 and September 30, 1980 must be filed by December 31, 1981.

Part B—Doctors' Services Covered[13]

— Medical and surgical services by a doctor of medicine or osteopathy
— Certain medical and surgical services by a dentist (see following section)
— Chiropractic by licensed and Medicare-certified chiropractors limited to manual manipulation of the spine to correct a subluxation
— Services, except routine foot care, by podiatrists for which they are legally authorized by the state in which they practice
— Other services ordinarily furnished by the doctor's office and which are included in his bill, such as: diagnostic tests and procedures; medical supplies; services of the office nurse; and drugs and biologicals which cannot be self-administered
— Services by radiologists and pathologists to hospital inpatients will be paid 100 percent of reasonable charges
— Doctor's services for outpatient treatment of a mental illness will be paid to extent of no more than $250 in any one year

Part B—Dental Services Covered[14]

The medical insurance of Part B covers services of dentists only when surgery of the jaw or related structures, or setting of fractures of the jaw or facial bones is involved.

---

[13]Services not covered include: routine physical check-ups; routine care of flat feet, sprains or partial dislocations of the feet; eye refraction and examinations for prescribing, fitting, or changing eyeglasses; hearing examinations for prescribing, fitting, or changing hearing aids; immunizations unless directly related to an injury or immediate risk of infection such as antitetanus injection given after an injury; those of certain practitioners such as Christian Science practitioners, and naturopaths.

[14]Medical insurance of Medicare Part B does not pay for dental services such as filling, removal, replacement, or other care of the teeth, or for the treatment of gum areas, or surgery or other services related to these kinds of dental care.

Part B—Laboratory and Radiology Services by Doctors for Hospital Inpatients

Medicare Part B insurance pays 100 percent of all reasonable charges by doctors for radiology and pathology services for Part B inpatient beneficiaries in a participating or otherwise qualified hospital. Since these fully paid expenses for the services of radiologists and pathologists are an exception to the coinsurance feature of Part B insurance, these expenses cannot be counted toward the $60 deductible.

Part B—Ambulance Service Covered

Medicare medical insurance will help pay for ambulance transportation of a Part B beneficiary by an approved ambulance to a hospital or a skilled nursing home only when:

—The ambulance, its equipment and personnel meet Medicare requirements
—Transportation by other means would endanger the patient's health
—The patient is taken to a facility serving the locality, or is the nearest facility equipped to take care of the patient

Part B—Outpatient Hospital Benefits

The following are outpatient hospital services which Part B medical insurance helps pay for:[15]

—Laboratory and other diagnostic services
—X-ray and other radiology services
—Emergency room services
—Medical supplies, such as splints and casts
—Other diagnostic services
—Blood (except for first three pints)

Under the 1972 SSA Amendments covered speech therapy services may now be provided to inpatients of hospitals and SNFs under Part B Medicare medical insurance as outpatient services if the patients have exhausted their inpatient days or are otherwise not entitled to hospital insurance Part A.

Part B—Outpatient Physical Therapy

Physical therapy services are covered when they are furnished by a qualified hospital, SNF, home health agency, clinic, rehabilita-

---

[15]Part B medical insurance does not help pay for: tests given in a routine checkup; eye refractions and examinations; immunizations, unless directly related to injury; or hearing examinations for hearing aids.

tion agency, or public health agency, and they are furnished under a plan established and periodically reviewed by a physician.

A hospital or SNF may now provide covered outpatient physical therapy services under Medicare Part B medical insurance to its own inpatients if they have exhausted their inpatient days under Medicare Part A or are otherwise not entitled to Part A coverage of these services.

Part B—Home Health Benefits

Under Part A the Medicare hospital insurance helps pay for home health benefits after a stay in a hospital and/or a skilled nursing facility. Part B covers home health care without the necessity of the beneficiary previously having been a bed patient of a hospital or a SNF in the same benefit period.

Up to 100 visits by home health personnel within a calendar year to a beneficiary are benefits under Part B if all the following conditions exist:

—The beneficiary needs part-time skilled nursing care or physical or speech therapy services
—The beneficiary is confined to his home
—The physician signifies that the beneficiary needs home health services
—The physician sets up and periodically reviews the plan for home health care
—The home health agency is participating in Medicare

The services provided under home health care which Medicare helps pay for include:[16]

—Part-time nursing care
—Physical, occupational or speech therapy
—Part-time services of home health aides
—Medical social services
—Medical supplies furnished by the agency
—Use of medical appliances

Part B—Other Medical Services and Supplies

When any of the services listed below are furnished by a participating hospital, a skilled nursing facility, or a home health agency, that institution will file a claim with the carrier and will also bill

---

[16]Home health services not paid for under Part B include: full-time nursing; drugs and biologicals; personal comfort or convenience items; noncovered levels of care; and meals delivered to the home.

the patient for his share under the coinsurance arrangement. Among the services Part B medical insurance helps pay for are:[17]

—Diagnostic x-ray and laboratory tests furnished by approved independent laboratories
—Radiation therapy[18]
—Portable diagnostic x-ray services in the home under a physician's supervision
—Surgical dressing, splints, casts, and similar devices[19]
—Rental or purchase of durable medical equipment prescribed by a physician for use in the home (wheelchair, hospital bed, oxygen equipment, for example)
—Services (other than dental) to replace all or part of an internal body organ. Included are corrective lenses after a cataract operation
—Certain ambulance services

Medicare (Part A) and the Hospital

For the Medicare program the federal government has set standards of certification and conditions for participation for the suppliers of institutional services, has established procedures for reimbursement of the suppliers, has specified that fiscal intermediaries[19] be selected for processing Part A Medicare claims, and has set up a nongovernment council of health and financial experts to act in advisory capacity.[20]

Under the law it is required that state or local health agencies

---

[17]Part B insurance does not pay for prescription drugs and drugs that are self-administered (insulin, for example), for hearing aids, eyeglasses, false teeth, orthopedic shoes, or other supportive devices for the feet.

[18]Medical insurance will help pay for these items in cases where Part A hospital insurance cannot pay.

[19]The fiscal agents for medical insurance claims under Part B, called "carriers," have somewhat wider responsibility than fiscal intermediaries of Part A. Carriers must be experienced in the health field to the degree that they are competent not only to accept and pay claims, but also that they can determine whether a provider's charge is reasonable, whether it is his customary charge for the service, and how it compares with customary charges in the community for like services. The carriers at the beginning of Medicare consisted of 33 Blue Shield plans, 15 commercial insurance companies, and one independent health insurer. These carriers serviced the 64 geographic regions into which the country was divided. Group prepayment plans are reimbursed on a reasonable cost basis directly by the Social Security Administration.

[20]The advisory body is called the Health Insurance Benefits Advisory Council (HIBAC). It is composed of nongovernment health and financial experts who advise the SSA on general policy for both Medicare and Medicaid.

(or other appropriate agencies) be used to certify that institutional providers of care and independent laboratories meet conditions for participation set by the federal government. The costs for this initial survey and for periodic rechecking are paid by Medicare. The details of the certification process and the conditions for participation are discussed in a section which follows.

Reimbursements for covered services provided by hospitals, skilled nursing facilities, and home health agencies under Part A are based on reasonable costs. Acceptable cost finding methods, allowable costs, and reporting methods for this reimbursement are discussed later in the chapter.

The intermediaries for Part A providers (hospitals, skilled nursing facilities and home health agencies) were originally nominated by groups of those institutions for consideration and judged for approval by the Social Security Administration. The intermediaries were chosen by SSA for the ability to act as a claims agent, payer of claims, and also on the ability to furnish consultative services on cost finding and accounting procedures so that the Part A providers will receive equitable payments for services rendered. However, if the provider chooses it may deal directly with SSA.

At the beginning of the Medicare program, the American Hospital Association nominated the Blue Cross Association as fiscal intermediary of its member hospitals. (A few of the member hospitals, however, chose other intermediaries.) Blue Cross was chosen by about 91 per cent of the hospitals, 54 per cent of the SNFs, and 78 per cent of the home health agencies.[21] The next largest group of intermediaries was of commercial insurance companies. A few other health organizations were chosen as intermediaries; a small percentage of providers chose to deal directly with SSA.

Certification of Hospitals (Part A)

The requirements of the Joint Commission on Accreditation of Hospitals (JCAH) or of the American Osteopathic Association (AOA) for approval of hospitals are generally accepted as satisfying conditions for participating hospitals under Title XVIII unless a state or region imposes higher restrictions for purchases of services. In practice, a state agency determines eligibility or ineligibility of an institution to participate in the Medicare program. The state agency certifies that the hospital:

---

[21]Robert J. Myers. *Medicare*, p. 179.

—Is accredited by JCAH or AOA
—Has established a utilization review plan meeting the requirements of the act; the plan is in effect, or will be in effect, the
first day of participation
—Has met the statutory requirements of the act, or if certain
deficiencies with respect to one or more conditions of participation have been found, that reasonable plans have been
made to correct the deficiencies; and, despite the deficiencies,
adequate care is being given, and without hazard to the health
and safety of the patients

Certification of a hospital by the state agency (acting under
agreement with the Secretary of HEW) as being in substantial
compliance will be for a period of two years. A list of deficiencies
of standards will be noted, and whether the deficiencies create a
serious hazard to health and safety, and whether the hospital is
making reasonable plans and efforts to correct the deficiency
within a reasonable period. Notice of eligibility or ineligibility for
participation made by the Secretary on the basis of the state
agency certification will be sent to the institution being considered by the SSA.

In like manner, the state agency will certify that an institution is
not in compliance, or is no longer in compliance. If on the basis of
the state agency's certification of noncompliance or no longer in
compliance the participation agreement is terminated, the hospital
can request that the determination be reviewed.

Special certification can be allowed in isolated regions where
the denial of certification would seriously limit the accessibility of
beneficiaries to hospitals. The special certification could be allowed only if the deficiencies noted did not place the health and
safety of patients in jeopardy. Resurveys would be required annually for specially certified institutions.

Another exception to general rules would allow payments to be
made for emergency services in nonparticipating hospitals under
special conditions.

Under the SSA Amendment 1972, a new mechanism for continued validation of the voluntary accreditation process was set up.
The Secretary of HEW was authorized to enter into an agreement
with any state to have the state certification agency survey hospitals accredited by JCAH on a selective sample basis, or a specific
hospital on the basis of substantial allegations and evidence of a
condition adverse to health and safety. If a survey institution is
found to have significant deficiencies relative to Medicare health

and safety standards, the institution may be terminated from participation in the program. An institution certified on the basis of JCAH accreditation must agree to authorize JCAH to release to the Secretary a copy of the most current JCAH accreditation survey if the institution is included in a certification survey.

Conditions for Participation of Hospitals, Part A

The conditions outlined for participation of the providers of services under Part A represent good organization and good practice. The conditions for participation of hospitals have been chosen for detailed description and discussion, but the same careful controls seem to have been used for all providers. An administrator could use Medicare conditions of participation guidelines as rules of practice.

The conditions for participation of hospitals under Title XVIII include:

Compliance with state and local laws. The participating hospital must meet all laws of licensure and standards; staff must be registered and licensed in conformity to laws; the hospital must operate in compliance with laws relating to fire and safety, to communicable and reportable diseases, to post-mortems, and to other relevant matters.

The governing body of the hospital. This body (or the legal body responsible for the conduct of the hospital) must be operated generally as follows:

(a) Under a set of written bylaws which stipulate the selection, term of office, and duties and requirements of the members and which bylaws specify to whom responsibilities for the operation and maintenance of the hospital are delegated.

(b) The governing body shall have regular meetings to plan for and evaluate the operation of the hospital and the care of patients.

(c) There shall be a committee structure consistent with the size and scope of the hospital. Principal among these should be: an executive committee to coordinate the activities and the general policies of the various hospital departments, and the special committees established by the governing board; a finance committee; a joint conference committee to liaison with the medical staff; and a building and maintenance committee.

(d) The governing body appoints members of the medical staff. This staff in turn works under written bylaws, rules and regulations which outline: procedures for submission and processing of staff applications; and definitions of physicians' privileges.

(e) The governing body appoints a qualified hospital administrator or executive officer, preferably one with formal training in a graduate program of hospital administration approved by the Association of University Programs in Health Administration. The administrator is to act as executive officer of the governing body in the management of the hospital and in providing liaison among the governing body, medical staff, nursing staff, and other departments of the hospital.

(f) The governing body must establish a policy requiring: every patient to be under care of a physician; a patient to be admitted to the hospital only on the recommendation of the physician; that a physician is on duty or on call at all times and available within 15 or 20 minutes at the most.

(g) The governing body is responsible for providing a physical plant staffed and equipped to provide services needed for patients.

The physical environment. Buildings should be constructed and maintained to assure safety and well-being of the patients as required by state laws and codes. Factors to be considered: facilities for the physical separation of isolation patients and for handling contaminated linens; at least 100 square feet floor space for a private room and 80 square feet area per patient in multiple rooms; facilities for emergency power, lighting, gas, and water; regular inspection and cleaning of all intake sources; proper waste disposal facilities, and generally good housekeeping. Fire control standards should be rigid and be enforced. A sanitary environment should be maintained by an infection committee and by infection control procedures. Also, the hospital should provide adequate diagnostic and therapeutic facilities to permit an acceptable level of patient care.

The medical staff. The staff, organized under bylaws approved by the governing body, should be responsible to that body for the quality of medical care provided patients of the hospital. The staff should work through a committee structure to carry out the policies of both the medical staff and the hospital. There should be enforced disciplinary procedures for infractions of hospital and medical policies.

The medical staff should attempt to secure autopsies in all cases of unusual deaths and of medico-legal interest and education. A minimum of 20 per cent of all terminal cases should be autopsied.

Standards should be set for consultations with qualified physicians under conditions where: the patient is not a good medical or surgical risk; the diagnosis is obscure; there is doubt as to the best therapeutic measures; and there is question of criminal action. The consultation should include an examination of the patient and a written and signed opinion to be included in the patient's medical record.

Medical staff appointments should be made by the governing board, with reappointments made periodically after reappraisal of the members' competence and character.[22] The staff membership or professional privileges should not be granted solely on certification, fellowship, or membership of a specialty body or society.

The active medical staff of the hospital performs the organizational duties of the medical staff: maintains proper quality of medical care in the hospital; adopts rules and regulations for governing the medical staff (with the approval of the governing body); elects its officers (or recommends appointments to the governing body if called for in bylaws); makes recommendations to the governing body about appointments to the staff and grants of medical staff privileges; and makes recommendations to the governing body about matters of concern to the medical staff.

Other staff categories which may be supplemental to the active staff, but which in no way reduce the responsibility of the active staff include:

(a) The honorary staff is usually composed of former active staff members, retired or emeritus, or other distinguished physicians the hospital desires to honor.

(b) The consulting staff is usually composed of recognized specialists serving in consulting capacity rather than as admitting or attending physicians.

(c) The associate staff category usually includes the members who use the hospital infrequently or who are less experienced or who are going through a period of probation before an appointment to the active staff.

(d) The courtesy staff members are usually those who want to attend patients in the hospital, but, for some reason, not disqualifying, are ineligible for appointment in another category of the staff.

---

[22]Appointments are made after consideration of recommendations of the credentials committee and of the medical staff voting membership.

The medical staff officers are usually elected by and from the active staff members (unless in rare situations, the officers are appointed by the governing board or by some other means).

The chief of staff as chief executive officer of the staff has the following responsibilities:

(a) To organize and administer the medical staff in accordance with terms of the staff bylaws and the rules and regulations
(b) To act in coordination and cooperation with the hospital administrator in all medico-administrative matters to carry out the policies adopted by the governing body
(c) To be responsible for the careful supervision over all clinical work in all departments of the hospital

Medical staff bylaws and rules and regulations. These regulations which have been adopted to enable the medical staff to carry out its responsibilities include:

(a) A descriptive outline of the medical staff organization
(b) A statement of qualifications of physicians necessary for staff membership, and the duties and privileges of each category of membership
(c) A procedure for granting and withdrawing of privileges of physicians
(d) A method of appeal from decisions affecting staff membership or privileges
(e) A specific statement forbidding the splitting of fees
(f) A provision for regular meeting of the medical staff
(g) Provisions for the keeping of complete and accurate clinical records
(h) A provision making the physician in charge of a surgical patient responsible for seeing that all tissue removed at an operation is delivered to the hospital pathologist, and that a routine examination and report is made at that time
(i) A rule permitting a surgical operation only on the consent of the patient or a legal representative, except in emergencies
(j) A statement providing that consultations be required except in emergencies
(k) A regulation requiring all physicians' orders to be recorded and signed
(l) If dentists and oral surgeons are to be accorded staff membership, necessary qualifications, privileges and rights of this group must be stated in the bylaws

Medical Staff Committees. Certain committee functions are required. In a small hospital the medical staff might work as a committee of the whole, but an organizational structure with at least two or three major committees would be a preferred method. Those major committees would probably include:

(a) An Executive Committee which coordinates the activities of the medical staff, receives and acts upon reports of other committees of the staff, and represents the staff as a whole where this is indicated

(b) A Credentials Committee to review applications for appointments and reappointments to the medical staff, and make recommendations to the Executive Committee on those applications and on the staff privileges connected with them

(c) A Joint Conference Committee composed of members of the governing body and medical and administrative staffs. The committee acts as a liaison among those groups

(d) A Medical Records Committee composed of staff members representative of a cross section of the clinical servies of the hospital supervises the maintenance of the medical records system

(e) The Tissue Committee reviews and evaluates all surgery done in the hospital on the basis of agreement or disagreement among the preoperative, postoperative, and pathological diagnoses and on the acceptability of the procedures followed

(f) A Utilization Review Committee composed of staff members representative of the clinical services to evaluate the quality of patient care under a regular utilization review plan

Medical staff meetings should be held at frequent and regular intervals to "review, analyze and evaluate" the work of the medical staff members. In addition, where the size of the hospital makes it feasible (all except the small general hospital of 75 beds or less), the medical staff should be organized in clinical services headed by a chief of service. The chief should be responsible for the administration of the clinical service and the quality of care given patients there.

The Nursing Department. The hospital must have an organized nursing department with a licensed registered professional nurse on duty at all times and with professional nursing service available for all patients at all times. Standards are given for supervisory personnel, for working relationships with physicians and with other departments of the hospital. Written nursing care procedures and written nursing care plans for patients are required as are constant review and evaluation of nursing care provided patients.

The Dietary Department. An organized dietary department under the direction of a qualified dietitian is required. Standards are set for written procedures, facilities, food storage, and therapeutic diets. Provision is made for contract food service from an outside management company as long as standards of trained personnel and other requirements are met.

Medical Records Department. A medical record must be maintained for every patient admitted for care in the hospital. Standards are given for the necessary contents of the record, its completion, its indexing and filing, and its preservation.

Pharmacy or Drug Room. The hospital must have a pharmacy under the direction of a registered pharmacist or a drug room under proper supervision. Standards are given for facilities, personnel, records to be kept, control of dangerous and toxic drugs, and a pharmacy and therapeutic committee to set standards and controls for drugs dispensed.

Laboratories. The hospital should have a well organized and adequately supervised clinical laboratory to perform those services commensurate with the hospital's needs. Anatomical pathology services and blood bank services should be available in the hospital or by arrangement with other facilities.

Medical Library. The library should contain modern textbooks and current periodicals relative to the clinical services offered by the hospital. The library should be easily accessible and available at all times to the medical and nursing staff.

Complementary Departments. Standards are listed for departments or services of surgery, anesthesia, dentistry, and rehabilitation as to effective policies and procedures, relating to the staff and the functions of the services to assure health and safety of the patients.

Outpatient Department. For hospitals which have outpatient departments there are stated effective policies and procedures relating to the staff, functions of the service, the facilities, and outpatient medical records.

Emergency Service or Department. The hospitals must at least be prepared to take care of an occasional emergency case even though the hospital does not have an organized emergency service. For the hospital with the organized service, there are effective policies and procedures relating to the staff, the functions of the service, the medical records kept for the emergency room, and the facilities deemed adequate.

Social Work Department. This department is not a requisite for participation in Medicare Part A. If such a department is in a participating hospital, standards are given for its organization, direction, personnel, and necessary records.

Utilization Review Plan. The participating hospital is to have a plan for utilization review which applies at least to services furnished by the hospital to inpatients who are beneficiaries under Title XVIII. An acceptable plan would review utilization on a sample basis (or another plan) of admissions, duration of stays, and professional services furnished. Also under the plan there must be provisions for a review of each case of continuous extended duration. Under section 238 of the 1972 SSA Amendment, if the utilization review committee of a hospital or skilled nursing facility in its sample or other review of admissions finds a case where inpatient care is no longer medically necessary, Medicare payment will be cut off three days after notice of the committee finding.

Psychiatric and Tuberculosis Hospitals. The conditions for participation of psychiatric and tuberculosis hospitals are similar in many ways to those for general hospitals, but with certain listed special requirements for medical records and for staff and facilities.

Reimbursement to Hospital Providers—Part A

The reimbursement to hospitals for services provided Medicare Part A beneficiaries is based on reasonable costs. The formula for reimbursement based on reasonable costs was established after extended consultations and on the advice of leading health organizations and individuals such as: American Hospital Association; American Nursing Home Association; American Association of Hospital Accountants (now Hospital Financial Management Association); Blue Cross Association and local plans; Health Insurance Association of America and private insurance firms; Health Insurance Benefits Advisory Council (HIBAC); and many hospital administrators and comptrollers.

The experience of third party payers such as the Blue Cross plans and various state and federal agencies was studied. The cost-based programs particularly were examined, and the AHA's *Principles of Payment for Hospital Care* was used as a guideline in considering allowable costs.

The objectives of the reasonable cost reimbursement formula to providers of hospital care under Medicare Part A included:

—To make the payments to providers as current as possible
—To make retroactive adjustments to cover increases in costs as they occur
—In making reimbursements, to take into account the percentage of total patients who are 65 years of age or older, to also account for the difference in rate of utilization and in length of stay in hospital for patients 65 and over
—To have flexibility at the beginning of participation to allow for the differences in record keeping in hospitals
—To attempt to accord equitable treatment to profit and nonprofit providers
—To recognize the needs of institutions to keep abreast of developments in the health sciences and the healing arts[23]

Two methods of apportioning costs have been used in the past: one based on Medicare beneficiaries' share of total charges figured by individual departments; the second method was a combination based on average cost per day for room, board and routine nursing charges plus the beneficiaries' share of the total charges of nonroutine and ancillary services. The methods will be discussed more fully in later paragraphs.

Payments, as stated, were to be kept as current as possible. A system was established of making interim payments at intervals of no less than once a month, with the payments based on estimates of costs. (This voluntary payment plan is sometimes referred to as Periodic Interim Payment or PIP.) In most cases experience with other third party payers had given an accounting basis for estimate of cost. A retroactive adjustment was scheduled for the end of each accounting period.

Annual costs reports and other financial data are required of hospital providers under Part A. Definitions, statistics, reporting and accounting practices are those standard for the hospital field.

Authority to place a limitation on provider costs to be recognized as reasonable under Medicare was given to the Secretary of HEW under the 1972 SSA amendments. The limitation will be based on comparisons of the costs of covered services by various classes of providers in the same geographic area. Providers of ser-

---

[23]At the beginning of Medicare a 2 percent "plus factor" was allowed for keeping abreast of developments and for other contingencies. This was dropped a year or two later.

vices will be allowed to charge beneficiaries for the unreimbursed costs of services in excess of, or more expensive than, services necessary for the efficient delivery of needed health services. (The exception to this rule would be in cases where the physician who admitted the patient had a financial interest in the facility.) The provider would be required to notify the beneficiary of the charges for expensive or luxury services prior to admission. One overriding provision was that SSA would always pay the lesser of costs or charges.

Principles for Specific Reimbursable Costs

One of the key points stressed in Chapter 4 was that the debatable areas of cost were critical areas to the operation of a solvent hospital. Considerable space was given to consideration of items such as depreciation, bad debts, education, and research. The position of the A.H.A., both early and current attitudes, was examined in detail. The same critical area must be considered again, this time from the standpoint of health insurance for the aged as it affects providers of hospital care. The federal government also has a set of "principles" on this gray area of debatable costs. Each of them will be considered briefly.

Depreciation. An allowance for depreciation as a cost is given when it is based on historical cost or on market value at time of donation for donated items. The method of computation can be: straight line; double declining balance; or sum-of-years' digits. However, accelerated depreciation is no longer allowed on new assets, is limited to 150 percent of straight line when allowed, and is allowed only when it is proved necessary to supply the capital account. Medicare allows depreciation and interest expense on capital planning for amounts over $100,000 only when approved by an area planning agency. One favorable ruling is the allowance of depreciation on assets being used by the provider at the time it enters the program, even if already wholly or partially depreciated on the provider's books.

Interest Expense. The Medicare principle is that necessary and proper interest on current indebtedness is an allowable cost. Interest on loans which result in surplus funds or on loans not reasonably related to patient care would not be considered allowable cost. Interest expense to be an allowable cost would first be reduced by the amount of interest earned on investments, except for interest earned on gifts and grants, restricted or not restricted, but held separate and not commingled with other funds. Although depreciation funding is not required, it is encouraged by the provision that interest earned on the invested depreciation fund is not deducted from the interest which is considered an allowable cost.

Bad Debts, Charity, and Courtesy Allowances. All three of these items are considered deductions from revenue and not to be included in allowable costs. One exception is made about bad debts. If beneficiaries under Medicare fail to pay the deductible and coinsurance amounts they have incurred, those amounts can be included by the provider in the Medicare program's share of costs after reasonable collection efforts have been made.

Educational Costs. An appropriate part of the net cost of educational activities is an allowable cost. The appropriate part, of course, is the Medicare program's share according to the reimbursement formula chosen. The educational activities include medical, osteopathic, dental and podiatric internships and residency programs, other recognized professional and paramedical educational training programs either licensed by the state or conducted by professional and technical societies and associations, and approved by the Social Security Administration. The "net" educational cost refers to the stipends of trainees, teacher salaries, and other costs less any reimbursements from grants, tuitions or directed donations.

Research Costs. Costs incurred for research purposes "over and above usual patient care" are not considered allowable costs. This ruling is based on the fact that federal research grants and funds from foundations and private donors are sufficient to finance most research. However, the provider is allowed to include expenses of studies, surveys, and analyses necessary to the provider's administrative and program needs.

Grants, Gifts, and Income from Endowments. Unrestricted grants, gifts, and income from endowments should not be deducted from operating costs in computing costs under the reimbursement formula. However, if the grants, gifts, or income from endowments have been designated by the donor for paying specific operating costs, then those amounts should be deducted from the specific costs or category of costs.

Value of Voluntary Services. The principle covering voluntary services is similar to that of other third party cost reimbursement plans. The provider which has Sisters or other members of a religious order working in the hospital in positions necessary to normal patient care can include as an allowable cost for each of these volunteers an amount equal to that a lay employee of like training would earn in the community. The donated services of other individual volunteer workers cannot be included.

Purchase Discounts and Allowances, and Refunds of Expenses. All discounts, allowances, and refunds of expenses are reductions in the cost of goods or services purchased and are not income.

A Reasonable Allowance for the Compensation of Owners for Services is an Allowable Cost. In proprietary institutions the owner can be compensated for necessary duties which have to be performed at a rate comparable to that paid by comparable institutions. In addition, Medicare allows the owners of an institution a reasonable return on their investment.

Cost to Related Organizations. The principle relating to this point is stated: "Costs applicable to services, facilities, and supplies furnished to the provider by organizations related to the provider by common ownership or control are includable in the allowable cost of the provider at the cost to the related organization. However, such cost must not exceed the price of comparable services, facilities, or supplies that could be purchased elsewhere."

Plus Factor. As mentioned previously, a plus factor of two percent was originally allowed to cover contingencies, but was later dropped.

Differential on Nursing Wages. Recently a 8½ percent differential in nursing costs was allowed to compensate for the added care needed by Medicare patients. The cost base is salaries and wages of nurses and other personnel for nursing activities (not associated with nurseries or other services for which separate charges are made such as ICU, CCU, or other special inpatient units). Excluded from the cost base also are: administration; office personnel; nursing personnel in OR, central supply, recovery room, ER, delivery room, and nursery; employee health services; nursing in areas not for general inpatient use; payroll taxes; and employee benefits.

General Principles of Reimbursement

Costs Related to Patient Care. Payments to providers are based on "reasonable costs" which include direct, indirect, and standby costs for services covered under Medicare Part A and which are related to the care of beneficiaries. The provision for paying rea-

Table 7-5

Community Hospital*
Determination of Cost of Services of Beneficiaries
Departmental Method

Department	Charges to Medicare Beneficiaries	Total Charges (all patients)	Ratio of Beneficiary Charges to Total Charges	Total Cost	Cost of Beneficiary Services
			Percent		
Routine Services	$140,000	$ 600,000	23 1/3	$630,000	$147,000
X-ray	24,000	100,000	24	75,000	18,000
Operating Room	20,000	70,000	28⁴/₇	77,000	22,000
Laboratory	40,000	140,000	28 4/7	98,000	28,000
Pharmacy	20,000	60,000	33 1/3	45,000	15,000
Other	6,000	30,000	20	25,000	5,000
	$250,000	$1,000,000		$950,000	$235,000

*Source: "Principles of Reimbursement for Provider Costs," U.S. Department of Health, Education and Welfare, Social Security Administration HIM-5 (5-66), p. 25 (adapted).

sonable costs is intended to meet actual costs as they vary from one institution to another, or from one time to another.

Determination of Cost of Services to Beneficiaries. Formerly there were two methods for apportioning costs between the beneficiaries of Medicare Part A and other patients so that the share borne by the Medicare program was based on services received by program beneficiaries. The provider had the option of choosing either the departmental method or the combination method. In some cases, the provider might think one method was more favorable than the other for its situation. For cost reporting periods starting after December 31, 1971, any hospital (including a hospital-ECF complex) having less than 100 beds and all ECFs had to use the combination method; all other hospitals had to use the departmental method of apportionment. The combination method of apportionment was eliminated under regulations published in January 1979 and effective July 1, 1979. All hospitals, even those having fewer than 100 beds, were required to use the departmental method after that date.

(a) The departmental method apportions cost by a formula based on the ratio of beneficiary charges to total patient charges which is applied to cost on a departmental basis. In Table 7-5 under "Department" are six revenue centers of Community Hospital. For routine services the charges to Medicare beneficiaries were

$140,000, the charges to all patients $600,000. Thus, the beneficiaries charges were 23 1/3 per cent of all routine charges. The total cost of all routine services was $630.000. Using the 23 1/3 percent ratio of $630,000 as the beneficiaries' share of cost of routine services, the result is $147,000. When each of the six departments is computed on the basis of ratio of beneficiaries' charges to total patient charges to total cost, the beneficiary costs arrived at by the departmental method in this example are $235,000.

(b) The combination method embodies two formulas: (1) the cost of routine services (room, board, routine nursing, and floor stock drugs and supplies for which no extra charge is made) is computed by using the average cost per patient day for those services for all patients; and (2) the cost of ancillary services is computed on a departmental basis on the ratio of charges to charges to costs as used in the departmental method illustrated in Table 7-5. In Table 7-6 the combination method is illustrated by using the same example as used in Table 7-5 plus the added data on total days of inpatient care needed to illustrate the combination method. The total cost of beneficiary care computed by the combination method was $245,500.

The examples given do not necessarily prove that the combination method is more advantageous to the provider than the departmental. The provider must consider the patient mix (Medicare versus non-Medicare), length of stay for the two groups, the patterns of ancillary service in the hospital and community, as well as any other variables which might affect the two methods of computation.

Adequate cost data and cost finding. Cost data must be based on an approved method of cost finding and on the accrual basis of accounting. Either the step-down method or the double apportionment method may be used. More sophisticated algebraic and computerized methods may be employed with the approval of the intermediary. When a provider has elected to use the double apportionment method it may not thereafter use the step-down method without the approval of the intermediary.

Utilization of Medicare

Nearly all persons 65 years of age or older are eligible and have enrolled under Medicare Part A Hospital Insurance and only a slightly smaller number in Medicare Part B Supplementary Medical Insurance. States are allowed to enroll and pay the premiums for Part B Supplementary Medical Insurance (SMI) for public as-

Table 7-6

Community Hospital
Determination of Cost of Services to Beneficiaries
Combination Method *

Routine Services (based on 30,000 inpatient days of which 7,500 were applicable to beneficiaries)

Total cost of routine services = $630,000
Total inpatient days for all inpatients = 30,000
Average cost per day for routine services—$630,000 ÷ 30,000 = $21 per day
Cost of routine service for beneficiaries = 7,500 × $21 = $ 157,500

Ancillary Services (all ancillary services from Table 7-1)

Charges to Medicare Beneficiaries	Total Charges	Ratio beneficiary charges to total charges (percent)	Total Cost	Cost of Beneficiary Services
$110,000	$400,000	27½	$320,000	$ 88,000

Total Cost of Services to Beneficiaries

Routine services	$157,500
Ancillary services	88,000
	$245,500

*Dollar and percentage totals from Table 7-2.

sistance recipients. As of December 31, 1968, 39 states, Guam, and the Virgin Islands had active agreements under which approximately 1.6 million public assistance recipients were enrolled for SMI. In 1972 there were 20.9 million persons enrolled for Part A Hospital Insurance (HI). Over $6.1 billion were reimbursed for HI benefits that year. For that same period there were over 20.1 million persons enrolled under Part B SMI; over $2.5 billion were paid in SMI claims during the year.[24]

More recent data are available on participating health facilities. As of July 1973 the number of providers of services certified to participate in the Medicare program was:[25]

—6,757 hospitals with 1.148 million adult beds
—3,977 SNFs with 291,000 nursing beds
—2,211 home health agencies
—2,929 independent laboratories

The total number of general adult beds in participating short-stay hospitals represented 42 beds per 1,000 enrollees, which ranged among the states from 31 to 101 per 1,000 enrollees. The participating SNFs provided 14.1 beds per 1,000 enrollees with a range among the states of 1 to 45 beds per 1,000 enrollees.

The financial impact of Medicare is very evident, for under this plan a large segment of the population with higher than average demand for services is being financed, in major part at least, by the federal government as third party. Supplementary insurance to pay deductibles and coinsurance not covered by Part A Hospital Insurance is being purchased by many Medicare recipients. Blue Cross alone sells policies to about one-third of them.

The Skilled Nursing Facility (Under Both Medicare and Medicaid)

The SSA Amendments of 1972 make provisions for using the term "skilled nursing facility" to replace the terms "extended care facility" used previously under Medicare (Title XVIII) and "skilled nursing home" used under Medicaid (Title XIX).

Care requirements of a skilled nursing facility have been defined in a U.S. government announcement of 1972 SSA Amendments as:

> A single common definition of care requirements for extended care services under Medicare and skilled nurs-

---

[24]*Medicare: Selected State Data, Fiscal Years 1968–1972.* DHEW (SSA) 74–1171.
[25]*Research and Statistics.* DHEW HI-55, April 2, 1974.

ing services under Medicaid is established as follows: Skilled nursing care provided directly by or requiring the supervision of skilled nursing personnel, or other skilled rehabilitation services, which the patient needs on a daily basis, and which as a practical matter can be provided only in a skilled nursing facility on an inpatient basis. The Medicare requirement that extended care services must be a continuation of treatment for a condition treated in a hospital is retained.

For Medicare patients this covers two classes of patients who may not have been covered before:

1. The patient who needs a variety of unskilled services on a regular daily basis, if the planning and overseeing of the aggregate of the unskilled services requires regular daily involvement of skilled personnel.
2. The patient who is in regular need of skilled rehabilitation services (other than nursing) which are essential to his recovery from an inhospital stay or to prevent his condition from worsening, and which as a practical matter should be provided in a skilled nursing facility.

A facility meeting the definition of skilled nursing facility (SNF) can participate in both Medicare and Medicaid provided it agrees to terms of participation. The definition of a skilled nursing facility is basically the former Medicare definition plus new provisions for submission of information on ownership, for adherence to certain fire and safety codes, for independent medical evaluation and audit of patients and patients' need for skilled nursing care, and for certain institutional planning requirements. The Secretary of HEW under present Medicare arrangments with state agencies will certify SNFs requesting participation in both Medicare and Medicaid. State agencies will continue to certify SNFs requesting participation in Medicaid only.

The Secretary is authorized also to waive the requirement for a registered nurse on one full shift seven days a week in certain rural areas where RNs are in short supply. Those rural institutions caught in shortage of help situation may be allowed to operate on a 40 hour per week five day coverage if the physician certifies patients can be without registered nurses for 48 hours, or if physicians or other nurses can cover the institution when patients need skilled help during the regular nurse's days away. Furthermore, the 1972 amendments say that SNFs cannot be required to provide medical social services as a condition of participation in either Medicaid or Medicare.

A further ruling affecting SNFs is one which authorizes state certifying agencies, subject to the approval of the Secretary of HEW, to provide such specialized consultative series to a skilled nursing facility as the facility may request and need to meet one or more conditions of participation.

Medicaid

Medicaid is the stepchild of political expediency, in fact, a kind of afterthought of Medicare. When the Social Security Amendments of 1965 were written, one of the pressing needs addressed was that of establishing a health care program for the elderly— Title XVIII, or, more commonly called, Medicare.

Other persons under 65 needing help were receiving some aid under a variety of federal, state, and county programs. It is likely someone in Washington thought it would be an excellent idea to lump together the blind, the disabled, the families of dependent children and others at the poverty level of all ages in one large Federal-state program supported in great measure by Federal funds. That became Medicaid, otherwise known as Title XIX.

The revenues from Medicaid (and Medicare) are important to hospitals, nursing homes, laboratories, physicians, pharmacies, home care services, therapists, and other providers, because the numbers of recipients of benefits from Federal and state funds is growing in percentage of revenue of those providers year by year.

Some people felt that Medicaid was a stopgap program which would aid the poor and medically indigent until Hubert H. Humphrey was elected President of the United States in 1968 and persuaded Congress to pass a national health insurance act. Of course, this did not come to pass.

In the years preceding Medicaid, the elderly, the blind, the disabled, and sick children had been aided through the Kerr–Mills Act and related legislation, but there was still a great need to be corrected.

Medicare was designed for those persons over 65 who might need hospital and medical care. It was an insurance plan which included many compromises: employee-employer financing as well as Federal general funds; hospital care and skilled nursing home care with deductibles paid by the patient; and a separate insurance plan (Medicare B) with costs shared by the beneficiaries and the Federal government to pay, at least partially, the fees charged by physicians for their services—to mention a few.

Medicaid may have been an afterthought to help the categorically needy previously mentioned (the blind, the disabled, children, the aged who needed assistance, the poor, etc.). Certainly there were many poor who were not receiving needed medical care, and there were many aged who could not pay the deductibles charged by hospitals and skilled nursing facilities (SNFs). Also many aged persons needed financial assistance to stay in intermediary care homes (commonly called nursing homes) after their discharge from a hospital or SNF. So Medicaid was structured as a means of taking care of this undetermined number of needy Americans.

Medicaid, or Title XIX, as it came out of Congress, was *not* a law which was put into action uniformly in all parts of the country. Again Medicaid was a compromise. Possibly only a compromise could pass Congress. The Hill–Burton Act of the 1940s may have been an example Congress followed. Hill–Burton was an act which provided for building hospitals in the postwar period and was heavily weighted in funding to the South and to rural areas. In administration the states operated in true states' rights tradition. Medicaid was and is heavily weighted to the poor states (the South).

Financing

Medicaid is a program to provide health care to the needy with the financing shared by the Federal government and the individual participating states. A state pays from 17 to 50 percent of the costs depending on the per capita income of the state in relation to the country as a whole. The Federal government pays the remaining costs, after the state's share, on an open-end basis.

Basic and Optional Benefits

Under Title XIX each state wishing to participate in Medicaid could enter into an agreement with the Secretary of Health, Education and Welfare to furnish at least certain basic mandated health services to a group of individuals in need of financial assistance and others considered categorically needy.[26] The state income level below which individuals were considered to be in need of financial assistance was set by the state.

The mandated services presently are:

---

[26]All states did not immediately apply for a Medicaid program. Nearly a decade passed before the last two states, Alaska and Arizona, began programs. The Arizona program was soon challenged in the courts.

- Inpatient hospital care
- Outpatient hospital care
- Physician's care
- Laboratory and x-ray diagnostic services
- Skilled nursing facility care
- Home health care
- Early and periodic screening, diagnosis, and treatment for needy children under 21

States were allowed also to include certain optional benefits, with the state paying its contracted share of costs. Optional services could include any of the following at a level and amount set at the discretion of the state:

- Medical care by a practitioner other than a medical doctor
- Private duty nurse
- Clinic services
- Dental services
- Physical therapy and related services
- Prosthetics and eyeglasses
- Other diagnostic, screening, preventive, and rehabilitative services
- Inpatient hospital, skilled nursing facility, intermediary care facility care for persons over 65 for tuberculosis or mental illness
- Intermediary care facility care
- Other medical care

Administration of Medicaid

Medicaid may be a financially shared program between the individual state and the Federal government, but the administration is primarily by the state (with a few basic guidelines set in Washington). From state to state the administrative body differs. Administration may be under the aegis of the state welfare department, the state health department, a combined health and welfare body, or, in at least one case (Mississippi), under a separate department. Whatever the administrative leadership, the Medicaid program retains aspects of a welfare program. In fact, welfare departments in most states determine eligibility of persons for Medicaid benefits.

The few basic guidelines set in Washington, as mentioned above, came through Medical Services Administration (MSA) of DHEW which has Federal oversight of the state programs. From the start of Medicaid this body has been trying to coordinate the effort. MSA was given only six months lead time at the beginning of Medicaid to negotiate and approve all the varied programs entered into with the states.

In the early 1970s Howard Newman became Commissioner and brought some order to MSA activities, but it would seem that the inherent weaknesses of Medicaid make an equitable program impossible.

Medicaid Eligibility

Certain persons are eligible for assistance in any Medicaid program. Basically these include anyone previously helped under assistance to the blind (AB), to the aged (OAA), to families of dependent children (AFDC), and to the partially or totally disabled (APTD)—the Kerr–Mills recipients, whose program was phased out in 1969 whether or not a state established a Medicaid program.

In addition, certain other individuals became eligible who formerly had been ineligible because of state laws with restrictive residence and age requirements. Under Medicaid these restrictions were removed.

Another large group became eligible because their family income was below the poverty level set in their state for a means test. The income level for qualification varies widely from state to state, more than 100 percent from lowest to highest. For example, when Medicaid became operative in New York State, an income of $6,000 for a family of four was set as a level below which Medicaid would apply. This figure for 1966 was a relatively good income. In fact, this $6,000 income for a family of four, and related levels for other sized families, affected nearly 45 percent of the state's population. Since New York is a comparatively high per capita income state, the state's portion of the Medicaid cost was 50 percent. The program was such a drain on the state treasury that a downward adjustment in the income level to qualify had to be made. MediCal (California Medicaid), which began with an eligibility level of $4,092 for a family of four, also found the program to be a tremendous financial burden.

Each state set its own level of income below which persons living anywhere in the state could qualify for Medicaid benefits. This often had a built-in inequity, particularly in states with extremes of metropolitan and rural areas. In New York State a $6,000 eligibility level had a much greater impact in upstate New York than in metropolitan and suburban areas. A great number of upstate residents were eligible for Medicaid who probably didn't consider themselves victims of poverty.

Besides including the so-called categorically needy—AB,

AFDC, OOA, APTD, and the low–income people—the states have the option of also including others who are sometimes called "medically indigent." Medically indigent persons can be described as those who have incomes over the means test level but who have incurred medical expenses which, if deducted from their incomes, would place them at the public assistance level. Usually in a case of this sort the person would spend for medical expenses down to the eligibility level and would then qualify for assistance. This spending down has sometimes been called the "notch effect." Only about half the states pay Medicaid benefits to the medically indigent.

Medicaid Costs

In the first years the states were attracted to Medicaid, particularly in regard to clients on public assistance, because some of the load which the state may have been bearing alone could now be shifted to Federal sharing of 50–83 percent of the expense. Hospitals began getting paid on the basis of reasonable costs for welfare and former charity patients, and this was a much better payment pattern. Nursing homes which had tried to negotiate rates that would cover costs for state or county supported patients, now found a better payment climate both in rates and in promptness. Physicians and other providers began to collect for their services according to negotiated rates based on usual and customary fees. Outside of the mass of paper work it seemed a good situation for the states and most providers, not to mention the people who were assisted.

What was not anticipated was the tremendous growth of the program both in numbers of recipients and in dollars spent. The actuarial figures used in projecting the cost of Medicaid were woefully under actual costs. What had been estimated as a $2 billion program became, within a decade, a $20 billion cost with about 24 million recipients.

To be fair, the program was hardly started before the effects of Vietnam and the attending inflation were felt. Many workers in the health field, particularly nurses and other hospital workers, were underpaid in comparison to workers in industry. The wage adjustments that had to be made were costly to the providers and therefore to Medicaid. Also the rapid rise of technology in health care increased costs through added capital expenditures and new patterns of utilization of the "machines."

Medicaid and Quality of Care

The states are responsible for the quality of care under the Medicaid program. Various devices have been used to oversee the programs; utilization committees, PSROs, and other types of peer review. Measurement of quality of care has always been a difficult task except for the most gross measurements. Researchers have always searched for but never found the perfect method. Some progress has been been made, particularly through utilization studies, but there is still a long way to go.

Medicaid Fraud and Abuse

Any agency or program that has a cash flow of $20 billion a year is going to attract the covetous. Unfortunately there are the covetous in all the strata and in all the professions of the health care arena, as there are in any cross section or sample of the American population. The Federal government has uncovered fraud and abuse among all kinds of providers and among recipients. There has been false billing, Medicaid "mills" where a patient gets a few seconds of attention, storefront laboratories working in collusion to defraud with those who refer work to them, and many other ingenious schemes to get a piece of the $20 billion. Unofficial estimates say that 5 percent of Medicaid expenditures is being drained off illegally. This figure may be optimistically low. Whatever the figure, vigilance is called for.

Medicaid and HMOs

Some states are experimenting by enrolling persons eligible for Medicaid assistance in local HMO programs. Originally it was believed that economies could be effected at the same time that quality medical care could be ensured. At this point the experiments cannot be fully evaluated.

Medicaid Utilization

The use of Medicaid services has risen much faster and to a much greater extent than expected, with more than 10 percent of the population currently being recipients. According to DHEW, the trend in the decade 1967–1976 showed some decrease in the use of inpatient hospital facilities, and an increase in outpatient care. There seems to be a greater demand for services by the elderly, particularly in intermediary care. Medicaid services are likely to change. This is discussed in the last chapter of the book.

Medicare and Medicaid Interrelationships

There has to be an interrelationship between the two programs because the insurance program which is Medicare cannot operate with deductibles to cover a population that can't pay deductibles.

There has to be a supplement to help those people who are medically indigent. If a person over 65 can't pay the Medicare B premium, then Medicaid has to be the assisting arm. There are many critics of Medicaid who complain about inadequate health care, inefficiency, fraud, and many other things. On balance, however, progress has been made.

Suggested Readings

Myers, Robert J. *Medicare*, selections.

Somers, Herman Miles and Somers, Anne Ramsey. *Medicare and the Hospitals: Issues and Prospects*, selections.

Stevens, Robert and Stevens, Rosemary *Welfare Medicine in America*, selections.

Stuart, Bruce and Spitz, Bruce *Rising Medical Costs in Michigan*, selections.

Appendix 7
1972 SOCIAL SECURITY AMENDMENTS

Listed alphabetically below under key words are items touched upon in the 1972 amendments to the Social Security Act which affect the Medicare and Medicaid programs. Many other changes under the 1972 amendments have already been incorporated in the revised text of Chapter 7.

Benefit Claims-Reassignment (Sec. 236). Payment for claims under Medicare can be made only to the patient, the physician, or the supplier who provided a covered service and accepted assignment except: (1) the payment may be made to the employer of the physican or supplier if he is required as a condition of his employment to turn over such fees to his employer; or (2) the payment may be made to the facility where the services are provided if the facility has a contractual arrangement with the physician or supplier giving it the sole right to bill Medicare for the services. Also, direct payment can be made to an organization administering a health care delivery system such as a prepaid group practice.

Capital Expenditures Limitations (Sec. 221). Certain amounts of reimbursement based on capital expenditures may be withheld or reduced to providers of health services and to health maintenance organizations under Medicare, Medicaid and child and maternal health programs by the Secretary of HEW when those expenditures are deemed inconsistent with health service or facility decisions made by designated state planning agencies. Procedures will be set up for the facility or organization proposing a capital expenditure to appeal an adverse decision.

Chiropractic Services in Treating a Subluxation of the Spine by Manual Manipulation (Sec. 273). The subluxation must have been demonstrated by x-ray. The practitioner must be licensed and meet certain educational requirements.

Colostomy Supplies (Sec. 252). Colostomy bags and necessary accessories are no longer classed as surgical dressings but as prosthetic devices. Coverage was extended to irrigation and flushing equipment and other items directly related to colostomy care, whether or not attachment of a bag is required.

Disclosure of Information Under Medicare and Medicaid (Sec. 249C). The Secretary of HEW will make available for public inspection: formal evaluations of carriers, intermediaries, and state agencies; comparative evaluations of the performance of contractors; and formal evaluations of the performance of providers of services. Such reports will not be made public until the contractor has had the opportunity (60 days maximum) to review the report and offer comments.

Also (in section 299D) the Secretary is required to make available to the public information from surveys of providers relating to the presence or absence of deficiencies in areas such as staffing, fire safety, and sanitation.

Durable Medical Equipment (Sec. 245). The Secretary of HEW was authorized to experiment in various geographic areas with reimbursement approaches intended to prevent unreasonable expenditures for prolonged rentals of durable medical equipment. Among methods to be considered were: lend-purchase arrangements; lump-sum payment when outright purchase would be cheaper for estimated period of use; and waiver of 20 percent coinsurance if beneficiary purchased used equipment at price at least 25 percent less than reasonable charge to purchase new equipment.

Health Maintenance Organization (HMO) (Sec. 249F). A HMO is defined as an organization which provides comprehensive health care on a per capita prepayment basis. Under the 1972 amendments established HMOs can qualify for an incentive reimbursement plan under Medicare by entering into a contract with the Secretary of HEW. The contract would specify the per capita amount the HMO would be paid in advance each month. The HMO would submit financial statements at the end of the fiscal year from which the Secretary would determine the average per capita cost for Medicare patients had the services been provided the beneficiaries under other health care arrangements. If the HMO's incurred costs were less than the other arrangments, the difference (savings) would be shared by the HMO and the Medicare Trust Fund under a stated formula.

Laboratory-Direct Billing (Sec. 279). The Secretary was authorized to negotiate a payment rate with independent diagnostic laboratories for covered laboratory services which, if the laboratory accepts assignment, would be paid in full by Medicare. No coinsurance would be collectible from the beneficiary because the rate accepted would be the full charge for the procedure.

Medical Insurance Hearing (Sec. 262). Enrollees, physicians, or suppliers who are dissatisfied with the determination or the promptness of action on a Medicare Part B medical insurance claim may file for a fair hearing if $100 or more is at issue.

Penalties for Fraud and False Reporting (Sec. 242). Certain acts, statements, or representations in connection with furnishing items or services, with program payments, or with certification of providers have been defined as subject to penalties under the Medicare program.

Physical Therapists (Sec. 251). Services of a licensed independently practicing physical therapist furnished in his office or the patient's home under a physician's plan, and meeting health and safety conditions specified by the Secretary were covered under Medicare medical insurance after July 1, 1973 up to $100 of incurred expenses in a calendar year (subject to medical insurance deductible and coinsurance).

Physicians' Charges (Sec. 224). Provisions have been made to set limits for physicians' charges in the Medicare, Medicaid, and maternal and child health programs by a formula relating to the charges of the previous fiscal year.

Planning (Sec. 234). Hospitals, skilled nursing facilities, and home health agencies are required under Medicare to have a written plan reflecting an annual operating budget and at least a three-year projected capital expenditures plan.

Professional Standards Review (Sec. 249F). The 1972 SSA Amendments authorize the establishment of independent professional standards review organizations (PSROs) under which practicing physicians will assume certain responsibility for reviewing the quality and appropriateness of care provided under Medicare, Medicaid, and maternal and child health programs. PSRO areas will be established throughout the country by geographic or medical service areas, each area generally containing a minimum of 300 practicing physicians. The PSROs will be responsible in their areas for assuring that services are medically necessary and provided in accordance with professional standards. PSROs will not be involved with reasonable charge determinations.

There is a review mechanism provided for reconsideration of a PSRO determination.

Proficiency Determination for Certain Health Personnel (Sec. 241). The amendment has made provision for the Secretary of HEW (in conjunction with professional organizations and state health and licensure agencies) to determine the proficiency of certain health personnel (experienced practical nurses, therapists, laboratory technicians, etc.) now excluded, or limited in responsibility, under Medicare regulations through December 31, 1977. After this date these health personnel must meet specific formal education, professional membership, or other requirements established by regulations.

Prospective Reimbursement Demonstrations (Sec. 222). Under the 1972 amendments the Secretary of HEW is directed to develop and carry out experiments and demonstrations in prospective reimbursement in Medicare. Experiments are authorized in testing changes in methods of reimbursement with performance incentives for intermediaries and carriers. Experiments can be tried with new types of providers (such as organizations providing comprehensive, mental, or ambulatory services, including ambulatory surgical centers), with the use of intermediate care or homemaker services by beneficiaries who could leave the hospital but are unable to maintain themselves at home unassisted. Also experiments can be tried for improving rehabilitation treatments of patients in long-term facilities and to determine if clinical psychologists should be more available under Medicare.

Provider Charges (Sec. 233). Payment for provider charges will be at the lesser of reasonable cost or customary charge. Where there is a public provider of service at no charge or at only a nominal fee, payment will be made on the basis of reasonable cost.

Reimbursement Appeals by Providers (Sec. 243). A five-member Provider Reimbursement Review Board will review appeals by providers when the intermediary makes a final cost determination with which the provider is dissatisfied. At least $10,000 must be involved and the provider must appeal within 180 days of the determination. Groups of providers may file an appeal on common issues when the aggregate amount is at least $50,000. The Secretary may, within 60 days, reverse or modify a Board decision favorable to the provider. In this event the provider has recourse to judicial review.

Services Outside the United States (Sec. 211). Inpatient hospital services furnished by a foreign hospital are covered for U.S. citizens under Medicare under certain conditions:

—If the foreign hospital is closer to, or substantially more accessible from, the beneficiary's residence than the nearest hospital in the U.S. that is suitable and available for his treatments;
—If the foreign hospital has been accredited by JCAH or a hospital approval program essentially comparable.

Coverage is extended in these cases to any ambulance or physician's service furnished. Benefits for these U.S. citizens are payable regardless where the illness or accident occurred or whether an emergency existed. Present provisions covering emergency inpatient hospital services outside the U.S. when the emergency arises in the U.S. are retained. Emergency coverage is extended to include beneficiaries who incur an emergency in Canada while traveling without delay on the most direct route between Alaska and another State. The reimbursement methods are essentially the same as for nonparticipating hospitals in the U.S.

Teaching Physicians (Sec. 227). The payment of teaching physicians under Medicare is to be on the basis of reasonable costs rather than on fee-for-service, unless:

1. a bona fide patient relationship exists between the physician and the patients for whom a fee-for-service charge is made; or
2. the hospital had, in the two-year period ending in 1967 and every year thereafter, regularly billed all inpatients for such physicians' services, and reasonable charges have been collected from at least 50 percent of patients in these periods.

Medicare payments will be authorized on a cost basis for services provided to hospitals by the staff of certain medical schools, but only in respect to services which would be eligible for cost reimbursement, if they were furnished by the hospital.

Payments for services donated by volunteer physicians can be paid into a fund designated by those physicians if the fund is to be used for educational and for charitable purposes.

Terminate Medicare Payments to Suppliers (Sec. 229). Under the 1972 amendments the Secretary was given authority to terminate payment, with public notice, for service rendered by an institutional provider of services, a physican, or any other supplier of health and medical services determined by the Secretary to be engaged in overcharging, furnishing excessive, inferior or harmful services, or making a false statement to obtain payment.

Therapy Services (Sec. 251). A definition of reasonable cost under Medicare for covered physical, occupational, speech or other therapy services or services of other health-related personnel (except physicians) is that the cost cannot exceed an amount equivalent to the salary which reasonably would have been paid, and any other costs which would have been payable, had the services been performed in an employment relationship. Any other reasonable expenses related to the service which an individual not actually working as an employee might have paid could be recognized. These other expenses might include such items as travel expense, office expense, and similar costs.

Withholding Medicaid Payments to Terminated Medicare Providers (Sec. 290). The Secretary was authorized beginning October 30, 1972 to withhold future Federal financial participation in state Medicaid payments to institutions which have withdrawn from Medicare without refunding Medicare overpayments or without accounting for Medicare payments to them.

Chapter 8
Charges and Rate Setting

The previous chapters have considered the two major sources of hospital revenues—Blue Cross and Medicare. However, a discussion of the sources of operating revenues would be incomplete without an examination of the matter of charges and rate setting. Admittedly, charges or revenues from self-responsible (self-pay) patients generally represent a relatively small segment of a hospital's total revenues. Nevertheless, it is a segment which, as will become clear, is critical to the total financial well-being of a hospital. Therefore, it is important for a complete understanding of hospital financial management that the reader be familiar with the techniques, mechanics, and philosophical issues related to the setting of rates for hospital services.

Background—The Problem

In Chapter 1 the objective of the manager of a commercial enterprise was stated as being that of maximizing owner's wealth, i.e., $W = E/R$. In order to achieve this objective, assuming that the capitalization rate (R) is constant and that earnings (E) are the difference between revenues and costs, the manager must not only minimize cost, but also set price at a level which will allow production to proceed to that point wherein marginal revenue equals marginal cost. Thus, the commercial manager is confronted with a two-sided problem.

In contrast, the hospital manager, though confronted with a substantial array of financial and economic problems, has not been forced to pay particular attention to the pricing problem. Due to the dominance of cost-based reimbursement agreements, concern has been focused, in the main, on cost as opposed to price. The hospital manager, therefore, primarily has concentrated his talents and abilities on controlling costs and assuring quality services.

For the most part, hospital managers have traditionally viewed revenues from self-responsible patients as the balancing factor in their revenue structure. That is, they have known, at least approximately, the hospital's financial needs and the amount of revenues which could be expected from third party and philanthropic sources. Given this information, the amount of additional revenues necessary to meet or balance any deficit occurring between financial needs and expected revenues becomes obvious. Knowing this amount, charges to self-responsible patients have then been set at levels which will generate revenues sufficient to balance financial needs and income. Thus, charges historically have been established not on the basis of cost, but rather on the basis of financial expediency. Table 8-1 illustrates this situation.

This approach to establishing charges has resulted in the hospital industry participating in what can perhaps be best described as overt price discrimination. As should be clear by this point, hospital prices discriminate in favor of patients covered by third party payers. These patients, in effect, pay for care at cost, while self-responsible patients pay for care on the basis of charges which are dictated by financial expediency and need, i.e., charges are established at levels designed to generate revenues equal to cost plus whatever additional funds are needed to meet the hospital's financial requirements.

In the case of commercial firms, such a pricing practice would likely violate antitrust laws and would be illegal. However, for whatever the reasons, the legality of this practice has not been questioned in the hospital industry until recently.[1]

It should be realized that there is nothing inherently or implicitly wrong with third party payers purchasing hospital services at cost. Third party payers argue, with some validity, that they are not only volume purchasers of care, but also that they are reliable and faithful purchasers. Therefore, they maintain that they should pay for care at a price which is less than that paid by an individual payer.

---

[1]The basic issues in question were tested in a recent court case (U.S. Dist. Ct. Western Dist. Pa.; Civil No. 68–69, January 6, 1972). In the case, the Travelers Insurance Company contended that Blue Cross of Western Pennsylvania violated the provisions of the Sherman Act. The court dismissed the suit, finding that Blue Cross' competitive status was not acquired by boycott or intimidation; it is not a monopolist, for it cannot control rate making or establish its own rates, has not violated the Sherman Act, and is entitled to McCarran Act exemption. In essence, the court concluded that Blue Cross has not established artificial restraint-of-trade practices.

Table 8-1

Charges Based on Financial Expediency

Step 1

    Revenues from Third Parties*
+ Revenues from Philanthropy
+ Revenues from Other Sources
    Expected Revenues

Step 2

    Financial Needs*
− Expected Revenues (from step 1)
    Revenue Deficit (Revenue needed from
    Self-Responsible Patients)

Step 3

$$\frac{\text{Revenue Deficit}}{\substack{\text{Expected Units of Service Provided} \\ \text{to Self-Responsible Patients*}}} = \substack{\text{Charges to Self-Responsible} \\ \text{Patients}}$$

*Assume that the values for these items are at least approximately known by management.

The first part of the above argument is basically the contention which all large volume purchasers put forth as justification for quantity discounts. This justification, while valid in some commercial and industrial instances, is not valid in the hospital setting. An industrial firm, due to the operational economies inherent in volume production, can offer a purchaser a quantity discount on large volume sales because its operating costs are less. Costs are reduced, for the firm can "tool up" for and run, in a single batch, a large quantity which it has neither to store nor to market. Unfortunately, these same conditions do not exist in the case of the third party purchaser of hospital services.

Admittedly, Blue Cross or the government purchases in total a large quantity of hospital services. However, these services are not purchased either all at the same time or all from the same hospital. Instead, the situation is one in which a large number of piecework purchases are made from various hospitals. Under these conditions, an individual hospital cannot reduce its production costs simply due to the fact that payment is derived from a single source. Thus, on pragmatic financial grounds the argument that third party payers should receive a quantity discount is neither justified nor valid.

In contrast, the notion that third party payers should receive a price discount because they are reliable and faithful payers can, to some extent, be justified. Historically, third party payers have not defaulted on their obligations, and hospitals generally can be assured of receiving payment. Thus, a hospital, when dealing with third party payers, incurs less of a business risk, for it can be confident of receiving payment and, hence, does not have to concern itself with the problems and costs of bad debts. The implication of this situation is that the economic costs, i.e., out-of-pocket plus intangible operating costs, of providing services to patients covered by third party payers are relatively less (by the bad debt cost element) than the cost of providing the same services to self-responsible patients (see Figure 8-1). Given this fact, it is reasonable for third party payers to pay less for services than individual payers, for their costs are less.

It is important to note that the foregoing does not imply that third party payers should not pay full costs. Due to reduced business risk, the full costs of providing services may be somewhat less for third party payer patients than for self-responsible patients. Third parties may thus pay somewhat less for services. However, if a hospital is to maintain a sound financial position, third party payers must pay at least their appropriate share of these costs. This approach to charging or billing for services is consistent with the common business practice of offering price discounts to reliable purchasers.

As was discussed in Chapter 4, third parties are not entirely satisfied with paying for services at their appropriate share of full costs. They want to exclude, by definition, several "real" operational cost elements from the items which are included in determining their share of cost. Thus, third parties, in effect, want more than just the price discount which should be available to any reliable purchaser. They want to pay for services on the basis of an adjusted cost, which obviously would be less than full cost.

Due primarily to both their bargaining power and the precarious financial position of most hospitals, third parties have been able to impose this adjusted basis of reimbursement on hospitals. The result of this has been that hospital have had to look at other revenue sources in order to obtain the funds necessary to meet the costs which have been excluded by third parties. Self-responsible patients have traditionally been the source to which hospitals have turned for these additional revenues.[2] The effect of this has

---

[2] Hospitals could also look to philanthropy and the government for these additional funds. However, neither of these sources is as easy to turn to as self-responsible patients. Philanthropy cannot be relied upon as a regular source of funds. Also, government is often either unwilling or unable to provide funds to nongovernmental hospitals.

Figure 8-1

Rate Setting—Theory

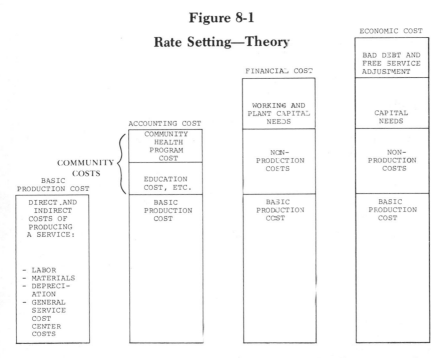

The Graphical Relationships in This Figure Are Only Illustrative. They Are Not Meant to Reflect the Relative Sizes of the Various Cost Premiums.

been that self-responsible patients—by paying more than their economic costs—have been subsidizing the care of third party beneficiaries.

At a time when hospital costs not only are increasing but also are increasing at a rapid, if not explosive, rate it is inequitable to charge any category of patients more than its "just" costs. Thus, this situation of self-responsible patients subsidizing other patients must be corrected. In order to accomplish this, two things must be done. First, third party cost-based reimbursement agreements must be renegotiated to include all economic costs of operation so that reimbursement will equal full economic cost and, secondly, hospital charges must be established on the basis of economic costs, not financial expediency.

If all payers for care are to be equitably treated, the need for the above actions is obvious. The matter of substantially changing the philosophy behind third party payment contracts is basically a political problem, which is beyond both the scope of this book and the power of an individual hospital. However, the problem of setting charges on the basis of economic costs is germane to this text.

Current Practice

As indicated earlier, charges or rates have historically been established on the basis of financial expediency. However, perhaps it would be more appropriate to describe the current practice of most hospitals as that of setting charges on a consensus basis which is then modified by financial expediency and need.[3]

The technique which is commonly used, except in those few states which have rigorous rate setting legislation can be defined as a consensus approach, for a hospital—in order to avoid public scrutiny of its rates and to be able to claim that its rates are reasonable—sets it own rates based upon the rates of other similar hospitals.[4] That is, an urban hospital would consider the rates of other urban hospitals and establish its charges at corresponding levels. Thus, to the extent that hospitals follow the patterns established by other similar hospitals, rate setting is done by consensus. However, to the extent that revenues from charges are used as a balancing factor in a hospital's revenue structure, the consensus is modified, i.e., rates are adjusted to meet financial needs. Thus, the approach which hospitals actually use can be most aptly described as a modified consensus approach.

This technique for establishing charges, along with the custom of setting the rates for routine services (room, board, and nursing services) at less than cost—so that they would be more comparable to hotel and restaurant charges—was probably initially adopted by hospitals as a defense mechanism against public opinion and pressure. Hospitals, however, are beginning to change their approach to setting charges.

The cost finding data which Medicare requires are providing hospitals with the basic quantitative information which is necessary in order to determine charges equitably. The impact of this increased knowledge is already apparent, as charges are now more closely corresponding to cost.[5] Additionally, the American Hospital Association's *Statement on the Requirements of Health Care Institutions* will, if and when operationally adopted, force third parties to pay for services on a cost basis which includes all economic costs in the reimbursement formula. If this is done, there

[3]Kaitz, Edward M., *Pricing Policy and Cost Behavior in the Hospital Industry*, Chapters 3 and 4.

[4]In these states, rates are based on cost or economic cost as is suggested in this chapter.

[5]Feldstein, Paul J. and Waldman, Saul "The Financial Position of Hospitals in the First Two Years of Medicare," *Inquiry*, Volume VI, No. 1, pp. 19–27.

will no longer be a need for hospitals to either view or use charges as the balancing factor in their revenue structures. Instead, hospitals will be financially able to establish charges on the basis of economic costs.

How, though, does one set rates so that the charges for services will correspond to the economic costs of providing those services? In order to answer this question, it is first necessary to identify those cost elements which constitute economic cost.

Rate Setting

Theory

The American Hospital Association, in its publication "Factors To Evaluate In The Establishment of Hospital Charges," states that:

> ... the rates charged for each individual service should reflect properly the operating expenses of the service rendered, plus an equitable share of the other financial needs for which the patient is responsible.[6]

The Association thus provides a reasonable and financially realistic philosophical guideline for establishing charges. However, it does not specifically indicate the cost elements which must be considered if charges are properly to reflect operating expenses and other financial needs, i.e., reflect economic costs.[7]

Perhaps the simplest approach to identifying and conceptualizing the costs which constitute total economic cost, and which should be included in setting rates, is to view a charge as being composed of a stack of premiums or cost elements. Figure 8-1 illustrates this concept.

As can be seen from the figure, the first cost element which should be included is the basic cost of producing the service. This cost is really nothing more than just the sum of the actual direct and indirect costs of production.

In addition to basic production costs, the hospital, if it is to

---

[6]American Hospital Association. "Factors To Evaluate In The Establishment of Hospital Charges," page 10.

[7]It is interesting to note that the concept of economic cost, first introduced in this text in 1971, is becoming increasingly accepted. The Blue Cross Association has recognized it in its policy on "Payment To Health Care Institutions." The federal government has recognized it in PL 93–641 (The Health Services Resources and Development Act of 1974) and state governments, such as the State of Maryland, have recognized it in their rate review laws. See Appendix A for a further discussion of legislated rate setting.

maintain a sound financial position, must also include premiums for community costs. That is, it should include cost premiums for services which it provides to the community but which are neither directly nor indirectly related to the actual production of any particular unit of patient service. Examples of costs of this nature are education, research, and community health program costs. The sum of these two categories of cost—basic production plus community costs—can be defined as accounting cost. This cost is simply just the total cost of a revenue or final cost center as determined through cost finding.

Economic costs, such as additional working and plant capital needs, should also be included as part of the stack of premiums. The inclusion of these cost elements is necessary in order to maintain both the quantity and quality of the hospital's capital stock. The total of these cost factors, plus accounting cost, can be identified as financial cost. This cost accurately reflects the financial requirements of the hospital, for not only are operating expenses considered, but also other financial needs are taken into account. Thus, if charges are to be equitable to both the payer and the hospital, they should be equal to the financial cost of producing a unit of service.

If a hospital were to set charges at the above rate, and if it were to receive payment on all its bills, it would generate revenues equal to its financial requirements. Unfortunately, hospitals do not always receive payment on all their patient billings. Therefore, financial cost must be adjusted for bad debts and free services. That is, an additional premium or cost element must be included in the charge structure. The inclusion of this last element sets the charge structure equal to economic cost. If a hospital were to charge for services at this rate, it would both receive revenues— billings less bad debts and free services—equal to its financial requirements and establish an equitable charge structure.

The foregoing reflects an implicit assumption that the institution is a nonprofit (Sec. 501-C3) hospital. As a result, a cost element to reflect a rate of return on invested equity has not been included in the model. If the hospital were investor-owned (proprietary) a rate of return on equity would be a real operating cost and charges would have to be set at a level sufficient to generate revenue to meet this financial requirement. This would be accomplished by adding another premium or cost element to the financial cost stack in Figure 8-1.

The question of whether hospitals should be organized for profit, and have the added cost of a rate of return, is a complex ethical, economic, and public policy issue. It must be recognized that investor-owned institutions are a significant and growing force in the hospital industry with over 1,060 hospitals and 105,657 beds. Moreover, the profit motive has proven in many phases of the economy to be a beneficial driving force requiring no apology. However, as a countervailing point, one must appreciate that, unless the profit motive produces compensating improvements in operating efficiency, the rate of return is an added cost—due to organizational form—which increases the price of hospital care.

Viewing the charge for a service as a stack of premiums is fine in theory. However, this theory, though hopefully increasing one's understanding of how charges should be established, does not explain how actually to establish charges. Therefore, let us turn now and examine the mechanics of rate setting.

Mechanics

The American Hospital Association has suggested three basic methodologies or techniques for determining the rates applicable to the products or services of the various revenue centers within a hospital. Each of these methodologies utilizes the notion of economic cost as the basis for establishing charges and attempts to apportion this cost—as reasonably as it is possible—to the particular units of service which are produced by the revenue center in question. The mechanics of each technique and the type of revenue center for which it is most appropriate are discussed below.

Weighted Procedure Rate Method. Those revenue centers, such as laboratory, radiology, and inpatient units, which produce various but relatively standardized services or products should determine their service charge in terms of average cost per weighted procedure or service. This technique requires that each different product which is produced by the revenue center be assigned a unit weight or value which is based upon the relative time, resources, and skill required to produce that product. That is, the unit value should represent the cost of performing a service relative to some other service which is used as a base, i.e., has a unit value of one. Table 8-2 illustrates the example relative value units suggested by the Connecticut Hospital Association for laboratory services.

Given a listing of unit values, the next step in calculating the service charge is to multiply the unit value for each service by the expected number of services which will be produced in order to

Table 8-2

Example Relative Value Units*

	Suggested Values		Suggested Values
1. CHEMISTRY EXAMINATIONS		Copper	100
		Cortisol, plasma	100
Acetone (serum)	20	Creatine	50
ACTH response test with administration	300	Creatine phosphokinase	50
		Creatinine, serum manual	40
Aldosterone	750	Creatinine, large volumes	30
Albumin	30	Clearance Calculation	10
Albumin & Globulin with total protein	60	Cryoglobulins with collection at 37°C	40
Alcohol, blood	100	Doriden	120
Aldolase	100	Electrophoresis, serum protein	80
Amino Acids, blood or urine	100	Electrophoresis, large batch	60
Amino Nitrogen	100	Electrophoresis, immuno	200
Aminotransfases (see transaminase)	50	Electrophoresis, lipoproteins	100
Ammonia	00	Electrophoresis, urine, CSF, protein	100
Amylase	40	Electrophoresis, haptoglobin	
Ascorbic Acid (Vit. C)	80		
Barbiturates, quantitative	50	**II. HEMATOLOGY**	
Barbiturates, specific identification	120	Anticoagulants, circulating	50
Bilirubin, direct & total	35	Bleeding time, Ivy	35
Bilirubin, micro or amniotic	50	Blood Counts	
Blood gasses-complete		Eosinophils	30
Blood gasses, Ph PCO_2 Cal. HCO_3	80	Platelets, smear estimate	20
Blood gasses, PO_2 alone	50	Platelets, quantitative	50
Blood gasses, O_2 Sat. calculated extra	10	RBC	15
		RBC, manual	15
Blood gasses with pH, PGO_2 and PO_2	100	Reticulocytes	30
		WBC, semi, large volume	10
Bromide	50	WBC, manual	15
BSP	50	WBC, differential, smear	20
Blood urea nitrogen (BUN)		Blood indices (math only)	5
Blood urea nitrogen, manual	25	Blood volume-Evans Dye	100
Blood urea nitrogen, large batch volumes	20	Bone Marrow (aspiration, H & E, Fe on clot and/or interpretation)	300
Blood Volume dye	100	Clot Retraction, qualitative	10
Calcium, manual	50	Coagulation time	
Calcium, large volumes	40	Coagulation time, Lee White	60
Catecholamines	200	Fibrinogen, quantitative	75
Carbon Dioxide, manual	35	Fibrinogen, quantitaative	75
Carbon Dioxide, large volumes	25	Fibrinolysins, qualitative	10
Carbon monoxide, qual, sean	50	Fragility of crythrocytes	150
Carotenes	50	G-6-P-D, Screen qualitative	50
Cephalin Cholest. flocculation	20	G-6-P-D, semiquantitative histochem	100
Chlorides, manual	30	Hematocrit	10
Chlorides, large volumes	25	Hemoglobin, manual	15
Cholesterol, total	50	Hemoglobin, large volume	10
Cholesterol, free and esters	100	Hemoglobin, plasma	50
Cholinesterase, typical	50	Hemoglobin, type F (Fetal)	60
Cholinesterase, debucane atypical	75		

* Source: Connecticut Hospital Association, Relative Value Schedule-Laboratory.

Table 8-2, continued

	Suggested Values		Suggested Values
Hemoglobin, electrophoresis	80	Phosphorous, large volumes	25
Hemoglobin, A2		Potassium, manual	25
Hemolysins, acid or cold screen	20	Proteins, total, chemical	30
Hemolysins, quant acid-Ham T	100	Proteins, refractometer	20
Hemolysins, auto	50	Salicylates, quanitative	30
L-E Preparation	100	Sodium, manual	25
Leukocyte alkaline phosphatase	100	Sodium, large batches	20
Malaria Smear	50	Sulfonamides	50
Methemoglobin	50	Thymol Turbity	25
Electrophoresis, hemoglobin	80	Transaminases, manual	40
Electrophoresis, A2	100	Transaminases, large volumes.	30
Placental estriols		Uric Acid, manual	40
Fatty Acid, total.		Uric Acid, large volumes	30
FSH		VMA	
Galactose Tolerance,		VMA, quantitative	100
see glucose per spec	30	Xylose, urine, no dose	100
Gamma Globulin salting out	30	17 Ketosteroids, total	75
Glucose, manual	25	17 Ketogenic, steroids	125
Glucose, large volume	20	ABO immune antibody screen	
Haptoglobin		& titer of infant	75
Hemoglobin, plasma free	50	RB Cells washed	150
Hydroxyindolacetic acid (5HIAA)	30	Platelets Concentrate	225
17 Hydroxysteroids (Porter-Siller)		Leukocyte poor blood preparation	50
Iodine, PBI alone	75	Open head workup-simple	375
Iodine, PBI large batch	50	Open head workup-complex	625
Iodine, BEI	150	Packed Cells preparation	25
T3 by column		Plasmaphoresis per event	600
T4		Phlebotomy	50
Iron, serum	50	Platelet Concentrate Preparation	150
Iron, binding capacity	100	Cryoprecipitate	225
LDH, manual	40	Antibody Technique Fluorescence	100
LDH, large volumes	30	Antistreptolysin O Titers	65
LDH, fractionation isoenzymes	80	Agglutinations (slide) febrile each	30
Lipase	50	Agglutinations (tube) Brucella only	60
Lipids, total	100	Agglutinations (tube) Coccydio-	
Lipids, triglycerides	100	myces	60
Lipids, phospholipids	60	Agglutinations leptosera, rubella,	
Lithium	50	tularemia, typhoid O silicosis	60
Macroglobulin, sia H2O test	20	Antibiotic sensitivity disc	30
Macroglobulin, electrophoresis		Antibiotic sensitivity tube	125
Macroglobulin, immunoelectro-		Autogenous Vaccine	300
phoresis		Cold agglutinins with titer	65
Magnesium, manual	50	C-Reactive Protein	40
Methemoglobin	50	Culture, general bact	50
NPN	50	Culture, general bact. with sensi-	
Osmolarity	25	tivity	75
Phosphatase, acid (total only)	40	Culture, blood with sensitivity	125
Phosphatase, prostatic & total	60	Culture, stool or urine with sensi-	
Phosphatase, alkaline manual	40	tivity	75
Phosphatase, large volume	30	Culture, fungi	75
Phosphorous, manual	30	Culture, fungus with definitive ID	100

Table 8-2, continued

	Suggested Values		Suggested Values
Culture, Tbc with smear.............	125	ABO immune antibody screen	
Dark Field............................	75	& titer of mother.................	75
Direct Smear clinical material		Osmolarity............................	15
including tbc....................	40	pH......................................	10
Heterophile, screen...................	30	Porphorins-screen.....................	15
Heterophile with absorption titer...	65	Copro, Uro, porphobilinogen.......	100
Immunoglobulins by diffusion		Phenylketonuria-(fe C13)...........	10
Ig G, Ig A, Ig M (all three)...........	100		
Latex fixation for slide R.A.F.			
with one dilution.................	40	**V. CLINICAL MICROSCOPY**	
Peripheral Smear for Parasites......	50	Phenolsulphonthalein (PSP).........	20
Plasma Clotting Factors		Porphobilinogen......................	35
Factor V..........................	125	Protein, qualitative...................	10
Factor VIII......................	125	Salicylates, screen (fe C13)..........	30
Factor IX........................	125	Sediment see mx......................	10
Factor X.........................	125	Specific Gravity, alone...............	10
Factor XIII......................	25	Sugar, qualitative.....................	10
Platelet Aggregation.................	10	Sugar, quantitative....................	25
Prothrombin time...................	25	Sulkowitch............................	10
Prothrombin consumption..........	50	Urinalysis, routine, complete........	30
Partial Thromboplastin time (PTT).	25	Urobilinogen..........................	25
Peroxidase stain......................	40		
RBC Morphology Only..............	20	**VI. MISCELLANEOUS**	
Sedimentation Rate...................	15	Gastric Analysis per specimen by ph	
Sickle Cell Preparation..............	20	Meter specimens fasting and	
Siderocyte Stain (Fe).................	30	max stim, pH and total acid out-	
Thrombin time, alone...............	30	put..................................	30
Thromboplastin generation test		Diagnex...............................	30
(TGT complete).................	50	Occult Blood..........................	10
Tourniquet test.......................	50	Sweat tests, plate....................	25
		Sweat tests, complete.................	
III. TRANSFUSION SERVICE		Sweat tests, Na or Cl.................	
ABO, cell grouping..................	20	Sweat tests, nails.....................	
ABO Grouping & Rh typing (rou-			
tine)................................	35	**VII. ADMINISTRATIVE**	
Rh cell typing (anti-D, Anti CD)		Stat collection only...................	40
slide................................	15	Night performance...................	20
Rh subgrouping (anti C, D, E, c, e)..	50	Routine Collection....................	20
Subgrouping other than common		Drawing separating and added	
Rh & ABO antigens..............	25	packaging, transportation and	
Crossmatch-routine (saline, albu-		record costs.....................	
min, antiglobulin)................	40	a. Simple, 1st class...............	25
Direct Antiglobulin (Coombs) test...	30	b. Complex (dry ice) also spe-	
Indirect Antiglobulin (Coombs) test.	35	cial..............................	100
		Local reduction (in a specific test)	
IV. SEROLOGY-BACTERIOLOGY		units...............................	
Antibody Titer (i.e., anti-Rh)........	65	because another institution as-	
Antibody Screen (simple).............	40	sumed drawing, sending and	
Antibody Identification..............	200	billing costs......................	10
Rhogam Workup with maternal		Local reduction of a specific test	
& infant screen...................		units as above but billing.........	5

Table 8-2, continued

	Suggested Values		Suggested Values
VIII. ISOTOPES		Brain, cisternograph with RISA	540
Au 198 microaggregate	340	Brain, technicium (te)	410
Blood Volume, dye	100	B12 Schilling, initial	140
Blood Volume, RISA first	25	B12 Schilling, with intrinsic factor	200
Blood Volume, RISA with repeats		Cardiac output with ISHA	
Blood Volume, Cr51 RBC's	140	Cardiac cisternograph with RISA	540
Blood Volume, Cr51 repeats with		Cardiac Scan (peripheral effusion)	220
same cells	100	Circulation Time	
Latex fixation for thyroid globulin		G-II 131 Triolein study	
antibodies	40	G-II 131 Oleic Acid study	
Pregnancy-chorionic gonadotrophins		G-II 131 Protein loss (PVP)	
Pregnancy-chorionic full titer	150	G-I Cr51 RBC intestinal blood loss	
Pregnancy-serologic slide test	40	Insulin Binding Index	100
Pregnancy-titers (3 tubes)	80	Insulin Immunoassay	100
Rubella hemagglutination inhibition	80	I 131 excretion, 48 hours	80
Serologic test for syphilis, VDRL	15	I 131 excretion, repeat 48 hours	40
Premarital VDRL	20	I 131 plasma descence	
Treponema Fluorescent antibodies	100	I 131 PBI	
Thyroid antibodies tube test	65	I 131 Uptake, single determination	
C. S. F. Tests		I 131 Uptake, multiple	150
Cell Count with differential	50	I 131 Uptake, with thyroid suppres-	
Fecal Tests		sion	150
Qualitative Stool Fat	20	I 131 Uptake with TSH stimulation	440
Microscopic examination of stool	25	I 131 Uptake with scintiscan	150
Occult Blood	10	Lung microaggregates	340
Ova & Parasites, complete	75	Pancreas scan, Se 75	125
Pin Worm Preparation	10	Placental scan	150
Urobilin, qualitative	25	Renal scan	380
Trypsin by titer	30	Renogram, Hippuranil I 131 or Hg	
Sperm Analysis		203	300
Sperm Count & Mobility	100	Rose Bengal, liver	220
Urinalysis		Rose Bengal, with scintiscan	
Addis Count	75	Spleen scan with sequestration	190
Routine & microscopic	30	T3 uptake with RBC	50
Acetone	0	T3 uptake with Resin sponge	60
Bence-Jones Protein Heat	25	T4 Murphy-Pattee	100
Bence-Jones Protein-Electro-		Phatmologram	20
phoresis	100	Ferrokinetics	400
Bile Ictotest	10	R3C Survival Cr51	200
Calculus Chemical Analysis	50		
Cell Count & Differential	75	IX. TISSUES & CYTOLOGY	
Fat Particles (free)	40	Gyn-Cervical & Vaginal	50
Hemoglobin (free)	10	Sputum, urine and cavity fluids	75
Hemosiderin	40	Gastric with collection	150
Hemogentisic Acid	20	Sex Chromatin determination	50
Melanin	25	Tissues	
Microscopic only (centrifuge)	15	Gross only includes pathologist	30
Myoglobin-screen	15	Gross & microscopic	300
Myoglobin-qualitative	100	Frozen section consultation	300
Body scan, whole	400	Bone Marrow	300
Bone, 1st section scan	260	Autopsy	5000
Bone, 2nd section scan	350		

determine the total number of weighted units.[8] Total economic
cost should then be divided by total weight units to determine
charge per weighted unit. Based upon these calculations, the
charge per service is determined simply by multiplying the charge
per weighted unit by the predetermined value of each service.
Tables 8-3 and 8-4 illustrate this technique for inpatient and laboratory revenue centers.

Admittedly, this technique for computing rates is relatively
complex. However, if the unit values assigned to each service are
appropriate, the resulting charge structure will be equitable to all
parties. Thus, the critical and, obviously, the most difficult factor
in this process is the selection of unit values. Various sources,
such as the American College of Pathology and the American College of Radiology, have developed listings of unit values which
may be appropriate to a particular hospital's needs.[9] However, a

---

[8]It should be noted that it is difficult, if not impossible, to establish equitable
charges without first developing accurate demand forecasts and expense budgets.
The basic principles underlying budgeting are discussed in Part IV. However, readers desiring additional information on these subjects should see *Operational Budgeting Systems,*H. Berman and P. Bash; *The Development of An Expense Budgeting
Procedure*, M. Lash; or *Quantitative Techniques for Hospital Planning and Control*,
J. R. Griffith.

[9]Remarks of Owen M. Johnson, Jr., Director, Bureau of Competition, Federal
Trade Commission. Mr. Johnson's remarks were made in April 1977 to the National
Health Lawyers Association.

"Another area of Commission concern is the promulgation and use of relative
value scales by professional groups. For those of you who are not familiar with the
relative value scale (or RVS), it is a listing of procedures or services with assigned
comparative values. Where the comparative values are expressed in dollar terms,
the publication and circulation of these schedules may constitute direct price-fix-
ing. Even where these procedures or services are ranked by some other numerical
index (for example, the recommended time for a procedure), physicians may, by
agreeing on a monetary conversion factor (for example, $75 per hour), produce a
price–fixing schedule.

"Promulgation of RVSs by members of a professional group can diminish price
competition in a number of ways. First, the scale, by its very nature, eliminates a
degree of independent choice for those who use it. Variation in overhead, direct
costs, and desired profits—the components of pricing in a competitive mar-
ketplace—are ignored by RVSs. More importantly, these scales make it difficult, if
not impossible, for the conscientious health care shopper to derive any benefits
from comparative pricing.

"In a series of cases the Commission has obtained consent orders from three
professional associations, the American College of Obstetricians and Gynecolo-
gists, the American College of Radiology, and the American Academy of Orthopae-
dic Surgeons; and a proposed consent settlement with a fourth association, the
Minnesota State Medical Association, is currently on file for public comment.
These orders require the organizations to withdraw all copies of RVSs and to
refrain from publishing or participating in the development of any such scales in
the future.

"One aspect of our RVS orders which has caused confusion has been the effect of hospital, before completely accepting any of these unit values, should first review them in terms of its own physical plant layout, processing techniques, capital and labor mix, and costs. If the proposed values are not suitable, the hospital should either subjectively modify them or, using industrial engineering techniques, develop its own value system. This latter alternative is quite costly and should only be used as a last resort when subjective modification does not provide workable results.

Hourly Rate Method. Those revenue centers, such as operating room, physiotherapy, and anesthesia, whose patient service is hours of use, should determine their service charge in terms of rate per hour. An example of the mechanics of determining charge per hour of usage for the operating room is presented in Table 8-5.

It should be noted that the operating room rate is expressed in terms of both rate per manhour and rate per operating room hour. The calculation of both rates provides the hospital with the flexibility necessary to assure that rates are as equitable as practically feasible. Thus, when a procedure is an average or typical procedure, i.e., the average number of personnel participate, the rate per operating room hour is appropriate. However, if a procedure is atypical, i.e., more or fewer than the typical number of personnel are involved, the rate per man-hour should be used. In this way, the hospital can "tailor" its rates to fit the actual service which was provided.

The charge for operating room use also can be calculated on the basis of the average cost per weighted procedure. However, due to the wide range of possible variation in the time, resources, and skill required to perform any given procedure, this technique is more suited to revenue centers which provide reasonably standardized services, such as those discussed above, than it is to the operating room. Therefore, hourly rates are recommended as the preferred basis for charging for operating room services.[10]

---

the Commission's actions on the value scales of third–party payers. It should be noted that these consent orders in no way restrict health insurers—whether private or government—from developing guidelines for assessing the reasonableness of charges. The Commission's concern has been confined to physicians' adoption of RVSs and efforts to ensure adherence to these schedules. Use of similar scales by third–party payers does not make them participants in price–affecting agreements of the type proscribed by the Commission's consent orders. In short, it is one thing for consumers to develop guidelines for evaluating fees, but quite another for competitors to publish and enforce pricing schedules. Despite this distinction, it is interesting to note that the Social Security Administration has directed private insurers who administer physician payments for Medicare to cease references to relative value scales banned by the Commission."

[10]Hourly rates, while an improvement over the weighted procedure method, are still not ideal, for they ignore the matter of personnel mix. Thus, to the extent that a rate can be adjusted for the actual mix of personnel used in any given procedure, it can be made more equitable.

Table 8-3

Laboratory Charges

I. *Assumptions:*

    A. Accounting costs for the laboratory = $150,000
    B. Financial and economic costs for the laboratory = a 20% addition
       or $30,000*
    C. Total economic cost for the laboratory (financial requirements) =
       $180,000
    D. Weighted Units Computation. (Example represents only a sample
       of all tests performed)

Amylase, blood	2,000	2.5	5,000
Bleeding time	2,500	1.9	4,750
Hematocrit	3,800	.8	3,040
Platelet count	3,900	1.0	3,900
Uric Acid	1,500	1.5	2,250

            Total Weighted Units: 120,000
            (All Tests)

II. *Calculation:*

Step A— (Total Economic Cost) ÷ (Total Weighted Units)
                                = Charge/Weighted Unit
            $180,000 ÷   120,000 = $1.50

Step B— (Charge/Weighted Unit) (Unit Value of Test) = Charge/Test
       ($1.50)(2.5) = $3.75 Charge/Amylase, Blood Test
       ($1.50)(1.9) = $2.85 Charge/Bleeding Time Test
       ($1.50)(.8)   = $1.20 Charge/Hematocrit Test
       ($1.50)(1)   = $1.50 Charge/Platelet Count Test
       ($1.50)(1.5) = $2.25 Charge/Uric Acid Test

---

*Premium for economic and financial costs should be based on historical ac-
counting data (bad debt and free service element), subjective estimates, and policy
decisions.
**These weighting factors are used just for purposes of illustration. Individual
hospitals should select weighting factors on the basis of their own unique physical
plants, processing techniques, capital-labor mix, and so forth.

Table 8-4

Inpatient Unit Charges

I. Assumptions:
A.

Type of Facility	Private Room	Semi-Private Room	Ward	Total
Expected Patient Days	2,000	6,000	2,000	10,000
Facility Unit Value	2	1 5	1	
Total Weighted Units	4,000	9,000	2,000	15,000

B. Costs

Accounting, financial and economic costs which are to be allocated on the basis of patient days = $350,000

Accounting, financial and economic costs which are to be allocated on the basis of unit value = $150,000

II. Calculation:

Step A — (Costs to be allocated on the basis of pt. days) ÷ (Pt. days) = Patient Day Charge Factor
$350,000 ÷ 10,000 = $35

Step B — (Costs to be allocated on the basis of unit values) ÷ (Total weighted units) = Unit Value Charge Factor
$150,000 ÷ 15,000 = $10

Step C — (Unit Value Charge Factor) (Unit Value of Facility) = Unit Value Charge Factor/Facility
($10) (2)   = $20 Unit Value Charge Factor/Private Room Bed
($10) (1.5) = $15 Unit Value Charge Factor/Semi-Private Room Bed
($10) (1) = $10 Unit Value Charge Factor/Ward Bed

Step D — (Pt. Day Charge Factor) + (Unit Value Charge Factor/Facility) = Charge/In-patient Unit
$35 + $20 = $55 Charge/Private Room Bed
$35 + $15 = $50 Charge/Semi-Private Room Bed
$35 + $10 = $45 Charge/Ward Bed

III. Explanation

A. Certain cost elements, such as nursing, dietary, medical records, and working capital needs, are, for the most part, used or applied uniformly to all patients. Thus, they should be allocated on the basis of patient days. Therefore, based on accounting data (budgets), the hospital should determine the total amount of costs which should be allocated on a patient day basis. This cost should then be divided by total patient days to determine cost per patient day.

B. Those cost elements which cannot be allocated appropriately on a uniform basis should be distributed on a weighted value basis. The mechanics of this distribution are basically the same as those depicted in Table 8-3. Cost elements which fall into this category are bad debts, plant capital needs, depreciation, housekeeping, plant operations, and so forth.

C. As the final step, the charges, as determined in items A and B above, should be combined to produce charge per type of facility.

Table 8-5

Hourly Rates

I. Assumptions:
    A. Accounting costs for the operating room = $100,000
    B. Financial and economic costs for the operating room = a
        30% addition or $30,000
    C. Total economic costs for the operating room = $130,000
    D. Expected hours of use = 2,000
    E. Average number of personnel per operation = 4
II. Calculation
    A. (Total economic cost) ÷ (Hours of usage) = Rate/Hour
        ($130,000) ÷ (2,000) = $65 Charge/hour
        This rate should be used when a procedure utilizes the
        average number of personnel
    B. (Hours of Usage) (Typical number of personnel) =
        Man-hours of usage (2,000) (4) = 8,000 man-hours
        1. (Total economic cost) ÷ (Man-hours of usage) = Rate
            per man-hour
            ($130,000) ÷ (8,000) = $16.25 Charge/Man-hour
        2. This rate should be used when a procedure involves
            more, or less, personnel than typical. For example,
            for a one hour procedure which utilizes 5 persons, the
            charge should be (5) ($16.25), or $81.25.

Surcharge Rate Method. Those revenue centers, such as pharmacy and central supply, which serve primarily a merchandising
function, should determine their rates in terms of a surcharge
which should be "added on" to the cost of the goods which they
supply. That is, those revenue centers whose function is that of
either handling or preparing goods for final distribution should
establish charges on the basis of the cost plus a surcharge for
handling and processing. An illustration of this method of determining charges is presented for pharmacy in Table 8-6.

Rate Setting Pragmatism

The above methodologies, with some minor modification such
as that necessary for inpatient units, will provide the hospital with
the techniques needed to establish charges equal to economic
costs for each of its revenue centers. However, determining or
knowing the theoretically ideal charge for each service is not
enough. For example, if the charge for a particular service based

Table 8-6

Pharmacy Charges

I. Assumptions.
  A. Accounting cost for pharmacy = $50,000
  B. Financial and economic cost for pharmacy = a 20% addition, or $10,000
  C. Total economic cost for pharmacy = $60,000
  D. Cost of drugs billed to patients = $45,000

II. Calculations:
  Step A — (Total economic cost) − (Cost of drugs billed to patients) = Total Surcharge
    ($60,000) − ($45,000) = $15,000
  Step B — (Total surcharge) ÷ (Cost of drugs billed to a patients) = Percentage mark-up
    ($15,000) ÷ ($45,000) = 33.3%
  Step C — (Percentage mark-up) (Cost of drugs*) = Surcharge
    (33.3%) ($12) = $4
  Step D — Surcharge + Cost of Drugs = Charge/drugs
    $4 + $12 = $16 Charge

* Assumed drug cost for a particular prescription.

on economic cost appears excessive management may, as a matter of policy, reduce the charge for that service and subsidize it by increasing the charges for other services.

Perhaps the best illustration of this type of situation was referred to earlier in regard to routine service rates. As was pointed out, hospitals, in order to avoid or at least to minimize public pressure and scrutiny, as a matter of policy set routine service charges at less than cost so that they will compare more favorably with hotel and restaurant rates. The obvious result of this practice is that inpatient units operate at a loss, i.e., costs exceed revenues. In order to recover this loss, "profits," i.e., revenues in excess of cost, must be generated by other revenue centers. Thus, it is common to find laboratory, radiology, and pharmacy producing "profits," while the operating room, the delivery room, and inpatient units operate at a loss.

In addition to adjustments in the rate structure for seemingly excessive charges, management may also be forced to alter rates due to third party payer attitudes and practices. As has been discussed, third party payers, in principle, should pay essentially the same rates as all other payers. However, as should be realized by this point, the simple fact is that they do not pay on the same basis. Accordingly, rate structures applicable to other payers must be adjusted if a hospital is to maintain a financially sound position.

The implications of these pragmatic factors, regardless of how distasteful, should be obvious. In order to maintain a financially viable position, management must adjust charges to meet financial realities. This fact, though philosophically repugnant, is a fiscal fact of life which intelligent management cannot ignore. The foregoing theory and techniques will provide management with the understanding and information necessary to determine the costs of these decisions, and hopefully will enable better decisions to be made. However, neither theory nor technique will change the fact that rate adjustment decisions are necessary.

Conclusion

Based on both the previous chapters and the above material, the reader should now have an understanding of the sources of hospital operating revenues, their philosophies, and the financial problems and considerations related to these sources.

Suggested Readings

American Hospital Association. *Cost Finding and Rate Setting for Hospitals.*

Berman, Howard J. and Bash, Paul L. *Operational Budgeting Systems.*

Dowling, William L. (ed.) *Topics in Health Care Financing,* "Prospective Rate Setting," Winter 1976.

Kaitz, Edward M. *Pricing Policy and Cost Behavior in the Hospital Industry.*

Lash, Myles P. "The Development of An Expense Budgeting Procedure."

Mueller, William J. and Soder, Earl. "Rate Setting," *Hospital Accounting,* December 1964.

Appendix 8-A*
Legislated Rate Setting

When the foregoing chapter was first written, the notion of economic cost was little more than a theoretical construct, whose

---

*Material for this Appendix has been drawn, in large part, from *Abstracts of State Legislated Hospital Cost Containment Programs* (HCFA Publ. No. 017 (5–78).

principal value lay in its usefulness in explaining desired management behavior. Similarly, the notions of third–party cost–based reimbursement agreements being renegotiated to include all economic cost, were little more than idealistic goals. However, in 1969 the State of New York enacted legislation giving the commissioner of the Department of Health the responsibility for certifying that proposed hospital rates were reasonably related to the cost of delivering efficient health care services. The Commissioner has implemented this responsibility through a formula approach to rate setting.

Since 1969, fifteen states have enacted legislation which requires the disclosure, review or regulation of hospital rates or budgets. Table 8A–1 summarizes the major characteristics of each of these fifteen state programs. Of the fifteen programs, five states (Colorado, Connecticut, Maryland, Massachusetts, and Washington) have rate–setting commissions with full authority to review and approve hospital budgets or rates. Two other states (New York and New Jersey) have given authority to state agencies to set Medicaid and Blue Cross rates.

The remaining eight states, with the exception of Wisconsin and Rhode Island, use a variety of organizational mechanisms to review and publicly comment on or to disclose findings as to the reasonableness of hospital rates. The Rhode Island program is carried out by Blue Cross. Wisconsin uses a joint committee of the Department of Health, Blue Cross, and the state hospital association. Both the Rhode Island and Wisconsin programs require hospital compliance with the findings of the review process.

Participation in each of the fifteen programs is mandatory for all non-governmental hospitals. Compliance with the programs is mandatory in all of the involved states except for Arizona, Maine, Minnesota, Oregon, and Virginia. It should be recognized, however, that states with voluntary compliance believe that public pressure and third–party contractual payment processes will result in actual compliance.

It is interesting to note that though support for (see Appendix 8–B), as well as the number of, legislated rate–setting programs is increasing, the cost containment effectiveness of such programs is still an open question. To begin to provide answers, the Health Care Financing Administration has recently financed the evaluation of six rate–setting programs; i.e., western Pennsylvania, upstate and downstate New York, New Jersey, Rhode Island and Indiana.* Of the six programs, four—western Pennsylvania, up-

---

*Hellinger, Fred J., "State Rate Review a Critical Assessment." *Hospitals* September 1, 1978.

state New York, New Jersey, and Rhode Island*—were shown not to have had a statistically significant impact on hospital costs. In contrast, the other two programs—Indiana and downstate New York—both showed a statistically significant cost impact.

This latter evidence does not, however, make it easier to draw firm conclusions about the effectiveness of legislated programs.** This is the case, for while the New York program is legislated, the Indiana program is just the opposite. It is a voluntary effort, established in 1960 by the Indiana Blue Cross Plan and the Indiana Hospital Association.

The Federation of American Hospitals (FAH), the national association of investor–owned hospitals, has also attempted to examine the effects of hospital rate regulaton. In 1970, the FAH financed a study, conducted by ICF corporation, which attempted to examine in eighteen states the impact of rate regulation on hospital costs and revenues. The eighteen states were grouped into three categories:

Mandatory Rate Regulation (Maryland, Connecticut, New York, New Jersey, Massachusetts)

Voluntary or Private Payer Operated Rate Regulation (Arizona, Indiana, Ohio, Pennsylvania, Wisconsin)

No Rate Regulation (Texas, Virginia, North Carolina, Florida, Illinois, Minnesota, California)

The findings of the study can be summarized as follows:

States with mandatory rate regulation exhibited performance similar to states with no rate regulation at all; however, two factors are relevant here:

—first, the only period in which mandatory rate regulation seemed to have a slight effect was in reducing hospital expenditures per case in the post ESP period (1974–75); however, this effect was more than offset by an increase in hospital utilization which produced higher expenditures per capita; thus, effective utilization controls appear to be an essential

---

*The New Jersey and New York programs are legislated programs. Indiana, Rhode Island and western Pennsylvania are voluntary efforts.

**There is very little indication that hospital rate regulation has a more significant effect than other factors on controlling hospital expenditures per case and per capita and in limiting hospital revenues per case and per capita; to the extent that any impact could be discerned, the states with voluntary rate regulation programs exhibited a 1–2 percent better performance than either of the other two groups on most measures over the period studied.

component of mandatory rate regulation; more research and consideration should be focussed upon whether PSROs are capable of such reductions or whether other approaches are required; and

—second, it is possible that socioeconomic factors might have produced higher rates of increase in the absence of mandatory rate–setting; however, our examination of states from the two groups with similar socioeconomic characteristics (Illinois and New Jersey) and in the periods before and after the introduction of rate regulation in other states (Maryland) provided little support for this possibility.

• States with voluntary programs might well form a good basis for further experimentation and research, despite the current emphasis on mandatory rate regulation programs, we found evidence that voluntary programs hold as much or more promise; thus, further consideration should be given during research and experimentation to disclosure–oriented programs (such as Arizona) and other voluntary approaches (for example, the use of competitive bidding to establish reimbursement levels).

• States considering development of rate regulation systems should consider the expected impact carefully; we were unable to identify any significant initial impact of rate regulation and the impact over time was greatly affected by other factors such as socioeconomic conditions, changes in utilization, and the Economic Stabilization Program.

In considering the above findings it is important to bear in mind that these evaluations focussed on so-called first generation programs. As rate-setting programs continue, it is likely that they will evolve into increasingly sophisticated and potentially potent cost containment programs. Whether such potency will accrue to the "community good"—or just fuel a regulatory agency's need to demonstrate that it can be "tough" regardless of the community cost—is, at the moment, a moot point.

The only conclusion which can be drawn now is one of uncertainty. Given the "state of the art," there is nothing inherently wrong with reaching this finding. Successive generations of legislated programs do, however, merit careful monitoring so that more reasoned and knowledgeable judgements can be made as to their ultimate usefulness and role.

Table 8 A-1*

Fifteen State Legislated Hospital Cost Containment Programs

State	Responsible Agency	Type of System	Voluntary vs. Mandatory	Payors Covered
Arizona	Department of Health Services: Local HSAs	Budget/Rate Review	Mandatory Review Voluntary Compliance	Charge-based including Blue Cros
California	Department of Health Facilities Commission	Disclosure	Mandatory Disclosure	Not Applicable
Colorado	Colorado Hospital Commission	Budget/Rate Review and Approval	Mandatory	All payors except Medicare and Medicaid
Connecticut	Commission on Hospitals and Health Care	Budget/Rate Review and Approval	Mandatory	Charge based
Maine	Health Facilities Cost Review Board: voluntary budget review organization	Budget/Rate Review Voluntary Compliance	Mandatory Review Voluntary Compliance	Charge-based
Maryland	Health Services Cost Review Commission	Budget/Rate Review and Approval	Mandatory	All payors
Massachusetts	Massachusetts Rate Setting Commission	Cost Rate Review and Approval	Mandatory	Blue Cross
		Budget/Rate Review and Approval	Mandatory	Charge-based
		Rate Setting	Mandatory	Medicaid

Health Care Financing Administration
Office of Policy, Planning, and Research
Office of Demonstrations and Evaluations
   *Abstracts of State Legislated Hospital Cost Containment Programs
HCFA Pub. No. 017 (S-78)
May, 1978

Revenue Control Method	Unit of Payment	Frequency of Review	Adjustments	Appeals
Total Revenue	Charges	Prior to any rate change	Not Applicable	Not Applicable
Not Applicable	Not Applicable	Annually	Not Applicable	Not Applicable
Total revenue; rates per admission by revenue center	Rate based charges	Annually	Volume and intensity	Public Hearings before Commission
Total revenue	Charges	Annually	Retroactive volume: unforeseen and material change in expense	
Not Applicable	Charges	Annually	Not Applicable	Not Applicable
Total revenue; departmental revenue or guaranteed revenue per case or maximum revenue per case	Rate-based charges	Annually and as necessary	Retroactive possible for volume and uncontrollable costs	Public Hearing before Commission
Cost-based	Routine per diem, Ancillary charges	Annually be denied	Excess costs may	Courts
Total revenue	Charges	Annually	None	Division of Hearing Officers
Cost-based	Per diem	Annually	Uncontrollable Costs	Division of Hearing Officers

Table 8 A-1 (continued)

State	Responsible Agency	Type of System	Voluntary vs. Mandatory	Payors Covered
Minnesota	Department of Health Minnesota Hospital Association	Budget/Rate Review	Mandatory Review Voluntary Compliance	Charge based including Blue Cros
New Jersey	State Department of Health	Budget/Rate Review and Approval	Mandatory	Medicaid and Blue
New York	State Department of Health	Rate Setting	Mandatory	Medicaid and Blue
Oregon	State Health Planning and Development Agency	Budget/Rate Review	Mandatory Review Voluntary Compliance	Charge based including Blue Cros
Rhode Island	State Budget Office: Blue Cross of Rhode Island	Negotiated Budget/Rate Review and Approval	Mandatory	Medicaid and Blue Cross
Virginia	Virginia Health Services Cost Review Commission: voluntary cost review organization	Cost/Charge Review	Mandatory Review Voluntary Compliance	Not Applicable
Washington	Washington State Hospital Commission	Budget/Rate Review and Approval	Mandatory	All payors Charge based
Wisconsin	State Department of Health: Rate Review Committee	Budget/Rate Review Approval	Mandatory	All payors except Medicare

Revenue Control Method	Unit of Payment	Frequency of Review	Adjustments	Appeals
Total revenue	Charges	Annually and when requested during year	None	DOH–Public Hearings before independent hearing examiner: MHA–hearing before appeals panel
Cost-based	Per diem	Annually	Retroactive: for volume, economic factors, pass-through items	Formal appeal before independent hearing officer
Cost-based	Per diem	Annually	Retroactive adjustment for actual economic factor: volume in downstate Blue Cross	Formal appeal before State hearing officer
Total revenue	Charges	Annually and when requested during year	Not Applicable	Not Applicable
Total revenue	Charges	Annually	Retroactive volume	Binding arbitration before independent mediation
Not Applicable	Not Applicable	Annual disclosure budgets as necessary	Not Applicable	Not Applicable
Total revenue rates per unit of service by revenue center	Rate-based charges	Annually	None Volume Volume	Formal hearing before commission or independent
Total revenue	Charges	Prior to any rate change at most once a year	None	Hearing before independent appeals board

Appendix 8-B*
State-Level Review and Approval of Budgets
For Health Care Institutions

In 1977, recognizing governmental and public concern regarding the rapidly escalating level of hospital expenditures and the resulting debate over the financial regulation of hospitals, the American Hospital Association's Board of Trustees and the Council on Financing directed the review of the Association's policy on regulation. The Special Committee to Reexamine AHA's Guidelines on Rate Regulation was formed to accomplish this task and to make recommendations for revisions in the Association's policy if necessary. As a basis for its policy review, the committee used the 1972 AHA policy document entitled "Guidelines for Review and Approval of Rates for Health Care Institutions and Services by a State Commission." The resulting document, which was approved by the House of Delegates of the American Hospital Association on February 1, 1978, is a revision of the 1972 version. The Association recognizes this policy document as reaffirming its position that the financial regulation of health care institutions be accomplished at the state level according to the prescribed method of prospective budget review and approval. Further, it recognizes this as a mechanism which will equitably contribute to cost containment within the health care industry while ensuring that health care services are provided in an efficient and effective manner.

I. Introduction

For many years, society in general and the government in particular have accorded top priority to making high-quality health care accessible to all. As a result, insurance coverage and governmental financing of care have increased to the extent that consumers of health services are largely insulated from the impact of their purchase decisions. In addition to these increased expenditures for services, there has been a massive infusion of government funds for facilities, manpower, and research programs to improve the distribution and availability of services. Both have contributed to extensive "demand-pull" inflationary increases in the cost of health care and growing financial problems for many health care institutions as well as for government. These pressures are further exacerbated by the inefficient method of retrospective payment determination that is currently employed.

The trend of spending an increasing percentage of the gross national product for health services presents a major problem for the nation's economy and for the federal budget. It is now evident that the effects of the public and private sectors' responses to the priority of health care will require compatible and comprehensive remedies in order to effect a moderation of the increases in expenditures for health care services.

The hospital industry recognizes the many reasons for the escalation of expenditures and, in a collective effort, is attempting to develop a rational system for regulating expenditures while maintaining quality and access. The industry has done this already by supporting planning and other regulatory mechanisms, such as utlization review and accreditation. The American Hospital Association advocates a system of payment regulation as described in sections II and III of these guidelines as a further effort in this direction.

This proposed system of payment regulation is supported by the American Hospital Association for the following reasons:

1. The proposed system is deemed the best method of moving to a prospective payment mechanism that apportions the payments equitably among all purchasers of services. The inadequacies of retrospective cost reimbursement have rapidly become more unsatisfactory to providers and payers alike.

2. Appropriate financing is essential to maintaining health care institutions' ability to continue to deliver high-quality services to their communities. The public support necessary to obtain financing for institutions at an appropriate level on a sustained basis depends upon public understanding of the reasons for cost increases related to new technology, quality improvements, inflation, and volume fluctuations. Because of this need, effective methods must be developed to inform the public of the nature of hospital costs and to assure the public about the efficiency and effectiveness of these institutions' expenditures and management.

3. The making of decisions on health service priorities and financing must be by a system that is publicly accountable and that balances the interests of consumers as well as third-party payers and providers.

4. The distribution of finite funds requires a highly flexible

regulatory system. The processes of the system must consider the following:

a.   The broad spectrum of local needs and circumstances
b.   The full variety of organizational and service configurations properly found in institutions
c.   The needs of all types of institutions from the small rural hospital to the large regional medical center

From year to year, the payment regulatory system must allow for payments as required not only for institutions that are adding expensive, complex services in response to planning decisions or incurring continual shifts in patient mix, volume, or scope of services, but also for institutions that are relatively stable in their operation or that are reducing their level of services.

5.   The payment regulatory system must be capable of integrating its decisions precisely with the decisions of other regulatory systems operating at the state and local level, such as planing, utilization review, or quality assurance controls, so that each regulatory system performs its intended purposes well and facilitates or complements the activities of each of the other regulatory systems.

6.   The payment regulatory system must be capable of identifying and impacting upon expenses that are considered excessive in health care institutions. This should be accomplished by prospectively denying recognition and payment of such expenses by promoting cost avoidance and by stimulating sound management through appropriate incentives.

7.   It is important to recognize that a health care delivery system must be consonant with the needs and desires of the community that is served. So, too, must all forms of regulation be consonant with the needs and desires of the community. In developing and implementing mechanisms that regulate the accessibility and utilization of health care institutions, the federal government has enacted P.L. 93-641 and P.L. 92-603 on the principle that administration and regulation at the state level is the most appropriate method to ensure community involvement. This principle has equal application to the mechanism for regulating health care expenditures, because the community's needs and desires relate directly to the level of health care institution expenditures. Therefore, the states, through appropriate public policy mechanisms, should have the responsibility to make decisions concerning the level of expenditures necessary to

ensure that the ends and desires they have determined for their institutions are met. A state-level regulatory mechanism provides greater access to the community and its institutions and thus an awareness of local issues that may impact upon them. These factors can then be considered in any determinations made.

Sections II and III of these guidelines are founded on the conviction that a federally mandated, state-administered or state-sanctioned prospective payment regulatory system, based on certain principles and characteristics described herein, has advantages over all other systems for accomplishing the above purposes. These guidelines would be implemented through federal legislation requiring government-regulated health care payment programs to recognize the payment decisions made by entities established at the state level. The federal legislation would also have to provide for the degree of national consistency among the state entities that would allow their role to be continued under any universal health insurance program. Thus, the federal legislation would be establishing another basic element in preparation for universal health insurance, compatible with the already established planning the Professional Standards Review Organization networks.

Several states now utilize some type of regulation of hospital payments. Most of these programs have not applied to all payers, and many use regulatory techniques that do not comply with the principles described herein. It is important, therefore, to distinguish between their very limited effectiveness and the greater potential for the system proposed in these guidelines.

As early as 1970, the probability of expanded payment regulation for health care was recognized by the American Hospital Association, and it initiated studies of other regulated industries in an effort to benefit from their experience. It established the Advisory Panel on Public Utility Regulation, whose recommendations became the basis for the "Guidelines for Review and Approval of Rates for Health Care Institutions and Services by a State Authority" that were approved in 1972.

In 1976, the Association established its Advisory Panel on the Regulation of Hospital Payment; its report is an addendum to the report of the Special Committee on the Regulatory Process. The advisory panel's findings were generally consonant with the earlier reports but emphasized the importance of integrating the payment regulation with planning and other regulations and avoiding the establishment of incentives for excessive utilization of patient services.

A succession of events has contributed to the growing support among health care institutions for federal legislation that places the responsibility and authority for administering payment regulation at the state level. One such event was the Economic Stabilization Program and the distortions in hospital economics it created. The latest impetus has been the introduction of federal legislative cost containment proposals. These proposals seek to regulate hospital expenditures with no recognition of the potential impact on the quality and availability of health care services or of the economic viability of institutions whose purpose is to serve patients.

II. The guidelines: purpose and concept

The basic objective of the guidelines delineated below is to promote the development of state-level regulation of hospital payments under which each institution would be paid its full financial requirements through a prospective payment mechanism that apportions the payments equitably among all the purchasers of its services. The realization of this objective will require that government and other payers accept nationally determined standards for the regulatory process. Flexibility must be built in to allow the state entity to use discretion in making decisions that will accommodate local considerations and provide management incentives.

In response to this need, the American Hospital Association proposes the following guidelines:

1. Each institution will establish its budget in accordance with the principle set forth in the American Hospital Association's statement *Financial Requirements of Health Care Institutions and Services* (AHA catalog no. S031) and related interpretations.

2. The budgets will be submitted to an entity established as described in section IIIC of these guidelines for reviewing and approving the budgets, using procedures and standards that are equitable to providers, payers, and consumers.

3. The review will be focused upon the institution's demonstrated financial requirements and projected volume at the department level. The approval will be of the budgeted gross and net revenue related to those financial requirements and volume. The charge schedule will then be required to be related to its approved aggregate gross and net revenue requirements. Individual charges will be subjected

to challenge only on the basis of their being discriminatory among classes of payers.

4. Charges will apply to all purchasers of services.
5. The approved revenue budget will apply for the following fiscal year, although the process will include an acceptable method for considering emergency adjustments of the budgets during the fiscal year.
6. The entity will receive fiscal year-end reports of the operating results of each institution. Its procedures will provide for retrospective evaluation of those results and prospective handling of substantial gains or losses due to major volume changes for the amounts projected.
7. Appropriate appeal mechanisms, including the right to direct judicial review, will be established to protect the rights of all parties.

III. Guidelines for federal delegation

A. Purpose. The purpose of the state regulatory process to be included in federal legislation is to approve budgets that promote quality and availability of service based on the health care institution's full financial requirements (as defined in the AHA statement *Financial Requirements of Health Care Institutions and Services*). The regulatory process must take into account the institution's community and regional role and its responsibilities as defined by the planning and other regulatory programs.

The process will cause those financial requirements to be allocated among all purchasers through equitable charge schedules. In any federal program of payment regulation that delegates a significant role to the states, the size of federal expenditures for health care services and the achievement of the national goals of such a regulatory program will require that provisions be made for federal oversight of the program. Therefore, to allow for effective delegation, certain criteria must be used to ensure the achievement of the desired goals and outcomes as well as equity among the programs conducted in the various states.

B. Plan. Under its authority, each state will be required to submit a plan and provide reports to the Secretary of Health, Education, and Welfare, showing that it meets the established criteria. Federal approval of those plans and reports will constitute federal delegation of the budget review and approval entity.

1. Budget review and approval will extend to all health care institutions that customarily charge for their services. For

health care institutions participating in a comprehensive prepaid health insurance program on a capitation basis of payment, the entity will review and approve the rate of payment for contracted institutional services under the capitation program and ensure that the institution's charge schedules are equitable for all purchasers, including those not participating in the capitation program.

2. After a public hearing process, it will promulgate and adopt standards for uniform reporting.

3. After a public hearing process, it will develop equitable criteria and methods for the review and approval of budgets including cost performance measurements and comparative evaluations that are equitably defined and uniformly applied.

4. The individual needs and peculiarities of health care institutions require it to recognize the individuality of the institutions it regulates, therefore precluding the use of standardized payment formulas uniformly applied to all institutions. It will review and approve institutions' budgets individually, based on their respective demonstrated financial requirements. The review will be on the institution's revenue total as opposed to line items. The approval decisions will be such that institutions rendering needed health care services and operating efficiently and effectively will have their financial requirements met and their financial solvency preserved on a current basis.

5. Its decisions should provide for financial incentives to institutions to encourage them to manage efficiently, and its decisions will encourage experimentation and innovation in institutional and financial management.

6. Its decisions will support the purposes of planning and other regulatory controls. It will facilitate the voluntary discontinuance of unneeded services and facilities by recognizing the costs associated with phasing them out as a financial requirement for the institution, and it will approve the budgets accordingly.

7. Its decisions will not encourage excessive volume of services and facilities by rewarding the increased use of services. It will use per patient day and per case costs only as a screen for selecting institutions for closer review, not as a unit for direct regulation.

8. It will monitor the decisions of other state regulatory agencies and legislative bodies and will inform them of the

economic impact of their decisions on the operation of
health care institutions.

9. It must be accountable to the public, the health care industry, and the state and federal governments. Public accountability requires it to operate in full public view. Further,
public accountability requires it to certify to the public as to
the reasonableness of the budgets established by the health
care institutions, therefore requiring it to explain to the public the nature of institutional costs, the reasons for those
costs, and the reasons for differences in costs among comparable institutions. In order to perform this function it must
require the public disclosure of health care institutions' financial condition, including balance sheets detailing assets,
liabilities, and net worth as well as detailed statements of
income and expense.

10. It is accountable to the public for ensuring the solvency of
institutions that operate efficiently and effectively and are
deemed necessary by the appropriate planning agency.

11. It is accountable to the state and federal government to periodically document its activities by presenting financial data
concerning the regulated industry.

12. Its budget approval decisions must be made on the weight
of the evidence in the record. In any budget review and
approval proceeding, it is the health care institution's responsibility to justify its budget. Potentially aggrieved
parties may appeal alleged arbitrary and capricious decisions to the courts. The courts must adjudicate based upon
the weight of the evidence in the record.

C. Organization and financing. In each state the budget approval entity may be organized in one of the following ways, but in
order to avoid conflict of interest and promote objectivity, the
entity must not engage in administering health service programs
or purchase institutional health services for either itself, its subscribers, or the state or federal government.

1. It may be organized as a full-time independent commission,
composed of three to five highly qualified, well-compen-
sated commissioners appointed by the governor to serve for
relatively long, staggered terms. Recommendations for commissioners shall be solicited from providers as well as other
interested parties. The commissioners should be chosen
with a view toward their ability to bring to the commission
broad-gauged, effective, and impartial policy direction. Dur-

ing their terms of appointment, commission members should not be permitted to engage in any other business, profession, vocation, public elective office or employment, or in any activity that would result in a conflict of interest with their duties as commissioner.

2. It may be organized as an independent commission, composed of five to nine highly qualified compensated or uncompensated commissioners, appointed on a part-time basis by the governor to serve for relatively long-staggered terms. Recommendations for commissioners shall be solicited from providers as well as other interested parties. They should bring to the commission broad-gauged, effective, and impartial policy direction, which may include a balanced representation from various interests.

3. It may be organized as a nongovernmental entity operating under a contract with the state and under sanction of state laws. Such an entity would have to be nominated or approved by two-thirds of the providers and the majority of major third-party payers subject to its decisions. The entity's actions would have to be generally authorized by state legislation so that its actions will be at least quasi-governmental or its decisions would have to be specifically approved by a government entity so that its decisions will be governmental in their effect. States should have wide latitude in the format for such entities, but they should follow procedures and principles that fulfill all of the requirements listed in these guidelines. Regardless of the manner in which it is organized, the entity must have a professional, well-qualified staff of adequate size. The staff will conduct ongoing activities including gathering and analyzing financial data and providing recommendations on budget approval requests.

    The entity's financing will be through assessments levied by the state legislature on an equitable basis against health care institutions or from general tax revenues. Assessments so levied must be used only for financing the direct and related expenses of the budget review and approval process. The financing, especially during the start-up period, may be augmented by grants from other sources. The cost of any assessment against the health care institution will be includable in its financial requirements.

D. Relationship with the planning process. The plan submitted by each state applying for federal delegation of the budget approval responsibility will include a protocol for the integration of payment regulation with other regulatory mechanisms within the state.

Decisions of the budget approval entity must be reached with the assurance that the health care institution's facilities are adequate and acceptable and do not unnecessarily duplicate other facilities and services within the community. Decisions related to the approved level of payments will be made in accordance with the established planning process and will finance the necessary provisions for changes in services and facilities in the region to achieve more effectiveness.

The entity's decisions should promote long-term efficiency and effective use of resources by facilitating voluntary discontinuation of unneeded services and facilities as approved by the planning process.

In addition, the protocol for the integration of planning regulation with budget review and approval will provide that:

1. The criteria used by the Health Systems Agency and the certificate-of-need agency in the review of the financial feasibility of applications will be jointly developed by the budget approval entity and the certificate-of-need agency.
2. On all applications for certificate-of-need agency approval, that agency will receive and consider financial analyses and economic impact studies provided by the budget approval entity.
3. The certificate-of-need agency's approval of a certificate-of-need application will be binding upon the budget approval entity to recognize the financial requirements associated with the service or facility.

E. Budget review and approval process

1. Grandfathering—At the time of the establishment of the entity and promulgation of its administrative regulations, the charges of all health care institutions than currently offered would be deemed reasonable, adequate, and proper; they will thus be constructively approved by the entity.
2. Budget approval process—Proposed budgets and charges, together with data for their justification, will be submitted by the health care institution within a specified period of notice prior to the beginning of the budget year. The institution could make a request more than 90 days in advance of the proposed effective date, but the notice should not be required to be longer than 90 days. During this notice period, the entity will perform the necessary approval process

and reach a decision on the propriety of the application. In the event that a decision is not announced by the 90th day following such application, the application will be deemed approved and may then be implemented by the institution. Where emergency situations arise under which changes might be needed to maintain the institution's ability to serve the community, the entity may reduce the specified notice period. This will be done under circumstances clearly defined in its regulations and after a prompt review of the institution's reasons for requesting emergency consideration.

In order to simplify the budget review and approval process, the entity will be authorized to permit changes in charges by the health care institution to be filed and implemented without the necessity for the formal hearing process in certain predefined situations, which are likely to be repetitive (such as allowances for routine inflation adjustments). The waiving of the advance notice requirements and the hearing process should apply to routine requests for changes in institutional health care charges when such changes are consistent with the approved budgeted gross and net revenue.

All institutional costs associated with the budget review and approval process will be considered appropriate elements of financial requirements.

3. Public hearing process—When budget applications are filed, the budget approval entity will cause public notices of the application to be given as specified in the entities' regulations. The notice will specify a deadline for filing written comment. In the event of protest, a formal public hearing on the merits of any substantial application may be ordered by the entity. In any case, where the application is being contested, the affected parties will have the right to present related evidence and arguments. The entity will prepare an official record, including testimony and exhibits, in each contested case and will follow appropriate rules of procedure for notice and hearing.

    All evidence, including records and documents in the possession of the agency of which it desires to avail itself, will be offered and made a part of the record in case, and no other factual information or evidence will be considered in the determination of the case. Documentary evidence could be received in the form of copies or excerpts or could be incorporated by reference.

    Whenever in a contested case the majority of the members

of the entity who are to render a final decision have not heard the evidence, the decision will not be made until a proposal for a decision, including findings of fact and conclusions of law, has been served upon the parties. In addition, an opportunity must be afforded to each party adversely affected to file exceptions and present arguments to a majority of the members who are to render the decision. Every decision and order rendered by the entity that is adverse to a party in a contested case will have to be in writing or stated in the record and be accompanied by findings of fact and conclusion of the law. The findings of fact will consist of a concise statement of the conclusions upon each contested issue of fact. A copy of the decision or order and the accompanying findings and conclusions will be delivered or mailed promptly to each party of record.

Any party aggrieved by a final decision in a contested case will be entitled to judicial review. In order to expedite its early determination, a matter under judicial review shall be given priority on the court dockets as a case of public interest. Any legal fees incurred by the institution in the budget review and approval process, as well as the appeals process, are justified elements of an institution's financial requirements. The entity, by regulation, shall provide for interim budgets and charge schedules to be used by the institution while the decision on its application is under judicial review.

IV. Implementation

In the legislation establishing the budget approval entity, there must be provisions for the implementation of the proposal with ample opportunity for the development of sound standards for reporting, criteria and methods for establishing the budget approval procedures, and implementation of the budget approval process. It is vital that deadlines be set as to how long the states have to initiate the entity and have the program become operational. Rather than setting different time spans for each stage of implementation, it is recommended that it be required that the program be enacted by law at the first legislative session subsequent to enactment and be implemented by submission of the plan for federal approval within one year after enactment. This allows flexibility for states in which the timing of the legislature's meetings does not coincide with a specified time period for setting up the entity.

The full implementation of the budget approval process should be approached with due consideration of the importance of developing a sound process as well as meeting the urgency of the timing. In order to achieve this, the need to educate health care institutions about budgets and the budgeting process must be met. While provisions for education are not the duty of the budget approval entity, it is imperative that all involved be aware of the need. This would then allow for the state hospital associations or some other body to fulfill the educational role.

Glossary

Full financial requirements. Full financial requirements, as differentiated from accounting costs, are defined as those resources that are not only necessary to meet current operating needs, but also sufficient to permit replacement of the physical plant when appropriate and to allow for changing community health and patient needs, education and research needs, and all other needs necessary to the institutional provision of health care services that must be recognized and supported by all purchasers of care.

Health care institution. The definition of health care institution as contained in the American Hospital Association's *Classification of Health Care Institutions* is: Establishment with permanent facilities and with medical services for patients, including inpatient care institutions, outpatient care institutions with organized medical staffs and home care institutions.

Independent commission. An independent commission is defined as an entity, established by law, whose sole purpose is the review and approval of budgets for health care institutions. It shall not be a subsidiary of any other agency or entity.

Major third-party payers. Major third-party payers are organized groups or governmental programs that usually pay hospitals directly for the hospital services provided to group members or program beneficiaries.

Oversight. The review of the implementation of a program, on a periodic basis, with specific attention to the regulations being promulgated and their consistency with the enabling legislation.

Parties. Parties are payers, providers, and consumers who have a direct or indirect interest in the activities and pronouncements of the budget approval entity.

Public hearing. A public hearing is an open forum for any member of the public as well as all other parties involved or interested in the budget review and approval process. Such hearings should be governed by the state's Administrative Procedures Act.

Volume changes. Volume changes, for the purpose of this document, are defined as changes in the number of patients treated as well as changes in case mix, intensity, and utilization patterns.

Part III
Working Capital Management

"The value of knowledge lies not in its accumulation but in its utilization."

E. Green

Chapter 9

General Principles

The previous sections have attempted to aid the reader in developing a feeling for the financial environment of a hospital and an understanding of it. The inclusion of this background material was necessary in order to provide a foundation for the following discussion of the financial subsystems of hospitals. The emphasis of this section will be on developing an understanding of the tools and techniques needed to guide and control the operation of these systems. In this chapter and the next we shall examine the general principles of working capital management. In the subsequent chapters, the management and financing of specific sysyems (cash, marketable securities, inventories and accounts receivable) will be discussed.

Introduction

The most appropriate way to begin a discussion of working capital management is to define what is meant by the term "working capital." Historically, there has been substantial disagreement between financial managers, accountants, and economists as to the exact definition of working capital. Some authorities have gone so far as to argue that the term is both misleading and inaccurate and that, in order to avoid confusion, it should not be used at all. However, the majority of authors and practitioners feel that working capital is an acceptable term and have defined it as being the total current assets of the hospital. Working capital, thus, refers to the sum of the hospital's investment in short-term or current assets—cash, marketable (short-term) securities, accounts receivable and inventories.

Net working capital is also a commonly used term. It should be noted, however, that net working capital and working capital are not synonymous. Net working capital is defined as the excess of total current assets over total current liabilities—accounts payable, accrued wages, and any other short-term liabilities. Thus, working capital equals total current assets, and net working capital equals total current assets less total current liabilities.

The important matter, however, is not the definitions of these terms. Certainly, it is necessary to start with an understanding of what is meant by the two terms. The critical question, though, is: What is the importance of working capital management? Why is sound working capital management needed for efficient "least cost" hospital operations?

Importance of Working Capital

In order to understand the importance of working capital management, it is first necessary to realize the significance of working capital to hospital operations. In the vocabulary of financial management, the word "capital" is a synonym for the term "total tangible assets", i.e., the capital of the hospital is equal to the sum of all of its assets. Total assets, in turn, can be classified into basically two categories—fixed or long-term assets, and liquid or current assets. Long-term (fixed) assets include such items as land, plant, equipment, and all other assets which are expected to be held for more than one year. Conversely, current (liquid) assets consist of cash and those other assets which are expected to be converted into cash within one year, e.g., accounts receivable, inventories, and short-term securities.[1]

Fixed assets are obviously needed if patient care services are to be produced. However, fixed assets alone cannot be productive. A hospital building cannot produce patient care. It holds the productive capacity or the potential to produce care, but unless another element or ingredient is combined with fixed assets this potential cannot be realized. Thus, if fixed assets are to be productive they must be combined with another type of asset or capital. Current assets or working capital is the element which must be combined with fixed assets if their productive potential is to be achieved.

---

[1]Deferred charges (prepaid expense) are not in the process of being converted into cash and, therefore, are not included in current assets. In normal operations, they are included as a separate item on the balance sheet and are periodically written off as expenses.

Working capital can be viewed as the catalyst which changes the productive potential of fixed assets into patient care services. Working capital, though it has no innate patient care potential of its own, is the means of converting buildings and equipment into patient care services. The obvious question, however, is how does working capital accomplish this? How is working capital able to make fixed assets productive?

In order to simplify the answer to these questions, it is helpful to view working capital as consisting just of cash. This view, while admittedly different from the foregoing definition, is not entirely unrealistic, for the other components of working capital (accounts receivable, inventories, and short-term investment) are just steps in the cash conversion process or cash cycle.

Figure 9-1 illustrates the cash cycle. If a wholesale firm is used as an example, it is relatively easy to visualize the steps in this cycle.

This example is quite simplified, nevertheless, it does illustrate both the cash cycle and the basic "cash" nature of working capital. Admittedly, as part of the productive process, working capital is converted into assets other than cash. However working capital begins and ends as cash and thus, at least for purposes of explaining its importance, can be viewed as cash.

Viewing working capital as cash, it is relatively simple to see how working capital is able to activate or bring out the productive potential of fixed assets. As cash, working capital can be used both to obtain and retain the factors of production which are necessary to make fixed assets productive. Cash can be used to obtain nurses, raw food, drugs, and all the other items which are needed if patient care is to be provided. Without working capital a hospital is just bricks, mortar, and metal. With working capital, it is a dynamic, productive community resource. Therefore, working capital is important, for it is a vital and necessary element in the production of patient services.

Importance of Working Capital Management

Given that working capital is necessary for hospital operations, it follows quite reasonably that management should devote some of its energies to the administration of that resource. However, because of the impact which working capital management, or lack of management, can have on costs, credit standing, financial solvency, and even the continued existence of the hospital, it is par-

Figure 9-1

Cash Cycle

(STEPS 1 & 4)

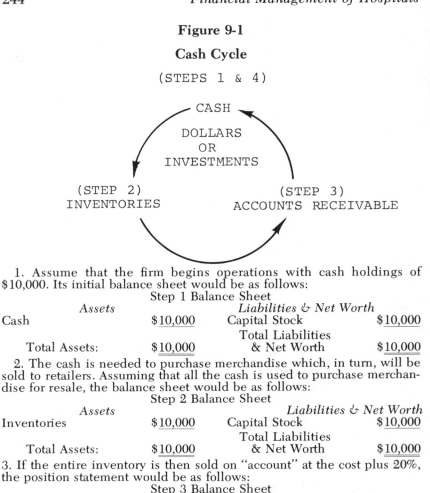

1. Assume that the firm begins operations with cash holdings of $10,000. Its initial balance sheet would be as follows:

Step 1 Balance Sheet

Assets		*Liabilities & Net Worth*	
Cash	$10,000	Capital Stock	$10,000
		Total Liabilities	
Total Assets:	$10,000	& Net Worth	$10,000

2. The cash is needed to purchase merchandise which, in turn, will be sold to retailers. Assuming that all the cash is used to purchase merchandise for resale, the balance sheet would be as follows:

Step 2 Balance Sheet

Assets		*Liabilities & Net Worth*	
Inventories	$10,000	Capital Stock	$10,000
		Total Liabilities	
Total Assets:	$10,000	& Net Worth	$10,000

3. If the entire inventory is then sold on "account" at the cost plus 20%, the position statement would be as follows:

Step 3 Balance Sheet

Assets		*Liabilities & Net Worth*	
Accounts Receivable	$12,000	Capital Stock	$10,000
		Retained Earnings	2,000
		Total Liabilities	
Total Assets:	$12,000	& Net Worth:	$12,000

4. The accounts receivable are all paid and the firm receives $12,000 in cash. However, management does not feel that it is necessary to hold all $12,000 in cash and, therefore, it invests $2,000 in short-term securities which readily can be converted back to cash. The balance sheet at the completion of these transactions would be as follows:

Step 4 Balance Sheet

Assets		*Liabilities & Net Worth*	
Cash	$10,000	Capital Stock	$10,000
Short-term Invest-		Retained Earnings	2,000
ments	2,000	Total Liabilities	
Total Assets:	$12,000	& Net Worth	$12,000

ticularly important that management carefully administer working capital.

Working capital management can be defined as the administration of both current assets and the liabilities incurred in order to finance or obtain those assets. This definition is broader in scope than the previous definition of working capital, for it includes both assets and liabilities. This broadening is necessary, however, because of the interdependence of assets and liabilities and the need to consider both factors if assets are to be properly managed.

This matter of interdependence may be somewhat confusing and should be clarified before proceeding. Liabilities (including equity) are the sources of funds used to obtain assets. For example, assume that a hospital purchases, on credit, drugs at a cost of $10,000. If this were the only transaction, the hospital's simplified balance sheet would be as follows:

Balance Sheet—After Drug Purchase

Assets	
Inventory—Drugs	$10,000
Total Assets:	$10,000

Liabilities	
Accounts Payable	
Drug Mfg.	$10,000
Total Liabilities	$10,000

The hospital has obtained an asset (inventory) but has also obligated itself to a liability (account payable) of the same amount. The account payable, therefore, has in effect financed or supplied the immediate funds needed to purchase the drugs. Obviously, at some point the account will have to be paid. For the moment, however, it is the source of financing and decisions in regard to the asset must also take into consideration the effect of the source of financing on the financial position of the hospital. Thus, if management is to properly administer current assets, it must consider not only the assets, but also the methods and alternative sources available for financing those assets.

The following chapters will discuss the management of current assets and liabilities in detail. However, in order to place this material in proper perspective, it is advantageous to consider first the cost minimizing potential of working capital management.

Quantity of Working Capital

It is axiomatic that if the total cost to the community of patient care is to be minimized, then the cost of working capital must also be minimized. In order to accomplish this, management must control two interrelated factors. It must determine both the level or quantity of assets and the proper asset financing combination so that these two factors, when taken together, will result in working capital costs being held to a minimum. Since this is a two-part problem, let us consider in this chapter the quantity aspect and in the next chapter the matter of financing current assets.

Perhaps the simplest approach to understanding how the level of working capital is determined is to return to the notion of working capital being cash. With this notion in mind, consider Figure 9-2.

Figure 9-2 pictures, in a rather elementary manner, two cash flow streams—a cash inflow stream and a cash outflow stream. The cash inflow stream represents the flow of cash payments to the hospital in return for services rendered. It can be viewed as consisting of two components: a production cycle and an accounts receivable cycle. The timing of cash inflows, i.e., the length of time between the initial production of a service and receipt of payment for that service, are hence a function of (1) how long it takes to produce the service (production cycle) and (2) how long it takes to receive payment for the service after it is produced (accounts receivable cycle). In this example, the cash inflow stream is assumed to consist of a production cycle of seven days and an accounts receivable cycle of 21 days. That is, the average length of stay is assumed to be seven days and the average delay in payment from the time the bill for services is submitted to the time the payment is received is assumed to be 21 days. Therefore, the timing of the cash inflow is 28 days.[2]

In addition to the cash inflow stream, the cash outflow stream must also be considered in determining the quantity of working capital. This is due to the fact that the minimum level of working capital which a hospital needs is equal to the difference between its initial cash inflow and outflow streams. The cash outflow stream represents the flow of payments which the hospital must

---

[2]Patient arrives on day 1 and stays until day 7. Therefore, the production cycle is 7 days. The bill for services is submitted on the day of discharge. Therefore, day 7 is the last day of the production cycle and day 8 is the first day of the accounts receivable cycle. If the accounts receivable cycle is assumed to be 21 days, then the sum of the two cycles is 28 days.

make in order to obtain labor, supplies, and other items needed to produce services. As was the previous case, it can also be viewed as consisting of two basic components: a salary payment cycle and a supplies payment cycle. The salary payment cycle represents the time period involved between salary payments. The supplies payment cycle represents the time period elapsed between the receipt of supplies and the payment for those supplies. In this example, for the sake of simplicity, it is assumed that salaries are paid biweekly and that supplies are paid for 28 days after receipt. Therefore, in a single cash inflow cycle (28 days) salaries are paid twice and supply expenses are paid once.

In the initial 28 day period there will be three cash outflow items. Offsetting these outflows will be one cash inflow. Due to the length of the production and accounts receivable cycles, on the 28th day the fees for the first seven days of production, i.e., for those patients entering the hospital on Day 1 and discharged on Day 7, will be received. Therefore, in the example 28 day period, the hospital (assuming charges are equal to costs) will receive payments equal to seven days' costs, but must make payments equal to 28 days' costs.[3]

Obviously, there is an imbalance existing here. Revenues equal to seven days' costs cannot possibly pay for the costs of 28 days of operation. Therefore, funds from some source other than revenues must be used to pay the costs which cannot be offset by the initial cash inflow stream. This "other source" of funds is the working capital or cash which the hospital must have available if it is to be able to meet its obligations and continue to operate until it achieves a self-sustaining position.

The amount of cash, or the quantity of working capital, which must be held is a function of the timing and amount of cash inflows and outflows. At a minimum, it is equal to the difference between the cash inflows received and the cash outflows paid during the initial cash inflow or, if it is longer, outflow cycle. Expressed algebraically, the minimum quantity of working capital which must be held is equal to $CO_j - CI_j$ where CO_j equals the cash outflows in period j, CI_j equals the cash inflows in period j, and period j equals the time period necessary to complete either a

---

[3]Again, for the sake of simplicity, assume that the term "costs" refers only to labor and supplies cost. Admittedly, there are other cost factors. However, inclusion of these other factors will not change the conclusions reached, but will greatly complicate the explanation. Therefore, it seems advantageous at this point to ignore these factors.

Figure 9-2

Quantity of Working Capital

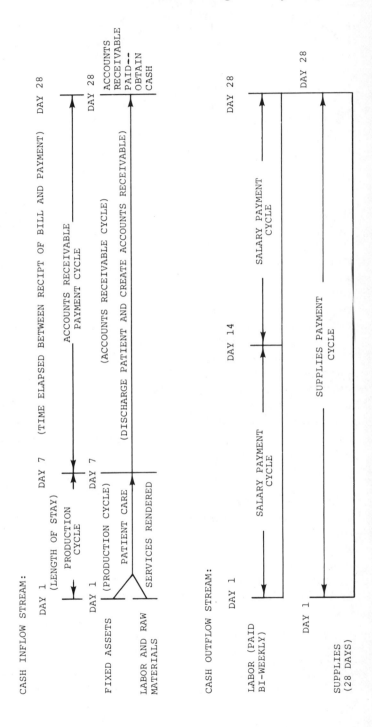

single cash inflow cycle or, if it is longer, a single cash outflow cycle, i.e.,[4]

$$CO_j - CI_j = \text{Minimum Quantity of Working Capital.}$$

This same concept can be illustrated in a somewhat different manner through the use of Table 9-1 and Figure 9-3. Table 9-1 is is based on the cycle timing assumption set out in Figure 9-2 and the following costs:

Cash outflows–
    salary cycles (2 cycles at $10,000) each=$20,000
    supplies cycle   =$ 2,000
                                $CO_j = \$22,000$

Cash inflows–
    cash receipts on the 28th day   =$5,500 $CI_j = \$5,500$

Using the formula described above, the quantity of working capital or the initial cash reserve which the hospital needs in order to be able to meet its cash outflows and attain a self-sufficient financial position is $16,500, i.e.,

    Quantity of Working Capital $= CO_j - CI_j$
                                    $= \$22,000 - \$5,500$
    Quantity of Working Capital $= \$16,500$

As can be seen from Table 9-1, if the hospital has an initial working capital investment of $16,500 it is able to meet all of its obligations.[5] The initial working capital investment acts as a pool or reservoir of funds which can be drawn upon, along with the cash inflows, to pay cash outflows. Figure 9-4 illustrates the reservoir conceptualization of working capital. Cash inflows of $5,500 are combined with a $16,500 reservoir of working capital to enable the hospital to pay costs of $22,000.

Figure 9-4 also illustrates how the timing and amount of cash inflows and outflows determine the level of the reservoir, i.e., the quantity of working capital which is needed. As can be seen from the figure, as cash inflows increase less working capital is needed.

---

[4]At this point the matter of uncertainty has not been considered. However, if the minimum quantity of working capital is to be determined accurately and realistically, the problem of uncertainty in regard to the timing and amount of cash inflows cannot be ignored. In the following chapters this matter will be discussed further.

[5]If volume or cost changes result in the absolute amount of cash inflows and outflows, changing then the quantity of working capital needed to achieve a self-sufficient financial position will also change at a corresponding rate. For example, if volume were to double causing labor expenses to increase to $40,000 and supplies expenses to increase to $4,000, then, all other factors being equal, the minimum quantity of working capital would also double to $33,000.

Figure 9-3

Quantity of Working Capital

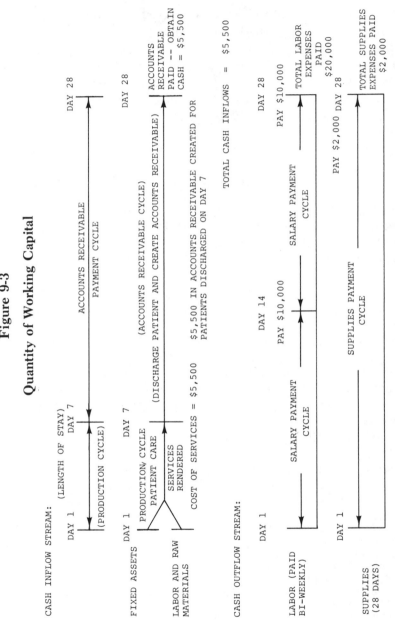

Table 9-1

Quantity of Working Capital

Day of Position Statement	Balance Sheet			Expenses
Day 0	Current Assets Cash =	$16,500	Current Liabilities Net Worth = $16,500	
Day 1	Cash = Inv. = Total:	$16,500 2,000 $18,500	Accts. Pay. = $ 2,000 Net Worth = $16,500 Total: $18,500	
Day 14	Cash = Inv. = Accts. Rec. = Total:	$ 6,500 1,000 11,000 $18,500	Accts. Pay. = $ 2,000 Net Worth = 16,500 Total: $18,500	Salaries = $10,000
Day 28	Cash = Inv. = Accts. Rec. = Total:	$ 0 0 16,500 $16,500	Accts. Pay. = $ 0 Net Worth = 16,500 Total: $16,500	Salaries = $10,000 Supplies* = $2,000
Day 35	Cash = Inv. = Accts. Rec. = Total:	$ 5,500 1,500 16,500 $23,500	Accts. Pay. = $ 2,000 Accrued Salaries = 5,000 Net Worth = 16,500 Total: $23,500	
Day 42	Cash = Inv. = Accts. Rec. = Total:	$ 1,000 1,000 16,500 $18,500	Accts. Pay. = $ 2,000 Net Worth = 16,500 Total: $18,500	Salaries = $10,000
Day 49	Cash = Inv. = Accts. Rec. = Total:	6,500 500 16,500 $23,500	Accts. Pay. = $ 2,000 Accrued Salaries = 5,000 Net Worth = 16,500 Total: $23,500	
Day 56	Cash = Inv. = Accts. Rec. = Total:	$ 0 0 16,500 $16,500	Accts. Pay. = $ 0 Net Worth = 16,500 Total: $16,500	Salaries = $10,000 Supplies = $2,000
Day N	Cash =	$16,500	Net Worth = $16,500	

Cash Receipts and Working Capital		Cash Outflows:	
Cash Inflows—Days 1–28	$ 5,500	Supplies	$ 2,000
Initial Working Capital =	16,500	Salaries	20,000
Total:	$22,500	Total	$22,000

*Attain financial self-sufficiency, i.e., cash inflows will equal outflows for any given period of "j" length.

Figure 9-5

Quantity of Working Capital

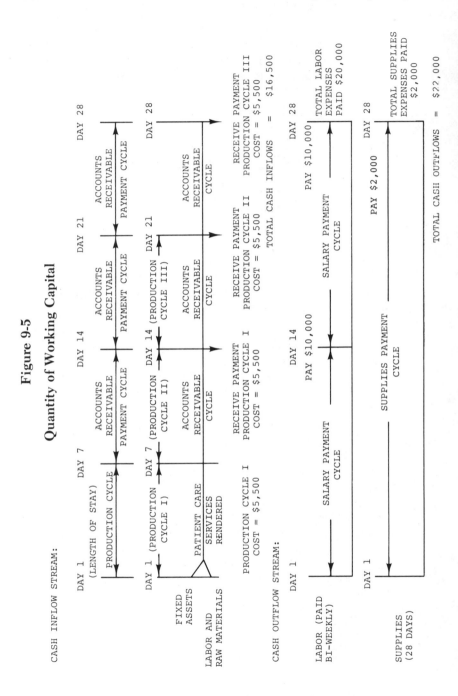

Figure 9-4
Working Capital Reservoir

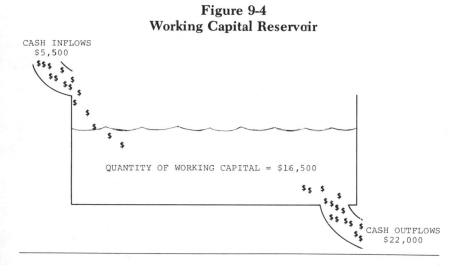

Conversely, as cash outflows increase more working capital is needed. Table 9-1 describes in numerical terms the effect which the iming of inflows and outflows can have on the quantity of working capital.

Table 9-2 and Figure 9-5 are based, with one exception, on the same cost and timing assumptions as were used in Table 9-1. The single exception is in regard to the timing of the accounts receivable cycle. In Table 9-1 the accounts receivable cycle was assumed to be 21 days. However, for purposes of Table 9-2, it is assumed that the cycle is accelerated from 21 days to 7 days. That is, the time period between patient discharge and patient payment is accelerated or shortened from 21 days to only 7 days.

Based upon these assumptions, in a single (28 day) cash outflow cycle, expenses, as was the previous case, will be $22,000. However, cash receipts for the same period will be greater than the $5,500 of the previous example. Due to the acceleration of the accounts receivable cycle, three cash inflows instead of only one will be available to offset cash outflows. Cash receipts of $5,500 will be received on the 14th, 21st and 28th days. Therefore, as is indicated in the table, receipts will be $16,500, payments will be $22,000, and $5,500 in initial working capital will be needed; i.e., CO_j =$22,000, CI_j =$16,500, and$_j$ =28 days:[6]

Quantity of Working Capital = $CO_j - CI_j$
Quantity of Working Capital = $22,000 - $16,500
Quantity of Working Capital = $5,500

---

[6]It should be noted, that since the cash outflow cycle is longer than the cash inflow cycle, that period is equal to the length of the cash outflow cycle—28 days.

Table 9-2

Quantity of Working Capital—Timing Factors

Day of Position Statement	Balance Sheet				Expenses
	Current Assets		Current Liabilities		
Day 0	Cash =	$ 5,500	Net Worth =	$ 5,500	
Day 1	Cash =	$ 5,500	Accts. Pay. =	$ 2,000	
	Inventories =	2,000	Net Worth =	5,500	
	Total:	$ 7,500	Total:	$ 7,500	
Day 7	Cash =	$ 5,500	Accts. Pay. =	$ 2,000	
	Accts. Rec. =	5,500	Accrued Salaries =	5,000	
	Inventories =	1,500	Net Worth =	5,500	
	Total:	$12,500	Total:	$12,500	
Day 14	Cash =	$ 1,000	Accts. Pay. =	$ 2,000	Salaries =
	Accts. Rec. =	5,500	Net Worth =	5,500	$10,000
	Inventories =	1,000			
	Total:	$ 7,500	Total:	$ 7,500	
Day 21	Cash =	$ 6,500	Accts. Pay. =	$ 2,000	
	Accts. Rec. =	5,500	Accrued Salaries =	5,000	
	Inventories =	500	Net Worth =	5,500	
	Total:	$12,500	Total:	$12,500	
Day 28	Cash =	$ 0	Accts. Pay. =	$ 0	Salaries =
	Accts. Rec. =	$ 5,500	Net Worth =	$ 5,500	$10,000
	Inventories =	$ 0			Supplies =
	Total:	$ 5,500	Total:	$ 5,500	$ 2,000
Day 35	Cash =	$ 5,500	Accts. Pay.	$ 2,000	
	Accts. Rec. =	5,500	Accrued Salaries =	5,000	
	Inventories =	1,500	Net Worth =	5,500	
	Total:	$12,500	Total:	$12,500	

Cash Receipts and Working Capital		Cash Outflows	
Cash Inflows	=$16,500	Supplies	$ 2,000
Initial Working Capital	= 5,500	Salaries	20,000
Total:	$22,000	Total:	$22,000

*Attain financial self-sufficiency; i.e., cash inflows will equal outflows for any given period of "j" length.

Accelerating the timing of the accounts receivable cycle thus, results in a reduction in the amount of working capital which is needed in order to attain a self-sustaining financial position. This is a critical point which should be kept in mind, for it will be referred to again later in the text. The question which still must be answered, however, is how does the quantity of working capital affect operating costs? What is the cost of working capital and how can this cost be minimized?

Working Capital and Operational Results

The relationship between the level of working capital and operational results can be seen clearly in the case of a manufacturing firm or any other commercial enterprise. Assume that both the absolute amount and the efficiency of managing accounts receivable and inventories are held constant and that the other current assets of the firm, cash and short-term investments, yield a lower return (profit) than that obtained on the firm's investment in fixed assets (land, buildings, and equipment). It is reasonable to make this last assumption, for cash earns nothing and if short-term investments earned more than fixed assets. then the firm should be in the marketable securities business instead of manufacturing.

Given these assumptions, management, in order to maximize profit and owner's wealth, must minimize the proportion of current assets to total assets. The more assets which can be channeled from current to fixed assets, with their higher rate of return relative to current assets, the greater will be the total profits of the firm. Table 9-3 illustrates this point numerically.

Investment in working capital thus represents an opportunity cost to the firm which is equal to the return lost by investing in current assets as opposed to fixed assets. The greater the quantity of working capital relative to total assets, the greater is this cost. Therefore, in order to both minimize the opportunity cost of working capital and maximize profits, management should attempt to reduce, as much as is feasible, the proportion of current assets to total assets.

The relationship of the level of working capital to operational results is somewhat more abstruse in the case of the hospital, for rates of return on various hospital investments are more difficult, if not impossible, to calculate. Nevertheless, it can be argued, at least on a subjective basis, that the rate of return on a patient service program on a lifesaving piece of equipment, or on just a piece of equipment which makes a patient more comfortable, is greater than that which could be obtained from an investment in

Table 9-3

Cost of Working Capital—Manufacturing Enterprise

Assume the following rates of return:

Cash	=	0%
Short-Term Investments	=	5%
Fixed Assets	=	10%

Case 1

Allocation of Assets		Returns
Cash	$ 100,000	$ 0
Short-Term Investments	$ 150,000	$ 7,500
Fixed Assets	$ 750,000	$75,000
	$1,000,000	$82,500

Case 2—Assume that assets ($150,000) are channeled from current assets—short-term investments—to fixed assets.

Allocation of assets		Returns
Cash	$ 100,000	$ 0
Short-Term Investments	$ 0	$ 0
Fixed Assets	$ 900,000	$90,000
	$1,000,000	$90,000

Conclusion:
The lower the proportion of current assets (working capital) to total assets, the greater is the firm's return on total investment.

cash or short-term securities. If this is the case, management should attempt to minimize the relative proportion of assets invested in working capital (cash and short-term investments) in order to maximize the return to the owner, i.e., the community.

The relationship of the quantity of working capital to operational results can also be viewed in another manner which may be somewhat easier to visualize. In this case, the matter of concern is the effect of the level of working capital on the costs which have to be borne by patients. In order to understand how the quantity of working capital affects the amount of costs which have to be borne by patients, it is necessary to view costs as net costs. That is, the costs borne by patients are equal to operating costs less nonoperating revenues. The costs of care borne by patients thus vary inversely with nonoperating revenues, i.e., as the amount of nonoperating revenues increases, the amount of revenues which have to be obtained from patients—the cost of care borne by patients—decreases.

This view of costs is not entirely contrived. As was discussed in previous chapters, third party payers offset nonoperating revenues against operating costs in order to determine the basis for computing reimbursable costs. Also, hospitals generally base their charge structure on the difference between their total revenue needs and the sum of both nonoperating revenues and revenues obtained from third party payers. Thus, in reality, the cost of care borne by patients is determined, at least in part, by the nonoperating revenues of the hospital.

Given this view of costs, consider once again the example described in Tables 9-1 and 9-2. With these examples in mind, assume that a hospital originally had $16,000 invested in working capital, but that it changed its credit and collection policies so that only $5,500 is now needed. If this were the case, there would be a cash surplus of $11,000. This cash would no longer be needed for day-to-day operations and therefore could be invested in revenue-generating securities. Assuming that it were invested in long-term corporate bonds earning 8%, this cash surplus would return an annual nonoperating revenue of $880.

Admittedly, $880 is not a great deal of money. However, it is sufficient to illustrate the point. A reduction in the quantity of working capital has enabled management to invest former working capital funds in revenue-gathering securities. These securities yield a nonoperating revenue which can be used to reduce the cost of care borne by patients. Eight hundred and eighty dollars is now available to meet operating costs which previously had to be met through funds provided by patients. Thus, by reducing the quantity of working capital, management is able to reduce the cost of care borne by patients.[7] Table 9-4 numerically illustrates this process.

As was the case with the commercial enterprise, investment in working capital represents an opportunity cost to the hospital. This cost is equal to the rate of return which could have been achieved if the hospital's working capital investment were reduced and the excess funds were invested in other assets. The greater the quantity of unnecessary or excessive working capital, the greater is this opportunity cost. Thus, in order to reduce the

---

[7] It should be noted that if the $11,000 had been invested in capital equipment instead of securities, the cost of care borne by patients would still be reduced. In this instance, the hospital would not have to build as much of a premium into the patient's bill for capital equipment. Thus, the patient's bill would be less.

Table 9-4

Working Capital and Cost of Care Borne by Patients

Assume: 1. Operating Costs = $100,000/year
           2. Working Capital Investment
              Original   =$16,500
              Improved Management   =$ 5,500
           3. Assets for Investment
              Original   =$ 0
              Improved Management = $11,000 (surplus funds
                                            created due to
                                            the decrease in
                                            working capital
                                            investment)
           4. Nonoperating Revenue
              Original   =$ 0
              Improved Management   =$ 880
              ($11,000 invested at 8%)

	Original Example	Improved Management Example
Operating Costs	$100,000	$100,000
Nonoperating Revenue	0	– 880
Cost of Care Borne By Patients	$100,000	$999,120

Conclusion:
A reduction in the cost of care borne by patients can be achieved by reducing the necessary quantity of working capital and investing the surplus funds in revenue-generating securities.

cost of care borne by patients, management must minimize the working capital investment of the hospital.

As has been seen in the above example, the quantity of working capital can be reduced if cash inflows are accelerated. Also, as will be discussed later, the quantity of working capital can be reduced by decelerating cash outflows. Therefore, if management is to reduce the cost of care borne by patients, it must minimize the quantity of working capital by accelerating cash inflows and/or decelerating cash outflows.

Conclusion

A word of caution should be expressed at this point. It should be clear now that the cost of care cannot be minimized if the hospital has an excessive amount of working capital. The operational rule or guideline which has been set out is that management should attempt to minimize the hospital's investment in working capital. However, this does not mean that the hospital should have a zero working capital investment. Just as too much working capital prohibits least-cost operation, too little can result in additional costs from not only such factors as having to borrow at inopportune times or having to forego purchase discounts, but also may result in insolvency and even—in the extreme—failure. Thus, management should strive not for the minimal, but rather the optimal quantity of working capital, i.e., that quantity which is sufficient but not excessive.

The following chapters will discuss the techniques for determining the optimal investment for each of the components of working capital. Given these techniques, the reader will be familiar with the tools needed to optimize the total quantity of working capital and minimize costs.

Suggested Readings

Beranek, William. *Working Capital Management*, Chapters 1,2.

Cleverly, William O. *Financial Management of Health Care Facilities*, Chapter 8.

Dewing, Arthur S. *The Financial Policy of Corporations*, Chapter 23.

Knight, W.D. "Working Capital Management—Satisfactory Versus Optimizing." *Financial Managment*, Spring 1972, pp. 33–40.

Lindsay, J. Robert and Sametz, Arnold W. *Financial Management, An Analytical Approach*, Chapter 3.

Weston, J. Fred and Brigham, Eugene F. *Managerial Finance*, pp. 439–445.

Chapter 10
Financing Working Capital

As has been discussed in the previous chapter, working capital management, by definition, is a two-part problem. In order to minimize the cost of working capital, administration must determine not only the proper level or quantity of assets, but also the proper asset financing combination. The foregoing chapter has examined the quantity aspect of the problem, or the relationship between the quantity of working capital and the cost of working capital. Therefore, this chapter will be addressed to the matter of financing working capital.

Source of Funds

Working capital can be financed from two basic sources of funds—equity and/or debt. Equity is the "owner's" investment in the hospital. It is the funds provided or contributed by the community both to obtain the hospital's physical plant and facilities and also to prime its operational pump, i.e., provide the initial working capital needed to sustain operations until the hospital reaches a self-sustaining position. Table 10-1 illustrates the manner by which equity can be used to finance working capital. The specific role of equity as a source of financing will be discussed below. For the moment, it should just be noted that equity is the owner's permanent investment in the hospital which can only be repaid or returned if the assets of the hospital are liquidated (see Table 10-1).

In addition to, or in place of, equity, debt can be used to finance working capital. Debt can be viewed as a temporary investment in, or loan to, the hospital which must be repaid. If the loan matures, or must be repaid within a year, the debt is considered to be short-term. If the period until payment is greater than one year,

Table 10-1

Working Capital Financing—Equity

Assumptions:

1. The community donates $3,500,000 to be used for the creation of Philanthrophy Memorial Hospital.
2. A 100 bed hospital is constructed at a cost of $3,000,000.

Balance Sheet 1
As of End of Construction.*

Assets		Liabilities and Net Worth	
Current Assets		Current Liabilities	$ 0
Cash	$ 500,000		
Fixed Assets		Net Worth	
Building and Equipment	$3,000,000	Owner's Equity	$3,500,000
Total:	$3,500,000	Total:	$3,500,000

*The $3,500,000 investment has been used to build and equip the building and provide working capital of $500,000. This $500,000 is needed to pay wages, supplies, and other expenses until that time when cash inflows become sufficient to meet cash outflows. Thus, the balance sheet after several months of operation may be as follows:

Balance Sheet 2
As of Several Months of Operation**

Assets		Liabilities and Net Worth	
Current Assets		Current Liabilities	
Cash	$ 100,000	Accounts Payable	$ 100,000
Accounts Receivable	$ 400,000	Net Worth	
Inventories	$ 100,000	Owner's Equity	$3,500,000
Fixed Assets			
Building & Equipment	$3,000,000		
Total:	$3,600,000	Total:	$3,600,000

**As is illustrated by balance sheet 2, the $500,000 in cash which was financed through owner's equity has been used to pay operating expenses and is represented by the cash of $100,000, and the accounts receivable of $400,000. As these accounts receivable are paid, the hospital should achieve a self-sustaining position.

the debt is generally categorized as long-term. The significance of the timing of debt maturity and its relationship to the cost of working capital will be discussed at a later point. Table 10-2 illustrates the manner by which debt can be used to finance working capital.

Table 10-2

Working Capital Financing—Debt

Assume the same situation as was described in Table 10-1 with the only difference being that $3,000,000 instead of $3,500,000 was contributed. Given these assumptions, balance sheet 1 would appear as follows:

Balance Sheet 1
As of End of Construction*

Assets			Liabilities and Net Worth		
Current Assets	$	0	Current Liabilities	$	0
Fixed Assets			Net Worth		
Building & Equipment	3,000,000		Owner's Equity	3,000,000	
Total:	$3,000,000		Total:	$3,000,000	

*The $3,000,000 has been used to build and equip the hospital. However, no funds are available to finance the working capital which is needed if the hospital is to actually operate. Therefore, assume that $500,000 is borrowed in order to finance working capital. The balance sheet, as of the first day of operations, would be as follows:

Balance Sheet 2
As of First Day of Operation**

Assets		Liabilities and Net Worth	
Current Assets		Current Liabilities	$ 0
Cash	$ 500,000	Long-Term Liabilities	500,000
Fixed Assets		Net Worth	
Building & Equipment	3,000,000	Owner's Equity	3,000,000
Total:	$3,500,000	Total:	$3,500,000

**The $500,000 is needed to pay wages, supplies and other expenses until that time when cash inflows become sufficient to meet cash outflows. Thus, the position after several months of operation may be as follows:

Position Statement 3
As of Several Months of Operation***

Assets		Liabilities and Net Worth	
Current Assets		Current Liabilities	
Cash	$ 100,000	Accounts Payable	$ 100,000
Accounts Receivable	400,000		
Inventories	100,000	Long-Term Liabilities	500,000
Fixed Assets		Net Worth	
Building & Equipment	3,000,000	Owner's Equity	3,000,000
Total:	$3,600,000	Total:	$3,600,000

***As is illustrated by balance sheet 3, the $500,000 in cash which was financed through long-term debt, has been used to pay operating expenses and is represented by the cash of $100,000 and accounts receivable of $400,000. As these accounts receivable are paid, the hospital should achieve a self-sustaining position.

Accounts Payable

It is also possible to finance working capital through the use of accounts payable or "trade credit." Technically, an account payable is a form of short-term debt. Accounts payable are debt obligations which arise out of the regular course of operational transactions—as opposed to being financial transactions such as the negotiation of a loan—and which must be repaid within a year. Normally, a buyer receives and uses goods before he is required to pay for them. This procedure represents the extension of trade credit by the seller and is reflected in the records of the buyer as an account payable.

Recall, for a moment, the example which was described in Table 9-1 of the previous chapter. In that example, it was assumed that in a single cash inflow cycle of 28 days, salaries of $20,000 were paid, supplies expenses of $2,000 were paid, and that $16,500 in initial working capital and $5,500 in cash inflows were needed in order to pay these expenses. However, if the timing of the supplies cycle changes, so that the payment for supplies is due in 56 days instead of 28, the initial working capital needs of the hospital also change. This situation is illustrated in Tables 10-3 and 10-4.

As is obvious from the tables, the extension of the due date for paying for supplies resulted in initial working capital needs decreasing by $2,000. However, under either set of assumptions, $22,000 in labor and supplies was needed during the 28 day period. Thus, if less initial working capital was needed under the second set of assumptions, financing or support from some other source, equal to $2,000, must have been obtained. As should be apparent from the example, the other source of support was the supplier who extended the payment period to 56 days, i.e., extended trade credit of 56 days. The extension of the payment period, therefore, is in effect a 56 day, $2,000 loan to the hospital.

The 56 day loan is a monetary obligation or liability of the hospital and should be reflected in the current liabilities section of the hospital's position statement as an account payable. Thus, through the use of accounts payable the hospital was able to support its cash outflows with less of its own cash. Accounts payable, therefore, have financed or supplied part of the hospital's working capital needs.

At first glance, this approach to financing working capital appears to be ideal. Through the use of accounts payable, the example hospital has been able to finance its working capital re-

Table 10-3

Effect of Timing of the Supplies Cycle on Initial Working Capital Needs

Original Assumption: (See Table 9-1)

Salaries Expense of $10,000 due 14th and 28th day	= $20,000	
Supplies Expense of $2,000 due 28th day	= $ 2,000	
Cash Outflows	= $22,000 = CO_j	

Cash Receipts on the 28th day	= $ 5,500	
Cash Inflows	= $ 5,500 = CI_j	
Quantity of Working Capital	= CO_j–CI_j	
	= $22,000–$5,500	
	= $16,500	

Chapter 10 Assumptions:

Salaries Expense of $10,000 due 14th, 28th, 42nd and 56th day	= $40,000
Supplies Expense of $2,000 due 56th day	= $ 2,000
Cash Outflow	= $42,000 = CO_j

Cash Receipts on the 28th, 35th, 42nd, 49th and 56th day	= $27,500
Cash Inflows	= $27,500 = CI_j
Quantity of Working Capital	= CO –CI
	= $42,000–$27,500
	= $14,500

quirements with less of its own funds. It would thus seem reasonable that the hospital should take advantage of trade credit whenever it is offered, i.e., incur an account payable whenever possible, for it provides the mechanism by which the hospital can reduce its investment in working capital and thereby free assets for investment in other areas. The decision rule, however, is not as clear-cut as the foregoing statement would lead one to believe.

Cost of Accounts Payable

Suppliers of goods realize that when they offer trade credit they are actually offering a loan. Additionally, they are aware of the fact that the granting of such a loan involves a cost to them, either in terms of an opportunity cost equal to the earnings which could have been obtained by using the loaned funds in some other manner, or an out-of-pocket cost equal to the interest expenses which have to be paid to some other source in order to obtain the funds needed to support the loan. Thus, suppliers are neither able nor inclined to provide trade credit for free and also realize that it is inconvenient, if not impossible, both for themselves and purchasers, to require cash payments. Therefore, they have adopted a compromise approach which allows for a variable price arrangement. That is, for the sake of convenience and business practicality, trade credit is offered for a limited period at no explicit cost.[1] Beyond the grace period, an explicit charge is made to the purchaser for the use of the credit.

The mechanism which is used to affect this variable price arrangement is one of selling on "terms" which allow for a purchase discount if payment is made within a specified time period. The exact nature of the sales terms which are offered varies with industry convention and the financial needs of the seller. Generally, terms are set at 2-10, net 30.

Terms of 2-10, net 30 mean that if a hospital pays for a purchase within 10 days of the date of invoice (the discount period) that the price of the purchased goods can be discounted or reduced by two percent. Thus, if a $100 purchase is made and paid for within 10 days, the hospital only has to pay $98 for the purchased goods. If the purchase is not paid for within 10 days, then the hospital has to pay $100 by the 30th day—the due date or the end of the net period.

The use of the foregoing sales arrangement means that the hospital is actually being offered the opportunity to purchase two different items. Obviously, it is purchasing goods. Additionally, if it does not exercise its option of paying within the discount period, it is purchasing credit. The purchase of credit, however, has a cost. Therefore, if a hospital is to minimize its costs, it should not incur the cost of trade credit unless it is the least cost credit or financing alternative.

Assuming that a $100 purchase is made and terms of 2-10, net 30 are offered, the cost of trade credit is $2.00 for the use of $98.00 for a 20 day period. On an annual basis, since there are approximately 18 twenty-day periods in a year, the cost of credit in percentage terms is 18 times $2.00 over the amount of money ($98.00) which

---

[1]As has been indicated, trade credit has a cost to the supplier. However, offering credit for at least a limited period is a necessary part of business and, therefore, represents a normal business cost which should be included in establishing the purchase price, as opposed to being set out as an additional explicit factor.

Table 10-4

Quantity of Working Capital

Day of Position Statement	Balance Sheet				
	Current Assets		*Current Liabilities*		
Day 0	Cash =	$14,500	Net Worth =	$14,500	
Day 1	Cash =	$14,500	Accts. Pay. =	$ 2,000	
	Inv. =	2,000	Net Worth =	14,500	
	Total:	$16,500	Total:	$16,500	
Day 14	Cash =	$ 4,500	Accts. Pay. =	$ 2,000	Salaries =
	Inv. =	1,000	Net Worth =	14,500	$10,000
	Accts. Rec. =	11,000			
	Total:	$16,500	Total:	$16,500	
Day 28	Cash =	$ 0	Accts. Pay. =	$ 2,000	Salaries =
	Inv. =	0	Net Worth =	14,500	$10,000
	Accts. Rec. =	16,500			
	Total:	$16,500	Total:	$16,500	
Day 35	Cash =	$ 5,500	Accts. Pay. =	$ 4,000	
	Inv. =	1,500	Accrued Salaries =	5,000	
	Accts. Rec. =	16,500	Net Worth =	14,500	
	Total:	$23,500	Total:	$23,500	
Day 42	Cash =	$ 1,000	Accts. Pay. =	$ 4,000	Salaries =
	Inv. =	1,000	Net Worth	14,500	$10,000
	Accts. Rec. =	16,500			
	Total:	$18,500	Total:	$18,500	
Day 49	Cash	$ 6,500	Accts. Pay. =	$ 4,000	
	Inv.	500	Accrued Salaries =	5,000	
	Accts. Rec. =	16,500	Net Worth =	14,500	
	Total:	$23,500	Total:	$23,500	
Day 56	Cash =	$ 0	Accts. Pay. =	$ 2,000	Salaries =
	Inv.	0	Net Worth =	14,500	$10,000
	Accts. Rec. =	16,500			Supplies =
	Total:	$16,500	Total:	$16,500	$2,000 *
Day N	Cash =	$14,500	Net Worth =	$14,500	

Cash Receipts and Working Capital

Cash Inflows—Days 1–56 = $27,500

Initial Working Capital = $14,500

Total: $42,000

Cash Outflows

Supplies $ 2,000

Salaries 40,000

Total: $42,000

*Attain financial self-sufficiency, i.e., cash inflows will equal outflows for any given period of "j" is being borrowed. The cost of trade credit, therefore, is 18 times 2 over 98 or about 37 percent. Trade credit is thus a relatively costly source of financing. Table 10-5 illustrates the mechanics of calculating the cost of trade credit.

The nature of the cost of accounts payable can be more clearly understood through the use of Figure 10-1. The vertical axis of the diagram measures the cost of credit in terms of an annual rate of interest. The horizontal axis represents time elapsed after the receipt of goods by the purchaser. During the discount period—day 1 to day 10—the cost of credit is not explicitly set out, and the credit can be viewed as being virtually an interest-free loan. This is the case due to the fact that the purchase price remains the same whether the goods are paid for on day one, day 10, or any day in between. Thus, while admittedly there is a cost for the use of credit during the discount period, the cost is buried or hidden in the purchase price and cannot be avoided.

After the expiration of the discount period—day 11—the hospital incurs an explicit cost for the use of the credit for the next 20 days, i.e., until the end of the net period—day 30. Whether the goods are paid for on day 11 or day 30, the cost is still the same. Thus, if a $100 purchase were made on terms of 2-10, net 30 and paid for on the 11th day, the purchaser would pay $2.00 for the use of $98.00 for just one day. Since there are 365, one-day periods in the year, the cost in dollars of using trade credit would be $2.00 times 365, or $730. In terms of an annual rate of interest, the cost of using trade credit would be 2 times 365 over 98, or 744.89 percent. As the graph indicates, as payment is delayed the cost of credit declines. The annual rate of interest is approximately 37 percent if the purchase is paid for by the due date, i.e., the 30th day. As payment is delayed beyond the due date, the annual interest rate will continue to fall. In fact, the annual rate can decline indefinitely.

Suppliers will attempt to prevent the cost curve from falling indefinitely by mailing past due notices, placing follow-up telephone calls, and taking stronger action, if necessary. These measures obviously increase the cost to the seller of offering trade credit. However, they do not raise the cost of credit to the purchaser for the invoice already outstanding. Failure to pay its obligation on time will raise questions about the hospital's ability to pay, the acumen of its management and, perhaps, even the trustworthiness of its management and governing board. These questions and doubts will not only make suppliers and other potential lenders less willing to offer credit to the hospital, but also will

Table 10-5

Cost of Credit

Cost of credit is a function of:
  1—the rate of discount;
  2—the discount period; and
  3—the net period.
Assume: hospital makes a $100 purchase and terms of 2-10, net 30 are
      offered:
  Rate of discount = 2%
  Discount period = 10 days
  Net period = 20 days
  Cost of goods = quoted price ($100) minus the discount.
        = $98 (This is the amount being borrowed.)*

*Under the above assumption, the hospital can obtain the goods for $98 by paying within 10 days. However, if it chooses not to pay until the end of the 30 day period, this decision will cost it an additional $2. Therefore, if the goods are not paid until the end of the 30 day period, the hospital has borrowed $98 for 20 days at a cost of $2. It should be noted that the loan is considered to be for 20 days because no explicit charge is made if payment is made before day 10.

Cost of credit on annual basis:

  1—$20 for every 20 day period, or $\frac{365}{20}$ = 18.25 × $2 = $36.50

  2—amount borrowed = $98

  3—interest rate = $\frac{\text{interest expenses}}{\text{amount borrowed}}$ = $\frac{\$36.50}{\$98.00}$ = 37.4%

---

probably increase the cost of future purchases, i.e., the hospital may have to pay cash in the future or may have to use vendors who charge more in order to compensate for the added costs of dealing with slow payers.

The nature of this future cost is illustrated by the dotted line in Figure 10-1. The line represents the indirect cost which is incurred by the hospital if payment is past due on the current bill, i.e., it represents the future costs that will be levied against the hospital if it defaults on its present obligation. Thus, if trade credit is used, the due date (the end of the net period) is the long-run, low point of the cost curve.

Given the nature of both the trade credit purchase arrangement and the foregoing cost curve, the use of accounts payable or trade credit as a means of financing working capital has some interesting managerial implications. In terms of financial management rules of thumb—the following guidelines can be set out:

The potential user of trade credit should choose one of two points at which to pay—
1. either the *end* of the discount period, or
2. the *end* of the net period.

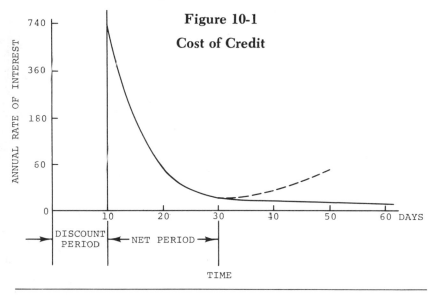

Figure 10-1

Cost of Credit

It should be noted that in both instances emphasis is placed on paying at the end of the period. This is the case, for if the hospital is going to take the discount, the cost of goods is the same regardless of whether the payment is made on day one, or the day on which the discount expires. If the hospital elects not to take the discount, then the cost of credit is incurred, but this cost is constant throughout the entire net period. Therefore, there is no financial incentive to force payment prior to the last day of the net period. Actually, the financial incentive lies in the direction of delaying payment. By delaying payment until the end of either the discount period or the net period, the hospital can more productively use its assets, for instead of committing funds to inventories, it can invest in revenue-generating securities which will provide a return.

Based upon the above guideline, the matter of when to pay under either alternative is clear. However, the critical question is how do you determine which alternative to select? In general terms, the answer to this question is simply that the best choice between the two is determined by the cost of credit from other available alternatives. If credit is needed, whether the discount is

Table 10-6

Decision Rule—Use of Trade Credit When Additional Financing Is Necessary

Basic Rule:
Whether the discount is taken or not depends on the cost of credit from the cheapest alternative. If the alternative rate lies below the low point of the trade credit cost curve, the financially prudent decision would be to take the discount and borrow from the alternative source in order to pay the invoice prior to the expiration of the discount period. If the alternative source of credit has a rate higher than the low point on the trade curve, then trade credit should be used.

Example I
A. Assumptions:
  1. $100 purchase on terms of 1-10, net 30
  2. Alternative source—factor or sell accounts receivable at a discount rate of 7% (see page 233)
B. Costs
  1. Dollar = $1 interest about 18%
  2. Dollar = $7 interest rate—none—have sold property
C. Decision
  1. Trade credit is the least cost alternative. Therefore, the discount should not be taken.

Example II
A. Assumptions:
  1. $100 purchase on terms of 1-10, net 30
  2. Alternative source A—factor accounts receivable at a discount of 7%
  3. Alternative source B—obtain a 30 day, 8% bank loan for $150 (note the added $50 is for the required compensatory balance)
B. Costs
  1. Dollar = $1 interest rate = about 18%
  2. Dollar = $7 interest rate = none
  3. Dollar = $1 interest rate = 8%
C. Decision
  On a cost basis it is a matter of indifference between trade credit and bank loan. Subjective factors should determine the choice.

Example III
A. Assumptions:
  Same as in II, except terms of sale are 2-10, net 30.
B. Costs
  1. Dollar = $2 interest rate = about 38%
  2. Dollar = $7 interest rate = none
  3. Dollar = $1 interest rate = 8%
C. Decision
  The bank loan is the least cost alternative. Therefore, the discount should be taken.

taken or not, should depend on the costs of the various alternative sources of credit. Thus, if an alternative source of credit is less costly than trade credit, the discount should be taken and the alternative source should be used as the means of financing working capital. Conversely, if trade credit is the least cost alternative, the discount should not be taken. It is only through this type of financing strategy that management can minimize the total cost of working capital.

The decision as to whether or not the discount should be taken may also depend on the alternative uses to which funds can be put. If funds are immediately available to pay a bill, then before they are used in this manner, management should compare the return which could be earned by investing the funds in some other manner versus the cost of trade credit. Thus, if the revenues which can be earned exceed the cost of trade credit, it would be financially imprudent to take the discount and forego the revenue.

Additionally, if the revenues are less than the cost of trade credit but exceed the cost of the least cost credit alternative, then the discount should be taken and the least cost source of credit should be used as the source of financing. Thus, the decision as to whether or not trade credit should be used depends, in the case where credit is needed, upon the cost of alternative sources of credit and, in the case where credit is not absolutely needed, on the revenues which could be earned from alternative uses of funds and the cost of alternative sources of credit.

One further point should be noted in regard to the cost of credit. Management, in determining the least cost credit alternative, should not only examine cost in terms of a percentage annual interest rate, but also in terms of absolute dollar costs. In the previous example, $98.00 could be borrowed for 20 days at a cost of $2.00. Thus, the cost of credit in absolute dollars would be $2.00, and in terms of annual interest rate, about 38 percent. As an alternative, however, assume that the hospital could also borrow $98 from its bank at an annual interest rate of 10 percent, but that it must hold the loan for at least six months.

At first glance, the bank loan appears to be the least cost source of credit—10% versus 38%. When absolute dollar costs are considered, trade credit is the least cost alternative—$2.00 versus $4.90. Thus, in order to minimize the total cost of operations, trade credit should be used as the means of financing working capital, for its "full" cost is less than the cost of the short-term bank loan (less any interest which may have been earned on the unused loan balances). Tables 10-6 and 10-7 contain numerical examples of the foregoing decision rules.

Table 10-7

Decision Rule—Use of Trade Credit When Additional Financing Is Not Necessary

Basic Rule

Whether the discount is taken or not depends on both the cost of credit from the cheapest alternative source and the return which can be earned by investing available funds in assets other than inventories. If the return which can be earned from investments in other than inventories is greater than the least cost credit alternative, then the financially prudent decision is to maintain the investment and finance inventories through the least cost credit alternative. That is, depending on cost, management should either take the discount and finance the purchase through an alternative source or if less costly, finance it through the use of trade credit. If the opposite is the case, then the financially prudent decision is to take the discount and finance the purchase (inventories) through available funds or assets.

Example I

A. Assumptions:
   1. $100 purchase at terms of 2-10, net 30
   2. Alternative source A—sell two short-term investments yielding 12% payable annually, payment due in 10 days if investment is still held.
   3. Alternative source B—obtain a 30-day 9% bank loan for $150 (note the added $50 is for the required compensatory balance).

B. Costs
   1. Dollars = $2.00 interest rate = about 37%
   2. Dollars = $12.00 (lose year's earnings due to the terms of payment interest rate = 12% yield (Alternative A)
   3. Dollars = $1.13 interest rate = 9% (Alternative B)

C. Decision
   The investment should be continued. However, the discount should be taken and the purchase financed through alternative source B.

Example II

A. Assumptions:
   Same as above, except earnings on investment are paid monthly.

B. Costs
   1. Dollars = $2.00 interest rate = about 37%
   2. Dollars = $1.00 interest rate = 12% (Alternative A)
   3. Dollars = $1.13 interest rate = 9% (Alternative B)

C. Decision
   The least cost alternative is to take the discount and finance the purchase through the sale of the short-term investment.

Short-Term Debt

As has been indicated above, short-term debt can be used as a substitute for accounts payable as a means of financing purchases and, therefore, it can be viewed as an alternative source of financing for working capital. In addition to its substitution role, short-term debt can also play a primary role in the financing of working capital needs. In order to understand the nature of this primary role, it is first necessary to consider the exact character of the hospital's working capital needs.

As is illustrated in Figure 10-2, the working capital needs of a hospital can be viewed as consisting of two components—a permanent segment and a temporary segment. Permanent working capital can be defined as the minimum working capital investment which the hospital must maintain if it is to be able to acquire the factors of production necessary for operations, i.e., it is the level of assets which is needed to finance the lowest expected level of operations. This quantity is represented by segment "AB" in Figure 10-2.

As is apparent from the diagram, the hospital's working capital needs fluctuate over time, but at no time do they fall below point "B." Thus, if the hospital is to be able to operate, it must have available on a continual basis a working capital investment equal to line segment "AB."

Working capital investment (volume and costs remaining constant) will be stable over time and can only be altered through changes in the cash inflow and/or outflow cycles. An example of how a change in the cash inflow cycle can affect permanent working capital needs was described in Chapter 9.

Given that permanent working capital is a permanent asset (investment), it should be financed through a permanent source of funds. This approach to asset financing is consistent with the general financial management decision rule which holds that the timing of assets and their sources of financing should be matched. Thus, long-term or permanent assets should be financed through equity or long-term debt.

In the case of the hospital, however, the above general rule is not as applicable as it is in regard to commercial industry. This is the case, for the hospital's ability to generate sufficient revenues to amortize any debt incurred for working capital purposes, due to the nature of cost based reimbursement agreements, is severely limited. Therefore, if the risk of insolvency and financial failure,

Figure 10-2

Working Capital Fluctuations

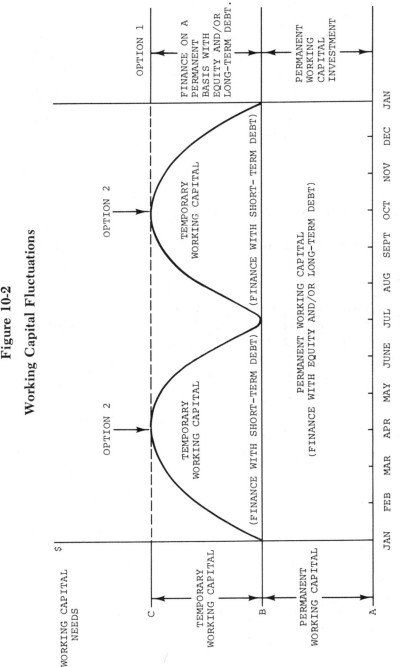

caused by defaulting on debt obligations, is to be minimized, the hospital must finance permanent working capital through equity.[2]

In addition to permanent working capital needs, the hospital, from time to time, will temporarily also have to increase its working capital investment in order to meet the financial demands generated by temporary or cyclical increases in service volume. These supplementary working capital needs are depicted by the curve lying between points "B" and "C" in Figure 10-2.

It is important to realize that these temporary working capital needs are a byproduct of increases in production volume and can be considered to be temporary because they are self-liquidating over the short run. The hospital, like almost all other industries, experiences certain periods during the year when the demand for services or products increases. In order to meet these increased demands, temporary additional peronnel and/or supplies are often needed. However, as the discussion of the previous chapter should have made clear, if additional personnel and supplies are to be obtained, then—as a prerequisite—additional working capital is needed to finance these temporary increases in the factors of production. Admittedly, as Figure 10-3 makes clear, these financial needs can eventually be met with funds derived from internal operations. Due to the lag between cash outflows and cash inflows, though, the need for these funds occurs before they are available. Thus, management is faced with the problem of deciding how to finance these temporary needs until that time when internally generated funds are available.

The potential sources of funds for financing temporary working capital needs are the same as those discussed earlier in this chapter, i.e., debt and/or equity. The decision facing management is that of determining which of these sources provides the least cost solution to the hospital's financing needs. Therefore, management must determine the costs of each of the financing alternatives.

Cost of Short-Term Financing

Given this problem, consider the cost of equity. If equity is used as the source of financing, then the accounting or out-of-pocket cost is zero, for no interest has to be paid. However, there is an opportunity cost if equity is used in this manner.

---

[2]It is worthy to note that even if debt is used to finance working capital, in the long run equity is the eventual source of financing. This is due to the fact that debt must be retired through either additional external equity contributions or retained earnings (internal equity contributions).

Figure 10-3

Nature of Short-Term Working Capital Needs

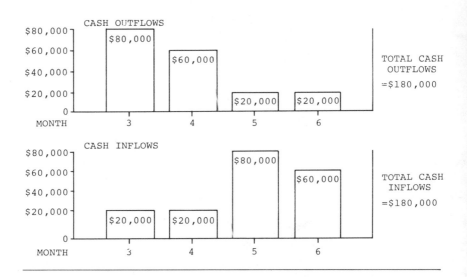

In a for-profit industrial firm opportunity cost can be viewed as the return foregone by investing equity in working capital, as opposed to the best alternative investment which is available. Given a listing of alternative investments, the firm can quite easily calculate the returns foregone and, therefore, the cost of equity financing. Based upon this cost, the firm can then compare the cost of equity to the cost of other financing alternatives in order to determine the least cost source of financing.

In the case of a hospital, the same opportunity cost notion exists, but because of the nature of the hospital's investment alternatives the value or magnitude of this cost is difficult to calculate. Nevertheless, the concept of opportunity cost can provide a useful approach to evaluating the relative cost of equity financing.

In the previous discussion of working capital financing, equity was recommended, for financially pragmatic reasons, as the most desirable source of funds for permanent working capital financing. The desirability of equity as the source of permanent working capital financing can also be justified in terms of an opportunity cost argument. The argument can be briefly stated as follows:

1. Permanent working capital funds are necessary if the hospital is to be able to operate.
2. Additionally, if the hospital is to be able to operate over the long run, permanently working capital funds cannot be obtained by means of debt financing, for at some point the debt must be repaid, and the hospital will be deprived of its permanent working capital funds.
3. Therefore, equity should be used as the source of financing, for it is the only permanent source of funds available and, thus, the only source that can ensure the continued availability of permanent working capital.
4. Consequently, the rate of return from investing equity in this manner is greater than that which can be obtained from an investment in any other alternative because the return is the hospital's ability to operate.
5. Therefore, the opportunity cost attached to not investing equity in permanent working capital is greater than the opportunity cost attached to not investing equity in any other alternative.
6. Thus, if management is to minimize costs, it must use equity to finance permanent working capital needs.

The same type of argument, however, cannot be made for the use of equity as the source of financing for temporary working capital needs. Temporary working capital needs are, over time, self-liquidating. Therefore, equity is not the only potential source of funds which can be used to finance these needs. Thus, the opportunity cost of not using equity as the source of funds is less in this case than it was in the previous one, for alternative sources are available and financially practicable. The decision as to whether or not equity should be used in this manner, therefore, should be based on an analysis of the cost of equity versus the cost of alternative sources.

If debt is used as the source of funds, then the cost can be said to be equal to the interest cost on the debt. If equity is used, then the cost is equal to the return foregone by not investing equity in another manner, such as lifesaving equipment or patient care programs. Admittedly, the rate of return on a piece of lifesaving equipment or a patient care program is difficult to determine. Intuitively, though, one would think that it is high and, certainly, at least higher than the interest rate on debt. If the rate of return from investing equity in other than temporary working capital is greater than the interest rate on debt, then the opportunity cost of

Table 10-8

Cost Advantage—Short-Term Debt

Assume:
1. Hospital needs $100,000 for only a single three-month period per year.
2. Long-term debt can be obtained for a period of three years at 8%.
3. Short-term debt can be obtained for a period of three months at 8%.

Annual Operating Costs—Assuming Excess Long-Term Funds Not Invested

1. Long-term debt: due to the nature of the debt contract—3 years—interest expense is incurred for the entire year. Cost, therefore   = $8,000

2. Short-term debt: interest expense is only incurred for the three months that the debt is used. Cost, therefore   = $2,000

3. Conclusion: operating costs can be reduced by $6,000 if short-term debt is used as the means of financing temporary working capital needs. Operating savings/ year   = $6,000

Annual Operating Costs—Assuming Excess Long-Term Funds Invested.
1. Long-term debt: gross cost   = $8,000
   Investment income (assuming invest for
      9 months @ 6%)   =   ($4,500)
   Net Cost   = $3,500
2. Short-term debt: gross cost   = $2,000
   Investment income   =   0
   Net Cost   = $2,000
3. Conclusion: short-term debt is still the least cost
   alternative. Operating savings/year   = $1,500

---

financing temporary working capital needs through equity is greater than the cost of financing through debt. Therefore, equity is not the least cost financing alternative and should not be management's primary choice as the means of financing temporary working capital needs.

Given that equity should not be the primary financing choice, the alternatives available to management are limited to just either long-term or short-term debt. Short-term debt is a feasible alternative in this instance, for the working capital needs are only temporary. The problem facing management is simply that of determining which of the two alternatives has the least cost.

If long-term debt is used as the source of funds then, as is depicted by Option 1 in Figure 10-2, total working capital funds are increased for the entire period. However, due to the seasonal nature of the working capital needs, funds are not needed for the entire period. Thus, if long-term debt is used as the source of funds, the hospital is paying for the use of working capital funds during periods in which they are not needed. It is therefore unnecessarily incurring additional operating costs.

Admittedly, the excess funds can be invested during the periods in which they are not needed for working capital purposes. It is unlikely, though, that the returns from such investments will equal the interest costs of the debt. The financial implication of using long-term debt, therefore, is that it results in unnecessarily increasing the cost of financing working capital, for it does not match the need for funds with the availability of funds. Consequently, if management is to finance temporary working capital at least cost, it must use short-term debt.

Table 10-8 illustrates the cost advantages of short-term debt as the source of temporary working capital funds. As is clear from the table, the cost advantage of short-term debt is due to the ability of management to synchronize the timing of the debt with the timing of the hospital's need for temporary funds.[3] One might conclude, therefore, that the management-decision rule for the financing of temporary working capital needs would be to finance these needs through short-term debt which has a maturity schedule matched exactly to the fluctuations in working capital. In theory, this decision-rule is basically correct. Unfortunately, in an actual operating situation this rule is inappropriate, for it does not take into account the matter of uncertainty in regard to the timing of cash inflows.

Debt, whether long- or short-term, represents a fixed obligation whose timing and amount are both certain, i.e., both the exact amount and the exact date of payment are known in advance. However, the cash inflows, which are the source of funds for servicing retiring debt obligations, are uncertain. The approximate timing and amount of cash inflows are known, but due to various factors, the exact timing and amounts cannot be accurately projected. Thus, the situation is one wherein a fixed obligation must be met through uncertain income flows.

---

[3] It should also be noted that, due to the term structure of interest rates, short-term debt is a less costly source of funds, for long-term rates are generally higher than short-term rates.

This type of situation presents a substantial and costly hazard to the hospital, for if the timings of working capital fluctuations and debt maturity are exactly matched and cash inflows are slower than anticipated, the hospital will be unable to pay its obligation and will be forced to default on the debt. Default is an expensive action, for at best it casts doubt on the hospital's credit standing and, at worst, it can result in failure and dissolution. Thus, the hospital must attempt to minimize the probablity of default.

This, however, does not mean that the hospital should forego the use of short-term debt. Rather, it means that managment should adjust or schedule the timing of the maturity of the debt in order to provide a margin of safety. This can be done by allowing the maturity date to overlap or extend a short period beyond the exact time for which the additional working capital funds are needed.[4] Figure 10-4 illustrates what is meant by this scheduling strategy.

In addition to scheduling debt maturities, management must also consider whether the debt must be secured or unsecured. Ordinarily, it is desirable to borrow on an unsecured basis, for in this way not only can the bookkeeping and administrative costs attached to a secured loan be avoided, but also maximum financial flexibility can be maintained.[5] However, if the hospital's credit rating is weak or if the hospital has other debt obligations outstanding, it may be necessary either to pay a premium (higher rate of interest) or to provide some assets as collateral or security in order to obtain the loan.[6]

Several different types of assets are acceptable forms of collateral. Marketable securities are generally considered excellent collateral as is real property, such as buildings and equipment. Unfortunately, most hospitals do not hold large portfolios of marketable securities and real property is usually reserved as security or

---

[4]The appropriate length of the overlap period varies with the degree of cash inflow fluctuations and management's willingness to accept uncertainty. Therefore, no meaningful general rule can be applied. Each instance must be determined individually based upon a study of historical cash inflows and estimates of future events.

[5]The hospital may elect to secure the loan if it finds that a secured loan will result in a lower interest rate. However, in making this choice the hospital should consider the trade-off between the reduced interest rate and the loss of financial flexibility.

[6]Generally, as part of the loan approval process a bank, or any other lender, will evaluate the hospital's capital structure, i.e., existing mix of long-term financing. Based on this evaluation, the bank may, at the extreme, refuse the loan, grant it only at a higher than usual rate of interest, or require that it be secured.

Figure 10-4

Short-Term Debt Maturity Schedule

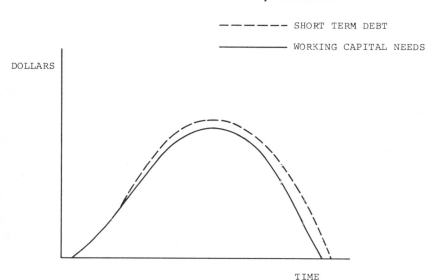

potential security for long-term debt. Thus, the bulk of secured short-term financing involves the use of short-term assets—accounts receivable or inventories—as collateral.

Accounts receivable, in addition to serving as collateral for short-term debt, can play another role in regard to short-term financing. The pledging of accounts receivable as security for a loan is commonly known as discounting accounts receivable. In this process, an agreement is made between the borrower and the lender wherein the lender takes the receivables, but has recourse to the hospital if a patient defaults on an account, i.e., the risk of default of an account remains with the hospital. Alternatively, in some instances accounts receivable, instead of being pledged, can be sold at a discount to the lender without recourse, i.e., the hospital is not responsible for defaults. This process is known as factoring accounts receivable and, although in legal terms it is not a loan arrangement, it can be conceptualized for our purposes, since cash is obtained for a price, as a hybrid form of debt.

While no statistics are available as to the number of hospitals which factor their accounts, it is unlikely that it is a large proportion. This is probably due to both the relatively poor quality of a hospital's self-pay accounts receivable and the adverse public relations effects which can arise if the purchaser of the accounts pursues collection too vigorously. Nevertheless, the existence of this source of short-term financing should be known.

It should also be noted that one other source of short-term financing may be available. Hospitals may obtain payment advances from third party payers in order to meet their temporary working capital needs. The nature and availability of these advances vary with the specific third party and the specific reimbursement contract. Thus, there is little value at this point in discussing this source of detail. It should suffice just to realize that advances may be available and that, if utilized, they represent a liability obligation or debt of the hospital.

Given the foregoing discussion, the critical point for management to understand is simply that, if costs are to be minimized, short-term financing (debt) must be used to meet temporary working capital needs. The form which this financing should take is a separate question which management can answer only after examining the cost of each alternative in order to establish which represents the least total cost to the hospital.

Conclusion

The discussion of the previous pages can be summarized into the following financial management decision rules:

1. Permanent working capital needs should be financed through equity.
2. Temporary working capital needs should be financed through short-term debt.
3. Trade credit (accounts payable) should be used as a source of working capital financing (either permanent or temporary) only when it is the least cost financing alternative.

Given these guidelines and the discussion in Chapter 9, the stage is now set for examining each of the primary components of working capital—inventories, accounts receivable, and cash. The management of each of these components is examined in the following chapters.

Suggested Readings

Cleverly, William O. *Financial Management of Health Care Facilities,* Chapter 8.

Healy, Sister Mary Immaculate. "An Analysis of Accounts Receivable with Emphasis on Factoring."

Lindsay, J. Robert and Sametz, Arnold W. *Financial Management: An Analytical Approach*, Chapter 6.

Van Horne, James C. *Financial Management and Policy*, Chapter 15.

Weston, J. Fred and Brigham, Eugene F. *Managerial Finance*, pp. 445–451.

Chapter 11
Inventory Management

The operating costs of a hospital can be segmented into the following expense categories[1]

Expense Category		Approximate Percent of Total Cost	
Personnel Costs			
Nursing	=	30%	
Other	=	33%	
Total:			63%
Nonwage Costs			
Supplies	=	12%	
Depreciation	=	5%	
Heat, light, maintenance, etc.	=	20%	
Total:			37%
		Total:	100%

Based on the above, it is clear that supplies expense is the single largest nonwage cost element and represents a significant cost factor. It is a factor which can result in not only the loss of nonoperating revenues, but also in unnecessary operating costs, if not properly managed.[2] Therefore, it is incumbent upon management to administer this element of cost carefully, if it is to achieve its operational goal.

---

[1] *Medical Care Prices, A Report to the President;* Department of Health, Education and Welfare, pp. 27–34.

[2] The Research Institute of America has found that the cost of having inventories ranges from 8.6 percent to 40.5 percent annually of the total value of the inventory.

The control of supplies expense lies to some extent in the areas of internal control, accounts payable management, and purchasing policies. However, the major potential for controlling this cost lies in the area of inventory management, for as basic accounting theory makes clear, supplies are current assets—inventories—until they are consumed in the production process. Thus, the control of supplies costs is actually a working capital management problem, for inventories are a basic component of working capital.

Why Hold Inventories?

Given that inventory management is a critical factor in controlling supplies expenses, how should management administer inventories in order to produce a least cost situation? That is, how does management determine the quantity or level of inventories which the hospital should hold? Before answering these questions, however, one should first examine why it is necessary to hold inventories.

In the case of a commercial enterprise, three basic factors are generally suggested as the causes or justification for holding inventories. These factors can be listed as follows.[3]

A. Time

The production process is not spontaneous; time is required to move goods through the process from raw materials to finished goods. Thus, at any single point in time the firm will hold some inventories in the form of "work or goods in process."

B. Discontinuities

The total production process can be characterized as consisting of various subprocesses, each of which must be coordinated with the others in order to produce a final product. It is impossible, however, to plan with sufficient precision such that goods will always move steadily from one process to another. Therefore, in order to prevent discontinuities in the production process from stopping the en-

[3]*Financial Management: An Analytical Approach*, J. Robert Lindsay and Arnold W. Sametz, pp. 51–54.

tire process, extra stocks or inventories must be kept available at the various stages of production.

C. Uncertainties

Due to the independent and segmented nature of the decision making process in the economy, an individual firm cannot always project with certainty the quantity of finished goods which will be demanded or the volume of raw materials which will be needed. Therefore in order to meet demands for goods and to ensure the continuation of the production process, buffer stocks or inventories of both finished goods and raw materials must be kept available.

The above causes for holding inventories appear to be more applicable to a manufacturing firm than to a retailing enterprise or a hospital. Factors "A" and "B" specifically relate to circumstances and problems inherent in the manufacturing process. However, factor "C"—Uncertainties—has a much wider applicability and is particularly germane in the case of the hospital.

The demand for hospital services has been shown to be highly unpredictable. Also, due to the lifesaving and/or health maintenance nature of hospital services, the cost of failing to meet demand can be quite high. Thus, management is confronted with both an uncertain situation and a situation wherein stopages in the production process, due to shortages of supplies, can be costly. Therefore, hospital management must hold a buffer stock or an inventory of needed supplies in order to assure the continuous provision of services.

Costs

Given the above need to hold inventories, management must determine both the quantity which should be acquired in any single order and the timing of that order if an optimal inventory is to be maintained and cost of supplies is to be controlled. If the size of the order quantity is to be knowledgeably determined, the costs involved in holding inventories must first be identified.

The economists, financial management experts, and business researchers who have studied inventory management have generally considered the following five categories or types of cost as relevant to determining the least cost order quantity size, i.e., the economic order quantity.

Purchasing Cost. The cost or price paid to suppliers for goods. This is an expense which cannot be avoided, for if the hospital is to be able to render services, goods must be obtained and be available. One might assume that this cost is not particularly relevant to the order size decision, since suppliers have to be paid their price and management has little option in this area. Even so, this cost may influence the quantity which should be ordered, for suppliers may offer quantity discounts which may make large order sizes attractive. Thus, this cost should not be ignored in determining the size of the order quantity.

For purposes of later reference, this cost will be referred to as "PD" where "P" equals the price or cost per unit and "D" equals the number of units purchased annually.

Order Cost. The administrative costs of obtaining the desired goods. This is the cost of such activities as writing specifications, soliciting and analyzing bids, preparing the order, receiving the goods, accounting for the goods, and paying the invoice. This cost may be large or small, depending upon the item purchased. If the item is standardized and the purchasing process routine, then the order cost will be relatively small. However, if it is the first time the item is being purchased or if the item is not standardized and specifications have to be written, bids taken, etc., then the order cost will be relatively large.

It should be noted that, regardless of whether order cost is large or small, it varies not with order size but rather with the number of orders placed: as the number of orders per year increases, total annual costs also increase. Therefore, the existence of this cost encourages large order sizes, for the larger the order size, the fewer the number of orders which have to be placed.

Order cost will be symbolized for later reference as "O." The average cost of placing a single order, therefore, is "O." However, the total annual outlay for order cost is "O" times the number of orders placed for the year. If "D" equals the number of units annually purchased and "Q" equals the order size, then D/Q equals the number of orders placed in a year. Total annual order cost thus equals "(D/Q)O."

Carrying Cost. The cost attached to holding inventories. This cost can perhaps be most easily understood if it is viewed as consisting of two interdependent segments: an opportunity cost segment and a holding or storage cost segment.

When a hospital decides to hold inventories, it is implicitly making a decision to invest some of its funds in inventories as opposed to some other investment alternative. This decision means that the hospital, at the very least, incurs an opportunity cost equal to the return which could have been obtained if the funds used to finance inventories had been invested in some other way. The size or amount of this cost varies directly with both the rate of return on the investment alternatives and the size of the inventory investment. The greater the inventory investment, the greater is the opportunity cost incurred by the hospital.[4]

In addition to opportunity cost, the carrying of inventories involves a holding or storage cost. If management is to avoid being accused of malfeasance or negligence, it must adequately protect inventory holdings. This means that inventory stocks must be stored, insured, and properly secured. Each of these items represents a cost which the hospital cannot avoid and which varies positively and incrementally with the level of inventory holdings. Thus, the holding of inventories involves a cost to the hospital which increases as the level of inventory stocks increase.

The existence of carrying cost supports an inventory decision which is exactly opposite to the decision which order and purchase costs encourage. Due to the relationship between the size of inventory holdings and the level of carrying cost, inventory stocks should be kept as small as possible if cost is to be minimized. This, in turn, means that order sizes should be small and that orders should be placed often. Thus, there is a conflict between order and purchase costs and carrying cost which must be resolved if a least cost solution is to be obtained.

Carrying cost, for purpose of later use, will be referred to as the quantity $(HQ + IP\frac{Q}{2})$. This approach to symbolizing carrying cost has been selected in order to make explicit its composite nature. The storage cost element of carrying cost is represented by the term "HQ" where "H" equals the cost of holding or storage per item and "Q" equals the order size which, as will be clear later, usually represents the maximum number of items that will be stored at any given time.

The opportunity cost element is represented by the expression,

---

[4]It should also be noted that if funds are borrowed to finance inventories, that a "cash" cost, as opposed to an opportunity cost, is incurred. This cost also varies directly with the size of the inventory investment and is equal to the interest expense due the lender.

"IP$\frac{Q}{2}$." That is, opportunity cost is equal to the highest alternative rate of return which could have been obtained times the average amount of funds which are invested in inventories. Thus, if
the highest obtainable alternative rate of return were 6% and the
hospital's average inventory holdings were $10,000, then:

$$\text{opportunity cost} = \text{IP}\frac{Q}{2}$$
$$I = 6\%$$
$$\text{P}\frac{Q}{2} = \$10,000$$
$$\text{opportunity cost} = (6\%)\ (\$10,000)$$
$$\text{opportunity cost} = \$600$$

As is indicated above, "I" represents the highest obtainable alternative rate of return. Generally, unless other information is available, "I" is assumed to equal the interest rate currently available in
the capital market. Average inventory holdings are represented by
"P$\frac{Q}{2}$" where "P" equals the price per unit and "Q" the order size. It
should be noted that $\frac{"Q"}{2}$ is the average inventory holdings, for,
in a case where demand is certain, at the beginning of a period
inventory holdings should equal "Q" and at the end of the period
they should equal "zero." Therefore, average holdings for the period
equals the initial inventory ("Q") plus the final inventory (zero)
divided by 2 or simply "Q/2." The rationale supporting this assumption is graphically illustrated in Figure 11-1.

Long or Overstocked Cost. The cost attached to holding unused
and/or unnecessary quantities of inventory stocks. This cost can be
most easily understood if it is viewed as potentially consisting of
two elements: a carrying cost component, and a perishability cost
component.

If goods are purchased for use in a particular period but are not
used in that period then surplus inventories exist, for more goods
than are actually needed are being held. In this type of situation,
the hospital is forced to hold or carry these surplus stocks (over-
stocks) until that period or time when they can be used. This
additional carrying of inventories, however, has a cost equal to the
extra carrying costs which must be incurred. For example, if goods
are obtained in period "one" but are not used until period "three"
then the hospital has held the goods for two periods longer than

Figure 11-1

Inventory Depletion

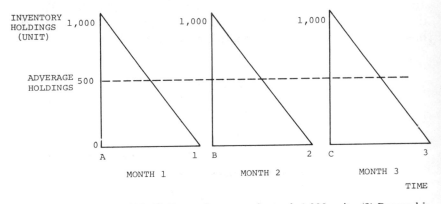

Assumptions: (1) Q = 1,000; (2) Demand per month equals 1,000 units; (3) Demand is constant over the month.

actually necessary. This means that additional unnecessary carrying costs are incurred, for funds invested in inventories are committed (opportunity cost) and storage costs are incurred for a longer period than is ideally necessary.

The nature of this component of overstocked cost can be seen by referring to Diagrams A and A' in Figure 11-2. Diagram A represents the total carrying costs of holding goods. If, as is indicated in the diagram, 100 units are held, but only 50 units are used in the first period and the other 50 are not used until the third period, then unnecessary carrying costs equal to the vertically shaded areas are incurred. These costs can be considered unnecessary, for if perfect information were available regarding demand, only 50 units would have been obtained for use in period "one." Therefore, no surpluses would exist and no costs would be incurred for holding extra goods which are not immediately needed. Thus, to the extent which surpluses do exist, their cost can be viewed as not being necessary for the continuance of operations.

Diagram A' depicts this same cost notion from a somewhat different viewpoint. In this instance, the increasing nature of carrying costs are shown over several time periods. As is indicated, if goods are obtained in period "one" and used in period "one," carrying costs per unit, at a maximum, will equal "OA." However, if goods are obtained in period "one" but are not used until period

Figure 11-2

Overstocked Cost

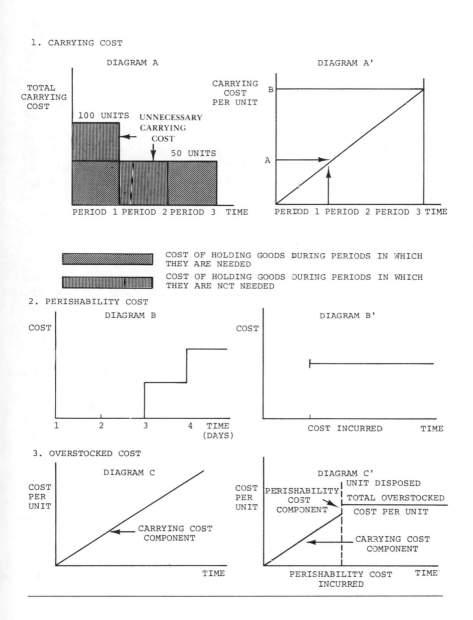

1. CARRYING COST

DIAGRAM A

DIAGRAM A'

TOTAL CARRYING COST

CARRYING COST PER UNIT

100 UNITS   UNNECESSARY CARRYING COST

50 UNITS

PERIOD 1 PERIOD 2 PERIOD 3   TIME

B

A

PERIOD 1 PERIOD 2 PERIOD 3 TIME

COST OF HOLDING GOODS DURING PERIODS IN WHICH THEY ARE NEEDED

COST OF HOLDING GOODS DURING PERIODS IN WHICH THEY ARE NOT NEEDED

2. PERISHABILITY COST

DIAGRAM B

COST

1   2   3   4   TIME (DAYS)

DIAGRAM B'

COST

COST INCURRED   TIME

3. OVERSTOCKED COST

DIAGRAM C

COST PER UNIT

CARRYING COST COMPONENT

TIME

DIAGRAM C'

COST PER UNIT

UNIT DISPOSED

PERISHABILITY COST COMPONENT

TOTAL OVERSTOCKED COST PER UNIT

CARRYING COST COMPONENT

PERISHABILITY COST INCURRED   TIME

"three," carrying costs per unit, at a maximum, will equal "OB."
Therefore, if overstocking or surplus inventories exist, the longer
these inventories are held, the greater will be the carrying cost
and, subsequently, the greater will be the overstocked cost.

The second component of overstocked cost—perishability—is perhaps not germane to all hospital inventory stocks. Nevertheless, it
should be discussed if the nature of overstocked cost is to be completely understood. Consider, for example, the case of a vegetable
peddler and his perishable inventory of fresh vegetables. Prior to
refrigeration, the peddler either had to sell his stock of vegetables
in a day or two, or throw them in the garbage and incur the cost of
the inventory which was disposed of as a loss. This loss, due to
spoilage or perishability, can be considered as an overstocking cost.

A similar situation can be found in the case of some hospital
pharmacy stocks which neither can be returned for credit nor dispensed after the expiration of certain time periods. In this instance, if the hospital is overstocked and unable to use the drugs
before the expiration date, it incurs a cost not only for carrying the
excess stock—carrying cost—but also a perishability cost equal to
the cost of the drugs which have to be discarded. Diagrams B and
B' in Figure 11-2 illustrate this cost.

It should be noted that, perishability cost is pictured in Diagram
B as a step-like curve due to the fact that the cost increases over
time as price is lowered in an attempt to sell the perishable goods.
For example, the vegetable peddler may on the second day, in
order to increase sales and avoid a "cash" loss, reduce the price to
just the cost of the vegetables. If surpluses still exist on the third
day he may, in order to minimize his losses, reduce the price to
less than cost. In this case, he will incur a perishability cost equal
to the difference between the cost of the goods and the price he is
charging. If, on the fourth day, surpluses still exist he may have to
discard the vegetables and thereby incur a perishability cost equal
to the full cost of the goods which are discarded. Thus, perishability cost increases in steps over time, as the differential between
price and cost changes.

Diagram B, however, is not an accurate representation of the
perishability cost curve in the hospital situation. In the case of the
hospital, the price of goods is not reduced in order to sell them
before they become completely spoiled and unusable. Thus, as is
shown in Diagram B', perishability cost for the hospital is a horizontal line. This is the case, for perishability cost is equal to the
cost of the goods which are no longer usable and this cost, once
incurred, does not change over time.

Total long or overstocked cost for any given item is equal to the sum of the carrying and perishability costs for that item. This total cost, for purposes of later reference, will be symbolized as "L" and is shown in Diagrams C and C'. Diagram C represents the case wherein overstocking does not involve a perishability cost component; e.g., unsterile dressings. In this case, overstocked cost is equal to just carrying cost. Diagram C' represents the case wherein overstocking involves both a perishability and a carrying cost component. In this instance, overstocked cost is equal to the sum of the two component costs.

Short or Stock-out Costs. The cost attached to holding an insufficient quantity of inventory stocks. This is the cost which a firm incurs when it is not able to meet demands for goods from its inventory supplies.

In the case of a commercial enterprise, stock-out cost can be viewed as consisting potentially of two types of costs—an immediate cash cost and an intangible cost due to lost future sales. Assume, that a customer demands an item which, at the time of his demand, is out of stock. If this is the case, the customer may be willing to wait a day or two for the item, but in all likelihood he will not be willing to wait as long as it would take to obtain the item through the normal delivery channels. Thus, the firm, if it is to avoid losing the sale, must go outside the normal delivery mechanism in order to obtain the desired goods. It may have to make special calls to its suppliers, assume the cost of an overtime production run, arrange for special transportation, etc. These activities represent a cash cost to the firm, which is reflected in terms of increased purchase and order costs and which cannot be avoided if the sale is to be saved. However, it must be realized that these costs arise due to a shortage of inventory stocks. Therefore, they can be considered to be the cost of stock-out or insufficient inventories.

Alternatively, a customer may not be willing or able to wait even a day or two for the goods. If this is the situation, stock-out has a cost equal to not only the current sale which is lost, but also to the discounted value (present value) of all future sales to that particular customer, which may be lost. Stock-out thus may also entail a future cost to the firm in terms of lost sales due to customer dissatisfaction. This cost, though difficult to measure, is nonetheless a real cost which must be considered in inventory decisions.

In the case of the hospital, inventory stock-out is just one aspect of the more general and basic problem of allocating resources. In order for a hospital to be able to provide patient care, it must obtain and have available certain supplies. However, if the hospital is to operate efficiently the quantities of these resources which are held available must be closely related to demand. The demand for hospital services, as has been indicated earlier, is highly unpredictable and the costs of failing to meet demand are high. Thus, in the case of inventories the cost of being unable to meet demand includes not only increased purchase and order costs, but also another far more significant intangible cost component.

The cost of inventory stock-out in the hospital situation should be measured both in terms of cash or monetary costs and also in terms of the intangible or non-monetary costs of illness, pain, and death. Unfortunately, for the decision-maker, a market mechanism does not exist for measuring these nonmonetary costs. Their magnitude, therefore, must be subjectively estimated.

Usually, due to the nature of these factors, a high value is attached to stock-out costs and the avoidance of any possibility of inventory shortages or stock-out is felt by many to be critical if not mandatory. However, from a pragmatic viewpoint it should be recognized that not only are there generally not enough resources available to guarantee that stock-out will never occur, but also that it is excessively costly to maintain inventory levels which will prevent any possibility of stock-out. Thus, a trade-off must be made or a balance found between stock-out costs, service demands, and overstocked costs if an optimal inventory management solution is to be obtained.[5]

Based on the foregoing, assuming stock-out is represented by "S," the total cost (TC) of obtaining and holding inventories can be expressed as follows:

$$TC = \underset{\underset{\text{Purchase}}{\downarrow}}{PD} + \underset{\underset{\text{Order}}{\downarrow}}{\frac{D}{Q}O} + \underset{\underset{\text{Carrying}}{\downarrow}}{(HQ + IP\frac{Q}{2})} + \underset{\underset{\text{Overstocked}}{\downarrow}}{L} + \underset{\underset{\text{Stock-out}}{\downarrow}}{S}$$

Purchase Order   Carrying Overstocked Stock-out
  Cost   Cost   Cost   Cost[6]   Cost[6]

---

[5]It should be noted that long and short costs involve a somewhat different type of management decision than order and carrying costs. Long and short costs require that management balance the need for inventories against the level of stocks. Order and carrying costs require that the size of orders be balanced against the frequency of orders.

[6]Due to the complex nature of these costs, they are expressed for the sake of simplicity of illustration as just L and S. The reader should note, however, that these costs are a function of such factors as order quantity and demand.

Given that these are the costs attached to inventories, the problem facing management is simply that of determining how to obtain the minimum value for TC. That is, determine the value of Q which will minimize TC.

Inventory Decisions—Certainty

In order to understand both how the above costs interact with one another and the approach which management can use to minimize total inventory costs, it is advantageous to begin first with a relatively simple set of circumstances. Assume, for the sake of illustration, that a particular hospital operates in a world of certainty. (The demand schedule facing the hospital is constant and known.) Also, assume that the delivery of ordered goods to the hospital is not instantaneous, but that the time lag between the placement of an order and the receipt of goods is constant and known.

Given these assumptions, the inventory total cost equation can be rewritten as follows:

$$TC = PD + \frac{D}{Q}O + (HQ + IP\frac{Q}{2})$$

The equation can be written in this form, for in the world of certainty overstocked and stock-out costs do not exist. Thus, these two cost factors for the moment, can be ignored. They will, however, be considered below as factors critical to the inventory management under conditions of uncertainty.

As indicated earlier, the first inventory decision which management must make is that of determining the quantity which should be acquired in any single order; i.e., determination of the economic order quantity. In the above equation, order quantity is represented by "Q." The problem facing management, therefore, is to determine the level of "Q" which corresponds to the lowest point on the inventory total cost curve; i.e., $TC_{minimum}$.

At first glance, this may appear to be a difficult task. However, $TC_{minimum}$ can be found by differentiating the above equation as follows to establish the optimal order size, i.e., "Q_E":[7]

$$Q_E = \sqrt{\frac{2DO}{IP + 2H}}$$

---

[7]Differentiation is a standard approach in calculus to solving a problem such as determining TC minimum.

"Q_E" is thus the economic order quantity or that order quantity which will result in total inventory costs being minimized. By solving the above equation management can determine the optimal order quantity for its own particular operational situation. Tables 11-1 and 11-2 illustrate the use of this equation.[8]

Once the economic order quantity (Q_E) is established, it is a relatively simple task for management to determine the solution to the second inventory decision; i.e., calculate the timing of when an order should be placed or the reorder point (R). Under conditions of certainty, the reorder point is simply equal to the number of units which will be demanded during the delivery time lag (D_L). That is, when the quantity of goods in stock is equal to the amount of goods which will be consumed in the time period between the placement and the receipt of an order then, the next order for additional goods should be placed.

The reorder point equation can be expressed simply as follows.

Reorder Point = Demand During Delivery Lag

or

$$R = D_L$$

Thus, if the delivery time lag is ten days and demand is 28 units per ten day period then the reorder point would be 28 units. Hence, returning to the foregoing example, when 28 units are left in stock an order for 58 units should be placed.

This same notion can be explained in a somewhat different fashion through the use of Figure 11-3. As is indicated in the figure, D (the slope of the curve) represents the rate of inventory use, line segment TE represents the time lag for deliveries, and E represents that point in time when inventory stocks are completely depleted. The inventory reorder date, therefore, is T and the inventory quantity which signals the need to reorder is R.

The data which management needs in order to develop a least cost inventory management policy are now available. If a hospital were to operate in a world of certainty, all of the information, i.e., how much to order and when to order, needed to minimize inventory costs and consequently supply costs, would be known. Unfortunately, hospitals do not operate in a world of certainty. Therefore, if it is to be realistic, the foregoing inventory decision model

---

[8]Persons wishing to read a discussion of a more complex economic order quantity problem should refer to the appendix of Chapter 11.

Table 11-1
Economic Order Quantity

Cost Factors:

P = price/unit = $100*
D = number of units purchased and used/year = 1,000
O = cost of placing a single order = $10

I = interest rate = 5%
H = storage cost/unit = $.50
TC = total cost
Q = order size
Q_E = economic order quantity

Equations:

$$TC = PD + \frac{D}{Q} O - (HQ + IP\frac{Q}{2})$$ where the minimum cost solution is

$$Q_E = \sqrt{\frac{2\ DO}{IP + 2H}}$$

$$Q_E = \sqrt{\frac{2(1,000)\ (10)}{.05\ (100) + 2.(.5)}}$$

$$Q_E = \sqrt{\frac{20,000}{6}} \quad \text{or} \quad Q_E = \sqrt{3,333.33}$$

Q_E = 58 units (approximately)

$$TC_{minimum} = (100)(1,000) + \frac{1,000}{58}\ 10 + [(.5)(58) + (.05)(100)\frac{58}{2}]$$

$$TC_{minimum} = 100,000 + 172 + (29 + 145)$$

$$TC_{minimum} = \$100,346$$

Conclusion:

Total inventory costs will be minimized if the order quantity is set at 58 units. Thus, 58 units is the economic order quantity.

* Changes in purchase price (P), due to quantity discounts, can be taken into consideration by simply using the lower value for "P" in the equation. However, the other cost factors in the equation must also be adjusted to reflect the impact of purchasing a larger quantity. Therefore, by solving a series of equations, each at a different purchase price, it is possible to determine the optimum quantity and price combination. It should be realized, however, since total demand is independent of inventory policy, that purchase price—including the amount of any quantity discount—is generally established at the outset and can be taken as a given.

must be expanded to take into consideration the uncertainty of actual hospital service demands.

Inventory Decisions—Uncertainty

In order to expand the inventory decision model to allow for uncertainty, the two relevant inventory costs which were ignored

Table 11-2 *
Proof of Table 11-1

Cost Factors: I=interest rate=5%
P=price/unit =$100   H=storage cost/unit
D=number of units purchased and used/year=1,000   =$.50
O=cost of placing a single order=$10   TC=total cost
Equation: Q=order size

$$TC=PD+\frac{D}{Q}O+(HQ+I\ P\frac{Q}{2})$$

*Solution:***

Order Quantity	Purchase Cost	+	Order Cost	+	Carrying Cost	=	Total Cost
40 units	$100,000	+	$250	+	$120	=	$100,370
50 units	100,000	+	200	+	150	=	100,350
56 units	100,000	+	179	+	168	=	100,347
58 units	100,000	+	172	+	172	=	100,346
60 units	100,000	+	167	+	180	=	100,347
80 units	100,000	+	126	+	240	=	100,365

Conclusion:
An order quantity of 58 units results in the least cost solution to the inventory total cost equation.

*The reader should note that the above technique can also be used as a trial and error approach to approximating the economic order quantity.
**Figures are rounded off.

---

in the previous model, i.e., stock-out cost and overstocked cost, must be considered. Admittedly, these costs are difficult to measure. However, if management is to be able to make rational and intelligent inventory decisions, an attempt must be made, even if it is only subjective, to measure these costs. Thus, for purposes of this discussion, assume that stock-out (understocked) cost is equal to $75 per unit and overstocked cost is equal to $2.00 per unit.

In the world of certainty, when inventory stocks reached quantity "R," management knew both that it was time to reorder and that the new order would arrive just as the last unit in stock was being consumed. In the world of uncertainty, however, the actual demand for goods after a new order has been placed may vary from the expected demand, leaving the hospital either over-or understocked.[9] Thus, the matter of concern is the variation in de-

---

[9]It must be emphasized that hospitals, as well as all other businesses, operate in the world of uncertainty and that in the "real" world constant and predictable demand is seldom, if ever, found. Thus, if realistic and workable inventory decisions are to be made, the approach described in this section should be used as opposed to the more pedagogical and introductory approach of the previous section.

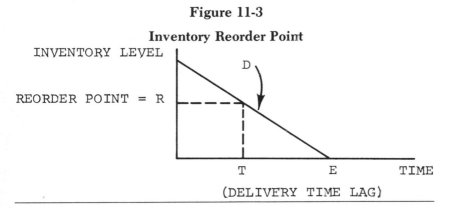

Figure 11-3

Inventory Reorder Point

mand after the reorder point, for it is in this period that the hospital is exposed to the dangers of uncertainty. This situation is illustrated in Figure 11-4.

As should be clear from the figure, the issue is one of finding a compromise or balance between overstocking and its subsequent cost, and understocking and its costs. In order to determine this balance knowledgeably, i.e., determine the optimum reorder point, management must first obtain two types of information: the probable variation in demand which can be expected during the reorder period, and the costs attached to being either overstocked or understocked. The costs attached to being overstocked and understocked were previously assumed Therefore, the problem is to develop some notion of the probable variation in demand which can be expected during the reorder period.

Assume—that based upon a study of historical records, information about future patterns of care, and subjective judgment—the following probabilities of various levels of demand can be developed.

Demand Estimates

Probability	.20	.25	.20	.15	.10	.10
Demand	27	28	29	30	31	32

Based upon this demand information and the previously assumed costs, management can now calculate the expected value or cost under each reorder point strategy and determine which strategy results in the least cost solution. Table 11-3 illustrates the mechanics of determining the least cost reorder point.

Given the least cost reorder point (32 units), management now has available the information needed to develop its inventory pol-

Figure 11-4

Demand Fluctuations and Inventory Stocks

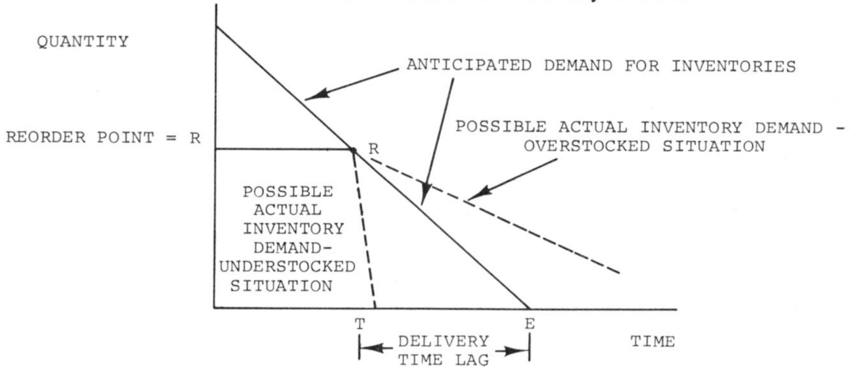

icy. From the previous discussion of the economic order quantity, the size of each order is known (58 units).[10] Also, from the above discussion and Table 11-3, the reorder point, and hence, the timing of orders is known. Thus, all of the information needed for managing inventories in a least cost manner under conditions of uncertainty is known.

Pragmatism

Admittedly, the foregoing model is a sophisticated management technique which necessitates not only a great deal of management skill and acumen in determining various inventory costs, but also which—if used indiscriminately for all stock items—can defeat its cost minimizing purpose. The problems involved in measuring costs were alluded to previously in regard to short and overstocked costs. These same problems also apply to other inventory cost components such as order and carrying costs. Order cost is usually a minor cost which is both difficult and costly to precisely measure. Thus, for the sake of expediency and practicality, this cost should be estimated. The same policy should be followed in regard to carrying and overstocked costs, for these items are also costly to accurately measure.

Short cost, due to the nature of the hospital's service, is perhaps both the most critical and the most difficult cost component to measure. It is difficult, if not impossible, in the case of a life-

---

[10]For our purposes, the economic order quantity can be considered to be the same under either conditions of certainty or uncertainty.

Table 11-3

Reorder Point—Uncertainty

Step 1—Assumptions:
  Understocked Cost = $75/unit
  Overstocked Cost = $2/unit
  Demand Distribution

Probability	.20	.25	.20	.15	.10	.10
Demand	27	28	29	30	31	32

Step 2—Overstocked and Understocked Cost Matrix—Unadjusted:

Reorder Point Strategy (units) \ Potential Demand	27	28	29	30	31	32
27	$ 0	$75	$150	$225	$300	$375
28	2	0	75	150	225	300
29	4	2	0	75	150	225
30	6	4	2	0	75	150
31	8	6	4	2	0	75
32	10	8	6	4	2	0

Step 3—Overstocked and Understocked Cost Matrix—Adjusted for Probability:

Reorder Point Strategy \ Potential Demand	27 (.20)	28 (.25)	29 (.20)	30 (.15)	31 (.10)	32 (.10)	Total Expected Cost
27	$ .00	$18.75	$30.00	$33.75	$30.00	$37.50	$150.00
28	.40	.00	15.00	22.50	22.50	30.00	90.40
29	.80	.50	.00	11.25	15.00	22.50	50.05
30	1.20	1.00	.40	.00	7.50	15.00	25.10
31	1.60	1.50	.80	.30	.00	7.50	11.70
32	2.00	2.00	1.20	.60	.20	.00	6.00

Table 11-3 (continued)

Step 4—Explanation:
Step 2—Unadjusted costs of various reorder strategies; for example:

Strategy	Demand	Cost
27 units	28 units	$75—1 unit short @ a cost of $75/unit
29 units	27 units	$ 4—2 units long @ a cost of $2/unit
31 units	31 units	0—supply equals demand

Step 3—Adjusted costs of various reorder strategies, i.e., adjusted by multiplying value obtained in Step 2 by the demand probability assumptions set out in Step 1. This step is necessary because of the unpredictable nature of inventory withdrawals.

Conclusion:
An inventory strategy utilizing 32 units as the reorder point, i.e., the quantity which signals reorder, will result in minimizing total inventory costs.

Explanation:
1. At point E, inventory stocks will be exhausted.
2. TE equals the delivery time lag where point T corresponds to an inventory level equal to R.
3. Thus, additional goods should be reordered when inventory stocks equal the number of goods which will be used during the delivery lag period.

saving item or service, to objectively determine the cost of being short. Thus, management must carefully evaluate both the patient care implications of stock-out for any given item, and the problems, possibilities, and expenses involved in obtaining an item on short notice. Based on this evaluation, the cost of being understocked should then be estimated as reasonably as is possible.

In addition to the cost measurement problems involved in using the inventory decision model, management must determine which stock items should be closely controlled. Indiscriminate application of the model to all inventory stocks will only result in increasing total cost. This is due to the fact that the expense of controlling low value items will exceed the expense attached to holding excess stocks of those items. Thus, the model should only be applied to those stock items which have a high potential for cost reduction. One technique which can be a useful aid in determining the appropriate application of the model is the ABC stratification of inventory items.

ABC stratification of inventories is a method of separating stock items into various categories in order to determine which items require close control.[11] Of the 1,000 to 3,000 items which a hospital typically carries in inventory, 10% to 15% of the total number represents 60% to 70% of the total inventory value. These high value items are the "A" classification and should be managed through the use of the above model.

Correspondingly, another 10% to 15% of the total number represent 20% to 30% of the total inventory value. These medium value, "B" classification items should be managed through the use of the economic order quantity component of the model. Reorder points, however, should be subjectively determined. The remaining 70% to 80% of the items, "C" classification should be managed through standardization and subjectively determined order quantities and reorder points.

Figure 11-5 illustrates the volume/value distribution of inventory items. The classification of any particular item, or group of items, should be based on an analysis of all inventory items in terms of item value, or cost per unit, multiplied by annual usage. The specific points of demarcation between "A" and "B" items and "B" and "C" items should be subjectively determined, based on management experience and the time and personnel available for inventory control.

Interrelationships

The techniques for inventory management should now be understood. Application of the foregoing financial management tools will help management to minimize not only the total cost of inventories and consequently total supplies expenses, but also the total quantity of working capital. This later result is due to the fact that the inventory decision model will enable management to determine the optimum inventory quantity or investment. Thus, use of the above techniques will aid management in minimizing the total cost of working capital (see Chapter 9). The least cost method of financing inventories should also be clear from the discussion of the previous chapter.

---

[11]Salling, Raymond C., "Can Your Inventory Control Be Scientific?" *Modern Hospital*, October 1964, pps. 34 and 36.

Figure 11-5

Inventory Volume/Value Distribution

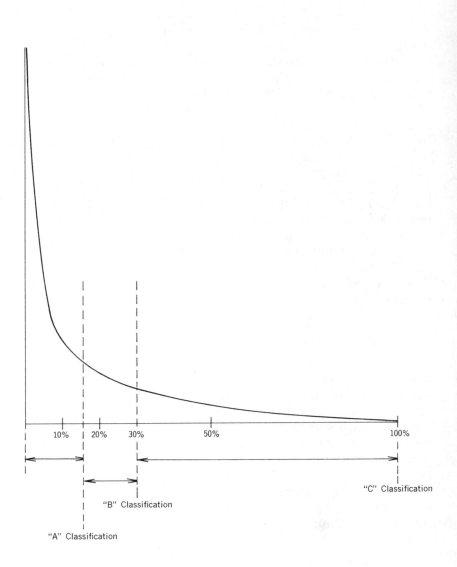

Suggested Readings

Bursk, Edward C. and Chapman, John F., editors *New Decision-Making Tools For Managers*, pp. 273–293.

Hillier, Frederick S. and Lieberman, Gerald J.. *Introduction to Operations Research*, Chapter 12.

Hopp, Michael, "Purchasing and Accounting Information System."

Lindsay, Franklin A. *New Techniques For Management Decision-Making*, pp. 114–118.

Lindsay, J. Robert and Sametz, Arnold W. *Financial Management: An Analytical Approach*, pp. 51–67.

Raitz, Robert E. "The Effect of Using an Economic Order Quantity Formula and Exponential Smoothing To Reduce Hospital Purchasing Costs."

Seawell, L. Vann. *Hospital Financial Accounting: Theory and Practice*, Chapter 12.

Appendix 11

Multiple-Item Orders—Joint Replenishment

The following material is adapted from *Production Planning and Inventory Control* by John F. Magee and David M. Boodman. It should be noted that while this material presents a more complex economic order quantity problem, the matter and technique of establishing reorder points are the same as discussed in the chapter.

Multiple-Item Orders

When an economical order is calculated, the controlling order cost may apply to the gross-order size which can be split among a number of items. For example, central supply may obtain a large number of items from a single source. It may be desirable, in this instance, to have any shipment from the source to the hospital equal, in total, an economical size.

In cases of this type, the economical order-quantity concept can be used to determine the size of the total order. Procedures can then be set up to determine (1) when to make an order and (2) how to balance the order among individual items. These procedures must meet the following requirements:

1. An order must be received before any individual item runs out.
2. The sum of the amounts of the individual items ordered must equal the total desired economical order size.
3. The quantity ordered should be balanced among individual items to delay need for the next order as long as possible.

An approach that can be used follows these lines:

1. A reorder point is set on each individual item. (This is set in the usual way to minimize total expected cost.)
2. A new order is made whenever the inventory on hand for an individual item reaches a reorder point.
3. The new order is distributed among items as follows:

Let I_i = inventory on hand of one item, the ith item

P_i = reorder point, the ith item

s_i = expected usage rate, the ith item

Q_i = amount of the order given over to the ith item

Q = total order size

I = total inventory, all items

P = total of the individual reorder points

S = total of the individual usage rates

Note that the quantities Q, I, P, and S must all be in common units. Then the amount of any individual product shipped would be

$$Q_i = s_i \; \frac{(Q + I - P)}{(S)} - I_i + p_i$$

This will result in an inventory on hand which will be balanced among all items in the following sense: the expected time before the inventory of an item reaches a reorder point will be the same for all items. This will put off the need for a new order as long as possible.

To illustrate how this procedure works, suppose an intravenous solution is available in three sizes: A, B, and C. Also, assume that the economic order quantity, as determined from the formula in the chapter, for total solution orders has been determined to be 400 quarts, total inventory on hand equals 270 quarts, total of individual item reorder points equals 240 quarts, and total usage is estimated at 150 quarts per week. Further assume that the inventory on hand for item B has reached the reorder point thus signaling the need for an order.

Based on the above the ratio

$$\frac{Q + I - P}{S}$$

can be calculated as follows:

Q = total amount of order   = 400 quarts
I = total inventory   = 270 quarts
P = total of individual reorder
    order points   = 240 quarts
S = total usage per week   = 150 quarts

$$\frac{Q+I-P}{S} = \frac{400+270-240}{150} = \frac{430}{150} = 2.87$$

Given the foregoing ratio and the following individual usage rates, inventory levels, and reorder points, the individual orders can be calculated from the formula

$$Q_i = 2.87_{si} - I_i + P_i$$

Item = (2.87) (usage rate) − Inventory + Reorder Point = Order

	Item	Quarts
A(½qt) = (2.87)	(100) − 32 + 20 = 275	137.5
B(qt) = (2.87)	(50) − 34 + 35 = 135.5	135.5
C(2qt) = (2.87)	(25) − 30 + 25 = 67.0	134.0
		407.0*

The order which would be placed would be as follows:

Item	Order/Units
A	138
B	136
C	134

The above procedure requires a calculation which can be added to the basic economic order quantity determination and which can be done in a straight forward way from data on the inventory record. Where balances of individual items are maintained on separate cards or records, a notation can be made on each record of the items to be ordered with it. In a mechanical system, using punched-card or internally programmed equipment, product codes designed to identify common-source groups are helpful in selecting the records for items to be ordered in conjunction.

---

*Difference between economic order quantity of 400 and 407 due to rounding error.

Chapter 12
Accounts Receivable Management

Accounts receivable, as Table 12-1 illustrates, is not only the largest single component of working capital but also, with the exception of certain fixed asset holdings, is a hospital's largest single asset investment.[1] The magnitude of a hospital's accounts receivable holdings is primarily due to two factors: (1) the nature and cost of hospital services and (2) the third party payer system. The significance of these factors will become clear as the discussion progresses. However, at this point, it is sufficient just to realize that these factors necessitate both that a hospital hold accounts receivable and that its holdings be a substantial segment of its total assets. Given this set of circumstances, it is incumbent upon management, if the quantity of working capital is to be optimized and actual operating costs are to be minimized, to control the size of this asset carefully.

The Nature of Accounts Receivable

Accounts receivable can be defined as the amounts or monies due from patients, or their agents, for services rendered to them by the hospital. As such, they can be considered to be the reciprocal of accounts payable, for the hospital's accounts receivable are a patient's or a third party payer's accounts payable. Furthermore, if accounts payable are viewed as business loans received (see Chapter 10), then accounts receivable must be viewed as business loans granted.

As was discussed earlier, accounts payable can represent a

---

[1]In the case of the commercial enterprise, the ratio of receivables to total assets centers on about 16 to 20 percent. However, wide variations are experienced among firms, particularly when non-manufacturing industries are included.

Table 12-1

Belden Mercy Hospital
Balance Sheet

October 31, 1968*

Assets

Current Assets		
Cash	$ 60,572	
Accounts Receivable (less allowance for collection losses of $84,149)	$569,299	
Inventories and prepaid expenses	$ 57,006	
Total Current Assets:		$ 686,877
Land, Buildings and Equipment		$3,296,627
Other Assets		
Deferred Financing Costs	$ 56,841	
Commercial Notes	$430,000	
Other	$199,490	
Total Other Assets:		$ 686,331
TOTAL ASSETS:		$4,669,835

Liabilities

Current Liabilities		
Current portion of long-term debt	$115,000	
Accounts payable and accrued expenses	$230,592	
Medicare payable	$ 98,943	
Total Current Liabilities:		$ 444,535
First Mortgage Bonds and Real Estate Contracts		$1,397,515
Deferred Contractual Adjustments		$ 67,000
Fund Balance		$2,760,785
TOTAL LIABILITIES AND FUND BALANCE:		$4,669,835

*Actual 1969 Balance Sheet of a 131 bed, nonprofit, general hospital. The name of the hospital has been changed.

---

costly source of financing to the borrower.[2] Conversely, if accounts payable are costly to the borrower, then accounts receivable should represent an attractive investment alternative to the lender. If this were the case, it would seem reasonable to assume that the lending firms not only would be eager to extend credit,

---

[2]See Chapter 10.

but also would gladly extend more if borrowers would want more accounts payable. However, this is not the case. The reason for this apparent inconsistency can be easily determined if one examines the business lending operations of a commercial firm.

Cost of Accounts Receivable

In Chapter 10, the interest rate on an account payable, with terms of 2-10, net 30, was determined to be, as of day 30, approximately 37%. This interest rate is obviously a substantial rate of return which lenders would be delighted to obtain. Unfortunately, 37% is not the actual rate of return which a lender receives, for the costs involved in granting credit are not considered. Thirty-seven per cent is a gross rate of return which must be adjusted if the net or "true" rate of return on accounts payable is to be determined.

Judging from the actions of most nonfinancial commercial enterprises, the net rate of return on accounts payable is insufficient to make the granting of credit a profitable investment alternative. Admittedly, financial enterprises, such as banks and commercial credit companies, find the granting of credit to be an attractive line of trade. However, for the nonfinancial firm there are costs attached to granting accounts receivable which a bank can avoid through economies of scale, specialization and expertise, but which make the granting of credit financially unattractive to the nonfinancial firm. The costs attached to accounts receivable can be identified and separated into three general types or categories: (1) carrying costs; (2) routine collection and credit costs; and (3) delinquency costs.

In the previous chapter, carrying cost was defined as the cost of holding inventories and was viewed as consisting of two independent cost segments—storage cost and opportunity cost. In the case of accounts receivable, the storage cost segment can be ignored for the most part, for elaborate warehousing and security mechanisms are not needed to hold or store accounts receivable. Carrying cost can thus be equated to the opportunity cost which arises due to the fact that the lending firm, in granting credit, is committing a part of its assets to an accounts receivable investment as opposed to some other investment alternative. Therefore, by definition, the lending firm incurs an opportunity cost equal to the return which could have been obtained if the funds invested in accounts receivable were invested instead in some other manner.[3]

---

[3]It should also be noted that if funds are borrowed to finance accounts receivable that a "cash" cost, as opposed to an opportunity cost, is incurred. This cost also varies directly with the size of the accounts receivable investment and is equal to the interest expense due the lender.

Table 12-2
Accounts Receivable and Carrying Costs

Assumptions:
    a. Firm makes two separate sales of $1,000 each
    b. Terms of purchase are 2-10, net 30
    c. If the discount is taken—cost to the purchaser is $980 each
    d. The highest available rate of return from an alternative
       investment is 12% per year.
    e. All receipts from sales are immediately invested.

Alternative A—Purchasers pay cash upon delivery.
  (No accounts receivable—firm is paid cash, which it invests
  at 12%)
    Cash Receipts = $1,960 (net receipts from two $1,000 sales)
    Income = $1,960 invested at 12% per year for 30
      days = $19.60 (approx.)

                Total Income $19.60

Alternative B—Purchasers pay at the end of the discount period.
  (Hold accounts receivable for 9 days—on day 10 firm is
  paid $1,960)
    Cash Receipts = $1,960 (received on day 10)
    Income = $1,960 invested at 12% per year for 20
      days = $13.07 (approx.)

                Total Income $13.07

Alternative C—One purchaser takes the discount and one pays at the end of the next period.

  Purchaser 1— takes discount. Therefore, firm receives $980 on day
              10 which it invests at 12% for 20 days = $6.53
  Purchaser 2— pays at the end of the net period. Therefore, firm
              receives a $20 return for the granting of cred-
              it = $20.00

                Total Income $26.53

Alternative D—Purchaser pays at the end of the net period.
  Firm receives a return of $20 on each purchase, i.e.,

                Total Income $40.00

Conclusion:
  Given the above discount terms, the granting of credit can be profitable, i.e., the return obtained from extending accounts receivable will exceed the opportunity or carrying cost if at least 25% of all purchasers elect not to take the discount.*

---

  *Determined by solving the following set of equations which assume:

A—100 sales at terms of 2-10, net 30
B—$980 = the opportunity cost of 100 sales (see Alternative A)
C—$6.53 = return on sales wherein discount is taken (see Alternative C).
D—$20 = return on sales wherein discount is not taken (see Alternative C or D)
E—X = number of sales on which discount is taken and Y = number of sales on which
    discount is not taken

$$980 = 6.5X + 20Y$$
$$100 = X + Y$$

It should be realized that carrying cost exists during the entire credit period, for the firm's funds are committed for the entire period. However, to the extent that some borrowers do not take the discount and prefer instead to pay for the use of credit, this cost is offset. In fact, as Table 12-2 illustrates, if carrying cost were the only cost attached to extending creidt, the use of accounts receivable could possibly be profitable for the lending firm. As was mentioned earlier, however, there are other costs.

In addition to carrying costs, the second major category of costs which are attached to the use of accounts receivable are routine collection and credit costs. These costs are operating expenses which arise due to the fact that if a firm is going to extent credit it must, in order not only to make knowledgeable credit decisions, but also to protect its revenue and operating position,

   a. operate a credit department—in order to identify those purchasers who are poor credit risks and, hence, should not be granted credit; and
   b. operate a collections department—in order to keep track of invoice, discount, and due dates; send payment reminders; and, when necessary, take follow-up action on unpaid accounts.

The operation of these departments can obviously be quite expensive. Therefore, since these departments are only needed if the firm extends credit, one can reasonably ask, Why should a firm extend credit? Why is it either necessary or advantageous to a firm to incur the additional costs inherent in offering credit? These questions can be answered in two ways.

First, it can be argued that credit exists due to business necessity. Consider, for a moment, the tremendous operational problems which would be created if credit were not available and all business transactions had to be conducted on a cash-and-carry basis. Without the existence and reasonable availability of credit, it would be impossible to either create or operate a diverse, multibillion dollar economy such as exists today. Admittedly, small items can be handled on a cash-and-carry basis; however, if constant production is to be maintained, if the economy is to grow, and if the wheels of commerce are to turn smoothly and efficiently, credit must exist. Thus, due to business and economic practicality, firms must extend credit if the economy is to operate and grow to its full potential.

The necessity and advantage of credit can also be explained in terms of sound and astute business practice. The extension of

Table 12-3

Impact of Credit Availability on Profits

I. *Assumptions:*

Situation A—Firm does not offer credit; all sales made on a cash basis.

1. Sales = 100,000 units
2. Profit Per Unit—$2 (cost per unit = $3; selling price = $5)
3. Total Profit = $200,000

Situation B—Firm changes policy and offers credit; terms net 30.

1. Sales = 150,000 units (100,000 units sold on a cash basis and 50,000 sold on credit)
2. Gross Profit Per Unit = $2
3. Total gross increase in profits due to the availability of credit = $100,000 (50,000 × $2)
4. Increase in costs due to policy change:
   a. *Carrying Cost.* Assuming the 50,000 additional units are sold on credit, the firm incurs a total annual production cost, due to these sales, of $150,000 ($3 × 50,000 units). In order to support this additional cost, assuming receivables are paid monthly and will be self-sustaining after the first month, i.e., the cash received in the second month for the first month's sales will support the second month's production, the firm must invest $12,500 or 1/12 of this total cost.* If the firm could earn 10% per year by investing these funds in some other manner, then the carrying cost (opportunity cost) attached to offering credit would be $1,250.
   b. *Routine Credit and Collection Costs.* The change in policy requires that the firm establish credit and collection departments. Assume the cost of these departments is $45,000.
5. Total additional cost = $46,250.
6. Net increase in profits due to credit availability—$100,000 less $46,250 = $54,750.
7. Total profit = $253,750.

II. *Conclusions.*
The availability of credit results in sales and profits increasing by more than the costs attached to the offering of credit. Therefore, if management is to increase total profits, it should make credit available.

*This assumes that sales are constant over the entire year.

credit obviously involves a cost to the lending firm. However, the availability of credit also widens the potential market for a firm's product, for both purchasers with ready cash and without ready cash can buy goods. The availability of credit can thus act to increase sales which, in turn, can increase profits. Therefore, if the availability of credit results in sales and profits increasing by more than costs, it is incumbent upon management, if it is to achieve its primary objective of maximizing owner's wealth, to offer credit. Table 12-3 describes this type of situation. The critical point to be realized is that firms offer credit not only because it is an operational necessity, but also because it is a potentially sound strategy for increasing profits.

In viewing the impact of the availability of credit on profits, a third cost to the lending firm must also be considered, if an accurate and complete analysis is to be obtained. In addition to carrying and routine credit and collection costs, the extension of credit carries with it another type or category of costs which can be identified as delinquency costs. These costs arise due to the uncertainties inherent in the credit screening and granting process.

It is unreasonable to believe that all purchasers will always pay their bills on time or even that all bills will always be paid. If buyers could be completely trusted to pay their accounts there would be no need for a credit department to screen applicants and identify poor credit risks. It is equally naive to believe that a credit department will be infallible in its screening process. Despite the most careful work and screening by the credit department, some purchasers will invariably fail to pay their bills. When this situation occurs, the selling firm must take certain steps in order to collect its past due accounts. It is at this point that delinquency costs begin to emerge, for the actions which the seller must take will add to the total costs of extending credit.

When an account becomes overdue, the first step which is generally taken is simply that of just allowing the collection department to follow-up on the account by reminding the purchaser that he is past due. If, as is often the case, this is all that is necessary in order to collect the account, then delinquency costs will not be significant.

However, if the reminders of the collection department are insufficient to cause payment, other, more costly, steps must be taken. For example, the account may be turned over to a collection agency which may charge 10–12% (or more) of the amount outstanding for its efforts, or a lawyer may be retained at a fee of at least 10% of the outstanding balance, or—as a last resort—the account may have to be written off as a bad debt with a resultant additional cost equal to the cost of the goods. Regardless of which specific step or steps are taken, the fact should be clear that delinquency costs can be quite expensive. In fact, it is largely due to this cost factor that credit extension, in and of its own right, is not an attractive businss opportunity for a nonfinancial firm.

Figure 12-1 illustrates the costs of credit to the lending firm and the potential impact of credit on profits. As is clear from the figure, the availability of credit can result in a large increase in gross profits while, at the same time, due to its costs, only have a limited effect on net profits and, subsequently, a relatively low rate of return. However, even with its low rate of return, a firm may choose to make credit available due to the necessities of business, or in order to protect its market position, or for other reasons. Whatever the specific reason, it must be realized that credit, though perhaps necessary, is costly, and, therefore, should be judiciously managed and controlled.

Management Guideline

Based on the foregoing discussion, the following guideline can be inferred for the management of accounts receivable.

General rule:

> The extension of credit is a costly undertaking for the lending firm and, hence, should only be utilized to the extent which it increases profits.

Interpretation:

> The extension of credit, while not in its own right an attractive line of trade for the nonfinancial commercial enterprise, can help to increase sales and can, therefore, act to enhance profits. However, if credit is granted indiscriminately, the costs incurred due to its extension can exceed the increased profits obtained due to an expanded sales volume. Thus, credit or accounts receivable should be kept to a minimum, with the minimum being that point where the marginal increase in profits equals the marginal increase in costs.

In summary, credit extension, though a costly operation to the lending firm, has a profit-increasing potential and therefore should be utilized to the fullest extent of that potential.

Figure 12-1
Credit and Profit*

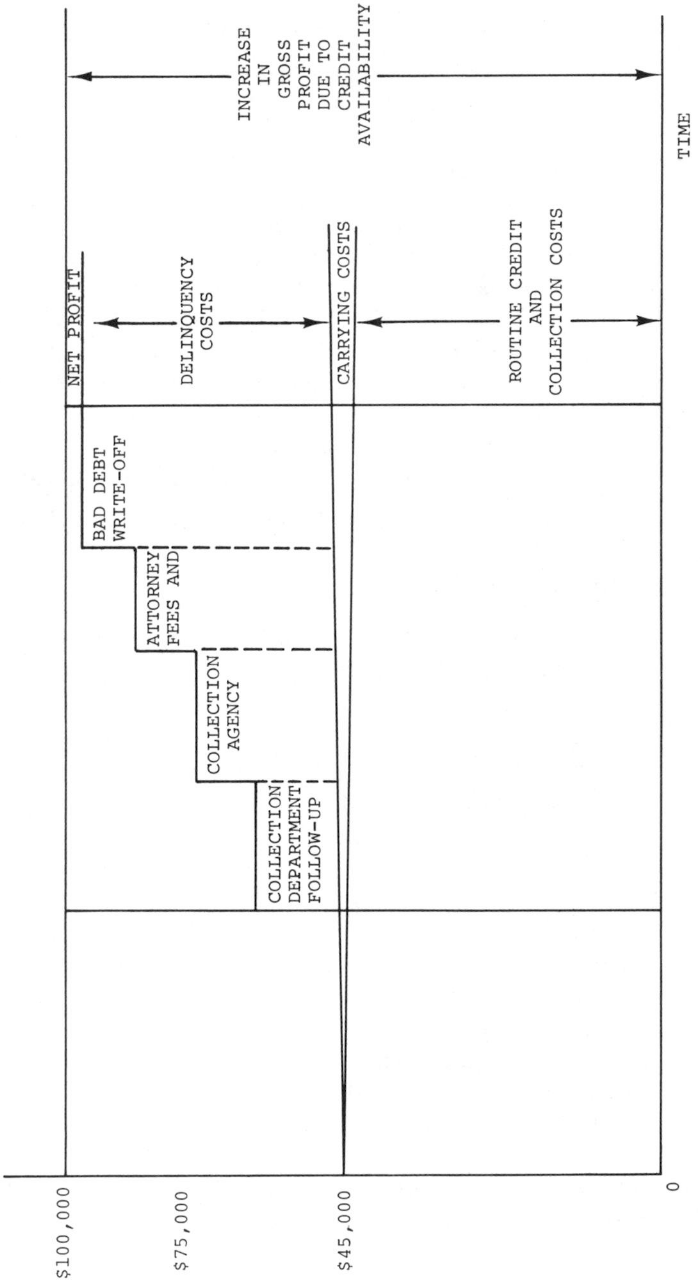

* RELATES TO TABLE 13-3

Hospital Accounts Receivable

Based upon the above material, the reader should now have a basic understanding of the potential and costs of accounts receivable in the commercial setting. With this understanding in mind, it is now possible to turn and examine the role of accounts receivable in the hospital setting.

As Table 12-1 illustrates, hospitals are in the credit business. A hospital, even if well managed, can typically expect to hold about 10% of its total assets and 75% of its current assets in accounts receivable. This is obviously a substantial investment. However, this investment is, at least in part, unavoidable.

A hospital is a community resource whose primary objective is that of providing the community with the services which it needs. In the strictest sense, this objective means providing services to any and all patients without regard to their financial situation or ability. In practical terms, from either a public relations or, as some courts are attempting to establish, a legal standpoint, a hospital cannot refuse care to a patient in need.[4] Given this fact, and the additional facts that hospital care is costly and that the need for hospital care is generally both emotionally and financially unexpected, it is not difficult to understand why a hospital cannot operate on a cash-and-carry basis and, hence, must extend credit to self-responsible (self-pay) patients.

The nature of hospital-third party payer relationships also forces hospitals into the credit business. It is impossible, if only due to the quantity of transactions and distance considerations, for hospitals to deal with third party payers on a cash-and-carry basis. Thus, credit granting is an intrinsic and unavoidable operational fact of life for hospitals.

Since hospitals are in the credit business, they incur the same credit extension costs as do commercial firms. However, unlike commercial firms, hospitals can neither use the profit-generating potential of credit to justify the costs of credit, nor have they chosen to offer their services on "terms" in order to offset the costs of credit.

The commercial firm can use the availability of credit to increase sales and, consequently, profits. A hospital, however, due to the nature of the demand for its services, cannot increase its patient days either by making credit available or by liberalizing its

---

[4]One could also argue this point in terms of the Internal Revenue Service regulations which require that a hospital, in order to retain its tax exemption, cannot be operated exclusively for those who are able to pay.

credit terms. Also, even if hospitals could increase their volume through the use of credit, this increase would not result in an increase in profits, for hospitals obtain the bulk of their revenues from cost-based reimbursement contracts which do not include an economic profit factor. Thus, the profit-increasing potential of credit does not exist in the case of the hospital.

Additionally, hospitals have traditionally felt that it would be unwise to charge interest, either in the form of offering services on "terms" or in the form of a lending or handling charge, on accounts receivable. Hospital managers have long held the position that charging interest will result in adverse public relations and also, due to the nondiscretionary nature of the bulk of hospital demand and the community resource position of hospital, that it is morally wrong. Recently, though, some managers have taken the position that charging interest is both justifiable and necessary if the hospital is to be competitive for the debtor's dollar. However, it is questionable, especially in light of the fact that in some states hospitals can only charge interest at the simple as opposed to the installment sales rate, if the revenues from these charges will outweigh the costs of extending credit.

Appendix 12 discusses the above matter in greater detail. Readers desiring additional information should refer to the appendix and the Suggested Readings at the end of the chapter. At this point, it should be realized that hospitals, for the most part, do not specifically charge for the credit which they make available to patients.

The implications of this situation are quite clear. Since hospitals cannot use the availability of credit as a mechanism for increasing sales and profits, the advantages or value of credit does not exist for the hospital as it does for the commercial firm. In the case of the hospital, the extension of credit only results in additional operating costs being incurred. Therefore, if part of management's goal or objective is to provide services at least cost, the operational guideline for managing accounts receivable can be stated simply as follows:

> Accounts receivable, and the granting of credit, should
> be kept to a minimum if costs are to be minimized.

Admittedly, as has been discussed, the holding of some accounts receivable is an unavoidable part of hospital operations. Management, however, can and must exercise some control over this amount if it is to minimize costs. Thus, the question which can be asked at this point, and the realistic problem which faces management is, What can be done in order to minimize the costs of accounts receivable? That is, given the constraint of operational necessity, what management actions can be taken to minimize the costs of accounts receivable?

Managing Accounts Receivable

The management of accounts receivable is a complex problem which begins not when a patient is discharged but rather with the preadmission of a patient and continues through until the account is paid or a decision is made to write off the account as uncollectable. Between these points, management is confronted with numerous internal and external operational problems and decisions, each of which requires definite management action if costs are to be minimized.

Basically, the problem of controlling the costs of accounts receivable centers on the matter of controlling the time or the length of the accounts receivable payment cycle. As was discussed in Chapter 9, the longer this payment cycle, the larger must be the hospital's working capital investment in accounts receivable. Consequently, the more assets which are involved, the greater will be the carrying costs. Also, the larger the amount of accounts receivable, the greater will be the routine credit and collection costs, for more people will be needed to keep track of the accounts and probably the greater will be the delinquency costs, for older accounts are less likely to be paid.[5] Thus, if costs are to be minimized it is imperative that the payment cycle be kept as short as is pragmatically feasible. The question confronting management is: How can this be done?

Viewing the problem realistically, hospital management, due to the presence of third party payers, is limited in regard to the amount of control which it can exercise over the accounts receivable payment cycle. It is unreasonable to believe that a single hospital can force a Blue Cross plan or the government (Medicare or Medicaid) to either reduce the amount of paperwork involved in billing for a covered patient or increase the speed with which they pay their debts, i.e., pay accounts receivable. A hospital, however, can improve its own "in-house" (internal) processing procedures and thereby accelerate the rate at which it is able to

---

[5]The Amercian Credit Indemnity Company suggests that an account which is 90 days past due will be diminished in value by 10%, an account 120 days past due 15%, etc.

submit bills to both third party payers and self-responsible payers. Obviously, to the extent to which a hospital can reduce its "in-house" processing time, it can reduce the amount of its accounts receivable holdings and carrying costs.

In order to accelerate "in-house" processing time, management must design an accounting system that ensures not only that all requests for services are registered, but also that all services rendered are *promptly* and *accurately* charged to the appropriate patient's account. The importance of these two factors should be clear. If extra time has to be spent in trying to identify services which have been rendered, internal processing time must increase. Also, processing time must increase if the correct charges are not promptly entered into a patient's account. The system should also be designed to ensure that adequate internal control checks and balances exist. A checklist of internal control requirements for accounts receivable is presented in Table 12-4.

The reader should realize that the design of the accounts receivable system is basically a systems analysis problem which should be solved by the hospital's industrial engineer, internal auditor, and controller. The role of general hospital management in this area is limited just to that of reviewing both the system design and its results, in order to ensure that it is functioning properly. Readers interested in further information on the design of accounts receivable systems should refer to the Suggested Readings at the end of this chapter.

The length of the payment cycle can also be reduced by improving the efficiency of the credit and collection function and by developing a systematic credit granting and follow-up procedure. Improving the efficiency of the credit and collection function will also reduce routine operating costs. Additionally, delinquency costs will be reduced by: implementation of a system for granting credit based on information necessary to evaluate a patient's credit status and a system with follow-up procedures for accounts receivable; proper organization and timing of collection efforts; use of collection agencies and legal assistance when necessary; and adoption of criteria for writing off an account as uncollectable.

The credit and collection function should begin, whenever possible, with the preadmission or preregistration processing of a patient. Through preadmissions, the hospital not only can obtain, prior to admission, the information necessary to confirm a patient's insurance coverage or systematically analyze his credit status, but also it can inform a patient of any required deposit or, if appropriate, request a credit review in order to arrange bank financing or a

Table 12-4

Accounts Receivable—Internal Control Checklist *

1. Are all charges made in accordance with the rate schedule?
2. Is a ledger account established for each patient admitted, and is it checked against the admission register?
3. Are satisfactory procedures followed in service departments to ensure the prompt reporting of *all* services involving charges?
4. Are charges for services checked for accuracy of:
   a. Period covered?
   b. Type of services?
   c. Rates used?
   d. Extensions?
5. Are control totals developed from the charge media and balanced against the accounts receivable posting?
6. If statistical data are maintained, are they correlated with recorded revenues?
7. Is a reconciliation of the total of the individual accounts in the accounts receivable ledgers with the general ledger control:
   a. Prepared periodically?
   b. Reviewed by a responsible person?
8. Are statements of all accounts receivable mailed regularly?
9. Are aging schedules:
   a. Prepared periodically?
   b. Reviewed and tested periodically by a responsible person?
10. Are the following functions handled independently:
    a. Posting?
    b. Credit?
    c. Development of control totals?
    d. Cash receipts?
    e. Allowance approval?
11. Do persons independent of accounts receivable personnel and credit department personnel confirm accounts by mail and by:
    a. Checking patients' statements with accounts?
    b. Keeping statements under control to assure mailing?
    c. Receiving reported differences directly?
    d. Investigating reported differences?

*Partial listing, adapted from American Hospital Association, "Internal Control and Internal Auditing For Hospitals" (American Hospital Association, 1969).

personalized payment plan. Preadmission is also particularly of value in identifying free service (charity) patients.

The fact that an account receivable goes unpaid does not, by definition, mean that the account should be classified as a bad debt. If, from the outset, the possibility of ever collecting on a particular account is zero, that account should not be classified as a regular or normal account receivable. Rather, the account should be classified as a free service account. The misclassification of free service accounts results only in wasted collection effort and expense, inflated accounts receivable balances, and a distorted picture of the hospital's collection efforts and results. Thus, if a true picture of the hospital's accounts receivable situation is to be obtained and if unnecessary collection efforts are to be minimized, free service accounts should be identified as early as possible.

Preadmission of patients can aid the hospital in the early identification of free service patients, for it enables the hospital to obtain the financial information needed to determine a patient's credit status. Based upon this information, the hospital not only can accurately identify such accounts, but also can attempt to find alternative sources of financial assistance in order to reduce the amount of free services which must be financed through internally generated funds.

Numerous texts and articles have been written on the specific mechanics of hospital credit and collection techniques and systems. Given the volume and quality of the existing literature, there is little value and insufficient space to either repeat or summarize that material in this text. Additionally, the mechanics of operating the credit and collections function should not be a primary concern of the hospital's administrator. Rather, it should be the concern of the hospital's credit manager, accountant, internal auditor, and controller. The administrator has neither the time nor the detailed knowledge necessary to involve himself in the day-to-day management of accounts receivable. His responsibility and concern lie instead in establishing policy, with the advice and guidance of the hospital's financial personnel, in such areas as bad debt write-offs, free service allowances, the use of service charges, and monitoring the functioning of the total accounts receivable system. The reports needed to monitor the system will be discussed in Chapter 14. However, before moving on to examine cash management, it would be worthwhile to consider two additional points.

Credit Cards

Commercial firms have found that the acceptance of bank and commercial credit cards can be a useful mechanism for accelerating the accounts receivable payment cycle. Credit cards, such as Visa and Master Charge are held by millions of persons and are accepted by over 600,000 businesses including some physicians and hospitals.

The advantage to a hospital of accepting these credit cards for payment of accounts centers on both the acceleration of the payment cycle and the reduction of collection efforts and subsequent costs. The key characteristics of a credit card acceptance agreement are that:

— the hospital agrees to accept the patient's credit card for payment of amounts owed;

— the hospital pays a fee—service charge—to the issuing bank for each charge submitted;

— the hospital must maintain an account at the bank issuing the credit card;

— the issuing bank agrees to pay all accounts to the hospital quickly by depositing funds in the hospital's account at the issuing bank, and;

— the bank determines the patient's credit worthiness and has no recourse for uncollectible accounts.

In essence a credit card acceptance agreement allows a hospital, for a fee, both to accelerate its payment cycle by shifting the problem of collection lags to the issuing bank, and to transfer a portion of its credit investigation and collection efforts (and costs) to the issuing bank.

Given the nature of the agreement, the financial decision rule as to whether or not to accept credit cards is quite simple. If the benefits (savings) in terms of reduced working capital needs and reduced credit investigation and collection costs exceed the sum of the costs of the fee and the tangible and intangible costs of either holding a subsidiary account at the issuing bank or transferring an entire account to the issuing bank, then, the hospital should consider more than just financial implications.

The use of credit cards by hospitals raises both public policy and philosophical issues. Stated simply, a hospital must weigh the internal financial implications against:

1. the potential increased cost of care to the patient, due to the interest charge which the bank or credit company adds to accounts which it finances over time, i.e., which patients pay in installments; and

2. its obligations, as a vital community resource, to not shift the burden of collection or of loss to another party (the card issuing bank or company) or, through the bank or company, to patients financially unable to pay for needed care. In addition to these factors the matters of "image and patient reaction" must be taken into account.

Obviously, each hospital must balance these issues in terms of its own environment and financial requirements. However, as a middle ground, it may be judicious management, if the acceptance of credit cards is financially justified, to limit acceptance either to certain services, e.g., emergency department or outpatient or to only charges which are less than a predetermined level—less than $100.

Credit and Collection Costs and Total Costs

Intuitively, it would seem that one approach to reducing the total costs of accounts receivable would lie in reducing credit and collection costs to a minimum. In some instances, however, the hospital may be able to decrease total costs by increasing credit and collection costs. It has been found, that as collection efforts increase, with an increase in credit and collection costs, that the average collection time and bad debt losses decrease, that is, carrying and delinquency costs decrease. Figure 12-2 illustrates this situation.

As can be seen from the figure, the initial increments in credit and collection expenditures (Y to Y_1) have no effect on carrying and delinquency costs. However, as more is spent (Y_1 to Y_2) carrying and delinquency costs begin to fall and continue to fall until a saturation point (Y_3) is reached. As the figure indicates, additional expenditures (Y_3 to Y_4), beyond the saturation point, have no cost reduction impact.

How much a hospital should actually spend on credit and collection efforts is an empirical problem which can only be solved by examining the costs and savings attached to different levels of expenditure. Ideally, funds should be invested until that point is reached wherein the marginal savings equal the marginal cost. That is, credit and collection expenditures should increase until that point wherein the savings from an additional expenditure just equal the cost of that expenditure. Table 12-5 illustrates this general rule.

Accounts Receivable and Financing

A discussion of accounts receivable management would be incomplete without an examination of the role and usefulness of accounts receivable in providing short-term financing for a hospital's temporary working capital needs. This material was discussed in part in Chapter 10. However, this topic is also important to accounts receivable management and, therefore, bears reiteration. The use of accounts receivable in short-term financing centers around either the pledging of accounts as security or collateral for a loan or the selling of the receivables. The pledging of accounts receivable is known as discounting accounts receivable. In this

Table 12-5

Credit and Collection Expenditures and Accounts Receivable Costs

General Assumptions:

Average account receivable holdings	=		$500,000
Cost of operating credit and collections department (annual)	=	$100,000	
Carrying cost per year (assuming opportunity cost at 6%)	=	$ 30,000	
Delinquency costs (average annual cost)	=	$150,000	
Total accounts receivable costs:			$280,000

Situation A

Employ an additional person in the collections department; cost=$12,000
Projected effects:

Cost of credit and collections department	=	$112,000
Carrying cost per year	=	30,000
Delinquency costs	=	150,000
Total:		$292,000

Decision: Do not hire additional person. Expenditure increases costs by more than the savings. This situation is similar to a move from Y to Y_1 in Figure 12-2.

Situation B

Develop and implement systematic credit and collection procedure which requires a staffing increase of three positions; cost = $50,000
Projected effects:

Cost of credit and collections department	=	$150,000
Carrying cost (reduce average accounts receivable holdings to $300,000)	=	18,000
Delinquency cost	=	100,000
Total:		$268,000

Decision: Implement the above actions. This situation is similar to a move from Y_1 to Y_2 or perhaps from Y_2 to Y_3 in Figure 12-2.

Situation C

Assume present situation is as described in Situation B above. Given this situation, the credit manager requests the hiring of an assistant credit manager at a cost of $15,000.
Projected effects:

Cost of credit and collections department	=	$165,000
Carrying costs	=	18,000
Delinquency costs	=	100,000
Total:		$283,000

Decision: Do not hire the assistant credit manager, for it does not produce a savings over Situation B. This situation is similar to a move from Y_3 to Y_4 in Figure 12-2.

Figure 12-2

Credit and Collection Expenditures and Carrying and Delinquency Costs

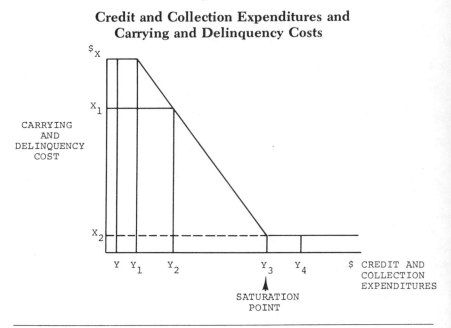

process the lender takes the receivables, but has recourse to the hospital (the borrower). That is, if an account is not paid, the lender can hold the hospital responsible for the account, and the hospital—not the lender—must absorb the loss.

In the case of hospitals, the discounting of accounts receivable can take one or both of two forms. The hospital may discount the accounts directly with a bank or finance company. In this instance, the hospital deals directly with the lender and the patient generally is unaware of the fact that his account has been discounted. If the patient defaults on the account, the lender obtains payment from the hospital and the hospital, in turn, attempts to collect from the patient.

As an alternative of the above, the hospital may develop an arrangement with a bank wherein the bank will make loans to patients for medical expenses. In the strictest sense, this arrangement does not actually involve the discounting of accounts receivable. However, it is similar to discounting in that the bank, in order to be agreeable to such an arrangement, will generally require that it have recourse to the hospital if the patient defaults on the loan. Thus, under either alternative the risk of default remains with the hospital.

A direct bank-patient loan arrangement is probably of most benefit to the hospital in regard to self-pay patients. Also, to the extent that it can provide a means of financing the self-responsible portion of a patient's bill, it can be of value relative to patients who are covered by third party payers. However, its use in regard to accounts due from third party payers does not appear to be practical. Alternatively, the discounting approach is practical for both third party and self-pay accounts and, depending on the costs, may be the most desirable short-term financing alternative if substantial amounts are needed.

Accounts receivable can also play another short-term financing role. Receivables can be sold or factored to a lender. In this process, the hospital sells, without recourse, its receivables to a bank or finance company. That is, the hospital not only transfers the receivables to the lender but also, transfers the risk of default to the lender. Generally, when receivables are factored, the patient is notified of the transaction and makes payment directly to the bank or finance company.

Accounts receivable factoring is a common practice in some hospitals. However, its value can be questioned. Factoring, due to the fact that the lender bears the risk of default, is more expensive than discounting. Also, if the lender harrasses the patient during the collection process, factoring can have adverse public relations effects. Thus, accounts receivable factoring is not recommended as a primary means of financing temporary working capital needs.

Conclusion

The role of accounts receivable in hospital operations should now be clear. It should be borne in mind that the granting of credit and the holding of some accounts receivable is a necessary and unavoidable part of hospital operations. However, the extension of credit and the holding of receivables are costly and, to the extent that the amount of accounts receivable can be reduced, the costs of operation can also be reduced. Therefore, the operational guideline for the management of accounts receivable is simply that, given the necessities of operation, accounts receivable should be kept to a minimum.

Suggested Readings

Barnes, E. H. *Barnes on Credit and Collection.*

Fritz, Michael H. "Collection Techniques."

Healy, Sister Mary Immaculate. "An Analysis of Accounts Receivable with Emphasis on Factoring."

Lippold, Ronald C. *Hospital Credit Training Manual.*

Markson, Thomas J. "Some of the Effects of a Service Charge on Hospital Accounts Receivable."

Markstein, David L. "The Pros and Cons of Credit Cards for the Hospital Field."

Massachusetts Hospital Association. "Follow Up Analysis: Methods and Procedure for Minimizing Financial Loss Risk and Accounts Receivable."

Seawell, L. Vann. *Hospital Financial Accounting: Theory and Practice,* Chapter 11.

Weston, J. Fred and Brigham, Eugene F. *Managerial Finance,* Chapter 13.

Appendix 12

Interest Charges and Accounts Receivable

I. Carrying Cost:

An opportunity cost equal to the revenue foregone by investing funds in accounts receivable as opposed to some other investment alternative. It should be noted, that carrying cost is an economic cost of operations. However, it is not an out-of-pocket cost since it is revenue foregone.

A. Current Status:

1. Third party payers

Presently, do not include carrying cost as an allowable cost.

2. Self-responsible patients

For the most part, hospitals do not presently charge interest on late charges. However, these charges could be added to the bills of self-pay patients who are late in payment and to the self-responsible portion of accounts due from patients who are covered by third party payers.

B. Conclusion:
1. This cost, though not an accounting cost, is an economic and "real" operational cost. Therefore, revenues to compensate for the income foregone (opportunity cost), due to the holding of accounts receivable for the usual or customary carrying period, should be obtained as part of normal operations.
2. Revenues to compensate for income lost (opportunity cost) due to payments which are delayed beyond the usual or customary carrying period should not be obtained from normal operations. This is the case, for these costs should be viewed as being due to unusual or abnormal events which are the responsiblity of particular debtors. Thus, they should be treated as abnormal and neither be aggregated into normal operating costs nor be offset through normal operating revenues. Instead, separate late or interest charges should be used to compensate for these costs. Such charges not only are economically justified, but also are mandatory if an economically sound financial position is to be maintained.

II. Credit and Collection Costs:
The routine operating costs incurred in the operations of the credit and collections department. As such, these costs are part of the normal day-to-day operations of the hospital.
A. Current Status:
1. Third party payers
An allowable cost which is included in the third party reimbursement formula.
2. Self-responsible patients
A "real" cost of operations which should be included in the hospital's charge structure.
B. Conclusion:
Revenues to compensate for these costs can and should be obtained as part of normal operations. Therefore, late or interest charges are not needed to provide revenue for these costs.

III. Delinquency cost:
The cost which arises due to patients' defaulting on their debt obligations. The magnitude of this cost, for each account which becomes delinquent, can range from just a small amount, for extra collection efforts on the part of the

hospital's collection department, to—at the extreme—the writing off of the entire account as uncollectable. Historically, third party payers have not defaulted on their agreed-to obligations. Therefore, this cost is attributable entirely to obligations which the patient has to pay himself.

A. Current Status:
   1. Third party payers
       A disallowed cost which is not included in the reimbursement formula. (As discussed earlier, Medicare allows bad debt costs [for its patients] as a reimbursable item, if a reasonable collection effort has been made.) It is, in effect, a price discount which is given to third party payers in recognition of the reduced business risk which they represent.
   2. Self-responsible Patients
       A "real" operating cost which should be recognized in the hospital's charge structure.

B. Conclusion:
       Revenues to compensate for these costs can and should be obtained as part of normal operations. Therefore, late or interest charges are not needed to provide revenues for these costs.

Chapter 13
Cash and Short-Term Investments

Most financial management authorities and practicing administrators would agree that cash is the lifeblood of the hospital. The
strong and steady circulation of cash is as critical to the good
health of a hospital as is the proper functioning of the circulatory
system to the health of a human organism. Given this importance,
it is incumbent upon management to manage cash effectively.
This chapter is devoted to examining cash management and the
investment of excess cash holdings.

Why Hold Cash?

The reason why a hospital, or for that matter why any other firm,
holds cash can be explained in several ways. Perhaps the most
sophisticated explanation is the Keynesian approach which identifies three motives for holding cash: transactions, precautionary,
and speculative.

The transactions motive can be defined as the need to hold cash
in order to meet payments (demands for cash) which arise out of
the ordinary course of conducting business, e.g., supplies purchased, labor costs, insurance costs. The precautionary motive explains the need to hold cash in terms of the necessity of having a
cash buffer or cushion available to meet unexpected cash demands
or requirements. Finally, the speculative motive can be defined as
the need to hold cash in order to be in a position to take advantage
of changes in security prices. According to the Keynesian hypotheses, all cash holdings can be explained and justified as being a
function or result of these three factors

If the Keynesian approach represents one extreme, the other is
represented by the practical businessman who would explain the

need for holding cash in terms of business necessity. Quite simply, if a firm is to be able to pay its bills as they come due, it must hold some cash balances. Regardless of which approach is used, the underlying reason is the same. Hospitals must hold cash due to the lack of synchronization between cash inflows and outflows.

If cash inflows and outflows could be synchronized, there would be no need for a hospital to hold any cash. In a synchronized situation, cash would just pass through the hospital. Cash, in effect, would go directly from the hospital's sources of revenue to its creditors. However, due to the uncertain character of cash inflows and the unexpected nature of some cash outflows, it is impossible, to either consistently or precisely synchronize the two flows. Thus, if management is to avoid having to default on obligations, it must hold a stock of cash available as a reserve.

Perhaps the simplest way to understand the effects of cash flow synchronization is to view cash holdings as a reservoir or pool into which flow revenues and from which drain payments to creditors. Figure 13 (Case 1) utilizes this approach to illustrate the implications of synchronization. The critical point to be realized is that, due to a lack of synchronization, hospitals must hold some cash balances.

Cost of Holding Cash

Given that a hospital must hold some cash balances, the obvious question is, "What are the costs of holding cash?" Generally, two types or categories of cost are associated with a hospital's cash holdings—a short cost and a long or carrying cost. As Case 2A in Figure 13-1 illustrates, short cost arises when a hospital's cash holdings are insufficient to meet all of its cash outflow demands.

The magnitude of short cost can vary markedly with the extent of the cash shortage and the frequency of occurrence. If the shortage is an occasional or infrequent event, it can be easily met, in most cases, at a small cost through either borrowing on an open line of credit or, if available, through the selling of short-term investments. If the shortages are either large or frequent, they will result in loss of discounts on purchases, short-term borrowing at high interest rates, a poor or deteriorating credit rating, or in insolvency. Any of these actions is obviously costly and should be avoided. Therefore, management should attempt to maintain a cash balance sufficient not only to meet routine transactions, but also to provide protection against unexpected cash requirements.

As was the case in regard to inventories, the existence of short

Figure 13-1

Cash Flow Synchronization: Implications

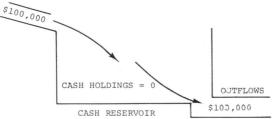

CASE 1 - CASH FLOW SYNCHRONIZED

INFLOWS - $100,000 RECEIVED ON DAY 20
OUTFLOWS - $100,000 DUE ON DAY 20

$100,000

CASH HOLDINGS = 0

CASH RESERVOIR

OUTFLOWS

$100,000

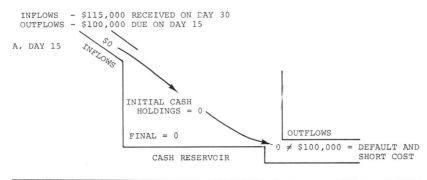

CASE 2 - CASH FLOWS UNSYNCHRONIZED

INFLOWS - $115,000 RECEIVED ON DAY 30
OUTFLOWS - $100,000 DUE ON DAY 15

A. DAY 15

$0

INFLOWS

INITIAL CASH
    HOLDINGS = 0

FINAL = 0

CASH RESERVOIR

OUTFLOWS

0 ≠ $100,000 = DEFAULT AND
                SHORT COST

costs argues for a hospital to hold a large cash inventory or balance. However, in addition to short costs, hospitals must also contend with long or carrying costs. These latter costs encourage a cash balance decision exactly opposite to the decision which short costs support.

Carrying or long costs can be defined as the opportunity cost attached to holding cash balances. When a hospital decides to hold any given amount of cash, it is in effect electing to invest some of its funds in cash holdings as opposed to some other investment alternative. This decision means that, at the very least, the hospital will incur an opportunity cost equal to the return which could have been obtained if the funds had been invested in some other way. The magnitude of this cost varies directly with

Figure 13-1 (continued)

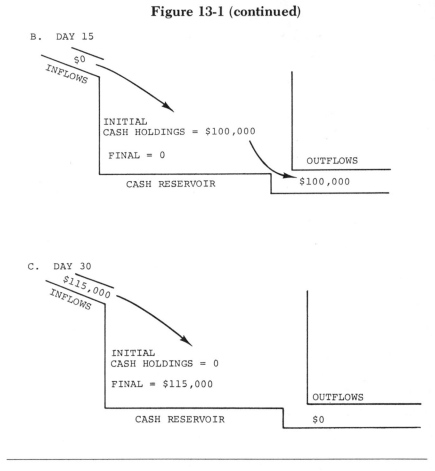

B. DAY 15

INFLOWS $0

INITIAL
CASH HOLDINGS = $100,000

FINAL = 0

CASH RESERVOIR

OUTFLOWS

$100,000

C. DAY 30

INFLOWS $115,000

INITIAL
CASH HOLDINGS = 0

FINAL = $115,000

CASH RESERVOIR

OUTFLOWS

$0

both the rate of return on the investment alternatives which are available and the size of the cash investment.

For purposes of analysis, the opportunity cost attached to cash holdings can be segregated into two components. As has been discussed, a hospital must hold some level of cash balances in order to be able to operate (see Case 2-B, Figure 13-1). This basic operational cash holding can be defined as the hospital's minimal cash balance. Since this minimal cash balance represents an investment it, by definition, has an opportunity cost which varies proportionately with the size of the minimal balance, i.e., the greater the balance, the greater the cost.

In addition to its minimal cash balance a hospital may, from time to time, due to the lack of synchronization between cash inflows and outflows, find itself holding cash balances in excess of the minimal level. An example of this situation is represented by Case 2-C in Figure 13-1. These excess cash holdings, like the minimal cash balance, represent an investment on the part of the hospital. Hence, they have an opportunity cost attached to them which varies directly with the magnitude of the holding.

Given that these are the costs attached to cash holdings, the issue facing management can be stated simply as that of determining how to minimize the total cost of holding cash. Actually, the problem can be most easily understood if it is viewed not as a single question, but rather as three interrelated problems. First, in order to minimize the opportunity cost attached to the minimum cash balance, management must develop the operating conditions necessary for minimizing the absolute amount of this investment. Secondly, based on the actual operating conditions, the magnitude of long and short costs, and the probability of incurring these costs, management must determine the optimal minimum cash balance, i.e., the amount of cash holdings which will minimize the total expected value of long and short costs. Finally, based on the minimum cash balance, management must determine both how to finance additional cash requirements and how to invest any excess cash holdings. Since this is a multi-part problem, let us first consider the matter of how to minimize the level or amount of the hospital's basic operational cash needs, that is, how to create the operating conditions necessary to minimize the absolute amount of the hospital's minimum cash balance.

Minimize Cash Holdings

As Case 1 in Figure 13-1 illustrates, it is not necessary for a hospital to hold any cash balances if cash inflows and outflows are synchronized. Therefore, if management is to minimize the size or amount of the hospital's basic operational cash requirements, it must attempt to synchronize cash flows. This point, while perhaps obvious, is much easier to logically deduce than operationally achieve. The difficulty lies in the fact that hospitals have relatively little control over either cash inflows or cash outflows.

The bulk of a hospital's cash outflows involve payments for personnel—salaries, taxes, fringe benefits. The timing of these payments is fixed either by the government, union contracts, insurance companies, or tradition and little can be done to alter the due dates for these payments. The remainder of a hospital's cash outflows generally involve payments for purchases of supplies and materials—food, drugs, electricity. The timing of these payments is, for the most part, fixed either by contract or convention. It is in regard to these outflows, however, that management may be able to exercise some discretion and thereby affect the timing of cash outflows. Therefore, to the extent possible, and from a cost minimization viewpoint desirable, management should attempt to decelerate or slow down the pace of cash outflows.[1]

Decelerating the pace of outflows is advantageous in that it allows more time for:

1. Cash inflows to be received—thus, increasing the probability of being able to match or synchronize inflows with outflows; and
2. Cash holdings to be invested—thus, reducing the opportunity cost attached to holding cash balances.

Management's strategy, therefore, should be simply that of carefully examining payment dates and alternative costs in order to decelerate cash outflows as much as is practical.

The control which a hospital may be able to exercise over cash inflows, though perhaps greater than that which can be exercised over outflows, is also limited. Due to its relative economic size and power, it is unreasonable to believe that a single hospital can bring sufficient pressure to bear on third party payers to force them to either accelerate or even change the timing of their payment schedules. Also, a hospital's influence over the payment schedules of self-pay patients, because of the restricted financial resources of these patients, is limited. However, though a hospital's ability to control cash inflows by influencing payers is restricted, it can—through its "in-house" processing and internal control procedures—still have a substantial impact on the timing of cash inflows. Figures 13-2 and 13-3 illustrate the impact which these two elements can have on cash balances.

It is axiomatic that the longer the "in-house" processing time, the longer a hospital must wait until cash inflows will be available to meet cash outflow demands. Conversely, the shorter the "in-house" processing time, the sooner cash inflows will be received and the greater is the probability that cash will be available to meet outflow demands. Management must attempt to accelerate the pace of cash inflows by reducing the length of "in-house" processing time, if it is to minimize its basic operational cash needs.

---

[1]As was discussed in Chapter 10, financing cash needs by foregoing the discount on accounts payable can be quite costly. Therefore, if total cost is to be minimized, financing should be obtained from the least costly source, which may not necessarily be accounts payable.

Figure 13-2

In-House Processing Time and Cash Balances

A. Case 1

Assumption: — Bill preparation and submission processing time = 14 days

           — Payor processing time = 21 days

           — Cash conversion processing time = 7 days

           — Cash outflows = $100,00 due on Day 30

           — Cash inflows — patients discharged, representing $100,000 in revenue, on Day 1

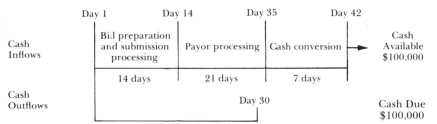

Cash Outflow = $100,000: Cash Available = $0

Implications:
    Due to the length of the "in-house" processing time, cash flows are not synchronized and the hospital is unable to meet its obligations. Therefore, a short cost is incurred.

B. Case 2

Assumption: same as above, except —

           — Bill preparation and submission processing time reduced to 6 days

           — Cash conversion processing time reduced to 2 days

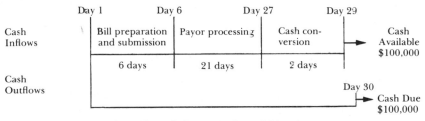

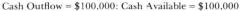

Cash Outflow = $100,000: Cash Available = $100,000

Implications:
    Due to the shortening of the "in-house" processing time cycle, the hospital is able to meet its obligations.

The shortening of the "in-house" processing time period can be viewed as a two-part problem. It involves not only the preparation and submission of patient bills but also the processing of revenues, once received, into cash. Both of these problems, and also the matter of internal control, are basically system design problems which should be handled by the hospital's industrial engineer, internal auditor, and controller.

As has been discussed earlier, general management's responsibility in areas of this nature should be limited. Primary responsibility for the development and the day-to-day operations of the "in-house" revenue processing and internal control systems not only is beyond the scope of general management's knowledge, but also is an inappropriate use of its time and unique talents. Management's responsibility in this area should be *just* that of ensuring that the hospital's revenue systems result in minimizing both processing time and revenue losses.

The management strategy for cash inflows can thus be summarized as one of attempting to both accelerate the pace of cash inflows, through efficient "in-house" processing systems, and protect revenue receipts through effective internal control measures. Accelerating the pace of inflows is advantageous in that it:

1. Increases the probability of being able to synchronize cash inflows and outflows, for inflows will be received at a faster rate; and
2. Provides the potential for reducing opportunity cost, for cash may be invested for longer periods.

The advantage of effective internal control lies in the fact that by preventing leakages or losses from the revenue system it increases the probability that cash will be available as needed. Hence, it enables management to maintain a smaller cash balance. Management, therefore, if it is to create the operating conditions necessary to minimize the absolute amount of the hospital's minimum cash balance, must both decelerate cash outflows and accelerate and protect inflows.

Determining the Minimum Cash Balance

Assuming that management has created the necessary operating conditions, its next problem is to actually determine the minimum cash balance. This problem is quite complex due to the uncertainty inherent in cash flows, the difficulties involved in accurately measuring long and short costs, and the numerous other factors which must be considered. However, it is a problem which must be solved if management is to administer its cash investment effectively.

Figure 13-3

Internal Control and Cash Balances

CASE 1

    INFLOWS - $100,000 RECEIVED ON DAY 20

    OUTFLOWS - $100,000 DUE ON DAY 20

    THEFTS - $2,000

    OTHER LOSSES - $3,000 = DUE TO NEGLIGENCE AND CARELESSNESS

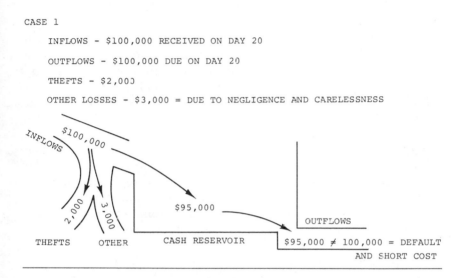

The size of a hospital's minimum cash balance can either be a function of a self-imposed or internal constraint or an externally imposed constraint such as a working capital agreement with a commercial bank. In this latter case, a formal or informal agreement may require the hospital to hold compensating cash balances, i.e., required levels of deposits in the bank as partial payment for services. Alternatively, a hospital may hold a cash balance in its bank in order to improve its banking relationships or to maintain an option for future borrowing. Regardless of the specific reason, the critical point is that a hospital's minimum cash balance may be established by an external constraint, such as a banking requirement. However, establishing a minimum cash balance on the basis of *just* external factors ignores the "real" issue in the cash management decision.

A decision about a hospital's minimum cash balance should depend primarily on the implicit or intangible return which is obtained from holding cash and the cost of holding cash. The return obtained from holding cash can be most easily understood if it is viewed simply as short costs which are avoided. Up to certain levels of cash holdings this return is quite high. Hence, up to certain levels the benefits obtained from holding cash—the avoidance of short costs—will exceed the opportunity or long costs attached to holding cash; i.e., the implicit return from holding cash is higher than any return which can be obtained by investing cash in an alternative manner.

As cash balances increase, the intangible return declines, for the probability of cash shortages and short costs is lessened. Consequently, at some point the opportunity cost of holding cash will exceed the benefits obtained from such holdings. The problem facing management is simply that of determining this "marginal" point.[2] Management must calculate that level of cash holdings which provides the optimal trade-off between long and short costs. This level of cash is, by definition, the minimum cash balance.

Since cash flows are uncertain, the approach which should be used for calculating the minimum cash balance is the same as that which was used for determining the inventory reorder point under conditions of uncertainty.[3] As was the case in regard to inventories, long and short costs are again difficult to measure. Nevertheless, if rational and intelligent cash decisions are to be made, management must attempt to measure these costs even if it is entirely on a subjective basis.

For purposes of illustration, it can be assumed that long or opportunity costs equal 5% of any excess cash balance, and short costs equal $200 per shortage occurrence plus, on average, 6% of the shortage. It should be noted that short costs are expressed in terms of both a fixed and a variable cost component. This has been done in order to reflect the fact that each time a hospital is forced to obtain a loan or defer payments, it must invest a certain amount of time and effort in soliciting and arranging the financing mechanism. This investment is approximately the same regardless of either the amount or the maturity schedule of the financing and, hence, can be viewed as a fixed cost. In addition to this fixed cost, the hospital incurs a cost for the use of the funds which it obtains. This latter cost, since it varies with the amount and maturity of the financing, can be viewed as a variable cost.[4]

---

[2]The "marginal" point is that where the additional or marginal return from holding another dollar of cash just equals the marginal cost of holding that dollar.

[3]Readers desiring a further discussion of the application of inventory techniques to cash management should refer to Appendix 13-A.

[4]In order to simplify the presentation, only an average variable short cost figure has been assumed. Some might argue tht this is inappropriate due to the fact that it does not specifically indicate the individual impact of both financing maturity and amount on variable cost. However, inclusion of both variable cost elements on an individual, as opposed to a consolidated average basis, not only greatly complicates the measurement aspects of the problem, but also the practicality of calculation. Thus, it is questionable if the benefit received from such a refinement would exceed its costs.

Table 13-1

Minimum Cash Balance

Step 1—Assumptions

Short Cost = $200 plus 6% of the shortage
Long Cost = 5% of any excess minimum cash balance
Net Cash Flow Distribution

Probability	.20	.30	.10	.20	.20
Net Cash Flow	+ 5,000	+ 3,000	+ 1,000	− 3,000	− 5,000

Step 2—Cost Matrix—Unadjusted (see Explanation—Step 4)

Minimum Cash Balance Strategy	Net Cash Flow + $5,000	+ $3,000	+ $1,000	− $3,000	−$5,000
$1,000	$ 50	$ 50	$ 50	$320	$440
2,000	100	100	100	260	380
3,000	150	150	150	0	320
4,000	200	200	200	50	260
5,000	250	250	250	100	0
6,000	300	300	300	150	50

Step 3—Cost Matrix—Adjusted for Probability (see Explanation—Step 4)

Minimum Cash Balance Strategy	Net Cash Flow + $5,000 (.20)	+ $3,000 (.30)	+ $1,000 (.10)	− $3,000 (.20)	−$5,000 (.20)	Total Expected Cost
$1,000	$10	$15	$ 5	$64	$38	$182
2,000	20	30	10	52	76	188
3,000	30	45	15	0	64	154
4,000	40	60	20	10	52	182
5,000	50	75	25	20	0	170
6,000	60	90	30	30	10	220

Step 4—Explanation

Step 2—Unadjusted costs of various minimum cash balance strategies, for example:

Table 13-1 (continued)

Strategy	Net Cash Flow	Cost
$1,000	+5,000	— Positive net cash flow; therefore, long $1,000 at a cost of 5% per $1,000 or $50.
$3,000	−3,000	— Negative net cash flow equal to the cash balance; therefore, cash needs equal available cash and cost is 0.
$3,000	−5,000	— Negative net cash flow which exceeds the cash balance; therefore, short $2,000 at a cost of $200 plus 6% of shortage; i.e., $200 plus 6% of $2,000 or $320.
$5,000	+1,000	— Positive net cash flow; therefore, long $5,000 at a cost of 5% per $1,000 or $250.

Step 3—Adjusted costs of various minimum cash balance strategies are obtained by multiplying the values calculated in Step 2 by the probability assumptions set out in Step 1. This step is necessary because of the unpredictable nature of cash flows.

Step 5—Conclusion
A Strategy involving a minimum cash balance of $3,000 will enable management to minimize total cash holding costs.

Along with estimates of long and short costs, management must also develop some notion of the probable variation in monthly net cash flows, that is, cash inflows less cash outflows, which can be expected during the year. Net cash flows are the critical factor, for the matter of concern is not the individual inflows or outflows, but rather the effect of these flows on the hospital's cash position. In order to determine this effect, it is necessary to consider both flows and this can be accomplished most readily and efficiently through an examination of the net flows.

Based upon a study of historical records, projections of future volume and patterns of patient care, estimates of third party payment practices and subjective judgments, assume that the following probabilities of various amounts of net cash flows can be developed.

NET CASH FLOW ESTIMATES

Probability	.20	.30	.10	.20	.20
Net Cash Flow	+ $5,000	+ $3,000	+ $1,000	− $3,000	− $5,000

Given this information and the previously assumed costs, it is now possible, by calculating the expected value or cost of various cash balance strategies, to identify the least-cost cash balance. Table 13-1 illustrates the mechanics of determining the least cost minimum cash balance.

Table 13-2

Cash Management Information Needs: Hypothetical Case

1. **Month 1**
   Operating Results:
   The hospital generates a positive net cash flow which leaves it with an excess cash balance, that is, a cash surplus over the minimum cash balance of $15,000.

   Action:
   Based upon an evaluation of available investment alternatives, management decides to invest the excess funds in a six-month bank note paying 12%. The terms of the note stipulate that interest will be paid only if the note is held to maturity.

2. **Month 2**
   Operating Results:
   The hospital incurs a negative cash flow which results in it needing $10,000 in order to meet its immediate cash obligations and restore its cash position.

   Action:
   After reviewing all available financing alterntives, management decides to redeem the bank note—incurring the early redemption interest loss penalty—and then proceeds to meet its obligations.

3. **Evaluation**
   At first glance, the Month 1 action appears to be reasonable. In the light of later cash flows, though, the inappropriateness of such action becomes obvious. If management had had more information available regarding future cash flows, it could have planned its investment strategy differently so as to maximize revenues while still being able to meet cash needs. For example:

   1. Hypothetical Case   Total Revenues = $ 0
   2. Possible Alternative—assuming management had projections of future cash flows, it could have invested its excess funds as follows:
      —$5,000 in the six month note
      —$10,000 in a Treasury Bill yielding 5% and due in 30 days

                                       Total Revenues = $342
   As the results of the alternative make clear, given information about future cash flows, management is better able to make cash decisions.

4. **Conclusion:**
   In order to wisely make cash investment or financing decisions, management must not only have data on the desired level of the minimal cash balance, but also on future cash flows.

As is indicated in Table 13-1, $3,000 is the least-cost minimum cash balance strategy. However, before management adopts this strategy it should consider several other factors. For example, if this strategy is accepted, there is a 20% probability that cash needs will exceed the available cash balance and that some type of financing will have to be arranged. Management should thus consider its willingness to bear the risk of being out of cash. Also, it should consider the governing board's attitude toward cash shortages and its willingness to borrow. Additionally, the previously discussed external factors or banking relationships and requirements should be included in the decision process.

The critical point to understand is that the cash balance decision should be made on the basis of various considerations. The most important of these is probably the least-cost minimum cash balance factor, for it indicates not only the least-cost strategy, but also the costs of other strategies. However, the final decision should not be made on *just* the basis of any *one* factor. Instead, it should be based upon an evaluation of the total situation—including, but not just limited to, the costs of the various cash balance strategies.

The Cash Budget

Once the minimum cash balance decision has been made, the stage is set for solving the third aspect of the cash management problem. Specifically, management must determine how to both finance additional cash requirements and invest any excess cash holdings. That is, if management is to minimize the total cost of needing and holding cash, it must determine not only the least cost method of financing cash needs, but also the most advantageous investment opportunities for any temporary excess cash balances. If these decisions are to be made knowledgeably, however, more information is needed than just data on the desired level of the minimum cash balance.

The necessity of additional information can be clearly seen in the hypothetical case described in Table 13-2. As should be apparent from the table, management must have information on both the desired minimum cash balance level and future cash flows. Information on the minimum cash balance can be obtained through use of the techniques discussed in the previous section and is necessary in order to determine if a cash surplus or, an additional cash requirement exists. Data on future cash flows can be obtained through the development of a cash budget. This latter information is needed in order to determine the appropriate investment—or financing strategy, if necessary.

A cash budget can be defined as a forecast or a schedule of future cash receipts and disbursements. Quite simply, it is a projection of future cash flows. It is designed to assist in controlling the hospital's cash position by enabling management to:

1. predict the timing and amount of future cash flows, net cash flows, cash balances, and cash needs and surpluses; and
2. systematically examine the cost implications of various cash management decisions.

The cash budget is thus an invaluable management tool, for it provides a substantial portion of the information necessary to both protect the hospital's cash position and ensure that it appropriately invests its assets.

A sample budget procedure, describing in detail the mechanics of preparing a cash budget, and an example of a cash budget's decision-making usefulness are presented in Appendix 13-2. This material should provide the reader with a thorough understanding of the nature and potential management value of a cash budget. The only additional point which is worthy of emphasis is the fact that a cash budget is not a primary budget. A cash budget is constructed from information obtained from the revenue, expense and capital budgets as opposed to being derived directly from basic operating decisions and forecasts.[5] Thus, the cash budget is actually a summary budget obtained by converting the foregoing budgets from an accrual to a cash basis. Figure 13-4 illustrates the relationship of the cash budget to the hospital's other budgets.

Investing Temporary Cash Surpluses

Based upon the desired minimum cash balance level and the information obtained from the cash budget, management now has available the data necessary to determine knowledgeably how to either finance additional cash needs or invest excess cash balances. The matter of financing additional cash or working capital requirements was discussed in Chapter 10. Thus, the nature of the available financing alternatives and the cost of those alternatives should be clear to the reader. The matter of investing excess cash balances, however, has not yet been examined. Therefore, before completing this discussion of cash management, the problem of investing excess cash balances should be considered.

---

[5]The accurate development of the hospital's expense, revenue and capital budgets is obviously critical to the construction of a sound cash budget. A discussion of the techniques and mechanics of preparing these budgets is included in Chapters 15–18 of this book.

Figure 13-4

Cash Budget

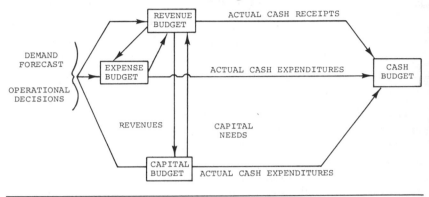

Due to any of a number of factors—seasonal occupancy fluctuations, delays in billings from suppliers, unexpected contributions, and so forth—a hospital may find itself with cash which is temporarily not needed for operations. These excess cash holdings represent an investment on the part of the hospital which, by definition, has an opportunity cost attached to it. Thus, if management is to minimize the cost of holding cash, it must invest its excess cash balances in revenue-generating securities as opposed to holding them as idle cash. The issue, therefore, is one of selecting the appropriate investment alternative—based on the amount of cash available, the length of time the excess will exist, and the financial situation of the hospital.

Numerous potential investment opportunities are available to a hospital. Marketable securities (short-term investments), however, generally present the most advantageous investment possibilities. This is due to the fact that these investment instruments, though producing a relatively low yield, provide an almost risk-less investment which is both highly liquid (marketable) and available in various maturities. These latter two points are particularly important.

Liquidity can be defined as the ability to sell an investment instrument rapidly without incurring a loss in principal. Due to the uncertain nature of cash flows, management may be forced to sell securities in order to meet unexpected cash needs. If the securities can be sold rapidly without a loss in principal, they obviously provide a better investment opportunity than alternatives which lack this characteristic.

The availability of numerous maturities is also advantageous. A wide range of maturity dates provides management with the flexibility needed to synchronize investment maturities with future cash needs. Such synchronization is vital if cash holdings are to be as productive as possible and if investment revenues are to be maximized. Thus, the guideline for the investment of excess cash balances can be set out as follows:

> Excess cash balances should be invested in marketable securities, with the actual investment selection based on the maturity schedules, yields, and risks which are most appropriate to a particular hospital's financial situation.

Table 13-3 lists the most common marketable security investment alternatives.

One additional point is worthy of note. The administration of a marketable securities portfolio is a complex and highly specialized task. A discussion of the specific techniques and mechanics of portfolio management are beyond the scope of this text. However, it is a task which is an integral part of the cash management process and as such should be the primary responsibility of the hospital's controller or financial manager. The role of general management in this area is limited to ensuring that the financial manager is carrying out his responsibility properly. This can be accomplished quite easily by comparing maturity schedules with the cash budget (in order to examine synchronization), by comparing the composite portfolio yield to yields available in the market (see Chapter 14), and by subjectively evaluating the portfolio in terms of the hospital's financial situation and willingness to bear risk.

Conclusion

The basic principles and mechanics of not only cash management but also working capital management should now be clear. The reader should now have a general understanding of both the factors which should be considered in arriving at working capital decisions and the techniques which financial managers can and should utilize as aids in making these decisions. Given this understanding, a manager needs only one other bit or type of information in order to evaluate a hospital's performance in these areas. He must have available certain informational reports. The following chapter is devoted to a discussion of the reports needed to evaluate the efficiency and effectiveness of a hospital's working capital performance.

Table 13-3
Marketable Security Investment Alternatives

Securities	Comments
Treasury bills: 91-day maturity, issued weekly.	These are the most popular investments since they combine security (as obligations of the U.S. government) with liquidity (because of the frequency and regularity of their issuance).*
U.S. Treasury notes, certificates of indebtedness, and tax anticipation certificates: More than 91-day but less than five-year maturities.	Also popular, these are useful for companies that wish to invest to meet specific cash requirements (dividends, taxes, and capital expenditures).
Federal agency securities: Offerings of five federally sponsored credit agencies (federal land banks, banks for cooperatives, federal home loan banks, federal intermediate credit banks, Federal National Mortgage Association) that issue their own securities and borrow directly from the public. Most corporate portfolios are restricted to nine-month to 1½ year maturities.	These securities are not guaranteed by the federal government, and their yield is generally just above that of Treasury securities. However, they are considered very safe investments.
Public Housing Authority notes: Issued to finance various government land development projects. Most corporate portfolios are restricted to one-year maturities.	These securities have the double advantage of being guaranteed by the federal government and of being tax exempt. The latter feature makes the effective yield to a corporation roughly double that quoted. The strong demand for these notes makes them very liquid in the secondary market.
State and local bonds: One-year and longer maturities. (A number of states will provide almost any maturity required by a corporate buyer.)	Those rated AA and AAA are considered very safe investments. Their tax-exempt status makes them the highest-yielding security in the money market. They are sometimes used to meet specific cash requirements.

Bankers' acceptances:

One-month to six-month maturities (usually three months).

A bankers' acceptance is a time draft, drawn on a large bank by a trader, that becomes a negotiable instrument and can be discounted for resale to investors. It is considered a very safe investment.

Commercial certificates of deposit (CDs):

Activity is generally restricted to prime certificates with a maximum maturity of 90 days. However, maturities of up to a year are available.

The CD is a receipt given by a bank for a time deposit of money. The bank promises to return the amount deposited plus interest to the bearer of the certificate on the date specified. The certificate is transferable and may be traded before its maturity date.

Because the denominations offered are large and Federal Deposit Insurance Corporation protection is limited** the size and reputation of the issuing bank are important.***

Finance company paper:

Short-term maturity, usually 90 days. (A number of finance companies will provide almost any maturity required by the corporate buyer.)

These obligations of companies financing consumer applicances and automobiles are reasonably safe, but much depends upont the reputation of the issuing company. They are traded on the secondary market, and maturity dates are usually very flexible. Yield is generally high.

Commerical paper:

Usually four-month to six-month maturities but sometimes as short as five days. (Purchasers usually intend to hold such obligations until maturity.)

Commerical paper today consists mainly of short-term, unsecured promissory notes issued by a relatively small group of highly rated companies. The yield is usually the highest of those that can be obtained from any short-term security, except tax-exempts.

Source: E.J. Mock. "The Investment of Corporate Cash," *Management Services,* Vol. 4, No. 5, (September-October 1967), pp. 55. Reprinted in E.J. Mock, et al., *Basic Financial Management* (Scranton, Pa.: International Textbook Company, 1968) p. 114.

*This rate changes quite frequently depending on the market's demand for money. In the mid-1970's the rate ranged from about $5^{1/2}$% to almost 12%.

**Insurance protection provided by the Federal Deposit Insurance Corporation was increased gradually from the original coverage of $10,000 for each depositor to the current limit of $40,000 for each.

***It may also be possible to obtain consumer certificates of deposit. These carry a lower yield, but may be available in denominations of as low as $500 with a maturity of six months.

Suggested Readings

Cash Management

Orgler, Yair E. *Cash Management and Models.*
Van Horne, James C. *Financial Management and Policy,* Chapter 16.
Weston, J. Fred and Brigham, Eugene F. *Managerial Finance,* Chapter 13.

Short-Term Investments

Cannedy, Lloyd L. "How Hospitals Use Money Market Instruments." *Hospital Financial Management,* November 1969, pp. 3–7 and 42.
Markstein, David L. "How to Make Short-Term Cash Work At Full-Time Rates." *Modern Hospital,* January 1970, pp. 63, 64 and 134.

Appendix 13-A[6]

Cash Management Models

Inventory control techniques dominated the early cash management models. The application of inventory theory to the management of cash was first explored by W. J. Baumol. The Baumol model is based on the assumption that payments are known and have to be made at a constant rate and that there are no cash receipts during the payment period. Additionally, the model is static in that it does not consider the interrelationships between subsequent time periods and is limited to the interval between two successive cash receipts. Consequently, this model is an oversimplification of reality and has limited applicability.

A second type of inventory model emphasizes the probabilistic nature of cash flows. An example of this type of model is the Miller and Orr model which assumes that net cash flows fluctuate in a completely stochastic manner as opposed to the deterministic cash outflows of the Baumol model.

The essential elements of both of these models are summarized below.

---

[6]Material for this Appendix has been adapted from: *Cash Management* by Yair E. Orgler and *Managerial Finance* by J. Fred Weston and Eugene F. Brigham.

The Baumol Model. The basic model is the standard inventory sawtooth model (see Figure 13-A-1). The inventory item is cash which flows out at a constant rate and is restocked instantaneously by borrowing or by withdrawing from an investment, i.e., selling the investment. Total cash outflows are assumed to be known and are made at a constant rate over a given period. The size and timing of cash inflows are completely controllable and are associated with a fixed cost per order and a variable cost per dollar (interest on a loan or the yield lost by selling securities). Since cash outflows are given, the only cash management decision is how much cash to obtain and at what frequency, assuming that the objective is to minimize total costs.

Based on these assumptions, which also underline the standard inventory model, Baumol solves his model and obtains the famous square-root formula for the optimal order size:

$$C = \sqrt{\frac{2bT}{i}}$$

where b is the fixed cost per order (transaction), T is the total amount of payments (cash flows), and i is the variable cost per dollar per period (interest rate). Since in this model the average amount in stock is half the order quantity, the average cash balance is:

$$\frac{C}{2} = \sqrt{\frac{bT}{2i}}$$

The Miller and Orr Model. The model is designed to determine the time and size of transfers between an investment account and the cash account according to a decision process illustrated in Figure 13-A-2.

Changes in cash balances are allowed to wander until they reach some level h at time t_1; they are then reduced to level z, the "return point," by investing h-z dollars in the investment portfolio. Again the cash balance wanders aimlessly until it reaches the minimum balance point, r, at t_2 at which time enough earning assets are sold to return the cash balance to its return point, z. The model is based on a cost function similar to Baumol's, and it includes elements for the cost of making transfers to and from cash and for the opportunity cost of holding cash.

The upper limit, h, which cash balances should not be allowed to surpass, and the return point, z, to which the balance is returned after every transfer either to or from the cash account, are computed so as to minimize the cost function. The lower limit is

Figure 13-A-1

Pattern of Cash Receipts and Expenditures—Baumol Model*

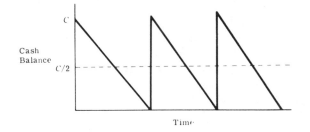

*Used with permission of *Quarterly Journal of Economics.*

---

assumed to be given, and it could be the minimum balance required by the banks in which the cash is deposited.

The cost function for the Miller-Orr model can be stated as E (c) = bE (N)/T + iE (M), where E (N) = the expected number of transfers between cash and the investment portfolio during the planning period; b = the cost per transfer; T is the number of days in the planned period; E (M) = expected average daily balance; and I = the daily rate of interest earned on the investments. The objective is to minimize E (c) by choice of the variables h and z, the upper control limit and return point respectively.

The solution is derived by Miller and Orr becomes

$$z^* = \left(\frac{3b\sigma^2}{4i}\right)^{1/3}$$

$$h^* = 3z^*$$

for the special case where p (the probability that cash balances will increase) equals .5, and q (the probability that cash balances will decrease) equals .5. The variance of the daily changes in the cash balance is represented by σ^2. As would be expected, a higher transfer cost, b, or variance, σ^2, would imply a greater spread between the upper and lower control limits. In the special case where p = q = ½, the upper control limit will always be three times greater than the return point.

Miller and Orr tested their model by applying it to nine months of data on the daily cash balances and purchases and sales of short-term securities of a large industrial company. When the decisions of the model were compared to those actually made by the treasurer of the company, the model was found to produce an

Figure 13-A-2

**Miller and Orr Cash Management
Model***

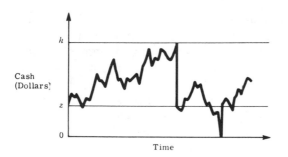

*Used with permission of *Quarterly Journal of Economics.*

---

average daily cash balance which was about forty percent lower ($160,000 for the model and $275,000 for the treasurer). Looking at it from another side, the model would have been able to match the $275,000 average daily balance with only eighty transactions as compared to the treasurer's 112 actual transactions.

As with most inventory control models, this model's performance depends not only on how well the conditional predictions (in this case the expected number of transfers and the expected average cash balance) conform to actuality but also on how well the parameters are estimated. In this model, b, the transfer cost, is sometimes difficult to estimate. In the study made by Miller and Orr, the order costs included such components as "(a) making two or more long-distance phone calls fifteen minutes to a half hour of the assistant treasurer's time, (b) typing up and carefully checking an authorization letter with four copies, (c) carrying the original of the letter to be signed by the treasurer and (d) carrying the copies to the controller's office where special accounts are opened, the entries are posted and further checks of the arithmetic are made." These clerical procedures were thought to be in the magnitude of $20 to $50 per order. In the application of their model, however, Miller and Orr did not rely on their estimate for order costs; instead they tested the model using a series of "assumed" order costs until the model used the same number of transactions as did the treasurer. They could then determine the order cost implied by the treasurer's own action. The results were then used to evaluate the treasurer's performance in managing the cash balances, and, as such, provided valuable information to the treasurer.

The treasurer found, for example, that his action in purchasing securities was often inconsistent. Too often he made small-lot purchases well below the minimum of h-z computed by the model, while at other times he allowed cash balances to drift to as much as double the upper control limit before making a purchase. If it did no more than give the treasurer some perspective about his buying and selling activities, the model was used successfully.

In addition to these inventory models, the techniques of dynamic programming and linear programming have been applied to the cash management problem. A discussion of these more sophisticated models, however, is beyond both the scope of this work and the typical needs of the operating hospital manager. Readers desiring information on how these latter techniques can be utilized, should refer to:

— Baumol, William, J., "The Transactions Demand for Cash: An Inventory Theoretic Approach," *Quarterly Journal of Economics*, LXVI, November 1952.
— Beranek, William, *Analysis for Financial Decision*, Homewood, Ill. Irwin, 1963, pp. 345–381.
— Calman, R.F., *Linear Programming and Cash Management: Cash ALPHA*. Cambridge, Mass: The MIT Press 1968.
— Miller, Merton H. and Daniel Orr, *An Application of Control Limit Models to the Management of Corporate Cash Balances*, Proceedings of the Conference on Financial Research and Its Implications for Management, Stanford University, Alexander A. Robichek, ed. New York: Wiley, 1967.
— Miller, Merton H. and Daniel Orr, "Model for the Demand for Money by Firms," *Quarterly Journal of Economics*, August 1966, pp. 413–435.

Appendix 13-B

Cash and Short-Term Investment

Part I—Cash Budgeting Procedure

Due to its operational importance, cash management is a complex problem which has attracted a great deal of management science interest in recent years. Various authorities have examined the problems involved in managing cash and have developed intricate analytical models designed to provide quantitative solutions for cash management problems. These models generally involve a large number of variables and constraints and require sophisticated computer knowledge and capacity if they are to be used. Also, these models, because of the abstraction requirements of constructing mathematical models, have limitations which restrict their operational application. It is the feeling of the authors at this point in time that the models are not appropriate hospital operational tools. Instead, the use of a cash budgeting technique which allows for the development of multiple budgets and the stimulation of various cash management decisions appears, at least for the present, to be a more feasible and practical approach to hospital cash management. A step-by-step description of such a technique is presented below.

Cash Budget Preparation

A. Step 1

The budget officer should obtain the information needed to determine to convert the accrual based primary budgets, from which the cash budget is derived (see Figure 13-4), to a cash basis.

1. *Information needed in order to convert primary budgets from an accrual to a cash basis*

    a—Revenue Budget
    — percent of total service revenue, both inpatient and outpatient, by source of payments, i.e., what percent of total revenues are received from Blue Cross, Medicare, self-pay patients, etc.;
    — average timing of accounts receivable cycle by source of payment, including self-pay patients, i.e., time period or lag between patient discharge and receipt of payment by source of payment;
    — percent of billed charges paid by the various third party payers, e.g., Medicare may pay 90% of billed charges, Blue Cross, 95%, etc.; and
    — timing of receipt of all other revenues, e.g., when income from investments will be received, when grants from the United Fund will be received, etc.

    b—Expense Budget
    — salary and wage payment periods;
    — timing of quarterly and other nonmonthly expense pay-

Figure 13-B-1
Sample Revenue Log Form*

Billing Data				Payment Data					Cash Receipt Data	
				Source of Payment						
Patient Name	I.D. No.	Date of Discharge	Amount of Bill (Total)	Primary Source	Amt.	Secondary Source	Amt.	Payment Amt.	Record Date	Source
Sample Entry Wilson, R. Dale	325362125	6-3-70	$891	Blue Cross	$800	Self-Pay	$91	$50 (cash)	6-3-70	Self-Pay
								$41	7-1-70	Self-Pay
								$800	8-5-70	Blue Cross

*This form can be used for recording both impatient and outpatient revenues. If it is used for outpatient revenues, the column headed "Date of Discharge" should be changed to "Date of Service."

ments, i.e., F.I.C.A. payments, insurance premiums, Federal Withholding Tax, etc.;
— percent of purchases for which "trade credit" is offered;
— average nature of trade credit terms;
— average payment "terms" for all other purchases; and
— timing of purchases; i.e., purchases made evenly throughout the month or on a specific day of the week.

c—Capital Budget (Plant and Equipment Budget)
— timing of plant and equipment expenditures, i.e., the month(s) in which a capital expenditure appropriation is actually to be paid.

2. *Technique for obtaining necessary information*
a—Revenue Budget
The data needed to convert the revenue budget should be obtainable from two sources—sampling study of revenues and the information available in the controller's office.
1) Sampling study of revenues
In order to determine the percent of total revenue by source, percent of total revenue paid in cash, and the timing of the accounts receivable cycles, a special study of both inpatient and outpatient revenues should be conducted, under the supervision of the budget officer, by the business office. The methodology for this study can be as follows:
— establish a log for recording all charges made for patient services (see Figure 13-B-1);
— each time a patient bill is prepared, an entry should be made in the log indicating the name and identification number of the patient, date of discharge or, for E.R. and O.P.D. services, the date of service, source of payment, and amount of bill.
— each time a bill is paid, an entry should be made in the log indicating the amount, date, and source of payment; and
— using the above information, the budget officer should determine the foregoing items.
A study of this nature should be performed annually for both inpatient and outpatient revenues and should encompass a period of at least three months.
2) Information available from the controller's office
The controller should have available information on the percent of billed charges paid by the various third

party payers. Additionally, the controller should have knowledge as to the timing of the receipt of investment income, United Fund grants, nursing school tuition, etc. Also the controller, based on historical experience, should estimate the timing and amount of any third party payment adjustment.

3) Other information
— Emergency room and outpatient revenues. These are patient service revenues and should be handled by means of the above special study.
— Deductions from revenues. See comment 2 above (A-2: a-2).
— Miscellaneous revenues, other operating revenues, and other revenues. If information in regard to the timing of the receipt of revenues budgeted for these items is not available from the controller, then, if acceptable subjective estimates cannot be made, sampling studies, similar to those described above, should be conducted.

b—Expense Budget
The data needed to convert the expense budget should be obtainable from two sources—sampling study of expenses and the information in the controller's office.

1) Sampling study of expenses
   In order to determine the percentage of purchases for which trade credit is offered, the average nature of trade credit terms, and the average terms for all other purchases, i.e., for purchases wherein trade credit is not offered, a special study should be conducted (under the supervision of the budget officer) by the purchasing department and any other departments which purchase goods directly. The methodology for this study can be as follows:
— establish a log for recording the receipt of all goods;
— whenever goods are received, an entry should be made in the log indicating: type of item, total cost of the goods, and the terms of purchase; and
— using the above information, the budget officer should determine the foregoing items.
   A study of this nature need be performed only annually and should encompass a two month period.

2) Information available from the controller's office
   The controller should have available information on

the timing of all regular nonmonthly payments and the salary and wage payment policies of the hospital.

c—Capital Budget (Plant and Equipment Budget)

The data needed to convert the capital budget to a cash basis should be obtained by the budget officer from the information available in the capital budget.

B. Step 2

The budget officer, in consultation with the controller and the director of the hospital, should determine the horizon or the planning period of the budget. Generally, cash budgets are prepared based on a planning period of one year which, in turn, is segmented into twelve monthly subperiods. This general approach is compatible with the hospital's other budgets, that is, they are also constructed using monthly subperiods and appear to be acceptable at this point in time. However, the budget officer should periodically review the length of the cash budgeting period and limit it to only that future time span beyond which additional information will not affect decisions made in the first subperiod.

C. Step 3

The budget officer, using the data determined in Step 1 and the revenues budget, should convert the revenue budget to the cash receipts segment of the cash budget. This is simply a mechanical task of applying the timing data obtained in Step 1 to the accrual based projections of the revenue budget (see Table 13-B-1).

D. Step 4

The budget officer, using the data determined in Step 1 and the expense budget, should convert the expense and capital budgets to the cash disbursements segment of the cash budget. This is simply a mechanical task of applying the data obtained in Step 1 to the projections of the expense and capital budgets (see Table 13-B-2).

E. Step 5

The budget officer should consolidate the data obtained in Steps 3 and 4 into the completed cash budget. A sample budget format is illustrated in Figure 13-B-2.

At this point, the cash budgeting process is completed. A comprehensive cash budget should now be available for management's use as a decision-making tool. An in-depth discussion of the managerial usefulness of the cash budget is beyond the scope of this text. However, Part II of this appendix briefly examines the decision-making potential of the cash budget.

Table 13-B-1

Conversion of the Revenue Budget to a Cash Basis

The conversion of inpatient revenue projections to a cash basis is presented below as a means of illustrating the mechanics of converting the revenue budget to a cash basis.

1. Assume the following inpatient revenue projection;

May	$100,000		
June	$ 90,000	August	$ 90,000
July	$ 80,000	September	$100,000

2. Based on the data presented earlier in regard to the percent of total inpatient revenue by source, the figure in "1" above can be recast to a cash basis as follows:

Revenue by Sources (Inpatient)

Source

Month	40% Blue Cross	20% Medicare	10% Medicaid	10% Comm. Ins.	15% Self-Pay	5% Other	Total
May	$40,000	$20,000	$10,000	$10,000	$15,000	$5,000	$100,000
June	36,000	18,000	9,000	9,000	13,500	4,500	90,000
July	32,000	16,000	8,000	8,000	12,000	4,000	80,000
Aug.	36,000	18,000	9,000	9,000	13,500	4,500	90,000
Sept.	40,000	20,000	10,000	10,000	15,000	5,000	100,000

3. Cash Receipts in September

Blue Cross	= 95%* of July billings** of $32,000 =			$30,400
Medicare	= 90%* of July billings** of 16,000 =			14,400
Medicaid	= 90%* of June billings** of 9,000 =			8,100
Comm. Ins.	= 100% of ½ Aug. billings**		$4,500	
	100% of ½ Sept. billings**		5,000	
				= 9,500
Other	= 100% of July billings** of 14,000 =			14,000
Self-pay	= 15% of Sept.billings of 15,000 =	2,250(cash)		
	20% of Aug. billings** of 13,500 =	2,700		
	40% of July billings** of 12,000 =	4,800		
	15% of Junebillings** of 13,500 =	2,025		
	5% of May billings** of 15,000 =	750		
				12,525

Total Cash Receipts Inpatient Revenue $88,925

*Adjustment made for the percent of billed charges paid.
**Adjustment made for timing of the accounts receivable cycle.

Table 13-B-2

Conversion of the Expense Budget to a Cash Basis

The conversion of supplies expense projection to a cash basis is presented below as a means of illustrating the mechanics of converting the expense budget to a cash basis.

1. *Assume the following supplies expense projections:*

    August = $10,000
    September = $15,000

2. *Based on the data presented earlier in regard to supplies purchases, the figures above can be recast to a cash basis as follows:*

Month	Purchases 2/10 net 30 Terms	Net 30 No Terms	Total
August	$4,000	$6,000	$10,000
September	$6,000	$9,000	$15,000

3. *If all purchase discounts are taken and supplies are purchased evenly over the month, then cash payments in September will be as follows:*

    August Supplies

    $1/3$ of supplies purchases for which terms are offered—
    supplies received on or after the 20th of the month = $ 1,333 (approx.)

    All of the supplies purchases for which no terms are
    offered = $ 6,000

    September Supplies

    $2/3$ of supplies purchases for which terms are offered—
    supplies received prior to the 20th of the month = $ 4,000

    Total Cash Disbursements Supplies: $11,333 (approx.)

Figure 13-B-2

Sample Cash Budget Format

Month	
Cash Balance (Beginning)	
Receipts	
Inpatient	
Outpatient	
Other Operating	
Nonoperating	
Total	
Disbursements	
Salaries & Wages	
Supplies	
Plant & Equipment	
Other	
Total	
CASH Balance (End of Period) Less: Minimum Cash Balance	
CASH surplus (shortage)	

Table 13-B-3
Example of a Cash Budget
(in thousands of dollars)

	Month 1	Month 2	Month 3
Cash Balance			
(Beginning)			
Receipts			
Inpatient	$ 750	$ 550	$ 825
Outpatient	360	300	300
Other operating	50	150	50
Nonoperating	25	20	0
Total Receipts	1,185	1,020	1,175
Total Cash Available	$1,635	$1,520	$1,675
Disbursements			
Salaries and wages	$ 600	$ 650	$ 650
Supplies	230	330	250
Plant and equipment	75	200	100
Other (notes payable)	0	0	160
Total	$ 905	$1,180	$1,160
Cash balance	$ 730	$ 340	$ 515
(Ending)			
Less: Minimal Cash balance*	500	500	500
Cash Surplus (Shortage)	$ 230	$ (160)	$ 15
Borrowing		$ 160	
Investment	$ 230		$ 15

*Assume that the minimum cash balance is determined through the techniques described in Chapter 13.

Part II

Decision-Making Potential of the Cash Budget

In order to examine the potential of a cash budget in aiding management to make cash related decisions, assume the following budget.

Based on the above assumptions, a $230,000 surplus exists in Month 1, a $160,000 deficit exists in Month 2, and a $15,000 surplus exists in Month 3. Implicit in the above is a sequential approach to cash management, i.e., a two step approach wherein the first step involves estimating the cash surplus or deficit and the second step involves an investment or borrowing decision. The sequential approach, however, is limited in that it fails not only to consider the interrelationship of the two steps, but also to use the information available in the cash budget to make least cost decisions. This point can be illustrated as follows:

Assume: return on investments = 6%
                                    cost of borrowing = 12%

Therefore: 1. $230,000 surplus in Month 1 can
                                    be invested at 6% for Months 2 and
                                    3. The resulting income will be
                                    $2,300.

                                    2. $160,000 will be borrowed at the
                                    beginning of Month 2, for Months 2
                                    and 3, at a cost of $3,200.

                                    3. The cost of managing cash in the
                                    above   manner   will   be $900
                                    ($3,200−$2,300 = $900).

However: Assume that management uses the
                                    foregoing budget as the means of
                                    simulating various cash manage-
                                    ment decisions in order to deter-
                                    mine the least cost decision, i.e.,
                                    use the foregoing budget as the ba-
                                    sis for developing alternative bud-
                                    gets which will reflect different
                                    cash management strategies.

For Example:

Alternative 1.

Based on the above budget, management decides to
change the timing of the capital expenditure tentatively
planned for Month 2 to Month 1. If this were done, then
the cash surplus in Month 1 would be reduced from
$230,000 to $30,000, the cash deficit in Month 2 would
be reduced from a deficit of $160,000 to a surplus of
$40,000 and the surplus in Month 3 increased, due to
not having to pay the note payable, to $175,000. Thus,
$30,000 would be available for investment in Months 2
and 3 and $40,000 would be available for Month 3. At
6% these surpluses would result in an income of $500
for the hospital as opposed to an expense of $900 as was
shown in the previous case.

Alternative 2.

Based on the above budget, management decides to invest only $70,000 of the Month 1 surplus and hold the

remaining $160,000 in cash. If this were done, then $70,000 would be available for investment during Months 2 and 3, the Month 2 deficit would be $0, and the Month 3 surplus would be $175,000. At 6% this cash management strategy would result in an income of $700, as opposed to the $500 income of Alternative 1 and the $900 cost of the original case.

Other examples could be used to explain the same point. However, the critical matter is not the exploration of various examples, but a realization that the cash budget is useful for more than just projecting cash surpluses and deficits. As has been illustrated, the cash budget not only can project surpluses and deficits, but also can be used as the basis for simulating various cash management decisions in order to determine the least cost management alternative.

Chapter 14

Management Reports: Working Capital

Hospital managers, like their counterparts in commercial industry, have found that as the scope of operations increases beyond the management capacity of a single individual that two steps must be taken if operational efficiency is to be maintained. First, in order to share the load and provide sufficient management coverage, the responsibility for the operation of certain areas or functions must be delegated to subordinates. Second, in order to judge how well or poorly these subordinates are carrying out their responsibilities, reports must be received from them. These two management principles are applicable to any area of hospital operation—including financial operations.

Financial reports are generally categorized as being either planning and informational reports or performance reports. Planning and informational reports can be described as statements designed to aid and enable management to both recognize overall trends and determine long-range policies and actions. Performance reports are documents designed to assist management in controlling current operations and expenditures. They can be conceptualized as consisting of two subcategories or types of reports—stock reports and flow reports.

Stock reports are statements which describe the performance of management in relation to the stock or inventory of values, i.e., the group of assets and liabilities that the hospital has at any particular point in time. Examples of this type of report are the hospital's balance sheet (position statement), aged accounts receivable report, and cash position report. Flow reports are statements which describe management's performance relative to the flow or movement of values, i.e., the stream of revenues and expenses which the hospital incurs over time. The best examples of this type of report are a hospital's income (operating) statement and its Hospital Administrative Services (H.A.S.) reports.

A discussion of flow reports is more germane to the matters of responsibility accounting and operational budgeting than to the topic at hand. Therefore, although they are important, flow reports will be left to another time and text. The focus of this chapter will thus be limited to the stock reports needed for the management of working capital.

Fundamental Principles

Before actually discussing the various financial stock reports which management should receive, it would be worthwhile to first review several fundamental reporting principles. These principles are basic not only to financial reporting, but also to management reporting in general. As such, they must be observed by the financial manager if he is to provide effective management reports. These basic reporting guidelines are presented below.

Timeliness. If reports are to be of value to management in controlling current operations, they must be current and up-to-date. A late report is almost as useless as no report at all. Hence, if reports are to be effective management tools, they not only must be prepared as frequently as necessary, but also must be promptly available. Only through timely reports can management obtain the information which it needs to control and guide operations.

Accuracy. The need for accurate reports should be obvious. If management is to have confidence in reports, and if reports are to act as an aid in controlling operations, they must be understandable, reliable, and valid. Late reports may be almost useless, but inaccurate reports are detrimental.

Clarity. Accuracy will create confidence in the reports which are provided. However, if reports are to be used to their fullest extent, management must feel comfortable with them. Reports should be clearly and simply designed, be expressed in language and terms familiar to the reader and, to the extent possible, be standardized. Through these considerations, reports not only can be tailored to management's desires and peculiarities, but also can be designed such that their usefulness will be maximized.

Figure 14-1

Comparative Reports

Part A—Simple Comparative Report

A and L Millstone General Hospital
Comparative Working Capital Report
As of February 29, 1972
(000)

Assets	1970	1971	1972	Liabilities	1970	1971	1972
Cash	$ 15	$ 17	$ 20	Accounts			
Marketable				Payable	$30	$32	$35
Securities	3	1	5	Salaries and			
Accounts				Wages Payable	10	12	5
Receivable	120	130	160	Accrued			
Inventories	17	13	15	Interest	5	3	3
Total:	$155	$161	$200	Total:	$45	$47	$43

Part B—Common Size Report

A and L Millstone General Hospital
Common Size Working Capital Report
As of February, 1972

Assets	1970	1971	1972	Liabilities	1970	1971	1972
Cash	9.7%	10.6%	10.0%	Accounts			
Marketable				Payable	66.7%	68.0%	81.4%
Securities	1.9	.6	2.5	Salaries and			
Accounts				Wages Payable	22.2	25.6	11.6
Receivable	77.5	80.7	80.0	Accrued			
Inventories	10.9	8.1	7.5	Interest	11.1	6.4	7.0
Total:	100%	100%	100%	Total:	100%	100%	100%

Comparability. Actual performance data alone usually are of
relatively little worth, for they do not provide management with a
frame of reference or a bench mark from which to base analysis
and evaluation. If management is to place actual performance in

the proper perspective, it must be able to compare it either to past performance or to reasonable standards. Only in this way is it possible to adequately judge current performance, identify trends, and determine the appropriate nature of any future actions.

Figure 14-1 presents examples of two types of comparative statements. Part A depicts a "simple" comparative report wherein current performance is presented alongside of either the previous year's performance or some standards. Statements of this type facilitate the identification of changes over time and enable management to readily discover trends which might otherwise go unnoticed. Thus, they improve the general usefulness of reports as a control device and should be used wherever possible.[1]

Part B illustrates another type of comparative report which can be helpful. In order to identify and evaluate relative changes in performance, managers, together with accountants, have developed "common size" reports. A "common size" comparative report differs from a "simple" comparative statement in that items are presented in terms of a percentage of the total instead of in absolute dollars. The advantage of this modification lies in the fact that it pinpoints relative changes and thereby allows management to evaluate the distribution of items and their implication.

"Common size" reports are not used as extensively as "simple" comparative statements. However, they do have some value for internal management purposes and should be used whenever they will add to management's decision-making capabilities.

Commentary. Reports are communication devices used to transmit information and ideas to management. In order to effectively accomplish this task, they should include explanatory comments designed to both direct the user's attention to important items and to interpret the significance and meaning of those items.

The commentary segment of a report should be aimed at expediting management by exception. It should distinguish between functions which are progressing satisfactorily and those which need management attention and concentrate on only the latter. This approach will result in both better reports and an improved utilization of management time and talent, for, hopefully, attention will be immediately directed and concentrated on only exceptional areas and problems.

---

[1]Comparative data are unquestionably of value. However, caution must be exercised in drawing conclusions from these data, for price level and volume changes can distort their validity.

Figure 14-2

Unger Memorial Hospital

Sample Balance Sheet as of December 31, 1970

Assets

Current Assets		1969		1970
Cash	$	125,000	$	27,000
Marketable Securities		20,000		115,000
Accounts Receivable—Patients		175,000		200,000
Accounts Receivable—Others		25,000		20,000
Inventory		40,000		45,000
Total Current Assets:	$	385,000	$	407,000
Fixed Assets				
Land	$	50,000	$	50,000
Equipment (net of depreciation)		825,000		875,000
Buildings (net of depreciation)		1,750,000		1,700,000
Total Fixed Assets:		$2,625,000		$2,625,000
Other Assets				
Endowment Fund A—Unrestricted	$	75,000	$	90,000
Endowment Fund B—Restricted		1,000,000		1,000,000
Total Other Assets		$1,075,000		$1,090,000
Deferred Charges				
Prepaid Insurance	$	5,000	$	7,500
Total Deferred Assets:	$	5,000	$	7,500
Total Assets:		$4,090,000		$4,129,500

Liabilities & Net Worth

Current Liabilities		1969		1970
Accounts Payable	$	138,000	$	150,000
Accrued Wages		22,000		30,000
Total Current Liabilities:	$	160,000	$	180,000
Long-Term Debt				
Mortgage—Building A		$1,000,000	$	950,000
Loan		300,000		300,000
Total Long-Term Debt		$1,300,000		$1,250,000
Net Worth		$2,630,000		$2,699,500
Total Liabilities & Net Worth:		$4,090,000		$4,129,500

Meaningfulness. The foregoing has pointed out the basic elements necessary for effective and usable reports. However, if the value of reports is to be maximized, one other overriding standard must also be met. They must provide meaningful and needed information.

Managers need performance data if they are to satisfactorily carry out their responsibilities. However, the case of the manager who receives so many reports that they must be delivered on a hand truck too often approaches reality. A data overload is just as counter-productive as insufficient data, for in both instances the manager will be inadequately informed. Hence, if reports are to be useful, they must concentrate on the critical or key variable which must be controlled—if the item under question is to be controlled—and not just provide a mass of words and figures which are either ill-focused or beyond a reader's absorption level.

This last standard is particularly important and merits careful consideration. Simply, reports must focus on problems as opposed to symptoms of problems. To accomplish this, they must provide data not on the elements of working capital per se, but rather on the process which underlies, and thereby controls, each element. This distinction should become clear through the following discussion.

Balance Sheet

Given an understanding of the above principles, the stage is now set for considering the various financial stock reports which management should receive. Of these reports, the most basic and comprehensive is the balance sheet or position statement, for it describes the total financial position of a hospital at any given point in time. Therefore, it is logical and reasonable to examine this report first.

A balance sheet can be viewed as being analogous to a photograph. A photograph depicts action, an event, or a subject at a particular point in time. Correspondingly, a balance sheet depicts the results of a number of financial events and actions at a particular point in time. It shows as of a specific date (point in time) the accepted monetary value of both the hospital's assets and obligations or liabilities. The difference between these two categories of items—assets and liabilities—is the hospital's capital or net worth. Due to the fact that the statement portrays a balance between assets and the total liabilities and net worth, it is commonly referred to as a balance sheet.

Figure 14-2 illustrates a sample hospital balance sheet. As can be seen, the statement is presented in the traditional corporate

Table 14-1

Ratio Analysis

The figures used in the following example were obtained from the balance sheet presented in Figure 14-2.

Ratio		*Actual*	*Approximate Guidelines**
Current Ratio = Current Assets to Current Liabilities			
$\dfrac{\$407,000}{\$180,000}$	=	2.3:1	5:1
Acid Test Ratio = Cash, Mkt. Sec., & Accts. Rec. to Current Liabilities			
$\dfrac{\$362,000}{\$180,000}$	=	2:1	4:1
Cash to Total Assets = Cash & Mkt. Sec. to Total Tangible Assets			
$\dfrac{\$\ 142,000}{\$4,129,500}$	=	3.4%	1.3%
Inventory to Total Assets = Inventory to Total Tangible Assets			
$\dfrac{\$\ \ 45,000}{\$4,129,500}$	=	1.1%	1.7%
Debt to Total Assets = Long Term Debt to Total Tangible Assets			
$\dfrac{\$1,250,000}{\$4,129,500}$	=	30%	-
Net Worth to Total Assets = Net Worth to Total Tangible Assets			
$\dfrac{\$2,699,500}{\$4,129,500}$	=	65%	-

*Approximate guidelines for a hospital with operating parameters representative of those found throughout the industry. For further reference see: "Ratio Analysis: A Technique For Financial Management in Hospitals," Berman, H.J., master's thesis, Program in Hospital Administration, University of Michigan. (Available as *Hospital Abstract* AC 1051 from University Microfilms, 300 N. Zeeb Rd., Ann Arbor, Michigan.)

finance format. The rationale for this approach should be clear from the discussion in Chapter 2. In addition to this basic change in presentation form, it should be noted that prepaid expenses are shown in an asset category entitled, "Deferred Charges." This was done in order to reflect the particular "near" expense nature of these assets and to distinguish them from current assets which can be readily converted into cash.

Balance sheets should be prepared for management's use no less frequently than annually and no more frequently than monthly. Monthly reports represent one extreme, for any period less than one month is generally too short a time span either for trends to appear or for management to act. Conversely, annual reports represent the other extreme, for if management is to avoid the allegation of fiscal negligence, it must review the financial position of the hospital at least annually. It is the authors' opinion that monthly or, at the extreme, quarterly reports are the preferable reporting frequency.

As indicated earlier, the balance sheet should be presented in a comparative form so that management can more readily evaluate its significance. Additionally, a technique known as ratio analysis can be used by management to evaluate a balance sheet.

Ratio analysis is a financial tool which is commonly used in commercial industry as a mechanism to aid management in interpreting a firm's balance sheet.

Quite simply, ratios are a means of expressing, in quantitative terms, the relationships which exist between various items in the balance sheet. These "actual" relationships can be compared to standard or "normal" ratios which can be used as guidelines to estimate financial performance and identify areas of inadequacy. The most frequently used balance sheet ratios are the following:

Current ratio	Ratio of current assets to current liabilities. Used as the basic index of liquidity and financial position.
Acid Test Ratio	Ratio of cash, marketable securities, and accounts receivable to current liabilities. Used to provide a more sensitive liquidity index than the current ratio, for it excludes inventories which are relatively illiquid.
Cash to Short-Term Debt	Ratio of cash and marketable securities to short-term debt. Used by

Figure 14-3

Sample Modified Daily Cash Reports

Havens General Hospital

Date_____

Beginning Daily Balance $_____
Cash Receipts

Source	Amount
Blue Cross	$_____
Medicare	$_____
Medicaid	$_____
Commercial	$_____
Self-Pay	$_____
Other	$_____
Total Receipts	$_____

Total Cash Available $_____

Cash Disbursements

Item	Amount
Payroll	$_____
Accounts Payable	$_____
Plant and Equipment	$_____
Other	$_____
Total Disbursements	$_____

Cash Balance $_____

Projected Cash Flows*
  Projected Receipts $_____
  Projected Disbursements $_____

Projected Cash Balance: $_____

*This segment of the report represents modification. Cash flows can be projected for whatever future period management feels is appropriate. Generally, the forecast period should not less than seven days nor more than a month.

creditors as an index of liquidity and ability to pay obligations.

Cash to Total
Assets

Ratio of cash to total tangible assets. Used to provide an index of both liquidity and asset allocation balance.

Inventory to
Total Assets

Ratio of Inventory holdings to total tangible assets. Used to provide an index of asset allocation blance.

Debt to Total
Assets

Ratio of total long term debt to total tangible assets. Used primarily by creditors as an index of the protection accorded their principal.

Net Worth to
Total Assets

Ratio of total net worth to total tangible assets. Used to provide an index of the risk attached to the firm's financial structure; i.e., the lower this ratio, the greater the risk.

Historically, the hospital industry has made limited use of ratio analysis. This has been primarily due to the lack of adequate ratio values which could be used as norms for comparative purposes. For the most part, hospitals have just adopted the standard ratios developed by other industries and have attempted to apply them directly to their own operating situation. Unfortunately, this approach has not been successful, for these borrowed guidelines have not been based upon either the unique operating parameters of the hospital industry or—and more importantly—the particular hospital in question. The norms which hospitals have traditionally used thus have been irrelevant, acting to confuse rather than to clarify balance sheet evaluation.

However, using the techniques which have been discussed in the previous chapters, a hospital can develop rate guidelines based upon its own operating situation. Using these standards, ratio analysis can become a meaningful and useful tool for hospital management. Table 14-1 presents examples of the mechanics of calculating various ratios.[2]

In addition to a balance sheet, management should utilize several other stock reports. These basic reports are examined in the following sections. It is important to realize that, depending on a hospital's particular operating situation and management's desires and style, reports other than those discussed may be utilized in some instances. The task of describing all possible working capital reports and their variations, however, is obviously beyond the scope of this text. Therefore, only those reports which are commonly used for working capital management will be discussed.

Cash Reports

Traditionally, daily cash reports have been used by administrators as their primary cash management report. These reports usually consist of just a summary listing of both cash receipts—by source—and cash disbursements by item. As such, their usefulness is quite limited, for they encompass too short a time span for management either to make an evaluation or to act. However, for hospitals with chronic cash shortages or with sharply fluctuating cash balances these reports, as modified by the addition of a cash flow projection, can be of valuable aid. Figure 14-3 illustrates a modified daily cash report.

Generally, comparative reports, which both contrast actual cash flows with the cash budget and estimate the next ending cash balance, are more useful to upper management than simple daily cash reports. This type of report is of more value, for it not only provides an analytical frame of reference for control decisions, but also, if prepared biweekly or monthly, allows management to both identify and evaluate trends. With this informtion, management can more knowledgeably select cash investment or financing strategies.

The usefulness of this type of comparative cash statement should be clear. In the author's opinion, this report should be used by most hospitals as their basic management report. Figure

---

[2]Based upon the techniques discussed in previous chapters and the particular hospital's operating situation, the ideal or standard amount of various asset and liability holdings can be determined for any given hospital. Based upon these quantities, "normal," i.e., standard, ratios can be calculated. It is particularly important to remember that each hospital's operating parameters and operating environment differs. Therefore, guidelines or normal ratios should be developed independently for each institution. Industry norms should be used only with caution and care.

Figure 14-4
Sample Monthly Cash Report
Lanoff County Hospital
For the Month Ending_____

	Actual	Budget
Beginning Cash Balance	$_____	$_____
Cash Receipts		
Inpatient	$_____	$_____
Outpatient	$_____	$_____
Other Operating	$_____	$_____
Nonoperating	$_____	$_____
Total:	$_____	$_____
Cash Disbursements		
Salaries and Wages	$_____	$_____
Supplies	$_____	$_____
Plant and Equipment	$_____	$_____
Other	$_____	$_____
Total:	$_____	$_____
Ending Cash Balance	$_____	$_____

Projected Cash Balance—Month Ending_____

$_____

Figure 14-5
Sample Investment Report
M. Cohn General Hospital
As of July 31, 1970

Security	Date Purchased	Cost	Market Value	Maturity Date	Yield	Income To Date
Hosp. Credit Corp.-Note	5-1-70	$10,000	$10,000	10-1-70	6%	$150
U.S. Treasury Bills	6-15-70	$19,750	$19,860	9-15-70	5%	-
Certificate of Dep.-Consumer	7-1-70	$ 5,000	$ 5,000	12-1-70	5.25%	-
Hosp. Credit Corp.-Note	7-15-70	$ 5,000	$ 5,000	3-1-71	5%	-
		$39,750	$39,860		5.04%	$150

Other Information:

Investment Balance Last Month	$45,000
Income This Month	$ 50
Total Investment Income (all investments) This Year=	$ 1,750

Figure 14-6
Sample Aged Accounts Receivable Report
Israel General Hospital
January 31, 1971

A. General

Time Outstanding	Amount Current Month	Amount Last Month
0-30 days	$12,500	$10,000
31-60 days	9,750	9,000
61-90 days	7,000	8,500
91-120 days	5,000	4,000
121-180 days	3,000	-
Over 180 days	-	-
Total Outstanding:	$37,250	$31,500

B. By Payer

Percentage of Revenue by Payer	40% Blue Cross		20% Medicare		10% Medicaid		30% Other	
Time Outstanding	Current	Last	Current	Last	Current	Last	Current	Last
0- days	$ 5,000	$ 4,000	$2,500	$2,000	$1,250	$1,000	$ 3,750	$3,000
31-60 days								
61-90 days	$ 3,900	$ 3,600	$1,950	$1,800	$ 975	$ 900	$ 2,925	$2,700
91-120 days	$ 2,800	$ 3,400	$1,400	$1,700	$ 700	$ 850	$ 2,100	$2,550
121-180 days	$ 2,000	$ 1,600	$1,000	$ 800	$ 500	$ 400	$ 1,500	$1,200
Over 180 days	$ 1,200	–	$ 600	–	$ 300	$ –	$ 900	–
	$ –	–	–	–	–	–	–	–
	$14,900	$12,600	$7,450	$6,300	$3,725	$3,150	$11,175	$9,450

14-4 presents an example of this statement. Hospitals with cash shortages or with rapidly fluctuating cash balances should also use the modified daily cash report as a supplement to this basic report.

In addition to the above, management should receive, at least monthly, a listing of the hospital's short-term investments. This report, as Figure 14-5 illustrates, should indicate the nature of the investment, date purchased, purchase cost, present market value, maturity date, yield, income received year-to-date, total investment balance for both the current and previous month, and composite portfolio yield. With this information, management can evaluate the quality and profitability of the hospital's short-term portfolio. Also, based on this report and the monthly cash reports, management can assess the appropriateness of both the short-term investment balance and the minimum cash balance.

Accounts Receivable Reports

As was indicated in Chapter 12, accounts receivable are the biggest single component of working capital. Hence, if for no other reason than just size, they should merit management's concern and attention. Accounts receivable, however, are critical for another reason. If receivables are not collected and are allowed to increase, it is not only possible but also likely that a hospital will not have sufficient cash available to pay its obligations as they come due. Thus, if management is to maintain the financial integrity of the hospital, it must be sure that the accounts receivable collection function is performed as effectively and efficiently as is possible.

The most basic of all accounts receivable control reports is the aged analysis of accounts or aged trial balance. This report can take numerous forms. In its simplest structure it is just a listing of the amount of receivables outstanding by the length of time for which they have been outstanding. Generally, the larger the amount of older accounts, the less efficient is the collection process and the greater is the danger of the hospital having an inadequate cash balance.[3] Figure 14-6 (Part A) is an example of an aged analysis of an accounts receivable report.

In addition to an aged trial balance, several other accounts receivable reports can be of value. Examples of such reports are:

Days of Service
Uncollected Report   A report indicating the number of days of service which have been rendered but for which payment is out-

---

[3]The research department of the American Collectors Association reported the following dollar values in delinquent accounts:

Age	Value
Current	$1.00
Two months old	.80
Six months old	.67
One year old	.49
Two years old	.27

The Association also reported that an overall recovery of 40 percent occurred during the first 90 days that the accounts were being worked on a collection basis.

standing. This statistic is calculated by dividing the accounts receivable balance by the average daily charge. The larger the number of days of service uncollected, the less effective is the collection process.

Accounts Receivable Summary Report

A report listing the amount of accounts receivable outstanding by source of payment and/or, if preferred, by type of patient. This is primarily an informational report designed to indicate where management attention should be concentrated. That is, attention should be focused on sources of payment whose accounts outstanding are increasing (see Figure 14-6; Part B).

Accounts Receivable Turnover Report

A report indicating the relationship between receivables and revenues. This statistic is calculated by dividing revenues for a specific period by the average accounts receivable balance for that same period. The smaller the turnover index number, the greater is the proportion of receivables to revenue and the less effective is the collection process. (For a further discussion of turnover, see "Inventory Reports" section of this chapter.)

Uncollectable Charge Off Report

A report indicating the details of accounts charged off, reasons why, and comparative monthly and year-to-date statistics. This is both an informational and a control report, for it enables management not only to obtain information of the collection process, but also to evaluate its final performance.

Based upon these reports, management has available the data necessary both to evaluate the overall effectiveness of the hospital's credit and collection efforts and to pinpoint any troublesome areas. Using this information, management should be able to assure that accounts receivable remain at acceptable levels.

Inventory Reports

The nature and mechanics of inventory management were examined in detail in Chapter 11. Given that material, the first step which must be taken is to assure that the hospital's actual inventory practices are as consistent as practicable with the ideal guidelines which were set out. In addition to this initial control step, management should receive reports, such as the inventory turnover report, which will aid it to continually evaluate and control the hospital's inventory practices and position.

Inventory turnover can be defined as the number of times during a given period, usually a month, that the existing inventory stocks would be depleted and replaced. This statistic can be calculated for each cost center by simply dividing the dollar amount of supplies and other inventory items which are expected to be used in a month by the dollar amount of inventories on hand. Generally, a low turnover rate indicates excessive inventory holdings and poor working capital management. A moderately high or high turnover rate usually indicates a desirable situation. An extremely high turnover rate often indicates insufficient inventory stocks. What a particular turnover rate specifically means can be determined either through an analysis of historical data and current operating conditions or through inventory control studies. Based upon these judgments, management can assess both a department's and the total hospital's inventory position. Figure 14-7 illustrates a monthly inventory turnover report.

Management may also find that other reports can be useful in evaluating a hospital's inventory position. For example, reports on actual and maximum inventories, on averages and shortages in physical holdings, or on comparisons between actual and budget may be of value. Therefore, the financial manager, in conjunction with administration, should determine the type of information needed, review the reporting options available, and provide these reports which will be of most value to management.

Figure 14-7
Lindsay General Hospital
Sample Monthly Inventory Turnover Report
May 31, 1974

(1) Cost Center	(2) Expected Monthly Usage	Inventory Holdings		(Col. 2 ÷ Col. 3A) Current Month	(4) Turnover Rate	
		(3A) Current Month	(3B) Last Month		Last Month*	Annual Average**
1. Central Supply	25,400	5,000	20,000	5.1	2.7	2.6
2. Dietary	102,700	32,000	45,000	3.2	3.2	3.0
3. Pharmacy	37,800	3,100	5,000	12.2	10.8	9.5
17. Nursing Unit-A	6,500	2,000	4,000	3.2	2.1	1.8

* From last month's report.
** Arithmetic average of turnover rates for the last 12 months.

Figure 14-8

Sample Purchase Discounts Lost Report

Anders General Hospital

Month Ending January 31, 1971

	Current Month		Last Month	
1. Total Purchases	$25,000		$30,000	
2. Purchases Offered with Discounts	$10,000	40%	$20,000	66.7%
3. Dollar Value of Discounts Available	$ 150		$ 400	
4. Dollar Value of Discounts Taken	$ 100		$ 400	
5. Dollar Value of Discounts Not Taken	$ 50		$ 0	

6. Explanation of Discounts Not Taken:

> *Cash shortage in the last quarter of the month—due to insurance premium payment—resulted in the need to defer payment on several large accounts.*

Accounts Payable Records

In contrast with the above items, control of both accounts and wages payable is not obtained through the direct management of the items per se, but rather through the controls exerted on the underlying processes which produce these liability accounts. Specifically, accounts payable are a function or a direct product of the purchasing process. Therefore, if the level of accounts payable is to be maintained at acceptable and manageable limits, the purchasing process must be controlled through the establishment of and the adherence to sound inventory and purchasing policies and procedures.

The same situation is also true in regard to wages payable. These payables are a function of the personnel process and can be controlled only through the proper management of that process. Thus, to maintain wages payable at financially reasonable limits, management must establish policies and procedures which assure that sound internal control exists over both hours worked and wage payments.

Hence, in order to control and evaluate the financial performance or position of the hospital relative to the above liabilities, management, for the most part, must examine the performance of the underlying processes. The balance sheet report and ratio analysis can provide some insight into the appropriateness of the relative size of these items. Also, a monthly report, indicating the amount of purchase discounts lost (see Figure 14-8), can be useful in evaluating the accounts payable payment function. It must be realized, however, that control over these items can be obtained only through the control of the processes of which they are a function.

Conclusion

Given the foregoing material, the discussion of working capital management is now complete. Based on the discussion in Chapters 9 through 13, the reader should have a sound understanding of the financial tools and techniques which can be of value in minimizing the size and, consequently, the cost of working capital. The discussion in this chapter has hopefully made clear the reports needed to evaluate a hospital's working capital position. Therefore, if all has gone according to plan, the reader should now have the knowledge necessary not only to evaluate a hospital's working capital performance and position, but also to correct any deficiencies.

Admittedly, there is more to hospital financial management than has been discussed in the foregoing chapters. The topics of operational budgeting, investment decisions, and responsibility accounting are all critical areas which are, unfortunately, beyond the introductory nature of this volume. The intent of this text has been only to provide an initial orientation to the financial environment of the hospital and to build a foundation for examining these more complex topics.

Suggested Readings

Choate, G. Marc. "Financial Ratio Analysis." *Hospital Progress*, January 1974.

Heckert, J. Brooks and Wilson, J. D. *Controllership*.

Seawell, L. Vann. *Hospital Accounting and Financial Management*, Chapter 11.

Van Arsdell, Paul M. *Corporate Finance: Policy, Planning, Administration*, Chapter 6.

Young, D.E. "Effective Presentation of Reports, Information for Understanding."

Part IV
Planning, Budgeting,
and Control

"Planning: the half science of breathing operational form and life into dreams; of applying the art of the possible to merge concept and operations into a single, cohesive, reality."—N.S. Hinkle

Chapter 15

Planning and Budgeting: Value, Prerequisites, Initial Decisions

Whether due to pragmatic considerations of operational need or to the legislative mandates of the Medicare program (Public Law 92–603) and/or state rate setting and review programs, the matters of the budget and budgeting are, and will continue to be, issues of central concern to management.[1] In the early 1960s, a study of Michigan hospitals found that " . . . budgeting is a management technique used by few hospitals in Michigan." Of the study's survey hospitals, only twenty-three percent (23%) prepared income and expense budgets. Moreover, of those hospitals preparing budgets, less than half involved the person responsible for the performance of a department in the development of the department's budget. Also, only about one-fifth (1/5) of the hospitals which prepared budgets supplied department heads with reports that compared actual and planned performance.[2] However, as was the case with cost analysis—where the study's findings were even

---

[1]Section 234 of Public Law 92–603:
An overall plan and budget of a hospital, extended care facility, or home health agency shall be considered sufficient if it—
(1) provides for an annual operating budget which includes all anticipated income and expenses . . . ;
(2) provides for a capital expenditures plan for at least a 3 year period . . . ;
(3) provides for review and updating at least annually; and
(4) is prepared, under the direction of the governing body of the institution or agency, by a committee consisting of representatives of the governing body, the administrative staff, and the medical staff (if any) of the institution or agency.
[2]W.J. McNerney et al., *Hospital and Medical Economics*, pp. 876–882.

less encouraging, i.e., only five percent (5%) of the hospitals performed cost analysis through use of any of the accepted methods (see Chapter 5)—the situation has markedly changed over the past fifteen years.

The importance of budgeting, as measured by the volume of the existing literature, is well recognized. The existing literature, however, is heavily oriented to the needs of the budget director; i.e., the financial officer responsible for preparing the budget. It concentrates, for the most part, on the technical and mechanistic aspects of budgeting and largely ignores the policy, organizational, and behavioral aspects. This literature, though certainly a necessary part of the total equation, is not designed to meet the fundamental needs of general management.

If management is to be able to capitalize effectively on the operational benefits of budgeting and the budget, it not only must be familiar with the mechanics but also must understand the management value and interpersonal dynamics of the process. While "forms" and "calculation techniques" will from time to time creep into the following chapters, the main thrust of this section will be on identifying and describing the principles and interrelationships which underlie operationally successful budgeting. This chapter will focus on the management usefulness of operational planning and budgeting as well as the prerequisite decisions which must be made. The following two chapters will address the process and the organizational dynamics of the process. The final chapter of the section will emphasize the value and operation of the management reporting or feedback process.

Perspective

Though this chapter addresses the managerial usefulness and initial facets of the budgeting process, it is important to understand the context in which the budget should exist. Too often, management falls into the trap of losing sight of or of forgetting the "real" reasons for preparing a budget. As emphasized below, "means" and "ends" can become confused if the budget becomes the "end"—as opposed to the "means"—of the corporate plan.

A hospital's budget exists and is only meaningful within the context of the institution's corporate plan. As is discussed in this and the following chapter, the budget is the monetary and operating reflection of the corporate plan. As such, it must always be borne in mind that the corporate plan "drives" the budgetary process. It is the budget which must be tailored to the plan—not the plan to the budget.

Given this perspective, the focus of Part IV is on the management mechanics of planning and the dynamics and process of budgeting and reporting. To the extent possible, the mechanics and the techniques of calculation will be left to the existing literature and other authors. Readers interested in exploring these topics in further detail should refer to the "Suggested Readings" at the end of each chapter and the bibliography.

Definition

Like other words in the English language, the word "budget" has, to some extent, been slandered. A negative connotation—emphasizing repressive control and also, in some instances, laborious and often useless preparation—has attached itself to the word. This connotation, while perhaps in some instances merited, is intrinsic neither to the definition of the word nor to its operational realization.

The word "budget" is derived from the Old English word "bougette." A "bougette" was a small bag or pouch which was used to carry items of value needed for daily business. When a trip was planned, the "bougette" was packed with the essentials for the journey. Thus, a budget is actually nothing more than a collection or list of items needed for carrying out some planned activity.

The traditional literature has been faithful to this definition. A budget is generally defined as a comprehensive operational plan or guide for some future period of time—usually, by convention, a year.

Operational plans can be expressed in a variety of ways, e.g., manhours, dollars, outputs, etc. A budget, however, is primarily a financial plan and is, therefore, expressed in dollars. Thus, the term budget might be more explicity defined as a comprehensive financial plan, based upon anticipated outputs and predetermined hospital goals and policies for future operations which is expressed in dollars of expense and corresponding dollars of revenue.

If one is really to appreciate what a budget is and understand how it can be of managerial value, it is necessary to go beyond either the historical or traditional definition. In its essences, a budget is both a definitive statement of corporate policy from an external perspective, and a potent management tool from an internal perspective.

Policy Statement

Each year, for the last several years, the Brookings Institution has published a book entitled *Setting National Priorities: The 19--*

Budget. These books have attempted to examine the nation's priorities and policies through the vehicle of the Federal budget. They have viewed the budget as the reflection of management's (the Administration's) choices in terms of objectives, strategies, and priorities. The nation's fiscal allocations and plans have been considered as simply a reflection of its policies and goals.

The fundamental principle applied by the Brookings Institution to the Federal budget is equally applicable in the "micro" or individual firm context. A hospital's budget is in actuality its primary statement of operating policy. If a hospital were publicly to express great interest in ambulatory care services, but budgeted only to increase the scope of its inpatient services, then, despite its rhetoric, its "real" policy is to emphasize inpatient care.

Admittedly, this kind of example is somewhat simplistic. It does, however, illustrate the general point. To the public, a hospital's budget is its statement of operating policy, for its budget depicts where the institution's interest and emphasis lie.

Realization that the budget is a policy statement also forces the recognition of a corollary principle. As a policy statement, a budget is a means to an end—not an end, in and of itself.

This principle should be taken as a warning signal. If preparation of the budget becomes the end—the goal which the organization is attempting to reach—then management has lost its perspective. At this point, management must act. Attention must be directed toward putting the process back in perspective by placing emphasis on the operational outcome as opposed to the "paperwork" effort of developing the budget. If management fails to heed this signal, then the institution may well become a captive of its budget process: producing instead of an operational plan, just reams of little used, or usable, paper.

Management Tool

From an internal perspective, the budget is a potent management tool. It is, perhaps, the best device available to management both for identifying those activities which will provide the greatest community benefit and for guiding the hospital in achieving the implementation and operation of those selected activities in the least disruptive manner.

Management is continually confronted with a variety of alternative activities and courses of action. Each of these alternatives has some cost attached to it and some corresponding related level of community benefit. If management is to meet its objective successfully, it must select from among the alternative demands for resources in such a manner as to produce a combination of activities which yields, in total, the greatest amount of community benefit (see Chapter 1).

In a "micro" economic context, management must move the institution to the margin.[3] Optimally, this would mean that expenditures for any particular activity should be continued until the point where the marginal cost—the additional cost—equals the marginal benefit to the community. In the less than optimal, but more realistic, instance, wherein resources are limited, the same principle of moving to the margin applies. However, in this case, management must place priority on those alternatives which produce the largest community benefits. It must fund projects in such a manner that, even though the marginal point might not be obtained for any particular project, the sum of "realized benefits" is maximized.

The budget and the budget process not only provide the tools to enable management to accomplish this but also provide an important part of the total mechanism needed by management to monitor the hospital's operational progress towards achieving its plan. How the budget and the budget process can be used in this manner can, perhaps, be better understood if one examines the relationship of the budget and budget process to each of the specific functions of management.

The literature traditionally defines the functions of management as those of planning, organizing, coordinating, and controlling operations and motivating employees. The budget and budgeting assist management in successfully carrying out each of these functions.

Planning

A budget, as defined previously, is a comprehensive operational plan expressed in dollars. The two-part nature of this definition should be recognized. The budget is not just an operational plan. Rather, it is the institution's operational plan expressed in dollars.

This point may at first glance appear to be just a bit of semantic manipulation. However, as will become clear, it is a critical distinction.

Planning is a management function. Budgeting is the conversion

---

[3]Readers interested in a detailed discussion of this concept should refer to any micro economics text such as, *The Price System and Resource Allocation* by Richard H. Leftwich.

of the management plan into dollars. It is a financial function. The primacy of the plan and the management function over the financial function must always be borne in mind, if the maximum value of the budget is to be obtained. If the order of importance is allowed to be reversed, then budgeting becomes a paper exercise fulfilling the imperatives of the finance staff but of little value to either general or line management. However, the budget process, if used with discretion and with a sensitivity to its proper purpose, can assist management in developing a comprehensive institutional plan.

Budgeting can aid management in planning in two ways. First, it provides the opportunity to plan. Systematic planning is often a task which does not require management's immediate attention. Therefore, it is often pushed aside in favor of more currently pressing operational issues. The budgeting process, however, requires that management both direct its attention to the future and plan for it. It, in effect, raises the priority of planning by making it a required component of the operational problem of developing a budget. By raising the priority of planning, the budget process not only forces management to devote attention to planning, but also provides at least one opportunity in the course of the year to plan.

The budget process also aids in planning by providing a structure in which to plan. The budget process forces management to view the future, and its subsequent plans for the future, in terms of operating expense, revenues, capital expenditures, and cash flows.

As pointed out in Chapter 13, a hospital's annual operating budget is the sum of four separate, but mutually dependent budgets: the expense budget, the revenue budget, the capital budget, and the cash budget. These four budgets, in addition to their critical role in assuring financial coordination, provide a framework for guiding the planning process, for they force management to consider each of its intended actions in terms of expense requirements, revenue-generating potential, capital needs, and cash flows.

Organizing

Budgeting is an aid to management both in organizing operations and in organizing resources. Effective budgeting and budgetary control—like effective cost analysis—require a clearly defined, responsibility centered organization structure with corresponding cost centers. In the case of cost analysis, the organizing of operations along distinct cost/responsibility center lines is necessary both to assure that the initial costs of each distinct function are correctly reported and to enable the accurate computation of the total costs of final cost centers (see Chapter 5). The reasons underlying the need for the same type of organization structure for purposes of budgeting and budgetary control are similar. It is only through this cost/responsibility center approach to the organization of operations that actual and planned performance can be meaningfully compared, evaluated—and most importantly—controlled.

Budgeting assists management in achieving this kind of organization structure by providing an incentive—in terms of the potential for improved operational control—for careful organization, with clear lines of control and responsibility. Additionally, the budget process aids management in organizing operations by providing documentation and a periodic opportunity for management to correct either overlaps or gaps in the allocation of responsibility.

The budget process is also the primary tool available to management for purposes of organized resources. As set out earlier, management must strive to move the hospital to the "margin", i.e., management must attempt to organize or allocate its resources such that the greatest total benefit is obtained. To accomplish this goal, alternative expenditure opportunities must be evaluated and funding priorities established such that the projects with the greatest benefits are funded first and, if need be, to the exclusion of other projects with lesser benefits.

In abstract, the necessity of this kind of conceptual approach to resource organization is easily understood. Moving from the abstract level to operational reality, however, creates somewhat of a problem. This is due to both the number of alternatives which must be compared and evaluated and the relative uniqueness of the benefits of each alternative. However, a tool is available which management can potentially use to move from concept and theory to operational implementation. This tool is known as a zero base budgeting.[4]

Zero base budgeting is an approach to budgeting which has been used successfully in both industry (Texas Instruments, Inc.) and government (State of Georgia). Essentially, zero base budgeting is a process wherein all expenditures are evaluated and rank

---

[4]The following material has been drawn in the main from: *Zero Base Budgeting* by Peter A. Pyhrr. Readers interested in further information relative to the philosophy and mechanics of zero base budgeting should consult this reference.

ordered. In the traditional budget process, managers responsible for established (ongoing) activities generally have to justify only the increase which they are seeking over the previous year's appropriation. Customarily, what is already being spent is accepted as necessary and is implicitly approved as a continuing expenditure. Zero base budgeting differs from the traditional approach in that it requires every department to "make a case" and defend its entire budget request each year, just as if all its activities were entirely new.

By taking this perspective, zero base budgeting allows management to examine expenditure alternatives in their total, as opposed to just their incremental portion, and select those alternatives (organize its resources in a manner) which provide the greatest total benefit.

Procedurally, there are two basic steps in zero base budgeting:

1. *Developing Decision Packages*—This step involves the operating manager describing and evaluating each of the activities—both ongoing and proposed—for which he is responsible.
2. *Ranking Decision Packages*—This step involves senior management's analyzing and ranking, through cost/benefit analysis and/or subjective judgment, the decision packages developed in the first step.

Once decision packages are developed and ranked, management can accordingly allocate resources; funding the programs having the greatest net benefit, regardless of whether they are existing or new activities. The final budget is produced by taking the activities that have been accepted for funding, sorting them into their appropriate organizational units, and then summarizing the costs identified to produce the budget for each department as well as for the entire hospital.

An example of a decision package form and instructions is illustrated in Table 15-1. As can be seen, a decision package is composed of ten basic components which in total identify and describe a specific activity in such a manner that management can:

—analyze the activity and decide whether to approve or disapprove it; and
—if the decision is to approve, rank order the activity against other expenditure alternatives.

The matter of developing alternatives within decision packages is a critical part of zero base budgeting. This is the case for the identification of alternatives enables management to consider the full continuum of available choices, i.e., it expands the range of choices to include both intra- and interdecision package alternatives. Given a limitation on funds, if management is not presented with internal alternatives for an activity it might elect not to fund a particular activity as opposed to funding the activity—if it were performed at different level of effort or in a different manner. By either ignoring, or not being aware of, these internal alternatives, management makes less than the optimal choice and defeats, in part, the purpose of zero base budgeting. To avoid this pitfall, alternatives for accomplishing the desired objective, if they represent realistic options, must be presented as part of an activity's decision package.

As indicated, two classes or types of alternatives should be presented in each decision package. The first should examine alternative ways of accomplishing the same objective. The decision package should highlight the recommended way of performing the activity with the alternatives being identified and briefly explained.

A second category of alternatives focuses on different levels of effort. In this instance, a minimum level of effort should be identified as should the current and requested levels, presuming they are different. A separate decision package can be developed for each level of effort or a single package can be used with each level of effort being identified, briefly discussed, and rank ordered against the others.

Decision packages should initially be developed at the lowest practicable level within the organization. At a minimum, the manager accountable for each responsibility center should develop the decision package for the activities within that center. Ideally, however, the person responsible for each discrete activity, function, or operation within the responsibility center should develop the decision package for his programs. Details concerning the mechanics of preparing decision packages are set out in Appendix 15-A.[5] It should be noted that Appendix 15-2 complements 15-A by presenting a brief critique of the State of Georgia's zero base budgeting experience. This critique was prepared by Peter A. Pyhrr and is excerpted from his book, *Zero Base Budgeting.*

---

[5]The decision package described in the Appendix differs somewhat from that shown in Table 15-1. The difference reflects the needs of the involved organizations. The Appendix is an excerpt from the Zero Base Budgeting Manual used by the State of Georgia. The Table represents the same basic package, tailored to more appropriately fit the health environment.

Table 15-1

Lash County Hospital

Activity Decision Package

1) Program Area: ＿＿＿＿＿＿＿＿2) Activity: ＿＿＿＿＿＿＿＿＿
3) Objective ＿＿＿＿＿＿＿＿＿＿＿＿＿＿＿＿＿＿＿＿＿＿＿
＿＿＿＿＿＿＿＿＿＿＿＿＿＿＿＿＿＿＿＿＿＿＿＿＿＿＿＿＿

4) Activity Description: ＿＿＿＿＿＿＿＿＿＿＿＿＿＿＿＿＿
＿＿＿＿＿＿＿＿＿＿＿＿＿＿＿＿＿＿＿＿＿＿＿＿＿＿＿＿＿

　　　　　　　Starting Date ＿＿＿＿＿＿Completion Date ＿＿＿＿＿
5) Activity Benefit/Result:　　　6) Resources:
＿＿＿＿＿＿＿＿＿＿＿＿＿＿＿＿　　Man years　　Direct Expense
＿＿＿＿＿＿＿＿＿＿＿＿＿＿＿＿　　Mgmt.　　　Salaries
＿＿＿＿＿＿＿＿＿＿＿＿＿＿＿＿　　Super.　　　Travel
　　　　　　　　　　　　　　　　Tech.　　　　Other
　　　　　　　　　　　　　　　　Clerical
　　　　　　　　　　　TOTAL ＿＿＿　　　TOTAL ＿＿＿

7) Alternatives: Alternative Way of Accomplishing the Same Result
No.　　　　　　　　Alternative　　　　　Resource Requirement
　　　　　　　　　　　　　　　　　　　　Man years　　　　$

8) Alternatives: Alternative Levels of Effort
No.　　　　　　　　Alternative　　Benefit　Resource Requirement
　　　　　　　　　　　　　　　　　　　　Man years　　　　$

9) Ranking
No.　Alternative Number　Resource Requirements ($) 10) ＿＿＿＿＿＿
1　＿＿＿＿＿＿＿＿＿＿＿＿＿＿＿＿＿＿＿＿Identification of
2　＿＿＿＿＿＿＿＿＿＿＿＿＿＿＿＿＿＿＿＿Package Developer
3　＿＿＿＿＿＿＿＿＿＿＿＿＿＿＿＿＿＿＿＿
4　＿＿＿＿＿＿＿＿＿＿＿＿＿＿＿＿＿＿＿＿
5　＿＿＿＿＿＿＿＿＿＿＿＿＿＿＿＿＿＿＿＿Date ＿＿＿＿＿＿
6　＿＿＿＿＿＿＿＿＿＿＿＿＿＿＿＿＿＿＿＿

Table 15-1

Activity Decision Packages

(continued)

Instructions

1. *Program Department Area*
Identification by name of the program department area being addressed: Environmental Services, Administration, Outpatient Services, etc.

2. *Activity*
Identification of the activity being addressed: in Environmental Services it might be Heating and Cooling Plant; in Outpatient Services it might be Community Mental Health, etc.

3. *Objective*
Restatement of the program area's objective or that portion of the objective to which the activity applies: in Outpatient Services for the Community Mental Health activity the objective might be to provide the total service area with convenient access to mental health service.

4. *Activity Description*
Generic statement of the activity, with starting and completion dates from a process perspective when applicable. For example, under Environmental Services the description of the activities of a heating and cooling plant professional might be the licensed supervision, operation, and minor maintenance of the central heating and cooling system on an around the clock basis. This would be an ongoing activity.

5. *Activity Benefit/Result*
Statement in quantified terms of the benefit/result or output of the activity. Result *must* relate to the program area objective and be quantified. For example: Outpatient Services, Community Mental Health—through the use of outreach efforts—provide convenient access to mental health services for the total service area as measured by an increase in 5,000 visits by existing patients and the provision of services to at least 1,000 new patients.

6. *Resources*
Statement of estimated resource requirements. Expense information should just be direct costs.

7. *Alternatives:* Alternative Way of Accomplishing the Same Result
The purpose of this section is to force consideration of alternatives. In this instance, it is alternative ways of accomplishing the same result.
   The first alternative in this section should be numbered two (2) since the alternative indicated in item 4 is number one (1). Other alternatives should be ranked sequentially. Under the alternative heading, a

Table 15-1 (continued)

different approach to achieving the same end should be identified: hiring a consultant as opposed to doing the job yourself, or purchasing laundry services on a contract basis as opposed to operating the hospital's own laundry, centralizing OB on a community wide basis, etc. *If no visible alternative exists, then this section should be left blank.*

In the resource section the total man years and direct dollars of expense associated with each alternative should be set out.

8. *Alternatives:* Alternative Levels of Effort
The purpose of this section is to focus attention on alternative levels of investment and their resulting benefits. For example: for a $200,000 investment increase patient visits by 3,000 and new patients by 1,000; do eight reviews with a savings of $500,000; for $150,000 investment increase patient visits by 3,000 and new patients by 500. This section should just address alternatives to the level of activity of choice.

In the "No." column, the sequential listing of alternatives should be continued from the above section. Under "Alternative," the nature of the alternative should be briefly stated: 3,000 visits increase, 1,000 new patients, etc.

Under the "Benefit" column the benefit obtained from the alternative level of effort should be defined: convenient access to only 90 percent of the total service area.

The Resource column should be completed the same as is the case above.

If the alternative is to forego the activity, then the nature of the lost benefit should be set out.

9. *Ranking*
Identification of the ranking of each of the alternatives should be identified by its sequential number.

10. *Identification and Date*
Signature of the manager responsible on a day-to-day basis for the operation of the activity and the date on which the Decision Package is to be submitted for review.

The second step in zero base budgeting is the rank ordering of decision packages. The ranking process provides management with a vehicle for allocating its limited resources. Essentially, a rank ordering is simply a listing of all decision packages in order of decreasing cost/benefit to the total organization. Initial ranking selections should be made by the manager responsible for developing the decision packages. Managers at each succeeding level in the organizational hierarchy should consolidate the decision packages and rankings received from their subordinates and produce their own ranking for all the packages presented to them. Finally, senior management should consolidate all decision packages and rankings into a final total institutional ranking.

In theory, ranking decisions should be made on the basis of cost/benefit analysis. However, in the reality of the actual hospital operation environment, the role and value of the subjective judgment process should not be underestimated. For purposes of initial rankings, quantitative techniques can provide useful information. At the senior management level, however, the emphasis should primarily be on broad distinctions of relative order: assuring that package 5 is more important than package 35, and on determining the action to be taken in regard to discretionary, as opposed to required, activities. In both these regards, subjective judgment, honed by experience and a detailed knowledge of the environment is, perhaps, the best tool available. Figure 15-1 graphically illustrates the ranking process.

Before proceeding further, a final point is worthy of note. The foregoing discussion has approached zero base budgeting from the perspective of its being both a concept and a mechanical process. As will be reiterated in the following pages, hopefully to the point of understanding, a procedure—whether presented as a model approach or as the unique approach utilized by a particular organization—should never be arbitrarily superimposed upon an organization.

If operationally successful results are to be obtained, mechanical procedures must be tailored to the unique character, history, and style of the user organization. In some instances this tailoring may mean that some procedural components should be eliminated. Such deviance from a prototype procedural approach may be anathema to particular managers. It should be remembered however, that the emphasis must be on substance and results—not form and process. In the case of zero base budgeting, the important element is the basic concept of examining both the ongoing need for current activities and the alternatives available for conducting needed activities, not the process to be employed or the forms to be used.

Figure 15-1

Decision Package Ranking Process

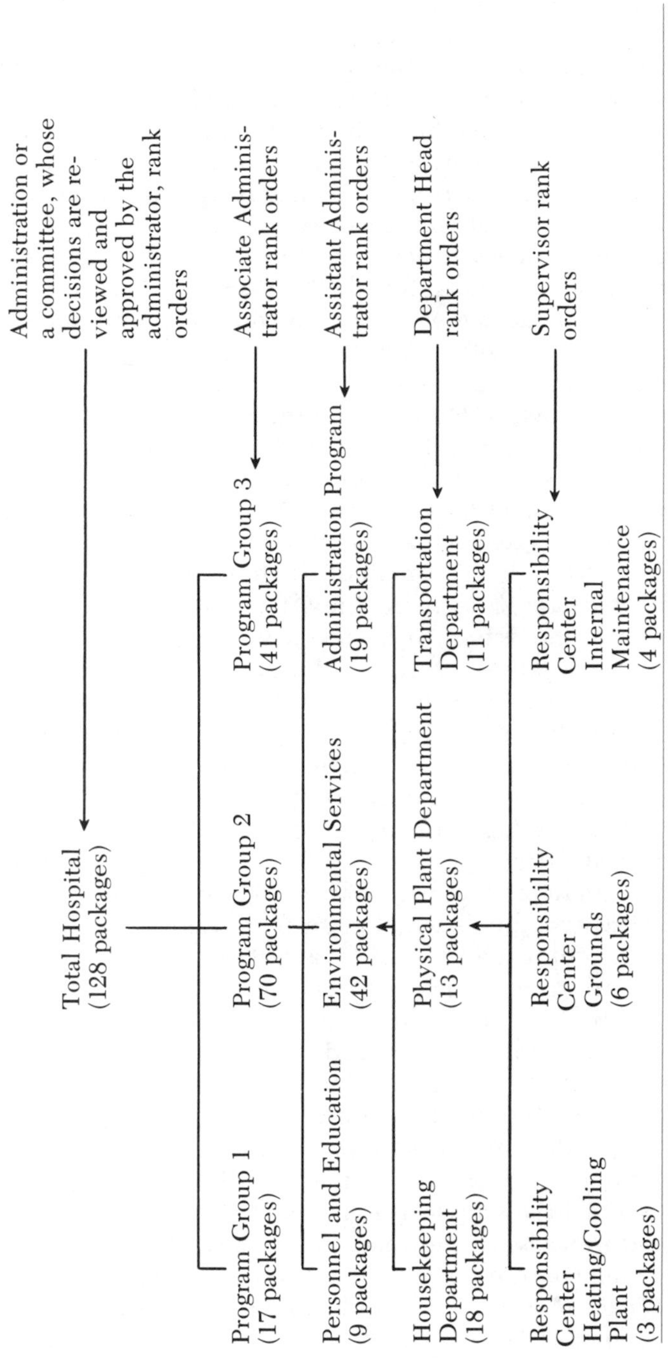

In addition to the foregoing, the reader should also note that zero base budgeting, though reasonable and probably acceptable in concept, will be a threatening set of ideas for some managers, particularly at the departmental level. Therefore, implementation of zero base budgeting ideas and procedures should reflect a careful appreciation and application of the principle of management of change.

This cautionary note is particularly germane in the application of zero base budgeting in the hospital setting. Clearly, there are a number of hospital activities wherein management's options to either expand, contract, or eliminate a function are limited. The existence of these activities does not invalidate the concept of zero base budgeting. However, it does require that the procedural mechanics of the concept be modified to reflect operational reality if the underlying concept is to prove useful.

The nature of the request modifications will obviously differ with the institution. In total, however, modifications should result in the "custom fitting" of the procedure to the needs and character of the particular institution. The underlying conceptual principles are, however, generally applicable to all institutions and to all resource organization problems.

Coordinating

Obviously, the budget and budget process, by providing a mechanism for comparing revenues and expenses are the key tools in assuring financial coordination. The budget process, however, is also a useful tool for assuring the coordination of operations.

As the discussion of Chapter 16 will make clear, the budget process provides the vehicle for establishing common goals and communicating those goals between and within operating programs. The process of common goal setting and communication provides the basis for operational coordination. Moreover, the budget process, by requiring that each responsibility center's plans be examined, allows management to evaluate planned operations critically (in terms of the common goals) and, if necessary, to make adjustments to assure that activity overlaps are eliminated, gaps are filled, and total operations are meshed into a coordinated result.

The budget process can also aid management in coordinating the allocation of resources among major expenditure areas. Just as zero base budgeting is useful in making micro level decisions (selecting between specific individual expenditure alternatives) a technique known as program budgeting is useful at the macro level for coordinating the allocation of resources among programs (coordinating the allocation of resources among groups of activities which are all directed toward the same goal or end result).

Program budgeting, gained wide recognition when it was introduced into the Department of Defense in 1962 by then Secretary of Defense Robert McNamara. It was later extended by Presidential directive to all other federal agencies in 1965.

As originally developed, program budgeting was intended to serve as a management tool for the purpose of systematically and rationally identifying the costs, consequences, and trade offs among alternative programs all directed to a similar objective.[6] For example, program budgeting could be used to examine and evaluate the relative benefits and consequent trade offs of inpatient care versus ambulatory care in terms of the hospital's objective of providing the community with needed patient care. It is by design a tool which is macro in nature and whose primary value lies in aiding management to achieve, over the long run, a rational balance (coordination) in the allocation of its limited resources.

Unfortunately, program budgeting has not realized all of its hoped-for value, at least in government operations. The reasons for this short fall are open to speculation. However, the difficulties and problems appear to have centered on implementation barriers and mechanical/procedural weaknesses. Deterministic program evaluation has proven difficult, if not impossible to accomplish. Also, implementation has been hampered not only by resistance to change but also by the need to fit the system into an often nonrationale (in an economic sense) political decision process. Nevertheless, program budgeting has produced some positive accomplishments in terms of improved information and decision making. Moreover, if used in a pragmatic manner, with a careful recognition of its limitations as a tool for detailed resource allocation decisions, it can be a useful management technique for evaluating and coordinating general resource expenditure choices.

The "fit" between zero base budgeting and program budgeting is discussed further below. At this point, it should just be recognized that the two techniques or approaches to budgeting are mutually reinforcing. Program budgeting is primarily of value in making choices between general areas of expenditure. Zero base budgeting builds on these decisions by examining, within each gen-

---

[6]Like zero base budgeting, the conceptual innovation in program budgeting is a simple idea, reflecting little more than basic common sense. In its essence, program budgeting is nothing more than disciplined thinking—in broad strokes—about what it is that an institution produces or does.

Figure 15-2

Zero Base Budgeting and Program Budgeting:
Decision Process Interrelationship

Step 1

Activity (Responsibility Center)[1]	Program[1]	Program Budgeting evaluation is used to determine the relative contribution and priority of activities toward achieving a specified objective. Once relative priorities are established the next step is to determine activity priorities, both within
Activity (Responsibility Center)[n]	Program[n]	and between programs. Zero base budgeting can be used for this.

Step 2

Program[1] Activity[1]	Zero base budgeting is used to rank activities based on costs and benefits. It focuses not on what will be done, but rather, on how
Activity[n]	it will be done. Program[1], Activity[1] would be funded first in priority to Activity[2], etc. Program[2], Activity[1] would generally be funded in priority to Program[3], Activity[1]. However, if analysis shows that Program[3], Activity[1] has the greater benefit, it
Program[n] Activity[1]	would be funded in preference. In this way, a check exists to both allocate to broad priorities and then to assure that within and between priorities activities of the greatest benefit are
Activity[n]	funded.

eral area, the specific expenditure choices. As a result of these two levels of decision, resources can be allocated in a manner which produces the greatest total benefit. This decision process is illustrated in Figure 15-2. Readers interested in more information on program budgeting should refer to the references listed in the Suggested Readings section at the end of this chapter and to the Bibliography.

Controlling

A budget is, perhaps, the most critical element in a management control system. As such, it acts as both an indirect and a direct aid in the controlling of operations.

In a simplistic sense, the budget is the key component of the monitor portion of a control system.[7] A control system can be

---

[7]The following material on control systems has been based on *Quantitative Techniques for Hospital Planning and Control* by John R. Griffith. Readers interested in more information on management control systems should refer to this work, particularly Chapters 1 and 10.

defined as a set of activities or devices which maintains, in terms of previously established goals, an ongoing assessment of the achievements of a process, and which attempts to correct the process when actual achievement is different from planned (expected) performance. Its purpose is twofold:

—to provide control of a process so that results are consistent with expectations

—to generate a warning signal when control is not being achieved

Mechanically, a control system can be viewed as consisting of three basic parts:

1. *Sensor*—the reporting mechanism which identifies the actual state of the process or operation under control; the output of the sensor is a reference signal.
2. *Monitor*—the process of comparing the reference signal (actual performance) against the expectations for the operation (the budget); the output of this process is an error signal— the measure of the difference between actual performance and expectations.
3. *Controller*—the mechanism for taking corrective action aimed at the reduction in the magnitude of the error signal, if the error signal exceeds a predetermined tolerance limit.

The interrelationship of the components is illustrated in Figure 15-3.

As the figure illustrates, the budget is the "expectations" portion of the control system. The budget provides the basis for management control, for it establishes the standard (the expectation) to which actual performance must be compared in order to identify out-of-control operational processes. Obviously, more than just a budget is needed if management control is to be successful. As discussed in Chapter 18, feedback or reports identifying—to the person responsible—the status of actual performance are needed at frequent intervals. It must be recognized, however, that operational control cannot be effective unless there is a standard—the budget— against which actual performance can be measured and evaluated.

In addition to the need for feedback, if maximum management control potential is to be obtained, the budget should be constructed on the basis of organizational responsibility centers. That is, it should be constructed as a responsibility budget, identifying performance expectations in terms of the individual responsible for the management of each activity and group of activities within the hospital.

Figure 15-3

Management Control Systems

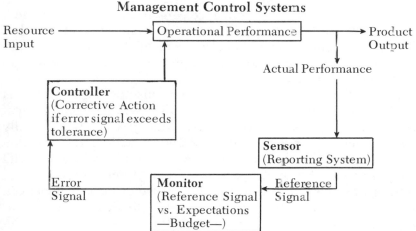

A responsibility budget, unlike either a zero base or program budget, is not an approach to resource allocation decisions. Rather, it is a way of organizing resource allocation decisions. The principle which underlies the construction of a responsibility budget is the same as that which guides the development of a chart of accounts (see Chapter 2) and which establishes the structure for cost analysis (see Chapter 5). The goal in all three cases is to categorize financial data in a manner which recognizes the hospital's organization structure and which consequently reflects the allocation of responsibility for operational performance.

The benefits of this approach to budget organization are three-fold. First, and most directly, it identifies performance expectations in terms of the person responsible for managing the operation and hence, allows any needed corrective action to be precisely directed. Second, it links the budgeting and reporting (chart of accounts and cost analysis) process by accumulating expected and actual performance data on the same basis. Finally, as is discussed below, it provides the steppingstone for motivating employees.

The budget is also an indirect aid to management in the control of operations. The indirect role which the budget plays can best be described as that of creating or adding to a sense of performance and cost consciousness. The managerial discipline and thought involved in budget preparation, together with the presence of the budget document, tend to make the entire organization think in terms of costs and to be sensitive to the relationship of current performance and actions to budget expectations. Moreover, by linking the budget preparation and performance reporting to the person accountable for the operation of a given responsibility center, the sense of performance consciousness is heightened. This is the case for not only is the entire organization captured in this sense of consciousness but also the focus of accountability and performance is directed to those individuals with the ability to guide and control actual outcomes.

A note of caution should be voiced at this point. The budget is obviously a potent tool for management's use in the controlling of operations. However, if, over the long run, its value is to be fully realized, management must use the budget with care and with a sense of empathy both for the reality of operations and the potential adverse effects of heavy handed management intervention.

To be effective, the budget must be viewed by management as an indicator of the relationship between expected and actual performance—not as a disciplinary mechanism or as an arbitrary whipping post. If management fails to use the budget with caution and sensitivity not only will its management benefits be negated but also, and more importantly, the budget will act to produce counter productive operational results. An improperly administered budget will result in an organization focusing on "beating" the budget—both in its preparation and actual performance phases—as opposed to meeting its responsibilities to the community.

Motivating

The budget and budget process present management with the opportunity to apply both positive and negative employee motivational stimuli. Certainly, as the previous discussion has illustrated, the role of the budget in controlling operations also involves motivational implications. For the most part, the stimuli produced by the control functions of the budget are negative: incorporating either real or imagined incentives to not exceed the budget. The strength of these negative stimuli should not be underestimated. It is because of their existence that management must, as emphasized above, administer the budget with a sense of caution and humility.

The budget process provides the opportunity for applying positive motivational stimuli. In fact, the budget process represents, perhaps, the simplest and easiest vehicle for implementing a program of management by objectives.

A responsibility budget is fundamentally nothing more than a statement of a performance goal expressed in dollars for a particular responsibility center and individual. The goal setting can be done jointly by the subordinate and his supervisor. The subordinate can prepare the budget, discuss it with his supervisor, and reach agreement with his supervisor as to its feasibility and his own commitment to achieve it. Under these conditions the subordinate has a considerable amount of motivation and pressure to perform in accordance with his own goals and commitments.

It should be emphasized that positive motivation is achieved by allowing subordinates to participate in the budget decision making process. The person who is going to be responsible and accountable for performance must be allowed to be involved in making the decisions and setting the goals by which his performance will be measured. It is only through this level of involvement that the subordinate will be both committed and motivated to perform in accord with the budget plan. If such involvement is not fostered, the value of the budget in motivating employees, and also to a large extent the usefulness of the budget in controlling operations, is substantially negated.

Budget Prerequisites

It should be clear, from the perspective of operational performance, why every hospital must have a budget. However, before a hospital can begin to prepare its budget, several internal operational prerequisites must be met and certain management policy decisions regarding the exact character of the budget must be made.

The operational prerequisites for budgeting are similar to those set out in Chapter 5 for cost analysis. Budget preparation, in common with cost analysis, requires:

1. A well designed organization structure which eliminates overlapping responsibility and clearly defines all accountabilities
2. A chart of accounts which both corresponds to the organization structure and allows for the accumulation of actual cost data by cost and responsibility center
3. An accurate accounting system capable of accumulating and appropriately assigning all financial data
4. A comprehensive management information system capable of collecting nonfinancial data relative to total volume of services demanded and cost center workloads

In addition to these similar prerequisites, budgeting requires several more, because it is both a time series process and a pro-

cess which should actively involve the entire management structure of the organization. Specifically these are:

1. Historical and current actual performance data for use in
   projecting future volumes and costs
2. A formal feedback reporting mechanism
3. A high level of management staff capability and sophistication

Historical and actual performance data are necessary for purposes of establishing the basis for projecting future workloads and
cost behavior. Generally, unless some phenomena are involved
which act to alter the historical relationships which characterize
the operations of any given environment, the best estimates of the
future are past performance and past performance trends. The
budget by its definition as a plan is future oriented. Thus, its
usefulness is heavily dependent on accurate estimates of the future. To attain these estimates with any degree of confidence historical data are a necessity.

A formal feedback reporting mechanism is also a prerequisite
condition for effective budget operation. The role of reporting in
the generic context of management control systems was discussed
above. In the specific case of budget operations the role of reporting is critical, for it is the "linking pin" between expectations (the
budget) and reality (actual performance).

Formal, detailed reports, incorporating responsibility reporting
and reflecting variances from originally budgeted activity should
generally be prepared, unless circumstances require increased
frequency, on a monthly basis. These reports should be provided
to all responsibility center managers. The level of detail provided
should be tailored to the level of management; with increasing
levels of supervision being given summary reports, unless they
request more detail. Management reporting, reporting procedures,
and report analysis are discussed in detail in Chapter 18.

The final prerequisite of staff capability is, perhaps, the most
important element in the successful preparation and use of a budget. As emphasized earlier, effective use of a budget requires that
management appreciate the subtleties of motivating employees
and maintain an empathy for the reality of day-to-day operations.
Only a sophisticated management team has the sensitivity necessary not only to avoid the potential pitfalls of budget use but also
to capitalize on the opportunities presented by both the budget
process and the resulting budget document. Without this sensitivity, the budget instead of being a productive tool may become just
a useless or even counter-productive paper exercise.

It is critical to recognize that while organization structures, data, procedures, and so forth are all necessary to effective budgeting, they are all of secondary importance when compared to capable management. Budgeting is fundamentally a people moving, as opposed to a paper moving, process. If it is to be successful, all levels of management must understand the value of budgeting, its limitations, how the budget is to be developed and used, and must understand their own specific roles and responsibilities. These latter items will be discussed in the following chapter. At this juncture, it is sufficient merely to appreciate the pivotal role which capable management plays in successful budget preparation and use.

Policy Decisions

In addition to assuring that the internal mechanics and management capabilities necessary for efficient budget preparation and effective budget use exists, management must also make a series of budget policy decisions, before undertaking actual budget preparation. These decisions are prerequisites to actual budget preparation, for they are the judgments which act to define the specific character of the budget. In broad terms, management, in addition to determining the basic structural design of the budget, must decide whether the budget is to be:

1. Comprehensive or limited in scope
2. Focused on only a fixed volume/workload estimate or be capable of accomodating varying levels of workload
3. A discrete or continuous process

Each of these major areas of management policy decisions is discussed below.

Structural Design. As is the case in architecture, the structural design decision is a fundamental choice in terms of determining the final shape and ultimate usefulness of the budget. Essentially, the design decision is composed of two parts. Whether the designer is an artist or a manager, he must determine:

—How to organize the materials, resources at his disposal. (In the case of designing a home, is it to be a colonial or a split-level? In the case of the budget, is it to be organized on the basis of discrete activities or programs?)
—How to put together, within the established organization, the various components involved. (In the case of a home, is it prefabricated or built on site? In the case of a budget, does

one adopt an incremental or a zero base approach to determining the allowable expenditure level of various responsibility centers?)

With respect to budget organization, management is confronted with the need to make both macro and micro level policy decisions. At the micro level, it must be decided how costs are to be grouped. Costs can be grouped on the basis of line items (natural cost accounts, such as salaries, medical supplies, drugs, laboratory supplies, travel, consulting fees) and/or on the basis of organizational work units. Also, within organizational work units, costs can be grouped on the basis of cost centers or on the basis of both cost and responsibility centers.

The need for some form of cost grouping should be clear. The magnitude of a hospital's budget operation is such that if all appropriation requests were treated in a disparate manner it would be difficult, if not impossible, for management either to obtain a realistic picture of the total operation or control ongoing operations. Hence, the question to be resolved is not the need for grouping but the method of grouping.

If costs are grouped on the basis of line items only, management can identify and control total hospital expenditures. It cannot, however, either identify or control cost and/or the result of the performance of a specific function, i.e., performance relative to the agreed upon objectives of any particular work unit. Therefore, in addition to grouping on the basis of natural account, management must design the budget so that costs are also categorized by work unit.

The basic work unit is a cost center. When cost and responsibility centers are synonomous, grouping on the basis of cost centers and natural accounts provides management with the information necessary both to clearly visualize and understand hospital-wide expenditure patterns and to control work unit and total hospital cost and performance. However, when cost and responsibility centers are not synonymous (which is the case more often than not) then, in addition to cost center grouping, responsibility center grouping is necessary. That is, the natural costs of the various involved cost centers must be grouped to show both total natural costs and the total costs of the responsibility center.

The importance of grouping costs on the basis of responsibility centers cannot be overemphasized. As the earlier discussion under "Management Tools" emphasized, organizing the budget such that it reflects the management allocation of responsibility for operational performance is essential if the control potential of the budget is to be realized. The only way the budget can be organized to accomplish this is to group costs on the basis of responsibility centers.

At the macro level, management is confronted with a similar problem. The question in this instance centers on how responsibility centers should be grouped or organized. Should they be grouped on an activity/department basis or should they be grouped by program area? The solution of choice is to organize ultimately along program area lines.

If the budget organization is limited only to an activity or departmental orientation, it is difficult for management to evaluate the scope and direction of the total hospital's planned activities in respect to either coordination of effort or conformance to stated policy objectives. Organizing the budget on a program basis, however, enables management to accomplish both these evaluative functions readily. Hence, in terms of organization, the structural design of the budget can be described as a program budget organized at the micro level by line item and responsibility center—with responsibility centers then grouped into programs at the macro level.

Management's choices are relatively limited in terms of how to put the budget together. Essentially the budget can be constructed either on a piecemeal basis wherein projects are reviewed and funded on their intrinsic merit with only passing regard to corporate direction and the merits of other projects, or on a wholistic (i.e., total entity) basis. Obviously the wholistic approach is the alternative of choice, because projects are viewed within the framework of program priorities and relative cost/benefit analysis. Also, the wholistic approach allows for resource allocation decisions to be made in a manner which increases the probability of the total benefit to the community being maximized (as opposed to the random probability of the piecemeal approach). The tools for implementing the wholistic approach, program and zero base budgeting, were discussed earlier.

As indicated, program budgeting is a tool whose primary value lies in aiding management to achieve, over the long run, a rational balance in the allocation of its resources. If used in a pragmatic manner—without overemphasis on requiring that all processes in the hospital, including those whose value is primarily subjective, be deterministically quantified—and with a careful understanding of its limitations as a tool for detailed resource allocation decisions, program budgeting can be a useful technique for evaluating and coordinating large resource expenditure choices.

Program budgeting is of little help to management in determining the allocation of resources within, as opposed to between, any given program areas. Because of this limitation, management must use another technique for determining allowable expenditure levels for their responsibility centers within each program areas.

Figure 15-4

Budget Design Decision Interrelationships

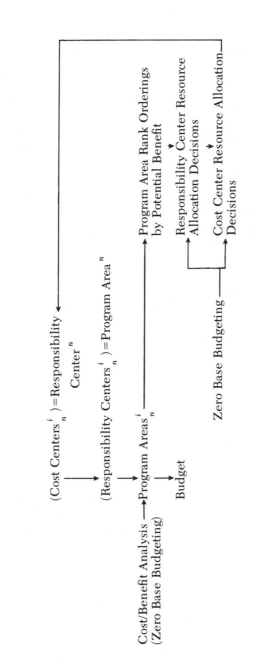

Typically, an incremental approach is used to resolve this problem. The weakness of this approach is apparent. The requirement that only the incremental expenditure request be evaluated and justified ignores the opportunity to evaluate all proposed expenditures and make the trade offs which will result in the greatest total benefit being achieved. To capitalize on this opportunity, a zero base approach to budget construction must be adopted.

In considering zero base budgeting the reader should bear in mind that, like program budgeting, it must be used in a pragmatic manner. Zero base budgeting was not designed primarily for a health services management application. Therefore, a too rigorous application of the principles requiring the presentation of alternatives for either services such as the emergency room and the general surgery operating rooms, where the possibility of implementing the alternatives is unlikely; or functions where the interchange of resources is impossible—will result in only unproductive and needless work and a loss of confidence and support of the staff for the budget program. If used pragmatically, however, it will provide management with a workable mechanism for evaluating alternative expenditure opportunities and selecting those which, in sum, produce the greatest total benefit.

Zero base budgeting also provides a tool which both complements and acts as a check and balance on program budgeting. It is important to recognize this relationship and the fact that all of the above design decisions build upon one another and are mutually supportive. Cost centers aggregate into responsibility centers which in turn aggregate into program areas.

Similarly, program budgeting is fundamentally a macro level application of the principles of zero base budgeting: the evaluation of the relative benefits of program areas as opposed to projects or specific activities. Zero base budgeting not only complements program budgeting by acting as a check or review mechanism on the priorities which have been determined, but also plays an independent part. That is, zero base budgeting is the basic tool for obtaining the specific expenditures which are to be undertaken within each responsibility center.

The relationship of the various design decisions is illustrated in Figure 15-4.

Comprehensive or Limited Scope. A comprehensive budget can be defined as a budget system wherein all planned capital and operating costs and all anticipated revenues are projected and then incorporated into a single, integrated budget document. In contrast, a limited scope budget is a budget system which includes only a particular element (or elements) of the total budget process. A limited scope budget, for example, may be a salary budget only—ignoring the other component costs of an expense budget—or it may be an expense and revenue budget, ignoring projected capital expenditures.

From the perspective of management efficacy it should be clear that a comprehensive budget is the budget system of choice. It is only through a comprehensive budget, wherein all phases of the hospital's production, physical, and financial operations are examined and planned that the full operational value and management usefulness of the budget and budgeting process can be realized.

Though the method of choice is clear (a comprehensive budget), recognition must be given to the problems inherent in the management of change when implementing a comprehensive budget system. In some hospitals, movement from a position of either no budget or a minimal budget to a comprehensive budget may well create too much organizational trauma to be accomplished effectively in one step. In such instances, a limited scope budget can play an important role as an evolutionary measure, providing management with the opportunity to control and spread the dislocation effect, intrinsic in any change, over a larger period of time. Whether such an evolutionary approach is necessary will depend on the history and current status of the organization and the skills and capacity of its management and supervisory personnel. In relatively weak organizations, and/or organizations which have just completed or are in the process of implementing other major change activities, an evolutionary approach may well represent the most desirable and pragmatic way of achieving an effective comprehensive budget system. In each instance, however, management must evaluate its own situation and accordingly design an implementation plan.

Fixed or Flexible. As its name implies, a fixed budget is one which is developed on the basis of a single estimate of expected workload or volume. Management, after considering past levels of workload, demographic factors, and changes in the hospital's range of services can estimate either a range of expected workloads or a single level of volume. If only a single volume estimate is made or if only a single volume estimate is used in preparing the budget, the resulting budget is said to be "fixed." To the extent that the single workload estimate is correct, a fixed budget is both an accurate budget and a highly reliable management tool. Even if projected and actual volumes differ, to the extent that a hospital's costs are fixed, i.e., do not directly vary with changes in workload, a fixed budget can be a reliable management tool.

Unfortunately, it is unusual in either a hospital or any other type of enterprise to find an operating situation which is so highly static that estimates of demand can be routinely made with perfect precision. Moreover, hospital costs are not entirely fixed. While no completely definitive data are available, it is generally agreed that over the near and long term as much as fifty to sixty percent of operating costs may be subject to variation. (The degree of short run variability may be quite limited—over a period of a month or several months only ten to twenty percent of total costs may either vary proportionately with volume or be susceptible to management efforts to vary with volume.) Given this kind of operating environment, a fixed budget, while of value, has certain implicit limitations. To correct for these limitations, a tool known as a "flexible budget" is available.

A flexible budget can be defined as a statement of expected financial performance which can be adjusted to reflect the efforts of operating at different levels of volume. Essentially, a flexible budget is a series of fixed budgets covering a specified range of volume alternatives. The size of the relevant range of alternatives will differ with each particular situation. However, as a rule of thumb, the accuracy of workload estimates for most hospitals should be within five to ten percent. Therefore, the range of a flexible budget should be no more than ten to twenty percent.

Also within the relevant range, budget alternatives should be developed only to reflect those changes in volume which will materially affect the budget. That is, if a one percent change in workload will neither significantly change unit cost nor materially influence the way management would plan or make decisions, then it is not necessary to prepare an alternative budget for each one percent change in volume. Typically, the traditional literature uses a five percent change in workload as the incremental volume change sufficient to justify the development of an alternative budget. However, the principle of a five percent volume change should not be taken as an absolute rule. The level of incremental change which should signal the need for an alternative budget varies in operating reality with each situation (production function) and must be determined for each hospital on the basis of an individual analysis and understanding of its cost behavior.

In theory, management must first analyze the cost structure of each department and identify: those costs which (over the budget period), regardless of volume, remain constant (fixed costs); those which remain constant relative to day-to-day volume but which can vary due to management decisions such as the opening or closing of a wing or nursing station (semifixed costs); those costs which vary on less than a proportional basis with volume (semi-variable costs); and those costs which vary directly with volume (variable costs). Given this analysis, management must then determine whether and to what extent the four categories of cost will change with various changes in volume. This analysis could begin by determining the minimum level of volume which could be expected with a high degree of confidence and then proceed to the maximum volume that could be expected reasonably. Based on this analysis, management can both identify the incremental volume levels requiring alternative budgets and determine the relative degree of cost variability from one level to the next.

The theoretical approach though accurate is cumbersome. Therefore, as an alternative, historical data can be reviewed and analyzed to determine at which levels of volume unit cost markedly changed, and to establish the relative amount of fixed and variable costs. Given these data, management can then identify the volume levels requiring alternative budgets.

Clearly, a flexible budget is the approach of choice. It provides a more valid and reliable internal management tool and is more defensible in terms of rate review, prospective payment, and external price control negotiations. A flexible budget, however, requires a degree of sophistication, knowledge, and skill which a hospital just beginning a comprehensive budgeting program may not possess. In such instances, an evolutionary approach, relying on a fixed budget and volume variance analysis, may be a more prudent choice.[8] As was the case earlier, in each instance, management must evaluate its own situation and design an implementation plan accordingly.

---

[8]Variance analysis is a technique for evaluating differences between actual and planned performance. Briefly, volume variance analysis is a device for identifying how much of a total variance is due to the difference between planned and actual volume. The calculation using assumed data can be illustrated as follows:

Budget = $10,000
Projected Volume = 5,000 units
Cost/Unit = $2/unit
Actual Cost = $12,000
Actual Volume = 5,500 units

(Actual Volume) − (Budget Volume) × Budget Unit Cost = Volume Variance
    5,500   −   5,000   × $2   = $1,000

Based on the above example, of the total variance of $2,000 ($12,000 − $10,000); $1,000 is due to an increase in volume. Therefore, presumably if unit costs do not decrease with volume, only $1,000 is due to increased supply prices or productive inefficiencies.

Continuous or Discrete. In addition to the foregoing, management must determine if it wants a continuous (rolling) or a discrete (periodic) budget. A discrete or periodic budget is one which is prepared at one point in time and applies to a fixed future period. Usually a periodic budget is a budget which is prepared annually and which encompasses in its projection a twelve-month time period. In contrast, a continuous budget is one which is updated routinely so that at almost any point in time the hospital is operating under a twelve-month plan. Typically a continuous budget is updated on a quarterly basis, i.e., as a quarter ends the remaining three quarters of the budget year are reviewed and, if necessary, revised and another quarter is added. However, a monthly updating cycle can also be used if the operating environment warrants budget review and revision on a greater frequency.

A continuous budget is the method of choice. Although in an absolute sense a continuous budget may require a bit more work, it:

—allows for a more even spreading of the budget workload;
—provides for the ongoing maintenance of a full twelve-month operating plan; and, most importantly;
—replaces the crisis environment that typically surrounds the budget preparation with an ongoing process which integrates budget preparation into routine general operations.

It should be recognized, however, that continuous budgeting involves both a high degree of familiarity with the process and mechanics of budgeting and a sophisticated management team. As was the case with other policy decisions, an evolutionary approach—beginning with a periodic budget and then proceeding to a continuous budget—may be the more pragmatic and effective decision. Again, management must make its decision based on the specific, unique operating situation.

As a related issue, management must also determine the period to be covered by the budget. The above discussion presumed a twelve-month budget period, for a twelve-month period is the generally accepted convention. A twelve-month period may not, however, be appropriate to all instances.

Probably the best answer, however inconclusive, to the question of how long the budget period should be is: long enough—but not too long. That is, presuming there are no statutory requirements, the budget period should cover a time span sufficient in length to allow for effective planning. Operationally, this means that it should be long enough to:

—discount for unusual short-term variations in demand and/or the nature of the operating environment; and

—take into account events in the future whose outcome will affect current decisions—extend to the planning horizon or that point in the future wherein additional information will not affect current decisions.

This last point is a key concept, for it acts to place a single period's budget preparation effort into a larger and longer term context and to emphasize the need for not only a current operating budget but also for a long-range plan.

Simply, if management is to be able to make sound decisions, it must weigh and evaluate those decisions against future needs in a prudent manner. Also, if management is to achieve the hospital's longer term goals successfully, it may have to begin to make preparations and take the initial steps toward those goals in the current period. Both these circumstances or requirements make clear the need for a long-range plan which can be used as a benchmark and an indicator of future direction.[9]

Such a plan need not be overly detailed. In fact, do to the difficulties and uncertainties of multi-year projections, the method of choice generally is a macro level approach, which identifies in broad terms the goals to be achieved and, in gross terms, the financial requirements associated with those goals.

Given the availability and use of a long range plan, the question of the period to be covered by the budget becomes somewhat of a moot point. A twelve-month period, synchronized with the hospital's fiscal year and set within the context of an overall longer range plan, generally should be an acceptable and workable period.

Conclusion

The foregoing discussion has attempted to define the nature and value of a budget and to identify the operational prerequisites and management policy decisions which must precede the effective preparation and use of a budget. The next step is actually to prepare a budget. To accomplish this step, one additional prerequisite is necessary. Management must select and implement a budget get preparation process, procedure, and organization. Chapters 16 and 17 address this last prerequisite.

---

[9]The development of a long range plan, aside from its financial implications, is an essential element of prudent management. Such a plan should be coordinated and consistent with the total communitywide health facilities and services plan, and should be reviewed, and ideally approved, by the local planning agency.

Suggested Readings

American Hospital Association. *Budgeting Procedures for Hospitals,* Chapters 1 and 2.

Brookings Institution. *Setting National Priorities: The 1977 Budget.*

Griffith, John R. *Quantitative Techniques for Hospital Planning and Control,* Chapter 1.

Hauser, Richard. "How to Build and Use a Flexible Budget," *Financial Management,* August 1974.

Hospital Financial Management Association. *Planning the Hospital's Financial Operations.*

Macleod, Roderick K. "Program Budgeting Works in Nonprofit Institutions." *Harvard Business Review,* September–October 1971.

Novick, David. *Program Budgeting.*

Pyhrr, Peter A. *Zero Base Budgeting.*

Silvers J.B. and Prahalad, C.K. *Financial Management of Health Institutions,* Chapters 4, 5, and 6.

Appendix 15-A

Example
Zero Base Budgeting Manual
State of Georgia

State of Georgia
Office of Planning and Budget

GENERAL BUDGET
PREPARATION PROCEDURES

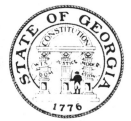

GEORGE BUSBEE
Governor

GENERAL BUDGET
PREPARATION PROCEDURES

FISCAL YEAR 1977 BUDGET DEVELOPMENT

Reproduced by courtesy of Governor George Busbee and the Executive Department of the State of Georgia.

F. Y. 1977 ZERO-BASE BUDGET

Procedures and Instructions

TABLE OF CONTENTS*

*Note: The following material has been excerpted from the complete budget preparation manual. As a result not all of the pages have been reproduced in this text. The complete table of contents is provided to give the reader a "feeling" for the scope of the total procedure manual.

ZERO·BASE BUDGET Procedures & Instructions

EXECUTIVE DEPARTMENT	
OFFICE OF PLANNING AND BUDGET – Budget Division	
SECTION	
F. Y. 1977 ZERO-BASE BUDGET INFORMATION	
SUBJECT	
A. BUDGET ACT PROVISIONS, B. CONCEPT AND PURPOSE, C. SIGNIFICANT MODIFICATIONS, D. SUBMISSION DATA	

A.   Budget Act Provisions

Code Section 40-4 of Georgia Laws (Budget Act) provides for estimates of financial needs to be submitted to the Office of Planning and Budget (OPB) each year by the Head of each Budget Unit by September 1.

The Budget Division of OPB has developed the Budget Procedures for the estimation of F. Y. 1977 financial requirements by State Departments of Georgia State Government.

A lot of work has gone into the revision of forms and procedures for the F. Y. 1977 Zero-Base process. The Governor feels that the changes will be useful to the Department as well as to OPB. No standard set of forms can be devised which will meet everyone's needs. OPB is prepared to review any form changes necessary.

B.   Concept and Purpose

The State of Georgia finds its budgeting responsibilities and needs best met by the budgetary process known as "Zero-Base Budgeting."

The concept of Zero-Base Budgeting is that all the financial requirements for a budget unit are justified and analyzed by decision makers and not just the increased or additional requirements. Managers are to assess benefits from ongoing operations, as well as needs for additional funds. The process identifies, to all levels of management, the cost, benefits and suggested operational improvements associated to reach their objectives. The objectives, as established by management, are communicated to the functional managers before the preparation of the budget begins.

The Zero-Base Budget process begins by identifying functions in the organization where cost data are maintained. The budget request for each function is developed in a series of "Decision Packages." Each Decision Package represents the fund requirement to support particular levels of the operations. The first package of a series of packages is developed at a Minimum Level of operations for the function. Additional levels of effort are Base Level, Workload, and New or Improved. See instructions for definitions of these levels.

The ranking of Decision Packages is completed by each Activity Manager and submitted to higher management. The final ranking is completed at the Department level. The ranking process offers each manager the opportunity to express service priorities at different funding levels. Refinements and modifications to the system are made from time to time, but the basic concept and purpose of Zero-Base remains intact.

C.   Significant Modifications

Significant modifications have been made to the Zero-Base Budget Preparation System. The more significant changes are as follows:

— 1.   Previously, one form was designed for use as a Decision Package. The levels of effort for each function were determined by each agency and the same basic form was used for each level of effort. The Zero-Base System as modified for this year defines each level of effort through the design of four (4) kinds of Decision Packages -- Minimum Level Decision Package, Base Level Decision Package, Workload Decision Package, and New or Improved Decision Package. Definitions of each are included in the instructions for the use of the forms.

— 2.   Functions, organizational cost units within an Activity, were previously defined exclusively by each agency. This year, OPB will request that each agency submit a list of functions at which a series of decision packages will be developed. The list will be reviewed and approved by OPB in order that planning and budget analysis can begin at an earlier date. Many budget functions in State Government have been defined as units much too large or much too small in the past. Our cooperative efforts in defining function units will be beneficial to both OPB and the Departments in insuring reasonable budget levels.

DATE Rev. 6/75	PAGE ¹	OPB · Budget · General

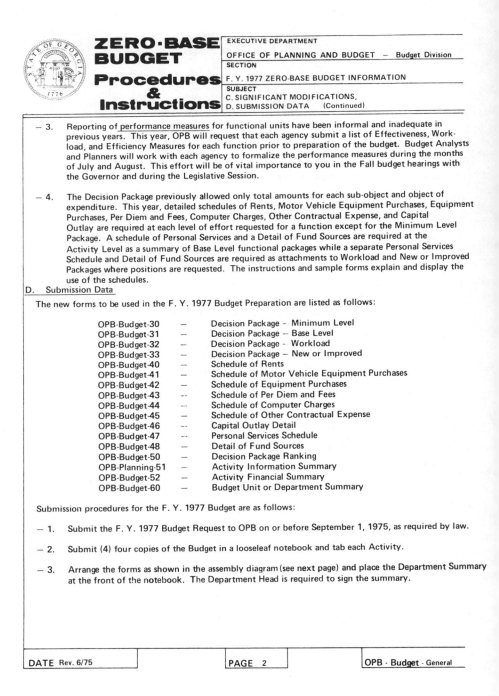

ZERO·BASE BUDGET Procedures & Instructions

EXECUTIVE DEPARTMENT	
OFFICE OF PLANNING AND BUDGET — Budget Division	
SECTION	
F. Y. 1977 ZERO-BASE BUDGET INFORMATION	
SUBJECT	
C. SIGNIFICANT MODIFICATIONS,	
D. SUBMISSION DATA (Continued)	

— 3.   Reporting of performance measures for functional units have been informal and inadequate in previous years. This year, OPB will request that each agency submit a list of Effectiveness, Workload, and Efficiency Measures for each function prior to preparation of the budget. Budget Analysts and Planners will work with each agency to formalize the performance measures during the months of July and August. This effort will be of vital importance to you in the Fall budget hearings with the Governor and during the Legislative Session.

— 4.   The Decision Package previously allowed only total amounts for each sub-object and object of expenditure. This year, detailed schedules of Rents, Motor Vehicle Equipment Purchases, Equipment Purchases, Per Diem and Fees, Computer Charges, Other Contractual Expense, and Capital Outlay are required at each level of effort requested for a function except for the Minimum Level Package. A schedule of Personal Services and a Detail of Fund Sources are required at the Activity Level as a summary of Base Level functional packages while a separate Personal Services Schedule and Detail of Fund Sources are required as attachments to Workload and New or Improved Packages where positions are requested. The instructions and sample forms explain and display the use of the schedules.

D.   Submission Data

The new forms to be used in the F. Y. 1977 Budget Preparation are listed as follows:

OPB-Budget-30	—	Decision Package – Minimum Level
OPB-Budget-31	—	Decision Package – Base Level
OPB-Budget-32	—	Decision Package – Workload
OPB-Budget-33	—	Decision Package – New or Improved
OPB-Budget-40	—	Schedule of Rents
OPB-Budget-41	—	Schedule of Motor Vehicle Equipment Purchases
OPB-Budget-42	—	Schedule of Equipment Purchases
OPB-Budget-43	--	Schedule of Per Diem and Fees
OPB-Budget-44	--	Schedule of Computer Charges
OPB-Budget-45	—	Schedule of Other Contractual Expense
OPB-Budget-46	--	Capital Outlay Detail
OPB-Budget-47	--	Personal Services Schedule
OPB-Budget-48	—	Detail of Fund Sources
OPB-Budget-50	—	Decision Package Ranking
OPB-Planning-51	—	Activity Information Summary
OPB-Budget-52	—	Activity Financial Summary
OPB-Budget-60	—	Budget Unit or Department Summary

Submission procedures for the F. Y. 1977 Budget are as follows:

— 1.   Submit the F. Y. 1977 Budget Request to OPB on or before September 1, 1975, as required by law.

— 2.   Submit (4) four copies of the Budget in a looseleaf notebook and tab each Activity.

— 3.   Arrange the forms as shown in the assembly diagram (see next page) and place the Department Summary at the front of the notebook. The Department Head is required to sign the summary.

DATE Rev. 6/75	PAGE 2	OPB - Budget - General

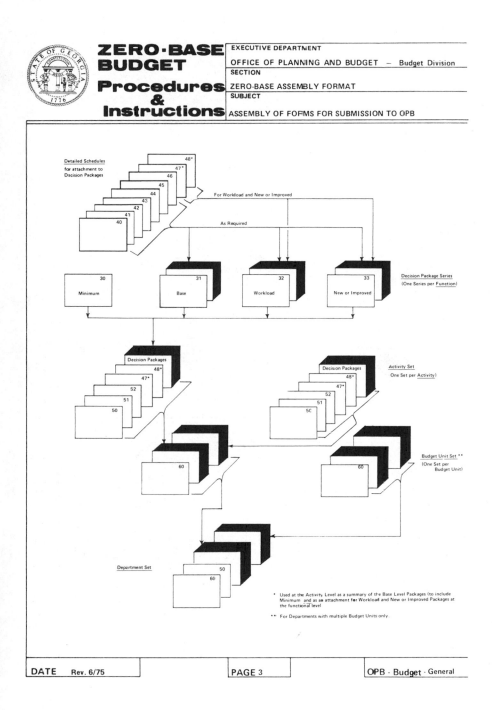

DECISION PACKAGE — MINIMUM LEVEL

OPB-BUDGET-30

OPB- Budget -30
(Rev. 6-75)

F. Y. 1977

ZERO-BASE BUDGET REQUEST
DECISION PACKAGE — MINIMUM LEVEL

Human Resources   Community Injury Control   Emergency Medical Health

Department   Activity   Function

	Function F.Y.76	This Pkg. F.Y. 77	Cum%
Describe the Function in terms of its objective County and City Medical Centers are charged to meet emergency situations such as sudden illness, injury, natural or man-made disasters, and poison cases. The centers do not coordinate their efforts across county and city lines nor do they have exposure to the latest techniques and equipment in the emergency medical field. Some centers are highly successful due to a special innovation that other centers do not share.	Positions This Package ___2___		
	A. TOTAL PERSONAL SERVICES	25,624	17,686	69
	1. Motor Vehicle Expenses and Repairs	900	600	
	2. Supplies and Materials	1,900	1,200	
	3. Repairs and Maintenance	500	300	
	4. Communications	400	280	
Describe the Function in terms of service provided in F. Y. 1976 Utilize a central staff to conduct medical emergency courses around the State to monitor the operations of the Injury Control Program. The courses will provide instruction to the centers on the latest medical emergency techniques and methods. The Base Level provides service for the 100 most populated counties by conducting one medical emergency course at each.	5. Power, Water, Natural Gas	250	200	
	6. Rents	273	273	
	7. Insurance and Bonding			
	8. Workmen's Comp. and Indemnities			
	9. Direct Benefits			
	10. Tuition and Scholarships			
Explain the Minimum Level of Service this Package provides Two positions and expenses to coordinate, develop, and conduct a medical emergency course in the 75 largest medical centers in the State. Two persons are required to conduct a course in each center and two persons can cover 75 medical centers annually.	11. Grants to Counties or Cities			
	12. Assessments by Merit System	132	88	
	13. Other Operating Expenses	450	206	
	14. Extraordinary Expenses			
	B.REG. OPERATING EXPENSES(Add 1-14)	4,805	3,147	65
	C. TRAVEL	800	550	69
	D. MOTOR VEHICLE EQUIP. PURCH.	4,680		
Explain the Impact of terminating the Service now provided that this Minimum Level Excludes	E. PUBLICATIONS AND PRINTING	1,350	1,000	74
One position and related expenses are deleted in the minimum level package. Approximately 25 medical centers will not have a medical emergency course in F.Y. 1977 that did have one in F.Y. 1976. Each excluded center would have to develop its own medical emergency plan. Some excluded centers would not choose to do so and an emergency situation in the area served by the center would not be met with the same efficiency as before.	F. EQUIPMENT PURCHASES	750		
	G. PER DIEM AND FEES	2,000	1,500	75
	H. COMPUTER CHARGES	2,900	2,000	69
	I. OTHER CONTRACTUAL EXPENSE	1,600	550	34
	J. AUTHORITY LEASE RENTALS			

Quantitative Measures (Effectiveness, Workload, Efficiency)	F. Y. 1976 Function	F. Y. 1977 Minimum Level				
			K. GENERAL OBLIGATION BONDS			
			L. CAPITAL OUTLAY			
Different Medical Centers Aided	100	75	M. LIST OTHER OBJECTS:			
Medical Emergency Courses conducted	100	75				
Cost Per Course/Total funds	$445	$352				
Cost Per Course/State funds	$245	$165	TOTAL EXPENDITURES (Add A-M)	44,509	26,433	59
			FEDERAL FUNDS	16,000	10,000	63
			OTHER FUNDS	4,000	4,000	100
			STATE GENERAL FUNDS	24,509	12,433	51

Package Name: Emergency Medical Health   Package 1 of 4

Prepared By: John Smith   Activity Rank 4

ZERO·BASE BUDGET Procedures & Instructions

	EXECUTIVE DEPARTMENT
	OFFICE OF PLANNING AND BUDGET — Budget Division
	SECTION
	DECISION PACKAGE PREPARATION – MINIMUM LEVEL
	SUBJECT
	INSTRUCTIONS FOR FORM OPB-BUDGET- 30

Form Purpose

A Decision Package Series identifies a function below the Activity Level where costs are recorded. You should generate a package or series of packages at the functional level approved by O. P. B. Each function you want to continue should have one or more Decision Packages, depending on how many levels of funding are requested for the function. The form OPB-Budget-30 is a Minimum Level Decision Package. For every function you will develop at least one minimum level below the F. Y. 1976 Budget for that function. The Minimum Level is a level of effort, expressed in terms of service and cost, below which it is not realistic or feasible to operate the function at all. For example, the Minimum Level in the sample shows two positions for conducting courses since one person could not efficiently conduct the particular coursework involved.

1. **Describe the Function in Terms of its Objective**

   — Explain the function by describing the need for the existence of the function in terms of a problem area or target group the function serves. The decision will be whether to fund the minimum level or not to fund the function at all.

2. **Describe the Function in Terms of Service Provided in F. Y. 1976**

   — Outline and explain the service provided by the function during F. Y. 1976. The service outlined should be explained in terms of solving the problem outlined in the objectives box. All services provided by the function in F. Y. 1976 should be outlined.

3. **Explain the Minimum Level of Service This Package Provides**

   — The Minimum Level Package represents a level of service below the level of service provided in F. Y. 1976 by the function. Explain the service provided by this level of effort in terms of which services can be provided at the minimum level.

4. **Explain the Impact of Terminating the Service Now Provided That This Minimum Level Excludes**

   — Outline and explain the services provided in F. Y. 1976 that the Minimum Level does not provide for. Item 3 and 4 together should total to Item 2 in terms of service provided.

Quantitative Measures (Quantitative Measures are required on the Decision Packages)

— Effectiveness data measures how well the services provided solve the problem and meet the objectives of the function both for F. Y. 1976 and for the Minimum Leve for F. Y. 1977.
— Workload data measures the effort required to deliver the services both for F. Y. 1976 and for the Minimum Level for F. Y. 1977.
— Efficiency data measures the cost per unit of workload both for F. Y. 1976 and for the Minimum Level for F. Y. 1977.

Financial Information

— Enter amounts budgeted for the function in F. Y. 1976
— Enter amounts requested for the Minimum Level under "This Pkg. F. Y. 1977".
— The Cum % is calculated by dividing the "This Pkg. F. Y. 1977" amount by the "Function F. Y. 1976" amount. Do not show Cum % for sub-classes of expenditure.

NOTE: Detailed forms 40-48 are not required on the Minimum Level Package.

DATE Rev. 6/75	PAGE 5	OPB - Budget - 30

DECISION PACKAGE — BASE LEVEL

OPB-BUDGET-31

OPB- Budget- 31
(Rev. 6-75)

F. Y. 1977

ZERO-BASE BUDGET REQUEST
DECISION PACKAGE — BASE LEVEL

Human Resources	Community Injury Control	Emergency Medical Health
Department	Activity	Function

	Positions This Package ___1___ **	Function F.Y.76	This Pkg. F.Y. 77	Cum%
Describe the Function in terms of its objective County and City Medical Centers are charged to meet emergency situations such as sudden illness, injury, natural or man-made disasters, and poison cases. The centers do not coordinate their efforts across county and city lines nor do they have exposure to the latest techniques and equipment in the emergency medical field. Some centers are highly successful due to a special innovation that other centers do not share.	A. TOTAL PERSONAL SERVICES	25,624	9,276	105
	1. Motor Vehicle Expenses and Repairs	900	326	
	2. Supplies and Materials	1,900	700	
	3. Repairs and Maintenance	500	200	
	4. Communications	400	176	
	5. Power, Water, Natural Gas	250	98	
	6. Rents *	273	77	
Describe the Function in terms of service provided in F. Y. 1976 (Base Level) Utilize a central staff to conduct medical emergency courses around the State to monitor the operations of the Injury Control Program. The courses will provide instruction to the centers on the latest medical emergency techniques and methods. The Base Level provides service for the 100 most populated counties by conducting one medical emergency course at each.	7. Insurance and Bonding			
	8. Workmen's Comp. and Indemnities			
	9. Direct Benefits			
	10. Tuition and Scholarships			
	11. Grants to Counties or Cities			
	12. Assessments by Merit System	132	44	
	13. Other Operating Expenses	450	244	
Explain the Cost Increase or Decrease in the Base Level over F. Y. 1976 Personal Services — Within-grade increases and annualization of a part-year position. Regular Operating Expenses — Primarily due to rental contract increase for office space. Travel — Increase in rate from 10 cents to 12 cents per mile. M. V. Equipment Purchases — Replacement vehicle. Equipment Purchases — 3 pocket calculators in addition to replacement of office equipment.	14. Extraordinary Expenses			
	B.REG. OPERATING EXPENSES(Add 1-14)	4,805	1,865	104
	C. TRAVEL	800	350	112
	D. MOTOR VEHICLE EQUIP. PURCH. *	4,680	5,112	109
	E. PUBLICATIONS AND PRINTING	1,350	500	111
	F. EQUIPMENT PURCHASES *	750	1,550	206
	G. PER DIEM AND FEES *	2,000	750	112
	H. COMPUTER CHARGES *	2,900	900	100
	I. OTHER CONTRACTUAL EXPENSE *	1,600	1,050	100
	J. AUTHORITY LEASE RENTALS			

Quantitative Measures (Effectiveness, Workload, Efficiency)	F. Y. 1976 Function	F. Y. 1977 Base Level		K. GENERAL OBLIGATION BONDS			
Different Medical Centers Aided	100	100		L. CAPITAL OUTLAY			
Medical Emergency Courses conducted	100	100		M. LIST OTHER OBJECTS:			
Cost Per Course/Total funds	$445	$478					
Cost Per Course/State funds	$245	$278					
				TOTAL EXPENDITURES (Add A - M)	44,509	21,353	107
				FEDERAL FUNDS **	16,000	6,000	100
				OTHER FUNDS **	4,000		100
				STATE GENERAL FUNDS	24,509	15,353	113

Package Name:	Emergency Medical Health	Package 2 of 4
Prepared By:	John Smith	Activity Rank 7

* Attach detailed schedule for F. Y. 1977 Base Level (Including Minimum Level) funds requested.
** Detailed schedule for the Base Level is to be developed at the Activity Level.

6

ZERO·BASE BUDGET Procedures & Instructions

EXECUTIVE DEPARTMENT	
OFFICE OF PLANNING AND BUDGET — Budget Division	
SECTION	
DECISION PACKAGE PREPARATION – BASE LEVEL	
SUBJECT	
INSTRUCTIONS FOR FORM OPB-BUDGET-31	

Form Purpose

The Base Level Decision Package is the next package developed after the Minimum Level Decision Package for a function below the Activity. The Base Level is a level of effort, expressed in terms of service and cost, that represents a <u>continuance of services or a reduction of services</u> provided in F. Y. 1976 and no more. Funds for additional service needs should be requested only on a Workload Decision Package or a New or Improved Decision Package. The Base Level Package costs will vary by function. Non-recurring expenditures should be excluded from cost as well as other funds budgeted in F. Y. 1976 but not needed in F. Y. 1977 to deliver the same level of service. Include increased costs for F. Y. 1977 (to deliver the same level of service delivered in F. Y. 1976) such as within-grade increases, postage increases, etc. The Base Level Package, then, will express only cost increases and decreases associated with the same level of services provided for in F. Y. 1976. Decreased service and corresponding decreased cost can be outlined in this package but not increased services.

1. Describe the Function in Terms of Its Objective

   — Repeat information displayed on the Minimum Level Package.

2. Describe the Function in Terms of Service Provided in F. Y. 1976

   — Repeat information displayed on the Minimum Level Package.

3. Explain the Cost Increase or Decrease in the Base Level Over F. Y. 1976

   — Assuming the same level of service (same or less, but not more) as provided in F.Y. 1976, outline the financial reasons why this package added to the Minimum Level Package costs less or more than was budgeted for the function in F. Y. 1976. Increases or decreases for the various object classes should be explained. Attach additional pages if more space is needed.

Quantitative Measures (Quantitative Measures are Required on the Decision Packages)

— Effectiveness data measures how well the services provided solve the problem and meet the objectives of the function both for F. Y. 1976 and for the Base Level for F. Y. 1977.
— Workload data measures the effort required to deliver the services both for F. Y. 1976 and the Base Level for F. Y. 1977.
— Efficiency data measures the cost per unit of workload both for F. Y. 1976 and for the Base Level for F. Y. 1977.

Financial Information

— Enter amounts budgeted for the function in F. Y. 1976.
— In the column headed "This Pkg. F. Y. 1977" enter incremental amounts requested above the Minimum Level and <u>not</u> the total requested for the Base Level.
— The Cum % is calculated by dividing "This Pkg. F. Y. 1977" amounts from both the Minimum Level and the Base Level by "Function F. Y. 1976" amounts. Do not show Cum % for sub-classes of expenditures.

NOTE: Detailed form 47 and 48 are not required at the functional Base Level but are required at the Activity Level by summarizing the functional Base Level Packages.
Detailed forms 40-46 are required to be attached to the Base Level Package for amounts requested in F. Y. 1977 where an asterisk appears on the Base Level Decision Package Form.

DECISION PACKAGE — WORKLOAD

OPB-BUDGET-32

F. Y. 1977

OPB-Budget · 32
(Rev. 6-75)

ZERO-BASE BUDGET REQUEST
DECISION PACKAGE — WORKLOAD

Human Resources	Community Injury Control	Emergency Medical Health
Department	Activity	Function

Describe the Function in terms of its objective   County and City Medical Centers are charged to meet emergency situations such as sudden illness, injury, natural or man-made disasters, and poison cases. The centers do not coordinate their efforts across county and city lines nor do they have exposure to the latest techniques and equipment in the emergency medical field. Some centers are highly successful due to a special innovation that other centers do not share.

Describe the Function in terms of service provided in F. Y. 1976 Utilize a central staff to conduct medical emergency courses around the State to monitor the operations of the Injury Control Program. The courses will provide instruction to the centers on the latest medical emergency techniques and methods. The Base-Level provides service for the 100 most populated counties by conducting one medical emergency course at each.

Explain the Workload Increase in terms of service provided above the Base Level Conduct a medical emergency course in each of the 63 centers not covered in the State. Every center in the State would receive one course annually. This additional workload is demanded by the centers not now being served.

Explain the Workload Cost Over the Base Level
Personal Services — Two new positions, including fringes, less one month delayed hiring factor.
Related Expenses — To cover 63 additional centers, the new positions will need additional expenses and office space renovations.
Computer Charges — Expansion of the system to add 63 centers. Federal funds are available to help cover the additional centers.

Positions This Package __2__

	Function F.Y. 76	This Pkg. F.Y. 77	Cum%
A. TOTAL PERSONAL SERVICES	25,624	15,810	166
1. Motor Vehicle Expenses and Repairs	900	150	
2. Supplies and Materials	1,900	600	
3. Repairs and Maintenance	500	100	
4. Communications	400	50	
5. Power, Water, Natural Gas	250		
6. Rents	273		
7. Insurance and Bonding			
8. Workmen's Comp. and Indemnities			
9. Direct Benefits			
10. Tuition and Scholarships			
11. Grants to Counties or Cities			
12. Assessments by Merit System	132	88	
13. Other Operating Expenses	450		
14. Extraordinary Expenses			
B. REG. OPERATING EXPENSES(Add 1-14)	4,805	988	124
C. TRAVEL	800	300	150
D. MOTOR VEHICLE EQUIP. PURCH.	4,680		109
E. PUBLICATIONS AND PRINTING	1,350	250	129
F. EQUIPMENT PURCHASES	750	100	220
G. PER DIEM AND FEES	2,000		112
H. COMPUTER CHARGES	2,900	300	110
I. OTHER CONTRACTUAL EXPENSES	1,600	200	112
J. AUTHORITY LEASE RENTALS			
K. GENERAL OBLIGATION BONDS			
L. CAPITAL OUTLAY		2,000	
M. LIST OTHER OBJECTS:			
TOTAL EXPENDITURES (Add A-M)	44,509	19,948	152
FEDERAL FUNDS	16,000	7,000	144
OTHER FUNDS	4,000		100
STATE GENERAL FUNDS	24,509	12,948	166

Quantitative Measures (Effectiveness, Workload, Efficiency)	F. Y. 1976 Function	F. Y. 1977 Base-Level	F. Y. 1977 Cumulative
Different Medical Centers Aided	100	100	163
Medical Emergency Courses conduc.	100	100	163
Cost per Course/Total funds	$445	$478	$415
Cost per Course/State funds	$245	$278	$250

Package Name: Emergency Medical Health   Package __3__ of __4__

Prepared By: John Smith   Activity Rank __10__

* Attach detailed schedule for F. Y. 1977 Workload funds requested in this package.

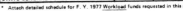

ZERO·BASE BUDGET Procedures & Instructions	EXECUTIVE DEPARTMENT
	OFFICE OF PLANNING AND BUDGET — Budget Division
	SECTION
	DECISION PACKAGE PREPARATION — WORKLOAD
	SUBJECT
	INSTRUCTIONS FOR FORM OPB-BUDGET-32

Form Purpose

The Workload Decision Package is developed only where funds are needed to meet increased workload at the functional level. Additional workload must be quantified and explained fully in terms of service and cost. A Workload Package must be documented in terms of additional funds needed above the Base Level. Additional workload which can be met without the need for additional funds should be included in the Base Level Package for the function.

1. **Describe the Function in Terms of Its Objectives**
   - Repeat information displayed on the Minimum Level Package.

2. **Describe the Function in Terms of Service Provided in F. Y. 1976**
   - Repeat information displayed on the Minimum Level Package.

3. **Explain the Workload Increase in Terms of Service Provided above the Base Level**
   - Explain additional workload which requires additional funds not provided for in the Base Level. The additional workload which can be met without the need for additional funds should be explained in the Base Level Package and not in the Workload Package. Workload must be quantified.

4. **Explain the Workload Cost Over the Base Level**
   - Point out the reasons why the additional workload will require more funds. The explanation should be expressed in terms of what the funds will be expended for to accommodate the additional workload above the Base Level.

Quantitative Measures (Quantitative measures are required on the Decision Packages)

- Show Quantitative Measures for "F. Y. 1976 Function." The "F. Y. 1977 Base Level" column will be repeated from the Base Level Package. The "F. Y. 1977 Cumulative" column will include the Minimum, Base, and Workload quantitative measures as a running total.
- Effectiveness data measures how well the services provided solve the problem and meet the objectives of the function.
- Workload data measures the effort required to deliver the services.
- Efficiency data measures the cost per unit of workload.

Financial Information

- Enter amounts budgeted for the function in F. Y. 1976.
- "This Pkg. F. Y. 1977" enter incremental amounts requested above the Base Level and _not_ the total requested through the Workload Package Level.
- The Cum % is calculated by dividing "This Pkg. F. Y. 1977" amounts summed from the Minimum, Base and Workload Packages by "Function F. Y. 1976" amounts. Do not show Cum % for sub-classes of expenditure.

NOTE: Detailed Forms 40-48 are required to be attached to the Workload Package for amounts requested in F. Y. 1977 where an asterisk appears on the Workload Decision Package Form.

DATE Rev. 6/75	PAGE 9	OPB - Budget - 32

DECISION PACKAGE – NEW OR IMPROVED

OPB-BUDGET-33

F. Y. 1977

OPB-Budget - 33
(Rev. 6-75)

ZERO-BASE BUDGET REQUEST
DECISION PACKAGE – NEW OR IMPROVED

Human Resources	Community Injury Control	Emergency Medical Health
Department	Activity	Function

	Function F.Y.76	This Pkg. F.Y.77	Cum%
Describe the Function in terms of its objective County and City Medical Centers are charged to meet emergency situations such as sudden illness, injury, natural or man-made disasters, and poison cases. The centers do not coordinate their efforts across county and city lines nor do they have exposure to the latest techniques and equipment in the emergency medical field. Some centers are highly successful due to a special innovation that other centers do not share.	Positions This Package __2__		
	A. TOTAL PERSONAL SERVICES * 25,624	15,810	229
	1. Motor Vehicle Expenses and Repairs 900		
	2. Supplies and Materials 1,900	500	
	3. Repairs and Maintenance 500		
	4. Communications 400	50	
Describe the Function in terms of service provided in F. Y. 1976 Utilize a central staff to conduct medical emergency courses around the State to monitor the operations of the Injury Control Program. The courses will provide instruction to the cneters on the latest medical emergency techniques and methods. The Base Level provides services for the 100 most populated counties by conducting one medical emergency course at each.	5. Power, Water, Natural Gas 250		
	6. Rents * 273	150	
	7. Insurance and Bonding		
	8. Workmen's Comp. and Indemnities		
	9. Direct Benefits		
	10. Tuition and Scholarships		
Explain the New or Improved in terms of service Conduct an additional 37 medical emergency courses. This improvement will provide 37 centers with at least 2 courses. The centers serving the greatest population will receive more intensive instruction and more specialized courses. Improved coordination for local services will mean better emergency medical health statewide.	11. Grants to Counties or Cities		
	12. Assessments by Merit System 132	88	
	13. Other Operating Expenses 450		
	14. Extraordinary Expenses		
	B. REG. OPERATING EXPENSES(Add 1-14) 4,805	788	141
	C. TRAVEL 800	200	175
Explain the New or Improved in terms of Cost Personal Services – Two new positions, including fringes, less one month delayed hiring factor. Related Expenses – To conduct 37 additional courses, the new positions will need additional expenses and office space rental. No additional Federal funds are available for expansion.	D. MOTOR VEHICLE EQUIP. PURCH. * 4,680		109
	E. PUBLICATIONS AND PRINTING 1,350	100	137
	F. EQUIPMENT PURCHASES * 750	100	233
	G. PER DIEM AND FEES * 2,000		112
	H. COMPUTER CHARGES * 2,900		110
	I. OTHER CONTRACTUAL EXPENSE * 1,600		112

Quantitative Measures (Effectiveness, Workload, Efficiency)	F. Y. 1976 Function	F. Y. 1977 Cumulative
Different Medical Centers Aided	100	163
Medical Emergency Courses Conducted	100	200
Cost Per Course/Total funds	$445	$423
Cost Per Course/State funds	$245	$289

J. AUTHORITY LEASE RENTALS		
K. GENERAL OBLIGATION BONDS		
L. CAPITAL OUTLAY *		
M. LIST OTHER OBJECTS:		

	Function	This Pkg.	Cum%
TOTAL EXPENDITURES (Add A-M)	44,509	16,998	190
FEDERAL FUNDS *	16,000		144
OTHER FUNDS *	4,000		100
STATE GENERAL FUNDS	24,509	16,998	236

Package Name: Emergency Medical Health   Package __4__ of __4__

Prepared By: John Smith   Activity Rank __14__

* Attach detailed schedule for F. Y. 1977 **New or Improved** funds requested in this package.

ZERO·BASE BUDGET Procedures & Instructions

EXECUTIVE DEPARTMENT	
OFFICE OF PLANNING AND BUDGET — Budget Division	
SECTION	
DECISION PACKAGE PREPARATION — NEW OR IMPROVED	
SUBJECT	
INSTRUCTIONS FOR FORM OPB-BUDGET-33	

Form Purpose

The New or Improved Decision Package is developed for a requested improvement of an ongoing operation of the function or for a requested new operation in a function. The New or Improved operation within an existing Activity must be quantified and explained fully in term of service and cost. Any complete new function under an Activity would be requested on a separate series of Decision Packages and not on the New or Improved Decision Package.

1. Describe the Function in Terms of Its Objective
   - Repeat information displayed on the Minimum Level Package.

2. Describe the Function in Terms of Service Provided in F. Y. 1976
   - Repeat information displayed on the Minimum Level Package.

3. Explain the New or Improved in Terms of Service
   - Explain the additional service provided which helps the function to better meet its objectives. An Improvement is an expansion of an ongoing operation of the function while a New operation is, by definition, an operation not conducted in the function for F. Y. 1976.

4. Explain the New or Improved in Terms of Cost
   - Point out reasons why the New or Improved service will require additional funds. The explanation should be expressed in terms of what the funds will be expended for to accommodate the New or Improved service.

Quantitative Measures (Quantitative measures are required on the Decision Packages)
- Show Quantitative Measures for "F. Y. 1976 Function." The "F. Y. 1977 Cumulative" column will include the Minimum, Base, Workload, and New or Improved Package quantitative measures as a running total.
- Effectiveness data measures how well the services provided solve the problem and meet the objectives of the function.
- Workload data measures the effort required to deliver the services.
- Efficiency data measures the cost per unit of workload.

Financial Information
- Enter amounts budgeted for the function in F. Y. 1976.
- "This Pkg. F. Y. 1977" enter incremental amounts requested above the previous level for function and not the total requested through the New or Improved Package Level.
- The Cum % is calculated by dividing "This Pkg. F. Y. 1977" amounts summed from the Minimum, Base, Workload, and New or Improved Packages by "Function F. Y. 1976" amounts. Do not show Cum % for sub-classes of expenditure.

NOTE: Detailed forms 40-48 are required to be attached to the Workload Package for amounts requested in F. Y. 1977 where an asterisk appears on the New or Improved Package Form.

DATE Rev. 6/75	PAGE 11	OPB · Budget · 33

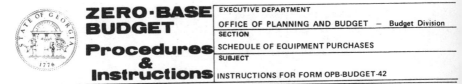

ZERO·BASE BUDGET Procedures & Instructions	
	EXECUTIVE DEPARTMENT
	OFFICE OF PLANNING AND BUDGET — Budget Division
	SECTION
	SCHEDULE OF EQUIPMENT PURCHASES
	SUBJECT
	INSTRUCTIONS FOR FORM OPB-BUDGET-42

Form Purpose

This form is a detailed schedule of Equipment for the function which will be attached to each decision package, except for a Minimum Level Package, where an amount is requested for Equipment in F. Y. 1977. The schedule, upon completion, should be copied and attached to each decision package, except Minimum, as a fully completed display.

— List the type of Equipment.

> Example: Office Equipment -- Typewriters
> Office Equipment — Adding Machines and Calculators
> Office Equipment — Furniture
> Lab and Medical Equipment
> General Equipment Furnishings

NOTE: Any one piece of equipment which costs over $500 must be listed separately.

— Show funds requested for Equipment Purchases for F. Y. 1977 divided into the three funding levels as requested on the decision packages.

— The F. Y. 1977 Equipment requests will be listed on this form from the individual decision packages where funds are requested for this particular object, with the exception of the Minimum Level which will be included in the Base Level for schedule purposes.

F. Y. 1977 ZERO-BASE BUDGET REQUEST SCHEDULE OF EQUIPMENT PURCHASES   Page 1 of 1   OPB-Budget - 42 (Rev. 6-75)

Human Resources _____ Community Injury Control _____ Emergency Medical Health
Department   Activity   Function

Type of Equipment (List Replacement then Additional)	F.Y. 1977 REQUESTED		
	Minimum and Base Level	Workload	New or Improved
Replacement:			
Office Equipment - Typewriters	450		
Office Equipment — Adding Machine	175		
Additional:			
Portable EKG Unit*	925		
Office Equipment — Adding Machine		100	100
* Any individual equipment item over $500 is to be listed separately.			
Total Equipment Purchases	1,550	100	100

DATE   Rev. 6/75   PAGE 15   OPB - Budget - 42

ZERO-BASE BUDGET Procedures & Instructions

EXECUTIVE DEPARTMENT	
OFFICE OF PLANNING AND BUDGET — Budget Division	
SECTION	
SCHEDULE OF PER DIEM AND FEES	
SUBJECT	
INSTRUCTIONS FOR FORM OPB-BUDGET-43	

Form Purpose

This form is a detailed schedule of Per Diem and Fees for the function which will be attached to each decision package, except for a Minimum Level Package, where an amount is requested for Per Diem and Fees in F. Y. 1977. The schedule, upon completion, should be copied and attached to each decision package, except Minimum, as a fully completed display.

— Categories for type of Per Diem is provided. List per diem not categorized under the caption "List Other."

— Identify the need for the Per Diem and Fee Categorized.

— Show funds budgeted for each type of Per Diem or Fee for F. Y. 1976.

— Show funds requested for Per Diem or Fees for F. Y. 1977 divided into the three funding levels as requested on the decision packages.

— The F. Y. 1977 Per Diem and Fees requests will be listed on this form from the individual decision packages where funds are requested for this particular object, with the exception of the Minimum Level which will be included in the Base Level for schedule purposes.

F. Y. 1977   ZERO-BASE BUDGET REQUEST / SCHEDULE OF PER DIEM AND FEES   Page 1 of 1   OPB - Budget - 43 (Rev. 6-75)

Department: Human Resources   Activity: Community Injury Control   Function: Emergency Medical Health

Type of Per Diem	Reason Service Needed	F. Y. 1976 Budgeted	F. Y. 1977 REQUESTED			
			Minimum and Base Level	Workload	New or Improved	TOTAL
Board/Commission Membs.	Local Board Members Per Diem	1,000	1,350			
Accounting/Audit						
Management Consulting	Study for Improving Special Medical Emergency Care	750	600			
Engineer/Architect						
Legal						
Educational	Medical Emergency Training Class at G. S. U.	250	300			
Medical						
Research						
List Other						
Total Per Diem and Fees		2,000	2,250			

DATE Rev. 6/75	PAGE 16	OPB - Budget - 43

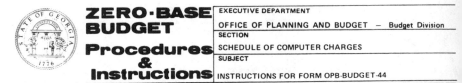

	ZERO-BASE	EXECUTIVE DEPARTMENT
	BUDGET	OFFICE OF PLANNING AND BUDGET — Budget Division
		SECTION
	Procedures	SCHEDULE OF COMPUTER CHARGES
	&	SUBJECT
	Instructions	INSTRUCTIONS FOR FORM OPB-BUDGET-44

Form Purpose

This form is a detailed schedule of Computer Charges for the function which will be attached to each decision package, except for a Minimum Level Package, where an amount is requested for Computer Charges in F. Y. 1977. The schedule, upon completion, should be copied and attached to each decision package, except Minimum, as a fully completed display.

— Show the account number of the system (assigned by DOAS).

— Show the narrative description of the system.

— Show the funds budgeted, by function, for F. Y. 1976 for each system and the funds requested for F. Y. 1977 as divided into the three funding levels.

— List new system development separately.

— The F. Y. 1977 Computer Charges requests will be listed on this form from the individual decision packages where funds are requested for this particular object, with the exception of the Minimum Level which will be included in the Base Level for schedule purposes.

NOTE: DOAS can **help provide the information you** need to prepare this form.

F. Y. 1977

ZERO-BASE BUDGET REQUEST
SCHEDULE OF COMPUTER CHARGES

OPB-Budget - 44
(Rev. 6-75)

Human Resources	Community Injury Control	Emergency Medical Health
Department	Activity	Function

		F. Y. 1976	F. Y. 1977 REQUESTED		
Account Number	SYSTEM DESCRIPTION	Budgeted	Minimum and Base Level	Workload	New or Improved
82121	Statistical system for county injury control	1,800	1,800		
92181	Payroll System	1,100	1,100	300	
	Total Computer Charges	2,900	2,900	300	

DATE Rev. 6/75	PAGE 17	OPB - Budget - 44

ZERO·BASE BUDGET Procedures & Instructions

EXECUTIVE DEPARTMENT	
OFFICE OF PLANNING AND BUDGET — Budget Division	
SECTION	
SCHEDULE OF OTHER CONTRACTUAL EXPENSE	
SUBJECT	
INSTRUCTIONS FOR FORM OPB-BUDGET-45	

Form Purpose

This form is a detailed schedule of Other Contractual Expense for the function which will be attached to each decision package, except for a Minimum Level Package, where an amount is requested for Other Contractual Expense in F. Y. 1977. The schedule, upon completion should be copied and attached to each decision package, except Minimum, as a fully completed display.

— List type of contract.

— Identify the need for the contract

— For each contract, show the amount budgeted for F. Y. 1976.

— Show funds requested for F. Y. 1977 for each contract, divided into the three levels of funding as taken from the decision packages.

— The F. Y. 1977 Other Contractual Expense requests will be listed on this form from the individual decison packages where funds are requested for this particular object, with the exception of the Minimum Level which will be included in the Base Level for schedule purposes.

F. Y. 1977 — ZERO-BASE BUDGET REQUEST — SCHEDULE OF OTHER CONTRACTUAL EXPENSES — OPB-Budget-45 (Rev. 6-75)

Human Resources (Department) — Community Injury Control (Activity) — Emergency Medical Health (Function)

		F. Y. 1976	F. Y. 1977 REQUESTED		
Type of Contract	Reason Service Needed	Budgeted	Minimum and Base Level	Workload	New or Improved
Ambulance Service	Emergency Ambulance Service for counties with no statewide system	1,600	1,600	200	
Total Other Contractual Expenses		1,600	1,600	200	

DATE Rev. 6/75 — PAGE 18 — OPB - Budget- 45

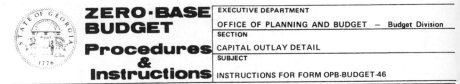

ZERO-BASE BUDGET Procedures & Instructions

EXECUTIVE DEPARTMENT	
OFFICE OF PLANNING AND BUDGET — Budget Division	
SECTION	
CAPITAL OUTLAY DETAIL	
SUBJECT	
INSTRUCTIONS FOR FORM OPB-BUDGET-46	

Form Purpose

This form is a detailed explanation of Capital Outlay for the function which will be attached to each decision package where an amount is requested for Capital Outlay in F. Y. 1977. Any additional information needed to explain the request should be attached.

— All sections of the form (A through G) should be completed for each project requested for each kind of decision package where applicable.

— All construction or project funds should be requested as Capital Outlay and not as General Obligation Bond or Authority Lease Rentals.

F. Y. 1977

ZERO-BASE BUDGET REQUEST
CAPITAL OUTLAY DETAIL

OPB-Budget-46
(Rev. 6-75)

Human Resources	Community Injury Control	Emergency Medical Health
Department	Activity	Function

A. THIS PROJECT: (Check One)

___ Is an Original Facility   _X_ Renovates an Existing Facility
___ Is an Addition to an Existing Facility   ___ Replaces an Existing Facility
___ Is part of a Master Plan (Previously Authorized) (Proposed)

B. LOCATION: Atlanta, Georgia
Size of Site Required _____
(Check where appropriate)
_X_ Site on Currently Owned Property   _X_ Utilities Already Available
___ Site to be Selected   _X_ Access Already Available
___ Site Already Selected

C. DESCRIPTION OF FACILITY:
General Description: (Attach Basic Layout, if possible)
Renovation of Offices in Atlanta, Labor Building, by adding partitions.

Functional Space Requirements: (in square feet) No additional square
feet needed
Special Standards or Requirements: Glass and metal partitioning bolted
to existing walls

D. JUSTIFICATION OF NEED:
This Renovation is needed to accommodate new positions requested
in the Workload Decision Package. Present office space can be
utilized if partitioned.
Number to be served by Facility ___2___
If new Facility, Indicate Alternatives Considered:
___ Leasing   ___ Renovation

E. ESTIMATED COST OF PROJECT:
Source of Estimate: J. M. Bennett, Building Supervisor

1. Design and Planning:	$	100
2. Land Acquisition:	$	
3. Construction: ___ sq. feet @ ___ per sq. foot	$	
4. Architectual Fees and Contingencies:	$	200
5. Utilities:	$	
6. Air Conditioning/Heating:	$	
7. Equipment:	$	
8. Other: Renovation Cost	$	1,700
TOTAL COST	$	

Less Other Funds Available
Source _____ $ _____
STATE FUNDS REQUIRED $ 2,000

F. ESTIMATED OPERATIONAL COST AT COMPLETION:
Expected Completion Date: January, 1977
Number of Additional Personnel Required None
Additional Funds Required when Project is in Full Operation $ None
Personal Services and Operating Expenses $ None

G. STATE FUNDS REQUESTED FOR ADDITIONAL YEARS:
If Funding will be extended over more than one year, explain and indicate the
amount required for each year: N/A

DATE Rev. 6/75	PAGE 19	OPB - Budget - 46

ZERO·BASE BUDGET Procedures & Instructions	EXECUTIVE DEPARTMENT
	OFFICE OF PLANNING AND BUDGET — Budget Division
	SECTION ACTIVITY OR DEPARTMENT DECISION PACKAGE RANKING PREPARATION
	SUBJECT INSTRUCTIONS FOR FORM OPB-BUDGET-50

Form Purpose

This form displays the Activity or the Departmental State Fund priorities for F. Y. 1977 for each decision package and the functional State fund cost for F. Y. 1976 for each first package in a series.

Rank

— Enter priority number of each package, starting with number 1 as the highest priority and ending with a number which equals the total number of packages. In any functional series of packages; e.g., 1 of 3, 2 of 3, and 3 of 3, Package 1 of 3 is always ranked higher than 2 of 3 or 3 of 3. However, Package 1 of 3 or 2 of 3 or 3 of 3 in one functional series can be ranked higher or lower than Packages in another functional series.

Package Name

— Enter package name of each Decision Package ranked and note the series number by it. Names of Decision Packages should be as descriptive of the function as possible, preferably the name of the function.

F. Y. 1976 Amount

— Enter the F. Y. 1976 Amount for State funds budgeted for the function and number of positions for each first package of a series; i.e., Package 1 of - will always have the F. Y. 1976 State funds and positions for the entire function shown. Package 2 of — or 3 of —, etc., will show a blank in the F. Y. 1976 amount column since the F. Y. 1976 amount was already shown by the first package of the series.

F. Y. 1977 Amount

— Enter the F. Y. 1977 amount for State funds requested and number of positions for each Decision Package ranked.

Cumulative Level

— Enter the Cumulative State funds, the percentage the cumulative amount represents to the Total F. Y. 1976 State fund total, and the cumulative number of positions.

Ranking Packages

— All Decision Packages are ranked even if Federal or Other funds finance the package.
— State fund amounts will be the only funds listed on the ranking sheet even if package is funded partially or fully by Federal or Other funds.
— Show positions for all ranked packages.
— Rank Decision Packages as to how effectively and efficiently each one contributes to the Departmental goals and objectives in terms of service.
— Decision Packages are ranked for each Activity and for the Department as well.

Debt Service Ranking

— Existing Authority Lease Rentals (A.L.R.'s) and General Obligation Bond (G. O. Bond) payments should be ranked with a high priority.
— DO NOT request new A.L.R.'s or G. O. Bond payments for construction in F. Y. 1977.
— Any request for construction in F. Y. 1977 shall be requested as Capital Outlay.

ACTIVITY RANKING

OPB-BUDGET-5(

F. Y. 1977

ZERO-BASE BUDGET REQUEST
DECISION PACKAGE RANKING

OPB-Budget - 50
(Rev. 6-75)

Human Resources — Department

Community Injury Control — Activity

R A N K	PACKAGE NAME	F. Y. 1976 BUDGETED		F. Y. 1977 REQUESTED		CUMULATIVE LEVEL		
		State Funds	Positions	State Funds	Positions	State Funds	% 77/76	Positions
1	Executive Adm. (1 of 2)	32,420	1	24,200	1	24,200	14.9	1
2	Planning (1 of 1)	34,121	2	30,200	2	54,400	33.5	3
3	Patient Appraisals (1 of 2)	24,946	2	11,748	1	66,148	40.7	4
* 4	Emergency Medical Health (1 of 4)	24,509	2	12,433	2	78,581	48.3	6
5	Food Service (1 of 2)	20,000	3	16,200	3	94,781	58.3	9
6	Housekeeping (1 of 3)	26,593	4	14,000	2	108,781	66.9	11
* 7	Emergency Medical Health (2 of 4)			15,353	1	124,134	76.3	12
8	Executive Adm. (2 of 2)			15,200	1	139,334	85.7	13
9	Patient Appraisals (2 of 2)			17,000	1	156,334	96.2	14
*10	Emergency Medical Health (3 of 4)			12,948	2	169,282	104.1	16
11	Capital Outlay (1 of 1)			2,000		171,282	105.3	
12	Food Service (2 of 2)			19,000		190,282	117.0	
13	Housekeeping (2 of 3)			11,000	2	201,282	123.6	18
*14	Emergency Medical Health (4 of 4)			16,998	2	218,280	134.3	20
15	Housekeeping (3 of 3)			15,000		233,280	143.5	20
	Activity Totals	162,589	14	233,280	20			
	* Decision Packages in Sample			233,280 — 143.5%				
				162,589				

Frank Doe — Approved By   Activity Manager — Title   August 18, 1975 — Date   Page 1 of 1

DEPARTMENT RANKING

OPB-BUDGET-5

F. Y. 1977

ZERO-BASE BUDGET REQUEST
DECISION PACKAGE RANKING

OPB-Budget - 50
(Rev. 6-75)

Human Resources — Department

Department Ranking — Activity

R A N K	PACKAGE NAME	F. Y. 1976 BUDGETED		F. Y. 1977 REQUESTED		CUMULATIVE LEVEL		
		State Funds	Positions	State Funds	Positions	State Funds	% 77/76	Positions
1	Executive Adm. (1 of 2)	32,420	1	24,200	1	24,200	3.3	1
2	Administrative (1 of 2)	44,200	4	32,000	3	56,200	7.7	4
3	General Obligation Bond (1 of 1)	200,000		200,000		256,200	35.1	
4	Authority Lease Rentals (1 of 1)	100,000		100,000		356,200	48.8	
5	Planning (1 of 1)	34,121	2	30,200	2	386,400	52.9	6
6	Emergency Facilities (1 of 3)	156,004	20	65,000	6	451,400	61.8	12
7	Housekeeping (1 of 3)	26,593	4	14,000	2	465,400	63.8	14
8	Administrative (2 of 2)			15,100	1	480,500	65.8	15
9	Patient Appraisals (1 of 2)	24,946	2	11,748	1	492,248	67.4	16
10	Emergency Facilities (2 of 3)			29,000	5	521,248	71.4	21
11	Food Services (1 of 2)	20,000	3	16,200	3	537,448	73.6	24
12	Staff Training (1 of 4)	62,200	6	7,000	1	544,448	74.6	25
13	Capital Outlay (1 of 1)	5,000		25,000		569,448	78.0	
*14	Emergency Medical Health (1 of 4)	24,509	2	12,433	2	581,881	79.7	27
15	Emergency Facilities (3 of 3)			110,721	9	692,602	94.9	36
16	Staff Training (2 of 4)			16,900	2	709,502	97.2	38
17	Housekeeping (2 of 3)			11,000	2	720,502	98.7	40
*18	Emergency Medical Health (2 of 4)			15,353	1	735,855	100.8	41
19	Executive Admin. (2 of 2)			15,200	1	751,055	102.9	42
20	Capital Outlay (1 of 1)			2,000		753,055	103.2	
*21	Emergency Medical Health (3 of 4)			12,948	2	766,003	104.9	44
22	Staff Training (3 of 4)			27,000	2	793,003	108.6	46
23	Housekeeping (3 of 3)			15,000		808,003	110.7	
*24	Emergency Medical Health (4 of 4)			16,998	1	825,001	113.0	47
25	Staff Training (4 of 4)			22,000	1	847,001	116.0	48
26	Food Services (2 of 2)			19,000		866,001	118.6	
27	Patient Appraisals (2 of 2)			17,000	1	883,001	121.0	49
	TOTALS	729,993	44	883,001	49			

Sam Doe — Approved By   Department Director — Title   August 26, 1975 — Date   Page 1 of 1
* Decision Packages in Sample

ZERO·BASE BUDGET Procedures & Instructions	EXECUTIVE DEPARTMENT
	OFFICE OF PLANNING AND BUDGET — Planning Division
	SECTION
	ACTIVITY INFORMATION SUMMARY
	SUBJECT
	INSTRUCTIONS FOR FORM OPB-PLANNING-51

Form Purpose

This form displays descriptive information about an Activity and shows specific data which indicates effectiveness of the Activity.

1. Activity Purpose

—Review and revise, if necessary, the statement of purpose for this activity found in Volume II, Program Display, of the Governor's Recommended Budget for FY 1976. Assure that the statement is consistent with expressed intent of pertinent enabling legislation or other source of authority. If at all possible, this statement should be expressed in terms that suggest measures of accomplishment.

2. Activity Description

—Review and revise, if necessary, the functional description of this activity found in Volume II of the Governor's Recommended Budget for FY 1976. Identify the service(s) being provided and categorize the recipients by service need. Indicate quantitatively the type and volume of service provided to each category of recipients.

3. Degree of Accomplishment of Activity Purpose

—Indicate quantitatively and qualitatively (where possible) the degree to which the activity is accomplishing its stated purpose. Use the measure(s) of accomplishment previously submitted to the Office of Planning and Budget.

4. Forecast of Substantive Changes in Scope of Activity

—Identify any expected (within the next five years) changes in the scope of activity purpose or in the functions performed. Identify the expected source of initiative for these changes and explain the expected effects of these changes on services being provided and on categories of recipients (examples: objectives accomplished thereby ending the need for that program; changing Federal program regulations).

DATE Rev. 6/75	PAGE 28	OPB - Planning - 51

ACTIVITY INFORMATION SUMMARY

OPB-PLANNING-51

F. Y. 1977	ZERO-BASE BUDGET REQUEST ACTIVITY INFORMATION SUMMARY	OPB - Planning - 51 (Rev.6/75)
Human Resources Department		Community Injury Control Activity

1. Activity Purpose

Plan and support the provision of emergency medical services to individuals in emergency situations such as sudden illness, injury, and natural or man-made disaster. Support and monitor the county operated medical emergency centers.

2. Activity Description

Conducts medical self-help courses and monitors operation of the injury control program. Plans for new EMS programs such as hospital disasters plans and exercises. Conduct medical emergency courses for county medical centers. The following is an indication of the types of services provided, categorized according to need:

	F. Y. 1975
Persons treated in injury control centers	32,000
Persons treated in poison control centers	1,200
Persons who have ready access to this service	2,500,000

3. Degree of Accomplishment of Activity Purpose

Of the estimated 70,000 individuals who needed emergency medical services during this program year, 68,000 received prompt and effective service through certified county EMS programs. One EMS training course was conducted in all 159 counties and 40 counties received 2 training courses thereby completing the total EMS instructional program. An estimated 90 percent of all poisonings were treated through poison control centers. Fatal injury/accident rates decreased by 1.2 percent.

4. Forecast of Substantive Changes in Scope of Activity

New Federal Health Planning legislation will bring about administrative and functional changes in the organization of EMS. These changes will affect the planning and funding of EMS in Georgia over the next 3 years.

ACTIVITY FUND SOURCES	Budgeted F. Y. 1976	Requested F. Y. 1977	DEPARTMENTAL ACTIVITY PROJECTIONS				
			F. Y. 1978	F. Y. 1979	F. Y. 1980	F. Y. 1981	F. Y. 1982
Federal Funds	16,000	23,000	50,000				
Other Funds	4,000	4,000					
State Funds	162,589	190,724	215,420	231,462	257,587	283,345	311,679
TOTAL FUNDS	182,589	217,724	265,420	231,462	257,587	283,345	311,679

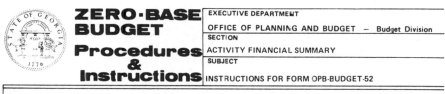

ZERO·BASE BUDGET Procedures & Instructions

EXECUTIVE DEPARTMENT	
OFFICE OF PLANNING AND BUDGET — Budget Division	
SECTION	
ACTIVITY FINANCIAL SUMMARY	
SUBJECT	
INSTRUCTIONS FOR FORM OPB-BUDGET-52	

Form Purpose

This form is a summary of sub-objects, objects, and fund sources of the Decision Package Ranking Forms, supported by the decision packages, for a entire Activity.

- Show amounts by categories listed for F. Y. 1975 Actual, F. Y. 1976 Budget, and F. Y. 1977 requested. F. Y. 1977 requested is divided into four funding levels summarized from the functional decision packages submitted.

- Amounts for F. Y. 1976 should represent the Annual Operating Budget to include amendments thereto approved by OPB since the beginning of the Fiscal Year.

F. Y. 1977

ZERO-BASE BUDGET REQUEST
ACTIVITY FINANCIAL SUMMARY

OPB-Budget-52
(Rev. 6-75)

Human Resources — Department

Human Resources — Budget Unit

Community Injury Control — Activity

OBJECTS/FUNDS	F. Y. 1975 Actual	F. Y. 1976 Budgeted	Minimum Level Packages	Base Level Packages	Workload Packages	New or Improved Packages	TOTAL All Packages
				F. Y. 1977 REQUESTED			
Number of Budgeted Positions	10	14	10	4	4	2	20
A. TOTAL PERSONAL SERVICES	110,024	148,200	92,100	27,544	27,200	21,400	168,244
1. Motor Vehicle Expenses and Repairs	900	1,500	1,000	600	250		1,850
2. Supplies and Materials	3,000	3,600	2,900	1,200	800	1,000	5,900
3. Repairs and Maintenance	700	900	600	500	200		1,300
4. Communications	600	750	490	600	100	100	1,290
5. Power, Water, Natural Gas	375	500	300	300			600
6. Rents	1,500	2,600	2,100	1,000		300	3,400
7. Insurance and Bonding	180	215	200	110		100	410
8. Workmen's Comp. and Indemnities							
9. Direct Benefits							
10. Tuition and Scholarships							
11. Grants to Counties or Cities							
12. Assessment by Merit System	360	574	440	176	176	88	880
13. Other Operating Expenses	1,000	1,200	900	400	100		1,400
14. Extraordinary Expenses	500	750	500	300			800
B. REG. OPERATING EXPENSES (Add 1-14)	9,115	12,589	9,430	5,186	1,626	1,588	17,830
C. TRAVEL	1,200	1,400	700	800	400	300	2,100
D. MOTOR VEHICLE EQUIP. PURCHASES	4,600	8,200	10,000				10,000
E. PUBLICATIONS AND PRINTING	2,000	3,900	2,000	2,200	400	200	4,800
F. EQUIPMENT PURCHASES	900	1,200		2,400	275	200	2,875
G. PER DIEM AND FEES	600	2,500	2,000	1,000			3,000
H. COMPUTER CHARGES	2,651	3,200	2,500	1,200	400		4,100
I. OTHER CONTRACTUAL EXPENSE	900	1,400	900	1,500	375		2,775
J. AUTHORITY LEASE RENTALS							
K. GENERAL OBLIGATION BONDS							
L. CAPITAL OUTLAY				2,000			2,000
M. LIST OTHER OBJECTS:							
TOTAL EXPENDITURES (Add A - M)	131,990	182,589	119,630	41,830	32,676	23,588	217,724
FEDERAL FUNDS	10,000	16,000	10,000	6,000	7,000		23,000
OTHER FUNDS		4,000	4,000				4,000
STATE GENERAL FUNDS	121,990	162,589	105,630	35,830	25,676	23,588	190,724

DATE Rev. 6/75	PAGE 30	OPB - Budget - 52

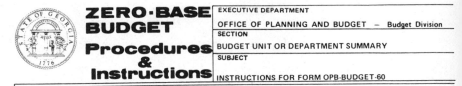

ZERO-BASE	EXECUTIVE DEPARTMENT	
BUDGET	OFFICE OF PLANNING AND BUDGET — Budget Division	
	SECTION	
Procedures	BUDGET UNIT OR DEPARTMENT SUMMARY	
&	SUBJECT	
Instructions	INSTRUCTIONS FOR FORM OPB-BUDGET-60	

Form Purpose

This form is a summary of objects and fund sources of the Activity Financial Summaries for each Budget Unit, if an agency has more than one Budget Unit, and for the entire Department. The F. Y. 1974 Actual Column should be per the Audit Report.

— Show amounts by categories listed for F. Y. 1974 Actual, F. Y. 1975 Actual, F. Y. 1976 Budget, and F. Y. 1977 requested. F. Y. 1977 Requested is divided into four funding levels summarized from the Activity Financial Summaries.

— Amounts for F. Y. 1976 should represent the Annual Operating Budget to include amendments thereto approved by OPB since the beginning of the Fiscal Year.

F. Y. 1977

ZERO-BASE BUDGET REQUEST
BUDGET UNIT OR DEPARTMENT SUMMARY

OPB-Budget - 60
(Rev. 6-75)

Human Resources — Department

Human Resources — Budget Unit

OBJECTS/FUNDS	F. Y. 1974 Actual	F. Y. 1975 Actual	F. Y. 1976 Budgeted	F. Y. 1977 REQUESTED Minimum Level Packages	Base Level Packages	Workload Packages	New or Improved Packages	TOTAL All Packages
Number of Positions	33	35	44	25	15	6	3	49
A. TOTAL PERSONAL SERVICES	315,786	330,124	430,493	306,171	151,126	42,126	32,126	531,549
B. REG. OPERATING EXPENSES	110,100	135,000	150,000	95,110	65,210	18,100	7,200	185,620
C. TRAVEL	7,048	8,100	8,900	7,210	2,010	1,000	500	10,720
D. MOTOR VEHICLE EQUIP. PURCH.	10,500	11,600	16,300	15,100	5,112			20,212
E. PUBLICATIONS AND PRINTING	1,530	3,686	4,200	4,100	900	400	200	5,500
F. EQUIPMENT PURCHASES	600	900	3,100	2,100	2,000	300	200	4,500
G. PER DIEM AND FEES	1,200	2,181	3,600	2,800	800			3,500
H. COMPUTER CHARGES	2,500	5,281	7,000	4,900	2,000	1,800		8,700
I. OTHER CONTRACTUAL EXPENSE	500	900	1,400	900	1,100	400		2,400
J. AUTHORITY LEASE RENTALS	75,000	75,000	75,000	75,000				75,000
K. GENERAL OBLIGATION BONDS	50,000	50,000	50,000	50,000				50,000
L. CAPITAL OUTLAY							2,000	2,000
M. LIST OTHER OBJECTS:								
H.E.W.-County Health Grants	800,000	875,000	1,000,000	1,010,000				1,010,000
TOTAL EXPENDITURES (Add A - M)	1,374,764	1,497,772	1,749,993	1,573,391	230,258	66,126	40,226	1,910,001
FEDERAL FUNDS	800,000	875,000	1,016,000	1,010,000	6,000	7,000		1,023,000
OTHER FUNDS			4,000	4,000				4,000
STATE GENERAL FUNDS	574,764	622,772	729,993	559,391	224,258	59,126	40,226	883,001

Official Signature
(Signature required only on Department Summary)

Commissioner
Title

August 29, 1975
Date

DATE Rev. 6/75	PAGE 31	OPB - Budget - 60

Appendix 15-B
Zero-Base Budgeting Critique
State of Georgia*

I. Purpose of Critique

The purpose of this critique was to analyze (1) the impact and effectiveness of zero-base budgeting in the preparation of the FY 1973 executive budget recommendation; (2) the problems encountered; (3) the changes desired to improve the process and the results obtained; and (4) the question of whether this process should be continued.

II. General Observations

1. The consensus is that zero-base budgeting can be effective and should be continued next year.
2. The quality of the decision packages and analysis is generally poor to mediocre (with several notable exceptions); however, these results are better than anticipated. The zero-base budgeting process significantly reduced (by about 50%) the amount of additional funds requested by the agencies, but major shifts (reductions) from current programs to high priority new programs did not take place, although there were some significant internal shifts within departments. In addition, the opportunities for reducing costs and improving effectiveness were not adequately identified and evaluated. This was to be expected, and quality improvements will come naturally as agency managers continue to use this type of analysis. [*Author's note:* My very critical observation of poor to mediocre quality of the analysis was based on Texas Instruments standards, which will probably never be achieved across a large government organization. However, the analysis was significantly better than any done previously and, after all, Rome was not built in a day!]
3. Most of the severe problems encountered this year can be avoided next year because of this year's learning experience as well as a few minor changes in the process. Also, the agencies should then be able to channel their efforts into improving the quality and depth of analysis.

---

*Phyrr, Peter A. *Zero Base Budgeting*, pages 130–136. © 1973, John R. Wiley and Sons. Reprinted with permission.

4. Some agency managers were negative about zero-base budgeting when they did not get the funds they desired.
5. This critique should be continued by working with each agency to identify those activities and operations that need substantial analysis and improvement so that the agencies can direct their efforts toward improving these areas before starting zero-base budgeting next year.

III. Implementation Problems

A. General
   1. There is little incentive in government to be cost effective, and most cost savings were made by agency directors or the Budget Bureau by eliminating packages rather than by improving the effectiveness of the operation.
   2. Some managers thought this would be a one-year exercise, with no budget decisions made from the packages, and package quality reflected this attitude.
   3. Many managers developed their packages and rankings to protect their people.
   4. The changes in the budget process every year confuse agency managers, put them at the bottom of the learning curve, force revisions in internal planning and control procedures, and reduce agency commitment to any given procedure.
   5. Large agencies and the Budget Bureau had mechanical problems of handling and analyzing the large volume of decision packages. (Next year more packages will be developed, since managers will do a more detailed analysis and will expand the process deeper into their field operations.)

B. Planning: There is a general lack of planning (including expenditure guidelines) across state government. Therefore, some of the effort that went into zero-base budgeting was wasted because some basic policy decisions had not been made before developing the packages and rankings.
   1. Policy decisions made at the Governor's review should have been made before developing decision packages.
   2. Many decision packages were prepared that had no chance of being funded.
   3. The dollar increments between the various levels of effort identified for many activities were too large. These packages were revised if time permitted, but in many

cases the packages were discarded and arbitrary decisions were made to determine the budget level. For example, an activity might have three levels of effort: 80, 105, and 130% of the current budget level. The 80% level might have been unrealistically low, with a 90% level being a realistic funding expectation, and the 130% level being unrealistically high, with 110% being a realistic level. (This is a common problem regardless of planning or expenditure guidelines, but it can become a major problem without guidelines, as it was this year in some agencies.)

4. The 80 and 115% expenditure guidelines were misunderstood by many agencies, which required that each activity have a minimum level of 80% or less, and often had one of the packages bring the level of effort to 115%.

C. Decision Package Formulation

1. Managers spend a great deal of time deciding the activities around which decision packages should be developed. This initial determination, with the many false starts and revisions, took about one month. This should not be a problem next year since agencies can determine before the start of the process exactly where they want packages developed—based on this year's experience.

2. Cost information was poor in many cases for several reasons:
   •Budget units encompass too many discrete activities, which makes cost allocation difficult and time consuming.
   •Many managers who prepared packages do not ever see budgets or actual costs.
   •Not enough detailed cost information was shown on the packages to evaluate the estimates, nor to evaluate line items such as travel or equipment purchases—which can be modified even if the package is approved.

3. Quantitative information was not identified and/or available, and it will probably take several years to develop adequate measures and data.

4. Alternative ways of performing each function were not adequately identified or examined; many managers did not seem to consider seriously any type of organizational changes.

5. Projections are probably not needed on the form since less than 1% of the packages actually commit the state to

increases in future years that exceed 10% (which was the guideline for identifying projections). These few packages that have projections can be readily anticipated and identified and reasonable projections could still be made if this section were not on the form.

6. There was no uniformity of approach in developing decision packages for·similar operations or institutions within each agency, much less among agencies.

D. Ranking
1. Agencies with large numbers of packages (exceeding 250–300) had difficulties in producing a single agency ranking. This problem was created primarily by sheer volume, but was compounded by a lack of detailed knowledge and understanding of the activities by middle and top level agency managers, and the lack of an effective ranking procedure.
2. The fragmentation of activities into detailed functions and levels of effort made it difficult for top level managers not intimately familiar with each program to understand each package and relate its importance to the program as a whole.
3. The final agency rankings were not evaluated or measured against any goals or objectives (since there was no planning) to evaluate the impact of various levels of funding, and some of the funding recommendations seemed to be a package-by-package accumulation of costs without framework or direction.

E. Governor's Review and Budget Bureau Management
1. Some agency directors had the impression that their rankings and priorities were sacred and were extremely unhappy about the changes recommended by the Budget Bureau.
2. Many agencies were not given enough lead time before the Governor's review to analyze and understand the Budget Bureau's questions and recommendations.
3. Packages and rankings were not discussed at all in some reviews (where the Governor concentrated on policy decisions and summary analyses prepared by the Budget Bureau—which based its analyses on the packages and rankings), and a few agencies had the feeling that zero-base budgeting was not really used.
4. The computer system had many start-up and maintenance problems that required a great deal of time from

the Budget Bureau analysts. These problems occurred because of the last minute haste in which the system was designed and programmed, and will be corrected before the beginning of zero-base budgeting next year.

IV. Recommendations for FY 1974

A. General
1. The state needs to outline a program for a comprehensive planning, budgeting, and control (detail budgeting, accounting, quarterly allotment, performance auditing, etc.) system. Such a total system would improve the effectiveness of each of the parts. There are current efforts in each area that need to be coordinated and planned if they are to be effective, and this planning problem is compounded since several efforts are not in the same stage of development or implementation.
2. The planning and zero-base budgeting procedures need to be firmly established and maintained for the remainder of the Governor's administration. Only minor modifications to the FY 1973 format and forms are needed, so that if the agencies know that the zero-base budgeting process will be continued with only minor modifications in format, they can make their plans accordingly. By the time the next governor is elected, agencies should produce a good product with reasonable efficiency, with the process standing a good chance of being continued in following administrations.
3. Programs and budget units need to be redefined in many agencies.
4. The agencies and the Budget Bureau need a compatible computer system to handle the volume of data and analyses. This system must meet internal agency needs, with the agency program feeding the Budget Bureau system. This system should also be compatible with the total planning, budgeting, and control concept.
B. Planning
1. There needs to be formal planning before zero-base budgeting to set basic priorities and policy decisions and provide agencies with an anticipated funding range.
2. The anticipated funding range should reflect the established priorities, have a 5 to 10% range, yet neither guarantee any agency the lower limit of the range if it cannot be justified by the decision packages nor limit the

agencies from requesting an amount in excess of the
upper limit of the range.

3. This planning process needs to be kept simple so that
we do not develop a full PPB system, which is being
abandoned by most states.

4. The agencies should be allowed to present their program objectives to the Governor, using discussions and
reviews rather than long text presentation as much as
possible. The Governor can then establish his priorities,
policy decisions, and anticipated funding ranges. We
must then ensure that the agencies establish internal
planning policy and guidelines for the managers who
will be preparing and ranking decision packages.

C. Decision Packages

1. Packages should be formatted to include detail cost information: personal services (salaries, benefits) plus operating expenses by account (19 accounts). This information can be computerized to produce the detailed budgets for the agencies as well as the Budget Bureau, with
the exception of the detail for personal services that can
be provided to a large degree from computer printouts of
the merit system.

2. More uniformity in package preparation, measures of effectiveness, and so on, can be achieved through Budget
Bureau coordination and internal agency planning and
management.

D. Ranking

1. The organizational level within each agency to which
the rankings are consolidated needs to vary by agency,
depending primarily on volume of packages. The volume problem experienced this year can be readily
solved by stopping the consolidation of rankings at a
manageable level, such as program or department.
Agency managers can then spend their time reviewing
these rankings, can identify their priorities among departments or programs, and can establish the cutoff levels for each ranking for several predetermined levels of
agency funding (corresponding to guidelines, goal expenditure level, etc.). This process will take about half
as much time as physically merging all packages yet will
not force the Governor to make trade-offs among 350
separate rankings, since each agency will have made
these trade-off analyses and recommendations for the

Governor's review. The final funding level can then be established, at one of the predetermined levels or some different funding level, with any desired modifications in packages and rankings.

2. More emphasis needs to be given to evaluating the impact that various funding levels have on program goals and objectives.

E. Governor's Review and Budget Bureau Management

1. The procedures to be followed in preparing the FY 1974 budget need to be established before January 1972 and communicated to the agencies so that they can prepare internally and develop the necessary planning and computer aids.

2. The Governor's review time can be shortened because of the planning process and the greatly improved quality of decision packages and rankings anticipated. A formal second review for all agencies probably will not be needed.

3. If the detail costing is shown on each package, the time required for this final step can be greatly shortened.

V. *Conclusion*

In summary, we believe that the pain and anxieties experiences this year can be greatly reduced in future years with the continuance of zero-base budgeting integrated with an effective planning process; and that great improvement in quality can reasonably be expected through the natural learning process and the improvements in agency and Budget Bureau management and analysis that will come with experience.

Chapter 16

Plan and Budget Preparation: Process, Organization, Accountabilities

Presuming that the value of a budget and the budgeting process are understood and the necessary operational prerequisites and policy decision exist, management should now be ready to begin to construct an operating plan and budget. This next step, as was indicated in Chapter 15, requires the existence of an additional prerequisite. Simply, if the budget is to be developed successfully, management must select/design and implement a budget preparation procedure.

Generally, a procedure can be defined as a system or a systematic way of accomplishing an identified objective. As is the case in most complex management processes, the budget preparation procedure involves two fundamental components. One part is essentially technical in nature: focusing on the mechanics and arithmetic of calculating budgeted costs. That is, it addresses the techniques and technology of such activities as:

—projecting workload (volume);
—converting volume estimates into resource requirements and revenue estimates;
—converting resource requirements into direct cost estimates;
—calculating indirect costs; and
—adjusting revenues and total costs to obtain the necessary equality.

The other component of the procedure can be viewed as being basically behavioral in character. It addresses both the organizational and interpersonal relationship aspects of the preparation process as well as the management of the entire process.

The technical aspects of budget preparation have been described in substantial detail by other authors. Therefore, the focus on this chapter will be limited to the behavioral part of the procedure, emphasizing the organization and management of the process. From time to time, the discussion unavoidably will touch lightly on a mechanism issue. However, readers interested in an in-depth knowledge of the technical aspects of budget preparation should go beyond these brief comments to the references provided in the Appendix, Suggested Readings, and Bibliography.

The Process

Due to both its general complexity and reiterative nature, perhaps, the most efficient approach to understanding the organization and management of the budget process is to begin by considering an overview of the entire preparation process. The individual steps involved in preparing an operating plan and budget, as well as the general sequence of effort, are listed in Table 16-1. Each of the identified steps is discussed below.[1]

The discussion of procedural process not only defines the anatomy of budget preparation but also provides the foundation and background for the examination of the related matters of budgetary organization and accountabilities. These topics are addressed in the latter portion of the chapter.

Phase I—Strategic Planning

1. Environmental Statement. The first step in a systematic corporate planning and budgeting process is the analysis of the hospital's present operating environment. Perhaps this analysis can be accomplished most effectively through the development of an environmental statement which sets out:

—the strengths and weaknesses of the institution;

—the nature of the institution's role within the community's health delivery system;

—the characteristics of, and any changes in, the population being served; and

—any other data which can be used to provide an objective "snapshot" of the hospital's current situation.

---

[1]It should be recognized that, though budget preparation is basically a sequential process, various steps in the process can be simultaneously accomplished. However, for purposes of simplifying the discussion of this chapter, the process is described in a step-by-step fashion.

Table 16-1

Sequential Steps:

Strategic Planning, Operational Planning and Budgeting Process

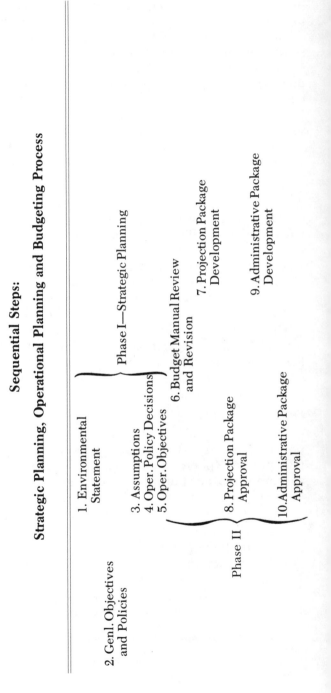

Table 16-1 (continued)

11. Genl. Budget Meeting

Phase III { 12. Technical Budget Meeting
13. Admin. Meetings
14. Decision Package Preparation
15. Admin. Meetings Ranking Decisions

Operational Planning Phase IV {
16. Revenue Budget Preparation
17. Detail Specification
18. Tentative Budget
19. Budget Integration
21. Budget Completion

Budgeting Phase V { 20. Administrative Review

22. Budget Approval } Phase VI

Phase VII { 23. Implementation
24. Feedback

The purpose of the environmental statement is to specify "where the hospital is." As such, it is necessarily the first step in the process, for it provides the benchmarks to be used in weighing all other budgetary decisions.

The environmental statement need not be a lengthy document. Its goal is simply to define succinctly those existent factors which will affect the hospital's operational performance and which, therefore, must be taken into account in planning and budgeting.

2. General Objective and Policies. Clearly stated and defined objectives and policies are a necessity for efficient and effective budgeting. General corporate objectives are needed to give the total budget effort a uniform direction. Without clearly stated objectives, each responsibility center and/or program area may attempt to follow its own internal imperatives, pursuing goals which, while perhaps not antithetical either to the goals of other program areas or the hospital as a whole, do not reflect the optimal use of available resources. The counter productivity of this kind of uncontrolled effort is obvious.

The rationale underlying the need for well defined corporate policies is not unlike the above reason for clearly stated objectives. Defined policies, like objectives, provide uniform direction. From the perspective of budget preparation, policies and objectives differ only in terms of their level of detail. Objectives assume a "macro view," focusing on broad goals. Conversely, policies have a narrower focus, aiming at clarifying the details of budget preparation and establishing basic internal operating parameters. Policies assure that the budget is developed with each responsibility center and program area utilizing the same information and preparation rules.

Operationally, the most convenient and efficient mechanism for setting general objectives and policies is the budget preparation process. Within this process, the definition of general objectives and policies flows from the environmental statement.

The setting of general objectives is:

—to provide the community with needed health services at an acceptable level of quality and at the least possible cost; and
—to provide needed care to patients regardless of their ability to pay.

The setting of policies is:

—to prevent restricting the use of the hospital to a particular group of physicians or surgeons; and
—to operate the hospital as a self-sufficient entity, etc.

This illustrates the sequential movement of activity which characterizes the entire budget preparation process. In setting objectives and policies, recognition must be given, if objectives and policies are to be realistic (capable of accomplishment) to the existent operating environment. Hence, general objectives and policies must be measured against the environment and tempered, as necessary, to produce a practical "fit."

A hospital's general objectives indicate what it is that the institution, as a whole, wishes to accomplish. Its policies act to modify its objectives by establishing the basic operating parameters within which the hospital's goals are to be accomplished. Typically, a hospital's objectives and policies will remain relatively constant from year to year. Nevertheless, since the operating environment is dynamic, these two factors should be reviewed and reaffirmed, at least on an annual basis.

3. Assumptions. The testing and setting of assumptions represents the first and the basic element of the planning and budgeting process. Assumptions can be described as statements which project future events and the resulting future environment. In this context, they can be operationally defined as statements describing future major developments which will affect hospital operations but whose occurrence is beyond the direct control of hospital management, e.g.,

—enactment of national health insurance or state rate review; or
—shift in the demographic character of the hospital's catchment area; etc.

Assumptions are, by definition, projections or estimates of the future. As such, they may well prove to be erroneous in the final analysis. At their inception, however, they represent management's "best judgment" as to what will happen. Hence their development should be based on a careful analysis and evaluation of objective and subjective data concerning both the local and national legislative and operating environments. Also, they should project events into the future up to the point of the hospital's planning horizon. That is, up to that point in the future, wherein the availability of additional information will neither improve nor change any current operational decision.[2]

---

[2]The length of a hospital's planning horizon will differ both with the nature of the hospital's environment and the type of assumption being considered. The general principle, however, is to limit the length of assumptions to that point in the future wherein additional input will not change current decisions. For example, if, in terms of day-to-day operational decisions, events four years into the future have no effect on current operating decisions, there is no need to project operational assumptions four years ahead. (Continued)

The notion of a planning horizon and the interrelationship of assumptions and operational decisions are two vital concepts which are often overlooked. The principal benefit of the assumption setting process is not the academic exercise—the hypothesizing, debating, and testing—of their abstract determination. Rather the value of assumptions lies in their conversion into a pragmatic statement of operational implications.

Operational implications can be defined, in working terms, as simply the recognition of the opportunities, threats, and the resulting actions which must be taken in order to capitalize on the environment which the assumptions predict. By translating assumptions into operational implications, the hospital is able to establish both the base line and the direction for all the decisions which follow in the budgeting process.

The notion of a planning horizon complements this "translation process" in that it sets the outer time limit for projections. Therefore, as opposed to setting assumptions as far into the future as the imagination can wander, one needs only to make projections and determine their implications up to the point of the planning horizon.

The existence of a planning horizon is also important in terms of long-range planning. The length of long-range planning cannot exceed the planning horizon, for no assumptions upon which to base the plan exist beyond the planning horizon. Hence, one can only plan ahead, i.e., develop a long-range plan, as far into the future as realistic and usable assumptions extend.

Presuming a hospital's planning horizon is three years, a long-range plan extending three years into the future could be developed. Based on the assumptions and their operational implications the results desired to exist three years into the future could be defined. These results would represent the objective or goal of the long-range plan. The activity, which must be undertaken in the first year of the plan if the objective is to be achieved by the third year, represents the current operational plan and budget. Thus, the operational plan and budget for any single year are a consistent part of a larger (longer) plan. This longer range plan extends as far into the future as the hospital's assumptions extends to the planning horizon and, if necessary, is modified as assumptions are modified and revised goals are established.

Two other factors should be recognized in regard to assump-

Typically, a hospital's planning horizon is three to five years. However, in the case of capital decisions the horizon might be longer. In each instance, assumption must be tested in terms of their impact on current decisions. If there is no impact then, at least at that point in time, the assumption is not needed.

tions. First, assumptions differ from either environmental statements or objectives. Assumptions are future-oriented. That is, they are predictions of events and circumstances which will take place and exist some months or years ahead. In contrast, environmental statements are oriented to the present. They are statements of conditions which exist now.

Assumptions also differ from objectives in that an assumption describes an uncontrollable event which is expected to take place. An objective represents just the opposite condition. It is a controllable event or result which is the desired outcome of a deliberate set of actions and which can be achieved through the successful performance of those actions.

The second point is that assumptions provide the first opportunity for the reiterative nature of the budget process to take effect. Based on the assumptions and their operational implications one might, in order to provide a better "fit" with the expected environment, "go back" and revise corporate objectives and policies. This opportunity for an "in process" revision should not be viewed as either wasted energy or as "sloppy workmanship" in the development of the previous steps. Rather, it is part of the "checks and balances" which are implicit in a sound budget preparation process and which should be taken advantage of both to verify previous steps and to provide a consistent total product.

4. Operating Policy Decisions. The next step in the process is an outgrowth of both the environmental statement and the determination of the operational implications of the hospital's assumptions. This step is actually composed of two substeps. The first is the setting of program priorities and the second is the establishment of a funding guideline.

The setting of program priorities can be viewed, in its most basic form, as a pragmatic application of program budgeting techniques. In Chapter 15, program budgeting was described as a mechanism used at the "macro" level, to assure the coordination of the allocation of resources among programs, i.e., to coordinate the allocation of resources among groups of activities which are all directed toward the same goal or end result. It was also pointed out that:

—program budgeting, for a variety of reasons, has not achieved all of its hoped for value; and

—if used in a pragmatic manner—without overemphasis on requiring that all processes in the hospital be deterministically quantified—and with a careful understanding of its limitations, program budgeting can be a useful management technique.

Possibly, the simplest and most pragmatic approach to applying the principles of program budgeting is to evaluate the environmental statement and operational implications of the assumptions in terms of identifying those activities (program areas) requiring priority attention. For example, the environmental statement identifies a lack of access to primary care in the hospital's service area and it is assumed that:

—the community's demand for primary care will increase, and
—the local health systems agency (comprehensive health facilities and services planning agency) will identify primary care as an underavailable resource and will link approval of nonprimary care projects to the availability of primary care.

Then, one could establish as an operational implication of the assumptions that there is need to establish primary care resources. Given the lack of such resources, as identified in the environmental statement, this need can be identified as a priority area.

The identification of a particular program as a priority area represents only part of the decision which must be made. The level of priority or the relative ranking, i.e., whether the program's priority is 1st, 2nd, or nth, must be determined. In traditional program budgeting relative rankings are determined in the main through quantitative and/or pseudoquantitative analysis. A substantially more simple and perhaps more appropriate approach, in view of the nature of the hospital's environment and product, is to make these same decisions on a subjective basis using such techniques as sensitivity analysis.

The matter of establishing relative priorities is, to a large extent, an abstract exercise unless the priorities are laid against a funding guideline. If adequate funds are not available to support activity in a particular program area, the identification of that program as a priority is operationally meaningless. Therefore, to avoid wasted effort and the adverse motivational effect of unmet expectations, general funding levels must be set along with priorities. The resulting product can be viewed as an "operational priority listing," i.e., that segment of the total rank ordering which actually will be undertaken.

The establishment of a funding guideline is a complex problem. If the hospital is located in a state which has implemented rate review, one distinct set of factors must be taken into account. If a large proportion of the hospital's revenues is generated through cost-based retrospective reimbursement, another, and different, set of constraints must be considered. The potential of using debt financing, as well as the institution's current and future general financial condition and surplus position, also must be evaluated.

Given the myriad of variables, it is an erroneous over simplification to attempt to define a set of general rules for the establishment of a funding guideline. All that realistically can be said is that:

—a funding guideline must be established;
—the guideline should be determined based on a careful evaluation of the hospital's financial condition, and its ability to generate constant or increasing amounts of funds, e.g., debt, philanthropy, grants; and
—based on the evaluation an estimate can then be made as to the level of funds available, the corresponding general increase in expenses which can be tolerated, and the particular program areas which can be given operational priority.

The difficulty inherent in establishing program priorities and funding guidelines should not be underestimated. However, the importance of accomplishing both these steps successfully cannot be over emphasized. Two of the "keys" to a meaningful budget effort are that the process be both creditable and streamlined, i.e., wasted effort is avoided. Neither of these requirements can be achieved unless the operational policy step in the budget preparation process is carried out successfully.

The setting (and communication) of operational priorities streamlines budget preparation, in that it provides, at the outset of the process, clear direction as to the scope of effort toward which each program area should plan. By providing this direction, it helps to prevent a nonpriority area from wasting energies in the development of an ambitious plan which will not be funded. Moreover, by providing a clear initial indication of the direction of emphasis and priority, it avoids the detrimental impact of false expectations.

The budget preparation, because of its reiterative and adjustment/balance nature, is a process which is so laced with intrinsic uncertainty that its credibility is almost always in question. Compounding this inherent credibility problem by not making operational priorities clear from the outset acts only to heighten the risk of the process being viewed as a "paper exercise." Obviously, this is a perspective which must be avoided in both image and reality. The setting and communication of operational priorities can be instrumental in avoiding both of these potential pitfalls.

5. *Operating Objectives.* The last step in Phase I is the setting of operating objectives. This step is a culminating step and as such is fundamentally a translation process.

Step 3, Assumptions and Operational Implications, defined what "needed to be done" in order to capitalize upon the hospital's future environment. Step 4, Operating Policy Decisions, refined the universe of "opportunities" to a subset of programs representing operational priorities, i.e., programs wherein actual operational activity will be undertaken. Step 5, Operating Objectives, translates operational priorities into specific, measurable goals which are obtainable within the budget period.

Recognition of two fundamental points is central to the successful completion of this step. First, operating objectives must be measurable in terms of objective indicator(s).

Without measurable objectives it is obviously difficult to determine either the resource inputs to be devoted to a given program or the inter- and intraprogram trade offs. Moreover, without measurable objectives the management control value of the budget process is substantially hampered. This is the case, for the measurable objectives represent the standard against which performance is to be judged. Without this standard, line management is in an uncertain position, subject to performance evaluation on the basis of only subjective judgment. Hence, measurable objectives are not only fundamental components of the entire budget preparation process, but also the critical variable which acts to "drive" the subsequent phases and steps in budget preparation.

Using the previous example, involving primary care, the operating objective for this program area could be assumed to be as follows:

—to provide the community with increased access to primary care as measured by the delivery of 50,000 primary care visits during the budget period.

This assumed objective is specific, quantified, and capable of measurement, i.e., a patient encounter tabulating system can be installed to accumulate data on the number of patient visits delivered. This objective thus meets management's needs in regard to both resource allocation decisions (it establishes the magnitude of effort), and operational control (it sets out the performance standard).

In terms of the conditions of the foregoing example, however, this objective is not acceptable, for it is not obtainable within the budget period. Recall, that one of the key factors supporting the operational priority for this program was the existing lack of access of primary care. Given this environmental condition, it is unreasonable to expect to move from a position of no or minimal activity to a large scale operation within a single budget period. Therefore, to set an objective reflective of large-scale activity is operationally unrealistic.

Rather than use the above objective, one should think in terms of a long-range plan. The goal of 50,000 visits may be the appropriate long-range objective. However, this goal can be achieved only through the successful completion of a series of sequential activities. The objective for the first budget period should be set within the context of the long-run goal, but should only "reach" to include those activities which can be accomplished within the budget period.

In this case, a more realistic objective might be:

—to provide the basis for increasing the community's access to primary care by developing a master plan of action and implementing phases 1 (Organization and Structural Requirements) and 2 (Facilities Development) of that plan.

This objective is obtainable as an initial effort and is thus a realistic performance standard. Also, it is measurable in that at the end of the period one can review progress and determine if the master plan exists and if its first two phases have been implemented.

Two additional points should be noted. First the operating objectives which are set at this phase of the budget preparation process are "macro" in nature, corresponding to the "program" level of activity. Detailed or "micro" level objectives should be set at a later stage and should involve a different level of management in the decision process. The goal at this point is not to eliminate line management discretion, imagination, and decision making. It is to refine the basic direction being taken by the hospital by setting out a specific program objective.

The second point which should be noted is that operating objectives should be tested and balanced against the General Objectives and Policies which were established in Step 2. The purpose of this testing is to assure consistency of the total operational plan and budget. It represents just one of the several checks and balances which can be imposed by viewing budget preparation as a reiterative process.

The foregoing discussion of Phase I has admittedly been detailed. This detail, however, is justified by the importance of this "front end" activity not only to the design of the final product but also to the usefulness and the success of the total effort. Often, there is a compulsion to rush into the "numbers" aspects of budget preparation with a resulting tendency to give the "strategic planning" (Phase I) aspect only a "light touch." This compulsion, while understandable within the context of an operating setting, must be carefully controlled if the budget effort is to be valuable. If it is not controlled, the hospital's plans will reflect its budget— as opposed to the more critical relationship of the budget reflecting management's plan.

Phase I lays the foundation for the construction of the actual operating plan and financial budget. While this phase is key to the success of the entire process, its actual accomplishments should not be overestimated. Phase I provides for the setting of corporate direction and the giving of a quantitative character or goal to that direction. However, it does not answer the basic operational question of how the institution "moves" to accomplish its goal. The development of this answer lies in the completion of Phases II through V. Its implementation lies in Phases VI and VII.

Phase II

Phase II can be viewed as being principally administrative in character. It is in this phase that the necessary materials (instructions, forms, data, etc.) for operational planning and budgeting are developed, reviewed, and approved.

6. Budget Preparation Manual: Review. Step 6, though the initial component of this phase, could be accomplished simultaneously with the foregoing steps. Essentially, this step involves the review and, if necessary, the revision of the hospital's budget preparation procedure.

Ideally, the budget preparation process should be set out in a procedure manual which describes the mechanics of preparing the operating plan and budget. In terms of content, the manual can be viewed as consisting of two basic components:

—a projection package; and
—an administrative package.

Each of these "packages" is discussed in detail below. At this point it should suffice to recognize that the projection package is simply a report of projected workloads for both the institution in total and the volume dependent responsibility center.[3] In its final form the projection package loses its independent package identity and is

---

[3] An example of a volume dependent responsibility center is inpatient dietary service, for its costs vary with volume; executive management is an example of a volume independent responsibility center.

subsumed within the administative package.[4] The administrative package, in turn, can be viewed as an "instruction book" which provides the forms, supportive data, and directions necessary for completing the forms and producing a plan and budget.

The purpose of this step, is not to examine and approve the materials which are being developed for future use. Rather, its objective is to review the previous years' material and process, and to identify areas where improvements could be made in terms of clarity, streamlining of the effort, usefulness of additional information, etc. These improvements, after their approval, are then to be incorporated into either the development of the current materials or in the operation of the process.

In simplest terms, this step provides the opportunity to learn from previous experience and errors. As such, it is basically a "stand alone" step which can be accomplished at any point in the annual budget cycle prior to the preparation of the administrative package.

7. Projection Package: Development. The concept of "packages" was first mentioned, as part of the discussion of the mechanics of zero base budgeting, in Chapter 15. It is a concept which will keep reappearing throughout the discussion for it is an integral component of the budget preparation. In this context, the notion of "packages" refers to groups (or packages) of information which are transferred for purposes of communicating either the raw data necessary for decisions or actual decisions between different levels of management.

The first of these packages is the workload projection package. This is the case, for the projection package provides the workload estimates necessary for the development of the details of the operating plan and the calculation of specific resource requirements.

In terms of content, the projection package consists of forecast of:

—total patient days;
—patient days per patient care unit; and
—workload for each of the other volume dependent responsibility centers.

Of these, the patient day forecast is, perhaps, the most critical projection. This is the case, for the patient day projection represents both an independent estimate of workload and, as Table

---

[4]It should also be recognized that the decision packages flow from the administrative package.

Table 16-2

Workload Forecasting*

Department	Workload Element	Forecasting Technique
1-Total Hospital	Total Patient Days	Regression Analysis
2-Patient Care Unit	Monthly Patient Day Projection	Exponential Smoothing
3-Dietary	Meals	Meals/Patient Day x Patient Days
4-Laundry	Pounds of Laundry	Pounds/Patient Day x Patient Days
5-Radiology	Relative Value Units (RVU)	RVU/Patient Day** x Patient Days
6-Laboratory	Relative Value Units (RVU)	RVU/Patient Day** x Patient Days
7-Housekeeping	Volume of Space	Subjective Estimate Based on Volume and Intensity
8-Emergency	Visits	Regression Analysis

*Readers seeking a more detailed discussion of forecasting techniques should refer to: Lash, Myles, P., "Development of An Expense Budgeting Procedure," thesis, University of Michigan Program in Hospital Administration (available from University Microfilms, Ann Arbor, Michigan as Hospital Abstract AC1-6955); and Griffith, John R., *Quantitative Techniques for Hospital Planning and Control;* Wheelwright, Steven, and Makridakis, Spyros, *Forecasting Methods for Management.*

**Relative value units/patient day should be adjusted to reflect changes in medical technology. This can be accomplished either subjectively and/or through trend analysis techniques.

16-2 illustrates, the base projection upon which many of the other responsibility center workload forecasts are built.

The forecasting technique utilized by any particular hospital will vary with that hospital's situation. The management principle is simply to identify a model or technique which consistently produces a "good fit." This can be accomplished by testing alternative forecasting approaches against historical data and evaluating the "fit" between actual volume and estimated workload. In evaluating "fit," the notion of relevant ranges, which was discussed in Chapter 15, should be borne in mind. In this instance the point is simply that if the estimate is consistently within the relevant range of actual, then the "fit" can be considered acceptable.

Table 16-2 lists, for several major responsibility centers, the workload element to be estimated and a possible forecasting technique. It should be recognized that other techniques—both more and less complicated in nature—can and should be used if they result in an acceptable "fit" with less effort or produce a better "fit" for either the same or a justifiable level of additional effort. Readers interested in additional information on forecasting should refer to the Suggested Readings and the Bibliography.

8. Projection Package: Approval. Prior to its incorporation into the administrative package, the projection package should be reviewed and approved. The organizational focus for review and approval will be discussed below. At this point it should just be recognized that, for purposes of accuracy, the volume estimates should be reviewed from the perspective of the impact of such factors as changes in the demographic character of the hospital's service area, technological changes in the practice of medicine, etc., and on historical trends. To the extent that such factors are operative, the mathematically forecasted workloads should be subjectively adjusted based on "best estimates."

As an aside, it should be noted that the projection package can be reviewed and approved together with the other portions of the administrative package in step 10. However, a separate review and approval step is suggested both to facilitate budget preparation by allowing activity to take place simultaneously whenever possible, and to simplify the review process.

9. Administrative Package: Preparation. The administrative package is the basic package for communicating budget preparation instructions and information to line management. It includes the data developed in the projection package—tailored to each hospital department. The total patient day forecast is provided to all departments; also, specific departmental workload estimates are provided to those departments having responsibility centers which are volume dependent—as well as:
—a cover letter from the administrator;
—a budget calendar;

—the materials developed in Phase I;

—decision package form and instructions;

—historical volume and cost data;

—personnel budget detail forms and instructions;

—current personnel complement, wage, and benefit data;

—supplies and other expense budget detail forms and instructions; and

—capital budget forms and instructions

Excerpts from an example administrative package are presented in Appendix 16.

In reviewing this Appendix it should be recognized that several departments contribute to its construction. The relative roles and responsibilities of the involved departments are detailed in later sections of this chapter.

10. Administrative Package: Approval. This step is the final step before direct line management involvement in budget preparation. Essentially, it is just a "sign off" step wherein the administrative package is reviewed to assure that approved revisions, as identified in Step 6, have been incorporated into the package and that the package is complete.

Phase III

Phase III can be characterized as being a communications phase. It consists of two staff meeting steps which interrelate in an additive manner.

11. General Budget Meeting. The first meeting is an introductory or general meeting which is designed for formally initiating the annual planning and budget preparation process for line management. The meeting should be "chaired" by either the hospital's chief operating or executive officer. Its agenda should focus on:

—reviewing and explaining the Phase I component of the administrative package;

—orienting line management to the basic budgeting procedure and process in a general fashion;

—reemphasizing the value to all levels of management of the budget preparation process and the budget document; and

—making clear the nature and the extent of the budget preparation support and aid which is available, upon request, to line management.

The tone of the meeting should tend toward informality and openness. Expository presentations should be as brief as practicable.

Questions from the floor should be encouraged and sufficient time should be allotted for an extensive question and answer period.

12. Technical Budget Meeting. The second communication meeting is substantially more technical in nature, focusing on the specific mechanics of the budget procedure and budget preparation. Operationally, this step may involve either a single meeting or a series of meetings. Moreover, the meeting(s) may be organized on either a total hospital basis or on the basis of program or subprogram areas. The logistics of these meetings should be shaped to complement the history, character, and budgetary sophistication of the hospital's staff. To the extent that operational planning and budgeting represent a new and/or complex undertaking, the number of meetings should be increased.

In terms of content, the technical meetings should concentrate on discussing the administrative package. Each section of the package should be reviewed; with particular emphasis placed on:

—explaining the mechanics and results and opportunities for revision of the projection package;
—clarifying the causal relationship of workload projections to personnel and supplies and other expenses budgeted;
—making clear the nature and the mechanics of each of the steps involved in preparing decision packages and detailed personnel, supplies and other expenses, and capital budgets; and
—reiterating the importance of properly meeting the due dates identified in the budget calendar.

As was the case with the general meeting, the tone of the technical meeting(s) should lean toward informality and openness. The meeting(s) should be "chaired" by either the director of the fiscal services division, the budget officer or a designated member of their staff.

In addition to providing information, the goal of the technical meeting(s) should be to establish and/or reinforce a feeling of mutual trust and problem solving between line management and the fiscal services division. To assist in accomplishing this, expository presentations should be secondary to answering questions from the floor. Also, the support services which the fiscal services division is ready to provide to line management should be clearly identified, with line management being encouraged to utilize these services whenever possible.

Phase IV—Operational Planning

As has been the case in the previous phases, Phase IV builds on the foregoing work. This phase, however, differs significantly from the others in two key respects.

First, it is an operational, as opposed to a preparational, phase. The previous steps have all contributed toward either specifying the design or laying the foundation for the development of the operating plan and budget. This phase draws together the outputs of these previous efforts and, using line management's imagination and initiative as catalysts, converts them into an initial or tentative operating plan and budget.

The second major distinction is addressed in more detail later in this chapter. At this point, it is sufficiently to recognize that it is in Phase IV that line management adopts an activist role. The work of Phases I and II could be accomplished largely apart from day-to-day line operations. Phase III involves the line manager. However, it is a passive involvement, centered on communications. It is not until Phase IV that the focus of activity shifts and line management becomes the principal factor in the process.

Table 16-3 is an expansion of Table 16-1. It identifies in more detail the specific steps which compose this phase. Appendix 16, the discussion of Chapter 15 (Zero Base Budgeting) and the discussion of Chapter 17 provide insight into the mechanics of each of the involved steps.

The point to be recognized is that the first segment of this phase, steps 13 and 14, produces the project and capital expenditure decision packages. These packages are then rank ordered in step 15. The final output of this phase is a ranked listing, which includes estimated costs of both approved capital expenditure and operating projects. This output, in turn, becomes the input for the next phase of the process.

Phase V—Budgeting

Phase V represents the detailed costing and financial data integration segment of the budget preparation process. With the exception of one step—20, Final Administrative Review—it is basically a computational and clerical phase, wherein the operational plan is converted into a traditional financial budget.

17. Detail Specification. The initial step in the phase involves two components. The first portion provides the basis for the metamorphosis of the operating plan into a financial budget by requiring that line management specify, in detail, the resources needed to carry out approved projects. In operational terms, line management should identify the number, position classification, and if appropriate, expected hiring date of all personnel (including the number and position classification of any personnel who will re-

Table 16-3
Budget Preparation Process: Phase IV Detail

13. Administrative Meetings 1–n: Responsibility Center/Department Level
(Objective of these meetings is to translate the hospital's environmental statement, assumptions, and operating policy and objective decisions into projects and activities at the responsibility center/department level. This translation process may involve a single meeting or a series of meetings. It is completed only when the responsibility center manager and his superior have, at least, reached general agreement as to the nature and direction of the budget period's operations and capital expenditures).

14. Preparation: Decision Packages
(Based on the decisions reached in step 13, line management develops decision packages which identify the activity—its benefits, costs, and alternatives. The nature of the activity and its benefits and alternatives should be defined in as much detail as is practicable. The cost of the activity should only be estimated with detailed costing pending further budgetary approvals.

Decision packages or decision forms should also be prepared for each potential capital expenditure.)

15. Administrative Meetings 1–n: Rank Ordering of Decision Packages
(This step involves a series of consecutive meetings wherein succeeding levels of management integrate and rank order decision packages prepared in the previous step. The general mechanics of this process were explained in Chapter 15.

It should be noted that, depending upon the budgetary experience of the hospital, this step may be preceded by another set of administrative meetings wherein the decision packages are reviewed for completeness, and, if necessary, revised prior to submission.

Capital expenditure decision packages also should be rank ordered at this point. As explained in Chapter 17, the process for ranking these expenditure alternatives may differ somewhat from the project ranking process. For example, the ranking process for small capital items—expenditures of under $x—may involve successive levels of management only up to the program level. Similarly, the ranking process for large items may involve an interdisciplinary committee, successive levels of management, a combination of the two, cr some other process).

16. Revenue Budget Preparation
(In conjunction with, but apart from, the above activities, the data from the projection package should be used to calculate the initial revenue budget. This budget is basically the product of the current charge structure, adjusted as appropriate for cost based reimbursement, multiplied by projected revenue center volumes of service).

ceive pay differentials) required for the project as well as the nature, timing, and amount of any other expenses, e.g., travel, consulting, printing, which are anticipated. In the case of capital expenditure projects, the amount of the expenditure and its timing should be identified.

Specification of project detail is deferred to this point in the procedure in order both to minimize wasted effort and to increase the credibility of the entire budgeting and operational planning procedure. If detailed project costing were allowed to take place at an earlier point, line managers would be required to invest substantial time and effort in specifying the resource requirements for projects which subsequently would not obtain approval. To the extent that this occurred, effort would be wasted and line management's acceptance of the budgeting and planning process would deteriorate. Both of these pitfalls can be avoided by delaying detailed project specification, at least, until the initial project approval decisions have been made.

The second component of this step is the conversion of line management's detailed resource specifications into actual dollars. This aspect of the process is basically a clerical and computational task and should be carried out primarily by the hospital's fiscal services division. Line management should be consulted, as necessary, to resolve questions and provide any needed additional detail. However, the prime accountability for converting the resource specifications into dollar costs should be the responsibility of the fiscal services division.

18. Tentative Budget Completion. The output of the above conversion process is the input for the generation of the hospital's tentative dollar budget. Organizing and aggregating the data developed in the foregoing step into the tentative budget are also basically clerical and computational tasks. Therefore, the fiscal services division should again have primary accountability for completing this step.

It is important to recognize that the budget which is produced in this step is only a tentative budget. This is the case because the budget, though consisting of approved projects, has not been matched against the revenue budgets. If in this matching process an imbalance exists which cannot be resolved through revision to the revenue budget, then obviously, either the expense and/or capital budgets must be revised. It is due to this possibility for adjustment and/or revision that the budget must still be considered as being tentative at this point.

19. Budget Integration. In step 16, the initial revenue budget was developed. It is identified as "initial," for it is essentially the product of the current charge structure multiplied by forecasted volume. In this step, the revenue budget of Step 16 is integrated with the tentative expense and capital budgets of Step 18.

The integration of these budgets is largely a mechanical task. It is done in order to determine if the necessary revenue/expense (both total dollar and cash) equalities exist. If they do, the budgets can be completed. However, if, as is more often the case, an imbalance exists then, an additional management judgment step is needed.

20. Final Administrative Review. Due to the accelerated rates of inflation in hospital costs, it is likely that there will be an imbalance between the initial revenue budget and the tentative expense and capital budgets. When such an imbalance occurs, senior management must make a series of decisions which will bring the two sets of budgets, i.e., revenue and expense, into balance on both a total and cash basis.

Generally, the first step in resolving any imbalance is focused on adjusting the revenue budget. The mechanics and pragmatics of setting charges have been discussed in detail in Chapter 8. These concepts should be applied in setting revised charges, at least, equal to economic costs. If, after adjusting the revenue budget an inequality still exists, then the expense and capital budgets must be revised. In this case, management must return to the rank ordering developed in Phase IV and defer a sufficient dollar amount of previously approved projects to bring expenses and revenues into equality.

Admittedly, deletion of a project at this point is a painful decision. However, it is a necessary decision to the financial health and perhaps survival, if the institution is to be preserved. Therefore, although the decision is necessary and justified it should be made with line management's full awareness of steps that have been taken to avoid it and the reasons why, even after these measures, it is still necessary. It is only with this kind of open communication and full understanding that the demoralizing effects of such decisions can be minimized.

21. Budget Completion. The final step in this phase is generation of the final revenue, expense, and capital budgets, based on the decisions of the previous step. The mechanics and accountabilities of this step are similar to those of step 18. Also included in this step is the conversion of these primary budgets into the final cash budget. The mechanics of developing a cash budget are discussed in detail in the Appendix to Chapter 14.

Phase VI and VII

By this point, the nature of Phase VI and VII can probably be intuitively deduced. Phase VI consists of a single step—22, board approval of the budget. If the above steps have been carefully carried out and the hospital's organizational system of financial checks and balances has been respected, with approvals being obtained at the necessary and appropriate times, then this step should present little problem being operationally no more than just a formality. Regardless of whether this step is a formality or a detailed line item review, it is a step which must be successfully completed if the budget is to have the institution's full legal support and commitment.

Phase VII is shown as consisting of only two steps, 23, Implementation and 24, Feedback. In theory, this characterization is correct. However, it must be recognized that each of these steps implicitly involves a multitude of substeps and tasks.

23. Implementation, refers to the operational function of carrying out the decisions made in the planning and budgeting process. Occasionally, effecting these decisions operationally may be a simple—or at least a relatively simple—matter. More often, however, it is a complex problem requiring the expert application of a variety of both general and technical managerial skills. An in-depth discussion of either the mechanics or the application of these skills is beyond the scope of this work. Readers desiring more information in this area should refer both to the Suggested Readings and the Bibliography.

24. Feedback, while perhaps not as technically complex as implementation, involves several aspects and subtleties. Moreover, as discussed in Chapter 15, the feedback process is, perhaps, the most critical contributing factor in realizing the full operational control potential of the budget. Due to the importance of this topic, it is discussed in detail in Chapter 18.

Organizational Structure

The foregoing has described the operational steps intrinsic to the development of a hospital's operating plan and budget. Admittedly, the content of any particular step, as well as the flow of steps, may be revised as the process is tailored to fit a given institution's operating environment and needs. However, as a generalized procedure, the above should serve as a valid baseline for the construction of an individual hospital's unique planning and budgeting procedures.

It is important to recognize that procedures, regardless of how well they may have been designed and drafted, are basically impotent. Like a road map, a procedure only identifies the route between points A and B; it does not, however, move one from point A to B. To transverse the route, a driving force is needed. In the case of planning and budgeting, the force that drives the process and implements the procedure is people.

Clearly, it is impossible to effectively develop and implement an operating plan and budget without the hospital staff at all levels cooperating and actively "working the problem." Equally obvious is the fact that if staff is to work efficiently, it must implement the planning and budgeting procedure within the framework of both a tightly designed organization structure and a carefully specified and coordinated set of staff accountabilities.

As was discussed in Chapter 3, a well managed hospital is generally the product of the efforts and intellects of a group of individuals who are organized to function both in concert and toward a common goal. Organization provides the mechanism for allocating responsibilities and channeling efforts such that the objectives of the institution can be efficiently and effectively achieved. Thus, sound organization in all areas of operation is one of the critical elements necessary for successful management.

Sound organization, however, can take a variety of forms.

Experience has demonstrated that while there is no single "right" organizational structure which can be recommended universally— certain patterns of organization have been found to be generally practicable. Moreover, certain principles can be applied with a high degree of uniformity. Specifically, the organization structure either should assist in assuring or provide the structure for:

—a system of management control checks and balances;
—complete allocation of all requisite duties;
—clear definition of responsibilites;
—coordination of responsibilities;
—operational decision flexibility; and
—a systematic policy decision process.

Utilizing these concepts, a prototype planning and budgeting organization structure can be defined. Figure 16-1 illustrates this prototype.

Figure 16-1

Prototype:

Planning and Budgeting Organization Structure

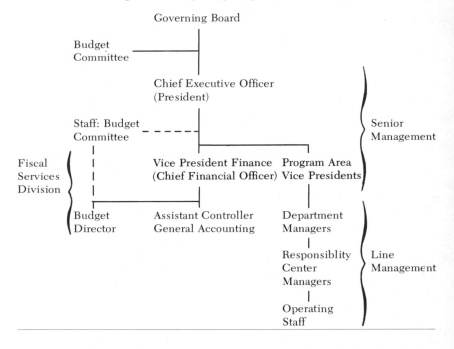

In considering this example, the reader should be careful to avoid the pitfall of adopting the proposed model as the universal answer to all planning and budgeting organizational questions. It is presented not as an "absolute solution" but rather as a benchmark or guideline for the tailoring of any particular institution's organization structure.

Accountabilities

The flow of authority is clearly documented in Figure 16-1. A final element, however is still missing.

To give the organization structure dimension, and to add the dynamics necessary to convert the process from paper procedure into actions, one must define staff accountabilities and relative roles. This step is needed not only to provide direction and control but also to provide a check and balance mechanism for assuring the coordination of all efforts.

Table 16-4 describes the accountabilities of the various staff levels and/or organizational units in terms of the itemized phases and steps of the process defined in the first part of this chapter.[5] The solid lines in the table indicate the staff group which carries the prime or principal accountability for the completion of a given step. Correspondingly, dotted lines indicate, where appropriate, the group(s) with a supporting or "staff" accountability for the same step.

While the table, for the most part, is self-explanatory, it may be of value to highlight several points.

Governing Board. As emphasized in Chapter 3, the governing board is vested by law with the ultimate authority and responsibility for managing all of a hospital's business. Therefore, the governing board is responsible for all phases of hospital operations, including financial operations.

In terms of operational planning and budgeting, this responsibility, at a minimum, is carried out through the review and approval of the final budget. In addition, the governing board, given the history and management style of the institution as well as its own prerogatives, may desire and have an ongoing involvement in the development of the plan and budget. From the perspective of obtaining expeditious decisions, increased governing board involvement—of a nonoperational, review and approval nature—is desirable. The points where this involvement should be focused are indicated (in Table 16-4) by dotted lines.

The organizational mechanics utilized to provide increased governing board involvement will obviously differ from one institution to another. However, as a guideline—if the board is large, meets infrequently, is uncomfortable or unproductive in dealing at its general meetings with operational details, etc.—the device of a Budget Committee (or Finance and Budget Committee) may prove to be quite useful. This committee should be board appointed and should consist of a membership which includes, at least, a majority of active board members. Its functions are to:[6]

—review annual and long-term budgets and detemine that forecasts are reasonably and accurately prepared;

---

[5]Table 16-4 is presented in the same design format as Table 16-1. This was done to allow both the authors and the reader to build upon the earlier material to produce a complete description of the planning.

[6]Cauana, Russell, A., *A Guide To Organizing The Hospital's Fiscal Services Division*, pages 12 and 13.

Table 16-4   Accountabilities: Operational Planning and Budgeting

Governing Board	Senior Management	Staff Budget Committee	Budget Director	Line Management	Fiscal Services Division
	1. Environmental Statement				
2. Genl. Objectives and Policies		Phase I			
	3. Assumptions				
	4. Oper. Policy Decisions				
	5. Oper. Objectives				
		6. Budget Manual Review and Revision			
			7. Projection Package Development		
	8. Projection Package Approval (Phase II)				
			9. Administrative Package Development		
	10. Administrative Package Approval				
	11. Genl. Budget Meeting				
			12. Technical Budget Mtg.	Phase III	
				13. Admin. Meetings	
				14. Decision Package Preparation	
				15. Admin. Meetings; Ranking Decisions	
		Phase IV	16. Revenue Budget Prep.		
				17. Detail Specification	
					18. Tentative Budget
					19. Budget Integration
	20. Administrative Review (Phase V)				21. Budget Completion
22. Budget Approval (Phase VI)				Phase VII	
				23. Implementation	
				24. Feedback	

Primary Accountability _____   Supporting (staff) Accountability - - - - - - -

—recommend budgets to the full board (or if appropriate the executive committee of the board) for their approval; and

—periodically review both operating results and, where significant budget variations are found, management's proposed of corrective action.[7]

Senior Management. The role of senior management can be summarized as consisting of the prime accountability not only for the generation of the Phase I materials but also, for:

—the approval of all subsequent general distribution planning and budgeting materials; and

—the determination of the specific components of the hospital's operating program.

In carrying out these accountabilities, it is vital that senior management recognize the necessity of its not acting in a vacuum. If the full motivational benefits of the planning and budgeting process are to be obtained, other components of the organization must be involved and contribute in a meaningful way to the development of these materials and the making of the requisite decision. The points of involvement and the groups to be involved in this participating approach are identified in the table by the dotted lines.

Staff Budget Committee. The creation and use of a staff level budget committee can be considered, perhaps, as an optional component of the budgetary organization. It is suggested as part of the prototype, for it both represents a logical extension of the principles of participatory management and it provides a vehicle which can yield operational as well as political dividends.

Ideally the committee should be multidisciplinary in nature, including in its composition medical staff representation as well as representation from nursing, administration, and the various general service and patient care departments. The committee's membership should also be designed to reflect a cross section of the institution's organization hierarchy. Selection of the specific committee members and the chairman should be done by senior management. In making its selections, management should focus on obtaining the involvement of individuals who can and will serve

---

[7]As was noted in Chapter 3, if this committee also serves as the Finance Committee, its functions are enlarged to include overseeing the financial operations and position of the hospital, ensuring that adequate working and long-term capital are available, and advising the board on all fiscal and investment matters.

not as parochial delegates but rather as representatives of the total institution.

The function of the committee, in addition to reviewing and suggesting revisions to the hospital's budget procedure manual, should be that of serving as an intramural review and advisory group. In this role it can provide useful operational insights into many of the decisions which senior management must make. Moreover, as the surrogate for the total staff, the committee can provide a workable mechanism for increasing staff involvement in the planning and budgeting process and subsequent commitment to the hospital's operating goals.

If increased commitment is actually to be obtained, it should be realized that the committee must be meaningfully involved in the decision process—even if in an advisory capacity. If the committee even appears to be being used as just "window dressing," its existence may well prove to be counterproductive. Therefore, prior to creating such a committee, senior management should carefully review its predilections and only establish the committee if it is committed to working with committee members in a participatory manner.

In addition to the foregoing, this committee can be of assistance in making capital budget decisions. The nature of the capital investment decision process and the role which a multidisciplinary committee of this type can play in this process are discussed in the following chapter. The possibility and benefits of including this additional role in the committee's charge should be carefully considered by senior management in determining whether to create such a committee.

Line Management. All too often, line management bears the brunt of the tedium which is inherent in converting operational planning into an operating budget. As a result, in many instances line management has come to view the planning and budgeting process as a "paper exercise" wherein clerical skills are of greater importance than either innovative thinking or management judgment.

When this becomes the case, either in reality or in line management's perception of reality then, as discussed in Chapter 15, the dangers involved in confusing "means" and "ends" may well be incurred. The risks in such instances are that the motivational and, to some extent, the control values of the budgetary process may be lost.

Obviously, the planning and budgeting process will always entail line management's carrying out some clerical tasks. However to the greatest extent practicable, these tasks should be limited both in scope and content. Line management's role should be primarily that of converting the governing board's and senior management's policy and operating objective decisions into a workable operating program. To the extent that this conversion process involves the completion of forms, tables, charts, and so forth, the responsibility for developing and submitting these materials should lie with line management.

The accountability for converting the operating program into the financial budget is not the responsibility of line management. Therefore, the line manager should not be burdened with the clerical tasks related to either this activity or any other activity which involves a process or set of decisions which are beyond his control, e.g., preparation of the initial revenue budget. To the extent that these clerical tasks are shifted to the appropriate point in the fiscal services division, not only will the total planning and budgeting process become more efficient but also, in the larger contexts of total organizational performance and control, management at all levels will be more effective.

In addition to its prime accountability, line management carries several supporting responsibilities. The nature of this "staff" role is identified in the table as was done in the previous instances, by dotted lines. The mechanisms for implementing this role will differ both from one hospital to another and from one task to another. For the sake of simplicity, it may well be most efficient to obtain line management's input to senior management through the vehicle of the staff conferences which should be an ongoing component of any hospital's management control system. Line management's input to the fiscal services division and the budget director should be obtained on an as-needed basis through generally less formal mechanisms, e.g., telephone calls and scheduled short meetings.

Fiscal Services Division

The fiscal services division's role in the planning and budgetary process has been alluded to in the above section. Essentially, it is accountable for the conversion of the planned operating program into dollar cost estimates and the aggregation of the individual cost estimates into a complete, integrated budget package. As such, the division plays a central role in the budgetary process. It is a role which must, however, always be kept in perspective. The planning and budgetary process is neither designed nor intended to function as a service to the financial manager and accountant.

Rather, the fiscal services division should and must function as a service and supporting agent to the entire organization and budgetary process.

Fiscal services division contributes in another way to the total process in addition to its multiple roles as a component of senior and line management, as a "staff" resource to the total hospital, and as a converter of the operating plan to the operating budget. Typically, the person who can be viewed as the project manager (the budget director) for the entire planning, budgeting, and feedback process is organizationally housed in the fiscal services division.

In many hospitals the role of budget director has traditionally been encompassed within the responsibilities of the controller or chief financial officer's office. Often the controller personally developed the hospital's budget. In some instances, this approach may have been—and may still be—appropriate. However, given the importance of planning and budgeting to the financial and operational health of the institution and the resources and time demands of an effective budgeting program, it is questionable if this approach to the allocational responsibilities is still the method of choice. In larger institutions, it clearly is not.

A full-time budget director, who is responsible not only for coordinating the planning and budgeting process but also for administering the mechanics of the feedback process, increasingly is becoming an operational necessity for both large and medium size hospitals. This need is particularly the case in those areas wherein either rate review or prospective payment programs have been implemented. Aside from the demands of the environment, the employment of a full-time budget director is a sound management decision which can produce savings and improvements in staff costs, if properly handled.

The budget director generally reports to the hospital's chief financial officer. His major accountabilities can be summarized as follows:

1. Establish written instructions for a formal planning, budgeting, and management reporting/feedback program.
2. Coordinate and provide assistance to activities of all levels of management in the development of their operating plans, as necessary.
3. Coordinate the activities of the fiscal services division in both providing support to management in the preparation of its operating plan and in converting the operating plan into a comprehensive financial budget.

4. Analyze major variances between actual and budget for management and department heads.
5. Establish procedure for accumulating accurate statistical data such as patient days, outpatient and emergency room visits, units of service provided by departments, etc.

Optional:[8]

6. Accumulate data for the filing of rate justifications and, if necessary, rate appeals.

The task confronting the budget director is, by way of an understatement, an interesting challenge. Not only must he possess technical skills in the areas of finance, accounting, and management but also he must have sufficient political skill to successfully tread the narrow path between a manager's legitimate, individual prerogatives, and the common needs of the institution. Given both the importance and demands of the job, the budget director, like the controller, must be more than just an accountant. He must have both the imagination and drive to breathe life, energy, and priority into a difficult task whose successful performance is beyond his direct control, and the skill to utilize and help others to utilize the resulting product as an effective management tool.

Conclusion

The foregoing has been an attempt to define the operational planning and budgeting process by first identifying the individual steps involved in the process and then by describing the organization structure and accountabilities which provide the process with driving force. The emphasis has been on providing both an anatomical and wholistic overview of the process.

By design, certain facets of the process have only been lightly touched and certain simplifying assumptions have been made. The first category of decisions reflects an appreciation of the existing literature and an attempt to avoid duplication. An exception to this rule is, perhaps, made in the following chapter which addresses capital investment decisions (capital budgeting). In this instance, a different type of balance—leaning more toward the analytic and quantitative—was sought with the existing literature.

The second category of decisions reflects the fact that for some questions there are no single right answers. In considering the material in the latter portion of the chapter, the reader should

---

[8]This accountability would apply in those jurisdictions which utilize some form of extramural rate review for purposes of establishing payment levels.

always bear in mind the essential principle that there is no universal solution to organizational questions. In the case of the budgetary organization, a variety of structural patterns can be effective, if they both: allow for a participatory approach to decision making; and allocate responsibility in a manner which enables each of the involved participants to feel that the job he is doing—the accountability he is assigned—is worthy of his time and efforts.

Suggested Readings

American Hospital Association. *Budgeting Procedures for Hospitals.*

Brown, Ray E. *Judgment in Administration.*

Caruana, Russell, A. *A Guide To Organizing the Hospital's Fiscal Services Division.*

Griffith, John R. *Quantitative Techniques for Hospital Planning and Control,* Part I.

Heckert, J. Brooks and Wilson, James D. *Controllership,* Chapters 6 and 7.

Lipson, Stephen H. and Hensel, Mary D. *Hospital Manpower Budget Preparation Manual.*

Schein, Edgar, H. *Organizational Psychology,* Chapters 4, 6 and 7.

Silvers, J.B. and Prahalad, C.K. *Financial Management of Health Institutions,* Chapter 4.

Sutermeister, Robert A. *People and Productivity.*

Appendix 16
Example
Administrative Package

INTER-OFFICE MEMORANDUM

TO: DEPARTMENT HEADS   DATE_____
     MANAGEMENT ROUNDTABLE

FROM: Ms. Martha Wolfgang, President

SUBJECT: FISCAL YEAR OPERATING PLAN AND BUDGET

Attached for your review and use is the Administrative Package which
will be used for the development of the fiscal year operating plan and
budget. As in previous years, the forms and instructions contained in this
package have been reviewed and approved by the Budget Committee.

Since this package contains both the information needed and the procedures
to be used in preparing the hospital's operating plan and budget, I urge
you to carefully review it and be prepared to raise any questions you might
have at either the general or technical budget meetings.

During the coming year, we estimate that our inpatient services and
census will remain at about their present level. Additional services,
however, will be added in the primary care area in order to respond to
the current need and future demand in our community. These services while
not increasing patient census can be expected to reduce emergency room
visits while simultaneously adding to the laboratory and radiology workload.

In developing your operating plan and budget, you should also carefully
review the assumptions and listing of operational priorities. These
factors should weight heavily both in your analysis of your own functions
and activities and in the design of your departmental operating plan.

You should, as a matter of standard operating procedure, discuss your
department's present operations and future plans with those persons who
are directly responsible to you. Staff should be briefed on the
hospital's financial situation and plans for the year, and their assistance
should be solicitied. Other department heads whose responsibility centers
affect your departmental operations can also be of immense value to the
preparation of your budget -- you are urged to consult with them.

To permit time both for consolidation of all budgets and for review of
the total budget prior to presentation to the Governing Board, you are
requested to begin preparation as soon as possible and to comply with
the due dates as set out in the budget calendar.

The Budget Officer and the Division of Fiscal Services are available to
provide you with any needed technical support or data. Call upon
them whenever they can be of assistance.

MW:g
Attachment

ADMINISTRATIVE PACKAGE
BRT GENERAL HOSPITAL

BUDGET CALENDAR

March 20	General Budget Meeting
March 22-29	Technical Budget Meetings
March 30-April 13	Administrative Meeting - I
April 13	Decision Packages Due
April 17-24	Administrative Meeting - II: Rank Orderings
April 25-May 2	Administrative Meeting - III: Rank Orderings
May 4	Final Rank Ordering and Specific Project Funding Decision
May 11	Personnel, Supplies and Other Expenses, and Capital Budget Detail Forms Due
May 23	Initial Integrated Budget Due from Fiscal Services
May 27-June 1	Administrative Meeting - IV: Budget Review and Adjustment
June 6	Budget Completed and Distributed to the Governing Board
June 15	Board of Governors Review and Approval of Operating Plan and Budget

BRT GENERAL HOSPITAL

STATEMENT OF GENERAL OBJECTIVE AND POLICIES*

In recognition of both its role as a community resource and its obligation to the community, the Governing Board of BRT General Hospital commits itself to using the resources entrusted to it:

> to provide the community with needed health care services, at an acceptable level of quality, and at the least possible cost.

In order to achieve this purpose, the Governing Board establishes the following general policies as parameters for purposes of guiding the operation of the corporation:

1. To the extent of its financial ability, the hospital will operate for the benefit of those not able to pay;
2. Consistent with the requirements for quality care, the hospital will not restrict the use of its facilities to a particular group of physicians or surgeons; and
3. Through the application of sound and imaginative management techniques and leadership, the hospital will not only protect its assets and income against subversion but also, assure that those assets are utilized in a manner which produces the greatest benefit to its service area.

---

* The following statement was initially approved by the Governing Board at their May, 1954 meeting and has been reviewed, as appropriate and as required by the hospital's operating environment, revised and reaffirmed annually, since that date, at the time of the annual meeting of the hospital corporation.

BRT GENERAL HOSPITAL

ENVIRONMENTAL STATEMENT

The following is an analysis of the hospital's present operating environment. This analysis describes the environment in terms of the strengths
and weaknesses of the hospital, the nature of its role within the community,
the nature of the population being served, and the general condition of its
operating milieu.

I. Internal Environment

Physical Plant: Average age of plant is 10 years. Plant is fully
air conditioned and meets not only State health
and fire codes but, also, Federal Life Safety
Code. Maintenance costs are stabilized but can
be expected to increase over the next 2 to 5
years.

Plant is presently utilized to capacity; grounds
will accomodate additional facilities, but addi-
tions to services will require new construction.

Patient Services: Currently, a full range of inpatient services
are provided. Hospital has also been designated
as an end stage renal center. Hospital has
operating and transfer agreements with the
regional medical center and with local skilled
nursing facilities and home health programs.

Ambulatory care program relatively weak; particularly in light of the community's lack of
primary care resources.

Radiology facilities also weak in terms
of special procedures capacity and capability.

Organization: Staff levels at 95% of table of organization
approved complement. Day care center program
has been successful in attracting RN's and
skilled technicians.

Staff turnover stabilizing and a maturing work
force developing.

Medical staff well organized and sensitive to both the hospital's and the community's needs. Open staffing in community has resulted in medical staff size being sufficient to support the hospital's capacity.

Financial:

Net margin has increased slightly over that experienced during the period of Federal price controls and is now at the 2.5% level. As a result, a modest reserve has been generated for purposes of new programs. Internal resources are not yet sufficient to support any large scale capital expenditure programs.

The development program effort has been underway for less than a year and it is still unclear as to amount - either the number or magnitude - of gifts which it will generate.

Quality of
Services:

Accreditation and licensure status in good standing.

Continuing medical education program becoming institutionalized with a resultant interlocking relationship developing between Director of Medical Education office and the Credential Committee.

A concurrent review program has been established. However, its efficacy as well as the efficacy of the entire quality control program will not be known until the PSRO conducts its review and determines if "designated" status is warranted. Currently, the hospital has obtained "waiver" status for purposes of Medicare.

II. External Environment

Community:

The hospital's primary service area currently has an estimated population of 120,000. This population has remained relatively stable in size. However, it has declined marginally in economic status while sometime polarizing into two demographic groups; one, aging and the other being young and relatively unskilled in terms of the labor market.

Health resource in the community has declined in proportion to the community's ability to incur out-of-pocket expenses. This decline has been particularly marked in the primary care area. As a result, community groups are placing increased pressure on the hospital to expand its emergency room and "walk-in" facilities.

Legislation: At the national level, the regulatory changes in
                          the Medicare program have placed, and will continue
                          to place, increased pressure on the hospital's
                          financial condition. For the present, these
                          pressures are being successfully accomodated.
                          However,continued lowering of the section 223
                          allowable cost ceiling may well result in some
                          Medicare costs having to be subsidized.

                          PL 93-641 is still in the process of implementation
                          and as of yet, has had no operational impact.
                          It is expected that, when implemented, it will
                          require that a more rigorous internal long range
                          planning and capital budgeting procedure be utilized
                          and that delays in capital expenditure decisions
                          be anticipated and planned for.

                          At the local level, rate review legislation has
                          not been enacted. The legislature while evidencing
                          frustration and disappointment with the performance
                          of the state's health care system, has determined
                          that the prudent course is to wait until experience
                          is gained with the various new federal Acts and
                          regulations.

III.Analysis

The hospital is in a sound operating condition and a relatively sound
financial condition. However, demand for both services and resources
is increasing particularly in terms of the provision of primary care.

The legislative picture in terms of the future is unclear. For the
moment, no further legislative intrusions into management decisions
are pending -- in terms of implementation in the next fiscal year.

BRT GENERAL HOSPITAL

ASSUMPTIONS*

The following assumptions represent management's "best judgement" as to the major phenomena which will affect hospital operations. These "macro level" assumptions should be carefully amplified through the projection of more detailed operational assumptions at the responsibility center level.

Legislation
1. A limited national health insurance program will be enacted by 1980; i.e., program limited in that it will focus in the main, on financing in patient care.

    Operational Implication:
    The program will eliminate some of the existing financial barriers to care and hence, will act as a catalyst for an increase in utilization. Current inpatient facilities should be able to accommodate the increase. Therefore, no operational implication beyond the need to continue normal maintenance and rennovation program.

2. State rate review/control legislation is not expected prior to national health insurance.

    Operational Implication:
    No direct implication as a result of legislative requirements. However, the potential of legislation requires that steps be taken immediately to dampen the possible intrusionary effect of regulation by increasing productivity and controlling costs.

Demand For Services
1. Demand for inpatient services in the coming fiscal year is expected to remain at about the same level as currently being experienced.

    Operational Implication:
    No new implication. Increased attention, however, must be focused on increasing the productivity of the inpatient production function.

2. As a result of being designated as an end stage renal center, demand for outpatient dialysis services will increase.

---

* Assumptions are defined as statements describing future events and/or developments which will affect hospital operations but whose assurance is beyond the direct control of hospital management.

Operational Implication:
An opportunity will exist for the hospital to better serve its extended
community. To successfully meet this opportunity, increased capital
and operating resources will have to be devoted to the renal program.

3. As a result of both the continued shift in the demographic composition
    of the community and the decrease in the "stock" of local physician
    services, an increased proportion of the hospital's service area
    will be looking to it as their principal source of primary care.

    Operational Implication:
    An opportunity will exist to better serve the local community. In
    order to capitalize on this opportunity, increased capital and operating
    resources will have to be devoted to primary care.

4. As a result of both technological advances and/or the increased
    demand for primary care, routine laboratory and radiology workload
    can be expected to increase. If properly channeled, the increase
    in primary care demand will result in a moderate decrease in emergency
    room visits.

    Operational Implication:
    Plant and equipment capacity in both laboratory and radiology is
    sufficient to accommodate a moderate to medium increase in workload.
    In view of the complimentary need to increase efficiency a moderate
    increase in workload in these areas should be accommodated through
    increased staff productivity. A medium increase in workload will
    require an increase in staff.

    The decrease in emergency room workload, while significant will not be
    sufficient to result in any major staffing pattern changes.

Other Considerations
1. Pressure will be increasingly placed on hospitals within the community
    to make better use of resources through consolidations and the sharing
    of services whenever practicable.

    Operational Implication:
    Public pressure, combined with the advent of PL 93-641, will reduce
    a hospital's ability to take unilateral actions. In the case of
    radiology special procedures this means that our activities
    will have to be carefully and explicitly coordinated with both our own
    and the community's needs and existing resources. Operationally, given
    the delays which can be expected from this kind of process, capital
    planning should be initiated and exploratory discussions - begun with
    other institutions. Also, complimentary steps should be taken in the
    financial area.

2. Labor and raw material costs are expected to increase at the rate
    of 12% per year. Intensity of services is expected to increase by 5%
    per year.

    Operational Implication:
    A seventeen percent increase in costs will result in both increased
    consumer and governmental pressure on the health delivery system and
    an increased willingness to impose stringent regulatory measures.
    To avoid arbitrary decisions, costs must be controlled. This can be
    achieved through increased productivity. Operationally, this means
    that work procedures, processes, and staffing patterns must be re-
    viewed at every level; with result oriented modifications made to
    increase efficiency.

BRT GENERAL HOSPITAL
Operating Policy Decisions

Program Priorities

Given the general objective of the hospital and executive management evaluation
of both the environmental statement and the statement of assumptions, program area
priorities have been established as follows:

1. Primary Care Program
2. Outpatient Patient Services Program
3. Radiology Program
4. Inpatient Patient Services Program
5. Ancillary Patient Services Program
6. Laboratory Program
7. Surgical Services Program
8. Environmental Services Program
9. Personnel and Education Program
10. Fiscal Services Program
11. Administrative Services Program

Funding Guideline

Revenue Estimates:
-20% of revenue obtained through cost based Blue Cross Plan payment.
   An 8% positive margin is generated through this class of purchaser.
-30% of revenue obtained through Medicare Program payments. A 1%
   positive margin is generated through this class of purchaser.
-15% of revenue obtained through Medicaid Program payments. This class
   of purchaser produces neither a positive or negative margin.
-25% of revenue obtained through patients having commercial insurance.
   A 3% positive margin is produced through this source of funds.
-10% of revenue obtained through self responsible patients. A 5%
   negative margin is generated by this source of funds.

Net margin about 2.5% or $200,000. Debt capacity is sound. However, this capacity
to be held in reserve against the contingency of either emergency needs or future
large scale rennovations. Philanthrophy is still an unknown factor; depending
on the results of the developmental program.

Program/Project Funding:

1. Existing patient care and environmental services programs to be funded at
    their present scope without improvements/expansion being obtained through
    productivity increases.
2. End stage renal and primary care projects to be given priority and to be
    expanded to a financially prudent level.
3. Radiology special procedures to be given, with the approval of the Governing
    Board, priority access to unrestricted philanthropic contributions.
4. Personnel and education, fiscal services, and administrative services programs
    to be reviewed with scope, to the extent possible, reduced. Funds made
    available through this effort, to be used to support primary care initiative.

OPERATING OBJECTIVES

Financial
          Continue to maintain a financially self-sufficient position through the
          generation of a positive margin of, at least, 2.5%.

Quality of Services
          Provide necessary and appropriate service at an acceptable level of
          technical quality as measured by the attainment of "designated" status.

Primary Care
          Provide the basis for increasing the community's access to primary care
          by developing a master plan of action and implementing phases 1 and
          2 of that plan.

End Stage Renal
          Provide adequate access to the community, to renal dialysis care as
          measured by elimination of the dialysis waiting list.

Operating
          Provide for improvements/expansion in services through increases in
          productivity as measured by a decrease in the ratio of full time
          equivalents to the weighted service index.*

---

* Note to the reader. The weighted service index is a subjective relative
  value system used by the hospital to aggregate inpatient days, outpatient
  visits, and ancillary services.

PROJECTION PACKAGE*

---

* Note to the reader: The projection package should be customized for each of
the volume dependent responsibility centers by providing both total patient
days and unique workload estimates for the particular responsibility center;
e.g., for a patient care unit: patient days/that unit; for dietary: projected
meals by type of diet.

TOTAL PATIENT DAY FORECAST*

Year	Patient Days	Approximate Occupancy
1	123,951	85%
2	138,375	95%
3	135,221	93%
4	138,011	95%
5	138,656	95%
Projected Year	138,300	95%

* Excludes Nursery Days

TOTAL PATIENT DAYS PER MONTH*

Year	Total	**	July	Aug.	Sept.	Oct.	Nov.	Dec.	Jan.	Feb.	Mar.	Apr.	May	June
1	123,951	3%	9,296	10,499	10,499	10,535	9,296	8,676	9,916	11,155	12,395	12,312	9,999	9,296
2	138,375	11%	11,051	9,686	11,761	11,089	10,379	11,010	11,071	13,144	13,145	14,529	11,130	10,378
3	135,221	-2%	11,494	8,789	13,523	11,493	10,817	9,465	11,495	11,493	10,818	13,524	12,169	10,141
4	138,011	2%	11,040	10,331	12,439	11,699	11,761	12,435	11,715	11,985	11,052	11,083	12,395	11,065
5	138,656	-0-	11,092	10,399	11,788	11,785	11,054	11,764	11,807	11,785	12,464	11,094	12,494	11,133
Proj.	138,300	-0-	12,406	10,372	11,796	11,755	11,041	11,061	11,778	11,708	11,777	11,780	12,447	9,681

* Excludes Nursery Days }
** Percent Change From Previous Year

The following table illustrates how the Projection Package is tailored
to needs of each responsibility center. All responsibility centers
would receive the foregoing patient day projections. Those responsibility
centers whose workload is volume dependent would also receive a projection, such as that shown for Hematology, which is unique to their
needs. The Administrative Package would also be similarly tailored --
in regard to historical cost data and current personnel complement
data -- to reflect the history and current situation of each particular responsibility center receiving the package.

WORKLOAD PROJECTIONS: TESTS
HEMATOLOGY DEPARTMENT

Year	July	Aug.	Sept.	Oct.	Nov.	Dec.	Jan.	Feb.	Mar.	Apr.	May	June	TOTAL
1	8,367	9,450	9,450	9,482	8,367	7,809	8,925	10,040	11,156	11,081	9,000	8,367	111,494
2	10,388	9,105	11,056	10,424	9,757	10,350	10,407	12,356	12,357	13,658	10,463	9,756	130,077
3	10,920	8,350	12,847	10,919	10,277	8,992	10,921	10,919	10,278	12,848	11,561	9,634	128,466
4	10,488	9,815	11,817	11,114	11,173	11,814	11,130	11,386	10,500	10,529	11,776	10,512	132,054
5	11,425	10,711	12,142	12,139	11,386	12,117	12,162	12,139	12,838	11,427	12,869	11,467	142,822
Proj.*	13,399	11,202	12,740	12,696	11,925	11,950	12,721	12,645	12,720	12,723	13,443	10,456	148,620

* Relative workload value/test in projection year 3.22

DECISION PACKAGE

FORM AND INSTRUCTIONS

PROJECT DECISION PACKAGE

1. Program Area:_____ 2. Activity:_____

3. Objective:_____

_____

_____

4. Activity Description:_____

_____

_____

Starting Date_____Completion Date_____

5. Activity Benefit/Result: 6. Resource Estimates
                                      Manyears   Expense
_____   Mgmt.____   Salaries
                                      Super.   Travel
_____   Tech.   Other
                                      Cler.   Cap.Costs
_____   TOTAL_____   TOTAL_____

7. Alternatives: Alternative Way of Accomplishing the Same Result

No.	Alternative	Resource Requirement	
		Manyears	$

8. Alternatives: Alternative Levels of Effort

No.	Alternative	Benefit	Resource Requirement	
			Manyears	$

9. Ranking

No.	Alternative Number	Resource Requirements($)
1		
2		
3		
4		
5		
6		

10. Identification of
    Package Developer

    _____

    Date:_____

PROJECT DECISION PACKAGE INSTRUCTIONS

1. Program Department Area
        Identification by name of the Program/Department Area being addressed; e.g.,
        Environmental Services, Administration, Outpatient Services, etc.

2. Activity
        Identification of the activity being addressed; e.g., in Environmental Ser-
        vices it might be, Heating and Cooling Plant; in Outpatient Services it
        might be Community Mental Health, etc.

3. Objective
        Restatement of the Program Area's objective or that portion of the objective
        to which the activity applies; e.g., in Outpatient Services for the Community
        Mental Health activity the objective might be: to provide the total ser-
        vice area with convenient access to mental health service.

4. Activity Description
        Generic statement of the activity, including starting and completion dates
        from a process perspective; e.g., for Environmental Services, Heating and
        Cooling Plant Professional, licensed supervision, operation, and minor
        maintenance, or an around the clock bases of the central heating and cooling
        system. Ongoing activity.

5. Activity Benefit/Result
        Statement in quantified terms of the benefit/result or output of the activity.
        Result must relate to the Program Area objective and be quantified; e.g.,
        Outpatient Services, Community Mental Health through the use of out-reach
        efforts, provide convenient access to mental health services for the total
        service area as measured by an increase in patient visits by existing
        patients of 5,000 and the provision of services to, at least, 1,00 new
        patients.

6. Resources
        Statement of estimated resource requirements. Expense information should
        just be direct costs. (NOTE: Detail resource estimates should be provided
        only after specific project funding decisions. Detailed estimates should
        be provided on the appropriate personnel, supplies, and other expenses
        and capital budget forms. These forms should be completed per the appro-
        priate instructions).

7. Alternatives: Alternative Way of Accomplishing the Same Result
        The purpose of this section is to force consideration of alternatives.
        In this instance, it is alternative ways of accomplishing the same result.
        The first alternative in this section should be numbered two (2) since
        the alternative indicated in item 4 is number one (1). Other alternatives
        should be ranked sequentially. In the alternative section, a differert
        approach to achieving the same end should be identified; e.g., hiring a
        consultant as opposed to doing the job yourself, or purchasing laundry
        services on a contract basis as opposed to operating the hospital's own
        laundry, centralizing OB on a community wide basis, etc. If no viable
        alternative exists, then this section should be left blank.

8. <u>Alternatives: Alternative Levels of Effort</u>
    The purpose of this section is to focus attention on alternative levels of
    investment and their resulting benefits; e.g., for $200,000 increase patient
    visits by 3,000 and new patients by 1,000, do 8 reviews with a savings of
    $500,000, for increased patient visits by 3,000 and new patients $150,000
    by 500. This section should just address alternatives to the level of
    activity of choice.

    In the "number" column, the sequential listing of alternatives should be
    continued from the above section. Under alternative, the nature of the
    alternative should be briefly stated; e.d., 3,000 visits increase, 1,000
    new patients, etc.

    Under the "benefit" column the benefit obtained from the alternative level
    of effort should be defined; e.g., convenient access to only 90% of the
    total service area.

    The "resource" column should be completed the same as is the case above.

    If the alternative is to forego the activity then the nature of the lost
    benefit should be set out.

9. <u>Ranking</u>
    Identification of the ranking of each of the alternatives should be identified
    by their sequential number.

    Resource Requirements are just a restatement of the above columns.

10. <u>Identification and Date</u>
    Signature of the manager responsible on a day to day basis for the operation
    of the activity and the date on which the Decision Package is to be submitted
    for review.

The remaining components of the Administrative Package:

>   historical cost data; and
>   current personnel and complement, wage, and
>   benefit data;

are generally included as part of the information provided - along with forms and instructions - in the personnel and supplies and other expense budgeting sections of the package. The forms and instructions for preparing the personnel budget and the supplies and other expense budget are typically quite involved in terms of both length and arithmetic manipulations. Therefore, instead of duplicating the work of other authors, reference is made to the following sources. Readers are urged to review these sources for a detailed explanation and examples of the process and mechanics of preparing these budgets.

>   American Hospital Association, <u>Budgeting
>   Procedures for Hospitals</u>
>
>   Griffith, John R., <u>Quantitative Techniques
>   for Hospital Planning and Control</u>
>
>   Hay, Leon E., <u>Budgeting and Cost Analysis for
>   Hospital Management</u>
>
>   Lash, Myles P., "Development of An Expense
>   Budgeting Procedure"
>
>   Lipson, Stephen H., and Hensel, Mary D.,
>   <u>Hospital Manpower Budget Preparation Manual</u>

An example procedure, including forms and instructions, for preparing the capital budget is presented in the appendix to Chapter 17.

Chapter 17

Capital Investment Decisions

Brief reference was made in Chapter 16 both to the development of capital expenditure decision packages and to the mechanics of the capital investment rank ordering and decision process.

Though the problems, goals, and general mechanics of capital budgeting are the same as those of planning and budgeting for general operations, the specifics of the budgetary process are somewhat different. In view of these differences, and as discussed below, the importance of these decisions, the anatomy of the capital budgeting process will be addressed in this chapter.

In considering this material, the reader should view it not as an entirely new subject but rather as simply an expansion of the discussion begun in reference to Phase IV in the previous chapter.

Importance

Of the myriad of decisions which will confront a hospital manager throughout his professional career, those involving capital investment choices are likely to be the most crucial. This is the case, for not only might these decisions involve the classic "life and death" trade offs but also, if an error in judgment is made, the costs of the decision error can be expected to be incurred over a considerable length of time. Given the importance of these decisions, hospital management should utilize carefully structured decision methodologies designed to minimize the probability of decision errors. Unfortunately, this has often not been the case.

Historically, the literature addressing hospital budgeting has been noted primarily for its paucity. Though recently the work of

511

several major authors has acted to fill many of the previously existing gaps, the current "state of the art" can be described, for most
hospitals, as still being primitive.[1] Based on a 1973 survey of 801
short-stay hospitals, it appears that:

—less than 12% of the hospitals use either of the more theoretically acceptable analytical techniques of internal rate of return or net present value analysis; and
—over a third of the hospitals use only subjective criteria for
capital decision making.[2]

When one considers the nature of a hospital's traditional financial
environment, the survey's results are not surprising. In an environment dominated by cost-based retrospective reimbursement
and private philanthropy, it can be easily understood why hospital
managers felt little pressure for rigorous investment decision
analysis and often opted for the safer, though perhaps more costly,
alternative of facilities and services expansion. Private philanthropy was eager to contribute funds and seldom questioned the
real need for additional hospital capital. Similarly, cost-based retrospective reimbursement by paying incurred costs neither questioned nor provided a "braking force" on the operating costs associated with unneeded capital expenditures.

The operating situation, however, can be expected to change
markedly over the next few years. The recent levels of inflation in
hospital costs, combined with a renewed understanding of the
relationship between cost and capital investment, have resulted in
increased consumer and governmental pressure for cost containment and capital rationing. Reinforcing these pressures has been
the enactment in 1972 of Public Law 92-603 (with its section 234,
Capital Budgeting, and section 221, Capital Approval provisions)
and in 1975 the enactment of Public Law 93-641 (The National
Health Planning and Resources Development Act) of federal legislation requiring more carefully evaluated capital decision. In response to these pressures, hospitals have begun using more rigorous capital investment analysis and decision techniques.

As indicated, the literature of the past several years has begun to
provide both a sound theoretical and pragmatic foundation for hos-

---

[1]Griffith, John R., *Quantitative Techniques for Hospital Planning and Control;*
Wact, Richard D., "Capital Budgeting Decision-Making for Hospitals," *Hospital
Administration,* Fall 1970; Silvers J.B. and Prahalad, C.E., *Financial Management
of Health Institutions.*

[2]Williams, John Daniel and Rakich, Jonathan, S., "Investment Evaluation In
Hospitals", *Financial Management,* Summer 1973.

pital capital budgeting. While a detailed duplication of this litera-ture would serve little value, a conceptual approach complements the previous material and also adds to the existing literature and state of the art. The following material utilizes such an approach. It is supplemented by a section focusing on the policy and me-chanics of evaluating, quantifying, and ranking the nonfinancial benefits of investment alternatives. Readers interested in a more detailed discussion of either the theory or mechanical techniques of capital budgeting should refer both to the Suggested Readings at the end of this chapter and to the Bibliography.

Process

To provide the basis for sound decisions, a hospital's capital bud-geting system must encompass the following major activities. These activities should be carried out in a sequential flow with all expen-diture alternatives progressing through the process as a group.[3] Appendix 17 illustrates this process from a procedural perspective.

a. Project Identification. The initial step in the process is the identification of all potential expenditure projects. This step should involve not only the formulation of proposals, but also the evalua-tion of proposals to assure that the potential expenditure is consis-tent with the hospital's objectives, assumptions, and priorities.

It is important to note that this evaluation step represents the first decision point in the capital rationing process. As such, it should be given careful management attention both as a device for sifting out inappropriate projects and as a mechanism for increas-ing the creditability of the entire budgetary process.

b. Cash Flow Identification. The second step begins to add quantitative definition to project proposals by requiring for each project the specification of all relevant cash flows.

Due to the nature of the hospital's business, it may be difficult—

---

[3]This wholistic approach to the decision process is necessary in order to reduce the possibility of benefit suboptimization. Presuming limited funds, if projects were considered independently on an "as ready basis" then all available funds might be spent on projects which, while having positive value, do not include alternatives which surface later in the period and which possess incremental val-ues greater than those of some of the funded projects. To avoid this pitfall, all expenditure alternatives should be identified and decided upon as a group. In this way the analysis not only can include both an absolute and relative evaluation but also can identify that set of projects which will yield the greatest total benefit for the available funds.

if not impossible—to definitively quantify all cash flows. To the extent possible, cash flows should be objectively projected. However, where quantitative objectivity is not practical, cash flows should just be estimated on a best judgment basis.

In developing estimates, projections of the magnitude as well as the relative timing of cash inflows and outflows should be made. These estimates, however, should only include the incremental costs which will be incurred as a result of undertaking the project. Previously incurred costs (sunk costs) and/or costs which would be incurred regardless of the investment decision (nonincremental costs) should not be included in the cash flow estimates.

Incremental capital and operating costs obviously should be treated as cash outflows. Any revenues which the investment is expected to generate plus any anticipated salvage value should be treated as cash inflows. Also, in those instances where the investment will not produce revenue but will result in decrease in operating costs, the expected savings should be viewed, for purposes of later analysis, as being a form of cash inflows.

c. Financial Analysis. Several alternative techniques are available for evaluating the financial implications of any given investment opportunity. Of the alternatives, net present value and internal rate of return analysis are the more theoretically acceptable approaches. These are preferred because both of these analytical techniques recognize the time value of money; i.e., a dollar today, because it can be invested and earn a return (interest), is worth more than the promise of a dollar a year from today. Between the two techniques, net present value is the method of choice, because it avoids the reinvestment bias which is intrinsic to the internal rate of return approach. (The internal rate of return approach assumes that cash inflows can be reinvested at the discount rate at least. To the extent that cash inflows can only be reinvested at lesser rates, the calculated rate of return is inaccurately inflated.)[4]

A detailed discussion of both the underlying theory and the mechanics of calculating a potential expenditure net present value (as well as present value tables for various interest rates) can be found in most general financial management textbooks. For purposes of this text, the example presented in Table 17-1 should provide a sufficient illustration and explanation of the mechanics of net present value analysis.

---

[4]Readers seeking a more detailed discussion of this point should refer to Van Horne, J.C. *Financial Management and Policy*, Second edition.

The calculations in the table are based upon the following formula:

$$PV = \sum_{t=1}^{T} \overbrace{\frac{CI_t}{(1+I)^t} + \frac{S}{(1+I)^T}}^{\text{cash inflows}} - \overbrace{\frac{C_t}{(1+I)^t} + \frac{CO_t}{(1+I)^t}}^{\text{cash outflows}}$$

where:

PV = present value
t = time period (usually a year)
T = life of investment
CI_t = cash inflow in period t (either revenue or savings)
S = salvage value
C_t = capital cost
CO_t = cash outflow in period t
I = interest rate (discount rate)

The input data for the above formula are obtained for the most part in step "b." The value for the interest or discount rate (I) is not, however, identified in the above step and presents somewhat of a unique quantification problem.

In the typical commercial setting the quantification of the discount rate factor is relatively simple and straightforward. Orthodox theory holds that the discount rate should be equal to the rate of return which the firm earns on its total assets. In the case of the hospital, this approach is of little use. Due to the preponderance of cost-based reimbursement and other intrinsic internal operating factors, hospitals typically have a relatively low operating margin.[5] As a result, their rate of return is low, providing an unrealistic benchmark for establishing a discount rate. An alternative approach must, therefore, be used.

An individual hospital in considering its expenditure opportunities might select one of the following three rates:

—the historic earnings rate on its investment portfolio;
—the interest rate which it would have to pay if it borrowed funds; or
—the rate of return allowed under Medicare for investor-owned hospitals.

or a rate somewhere between these alternatives. Unfortunately, no fixed decision rules are available. The specific discount rate

---

[5]In June of 1975, following the Economic Stabilization Program, the operating margin for the hospitals included in the American Hospital Association's Panel Survey was 0.88%. In the post-Economic Stabilization Program period, operating margin increased on the average to about 3.5%.

Table 17-1
Net Present Value Analysis:
Example

The following is an example of the calculation of the net present value for an assumed capital equipment investment. The basic financial facts can be summarized as follows:

PV = present value

T = useful life of 10 years

CI_t = $15,000/year for years 1 through 5; $14,000/year for years 6 through 10

S = $3,000

C_t = $25,000

CO_t = $9,000/year for years 1 through 5; $12,000/year for years 6 through 10

I = 7%

$$PV=\sum_{t=1}^{T} \frac{CI_t}{(1+I)^t} + \frac{S}{(1+I)^T} - \frac{C_t}{(1+I)^t} + \frac{CO_t}{(1+I)^t}$$

$$PV=\sum_{t=1}^{T} \frac{\text{Net Cash Flow*}}{(1+I)^t} + \frac{S}{(1+I)^T} + \frac{C_t}{(1+I)^t}$$

Present Value of Net Cash Flow

Year	CI_t	CO_t	Net Cash Flow (CI_t- CO_t)	Present Value Factor @ 7%	Present Value
1	$15,000	$ 9,000	$6,000	.934	$ 5,604
2	15,000	9,000	6,000	.873	5,238
3	15,000	9,000	6,000	.816	4,896
4	15,000	9,000	6,000	.762	4,572
5	15,000	9,000	6,000	.712	4,272
6	14,000	12,000	2,000	.666	1,332
7	14,000	12,000	2,000	.623	1,246
8	14,000	12,000	2,000	.582	1,164
9	14,000	12,000	2,000	.544	1,088
10	14,000	12,000	2,000	.505	1,016
					$30,428

Present Value of Salvage

Year	S	Present Value Factor @ 7%	Present Value
10	$3,000	.508	$1,524

Net Present Value of Investment

PV = Σ($30,428 = $1,524 - $25,000***)

PV = $6,932

---

*Net Cash Flow = CI_t minus CO_t

**Obtained from standard present value tables; see Tables 17-5 and 17-6.

***Present value is $25,000 due to the assumption that the expenditure is made in its entirety at the beginning of the period.

chosen by a particular hospital must be a subjective decision. The rate will, generally, fall between the extremes represented by the above listing; with the interest rate on borrowed funds serving as the discount rate floor. However, in selecting its discount rate, a hospital should not only evaluate its credit and general financial condition but also should seek expert financial advice as to both the condition of the capital market and the capital market's approach of an acceptable discount rate.

Benefit Analysis

d. Benefit Identification. The previous steps have concentrated exclusively on the financial aspects of capital decisions. Due to the nature of a hospital's business, analysis of only financial data is inadequate. If sound decisions are to be made, the financial evaluation must be complemented by the examination of the intangible factors, i.e., the patient care and services, or benefits which a particular investment will produce. The first step in this benefit evaluation is the identification of the benefits which accrue to any particular project.

Essentially, benefits must be identified in terms of two dimensions: from the perspective of both their qualitative and quantitative characteristics. The quantitative aspect of expected benefits refers to the volume of service anticipated from a particular project: the number of persons who will benefit. The qualitative aspect refers to the nature of the service which will be provided: life-saving with full recovery, life-saving with partial recovery, age of persons benefiting, disease prevention, etc.

Exhibit I describes a technique which can be used to categorize both the nature and the extent of a project's benefits. Readers should refer to this exhibit for a detailed discussion of benefit identification.

e. Benefit Evaluation. Benefit evaluation centers on the matter of converting, through the application of a systematic process, the data developed in the previous step into useful decision making information. In principle, this step is similar to step "c". However, in terms of mechanics it markedly differs.

The mechanics of benefit evaluation are addressed in Exhibit II. The material in the exhibit is presented as an example of a pragmatic benefit evaluation technique. It should be noted that it is not presented as the definitive answer to the benefit evaluation problem. Rather, it is shown as an alternative to less structured approaches and as a stimulus to the development of more effective techniques.

Table 17-2

Present Value of $1 Received Annually At the End Of Each "Year" For "N" Years

Years (N)	1%	2%	4%	6%	8%	10%	12%	14%	15%	16%	18%	20%	22%	24%	25%	26%	28%	30%	35%	40%	45%	50%
1	0.990	0.980	0.962	0.943	0.926	0.909	0.893	0.877	0.870	0.862	0.847	0.833	0.820	0.806	0.800	0.794	0.781	0.769	0.741	0.714	0.690	0.667
2	1.970	1.942	1.886	1.833	1.783	1.736	1.690	1.647	1.626	1.605	1.566	1.528	1.492	1.457	1.440	1.424	1.392	1.361	1.289	1.224	1.165	1.111
3	2.941	2.884	2.775	2.673	2.577	2.487	2.402	2.322	2.283	2.246	2.174	2.106	2.042	1.981	1.952	1.923	1.868	1.816	1.696	1.589	1.493	1.407
4	3.902	3.808	3.630	3.465	3.312	3.170	3.037	2.914	2.855	2.798	2.690	2.589	2.494	2.404	2.362	2.320	2.241	2.166	1.997	1.849	1.720	1.605
5	4.853	4.713	4.452	4.212	3.993	3.791	3.605	3.433	3.352	3.274	3.127	2.991	2.864	2.745	2.689	2.635	2.532	2.436	2.220	2.035	1.876	1.737
6	5.795	5.601	5.242	4.917	4.623	4.355	4.111	3.889	3.784	3.685	3.498	3.326	3.167	3.020	2.951	2.885	2.759	2.643	2.385	2.168	1.983	1.824
7	6.728	6.472	6.002	5.582	5.206	4.868	4.564	4.288	4.160	4.039	3.812	3.605	3.416	3.242	3.161	3.083	2.937	2.802	2.508	2.263	2.057	1.883
8	7.652	7.325	6.733	6.210	5.747	5.335	4.968	4.639	4.487	4.344	4.078	3.837	3.619	3.421	3.329	3.241	3.076	2.925	2.598	2.331	2.108	1.922
9	8.566	8.162	7.435	6.802	6.247	5.759	5.328	4.946	4.772	4.607	4.303	4.031	3.786	3.566	3.463	3.366	3.184	3.019	2.665	2.379	2.144	1.948
10	9.471	8.983	8.111	7.360	6.710	6.145	5.650	5.216	5.019	4.833	4.494	4.192	3.923	3.682	3.571	3.465	3.269	3.092	2.715	2.414	2.168	1.965
11	10.368	9.787	8.760	7.887	7.139	6.495	5.937	5.453	5.234	5.029	4.656	4.327	4.035	3.776	3.656	3.544	3.335	3.147	2.752	2.438	2.185	1.977
12	11.255	10.575	9.385	8.384	7.536	6.814	6.194	5.660	5.421	5.197	4.793	4.439	4.127	3.851	3.725	3.606	3.387	3.190	2.779	2.456	2.196	1.985
13	12.134	11.343	9.986	8.853	7.904	7.103	6.424	5.842	5.583	5.342	4.910	4.533	4.203	3.912	3.780	3.656	3.427	3.223	2.799	2.468	2.204	1.990
14	13.004	12.106	10.563	9.295	8.244	7.367	6.628	6.002	5.724	5.468	5.008	4.611	4.265	3.962	3.824	3.695	3.459	3.249	2.814	2.477	2.210	1.993
15	13.865	12.849	11.118	9.712	8.559	7.606	6.811	6.142	5.847	5.575	5.092	4.675	4.315	4.001	3.859	3.726	3.483	3.268	2.825	2.484	2.214	1.995
16	14.718	13.578	11.652	10.106	8.851	7.824	6.974	6.265	5.954	5.669	5.162	4.730	4.357	4.033	3.887	3.751	3.503	3.283	2.834	2.489	2.216	1.997
17	15.562	14.292	12.166	10.477	9.122	8.022	7.120	6.373	6.047	5.749	5.222	4.775	4.391	4.059	3.910	3.771	3.518	3.295	2.840	2.492	2.218	1.998
18	16.398	14.992	12.659	10.828	9.372	8.201	7.250	6.467	6.128	5.818	5.273	4.812	4.419	4.080	3.928	3.786	3.529	3.304	2.844	2.494	2.219	1.999
19	17.226	15.678	13.134	11.158	9.604	8.365	7.366	6.550	6.198	5.877	5.316	4.844	4.442	4.097	3.942	3.799	3.539	3.311	2.848	2.496	2.220	1.999
20	18.046	16.351	13.590	11.470	9.818	8.514	7.469	6.623	6.259	5.929	5.353	4.870	4.460	4.110	3.954	3.808	3.546	3.316	2.850	2.497	2.221	1.999
21	18.857	17.011	14.029	11.764	10.017	8.649	7.562	6.687	6.312	5.973	5.384	4.891	4.476	4.121	3.963	3.816	3.551	3.320	2.852	2.498	2.221	2.000
22	19.660	17.658	14.451	12.042	10.201	8.772	7.645	6.743	6.359	6.011	5.410	4.909	4.488	4.130	3.970	3.822	3.556	3.323	2.853	2.498	2.222	2.000
23	20.456	18.292	14.857	12.303	10.371	8.883	7.718	6.792	6.399	6.044	5.432	4.925	4.499	4.137	3.976	3.827	3.559	3.325	2.854	2.499	2.222	2.000
24	21.243	18.914	15.247	12.550	10.529	8.985	7.784	6.835	6.434	6.073	5.451	4.937	4.507	4.143	3.981	3.831	3.562	3.327	2.855	2.499	2.222	2.000
25	22.023	19.523	15.622	12.783	10.675	9.077	7.843	6.873	6.464	6.097	5.467	4.948	4.514	4.147	3.985	3.834	3.564	3.329	2.856	2.499	2.222	2.000
26	22.795	20.121	15.983	13.003	10.810	9.161	7.896	6.906	6.491	6.118	5.480	4.956	4.520	4.151	3.988	3.837	3.566	3.330	2.856	2.500	2.222	2.000
27	23.560	20.707	16.330	13.211	10.935	9.237	7.943	6.935	6.514	6.136	5.492	4.964	4.524	4.154	3.990	3.839	3.567	3.331	2.856	2.500	2.222	2.000
28	24.316	21.281	16.663	13.406	11.051	9.307	7.984	6.961	6.534	6.152	5.502	4.970	4.528	4.157	3.992	3.840	3.568	3.331	2.857	2.500	2.222	2.000
29	25.066	21.844	16.984	13.591	11.158	9.370	8.022	6.983	6.551	6.166	5.510	4.975	4.531	4.159	3.994	3.841	3.569	3.332	2.857	2.500	2.222	2.000
30	25.808	22.396	17.292	13.765	11.258	9.427	8.055	7.003	6.566	6.177	5.517	4.979	4.534	4.160	3.995	3.842	3.569	3.332	2.857	2.500	2.222	2.000
40	32.835	27.355	19.793	15.046	11.925	9.779	8.244	7.105	6.642	6.234	5.548	4.997	4.544	4.166	3.999	3.846	3.571	3.333	2.857	2.500	2.222	2.000
50	39.196	31.424	21.482	15.762	12.234	9.915	8.304	7.133	6.661	6.246	5.554	4.999	4.545	4.167	4.000	3.846	3.571	3.333	2.857	2.500	2.222	2.000

Source: Robert N. Anthony, *Management Accounting: Text and Cases* (3rd ed; Homewood, Ill.: Richard D. Irwin, Inc., 1964). Used

Table 17-3

Present Value of $1 Received At The End Of The "Year"

Years Hence	1%	2%	4%	6%	8%	10%	12%	14%	15%	16%	18%	20%	22%	24%	25%	26%	28%	30%	35%	40%	45%	50%
1	0.990	0.980	0.962	0.943	0.926	0.909	0.893	0.877	0.870	0.862	0.847	0.833	0.820	0.806	0.800	0.794	0.781	0.769	0.741	0.714	0.690	0.667
2	0.980	0.961	0.925	0.890	0.857	0.826	0.797	0.769	0.756	0.743	0.718	0.694	0.672	0.650	0.640	0.630	0.610	0.592	0.549	0.510	0.476	0.444
3	0.971	0.942	0.889	0.840	0.794	0.751	0.712	0.675	0.658	0.641	0.609	0.579	0.551	0.524	0.512	0.500	0.477	0.455	0.406	0.364	0.328	0.296
4	0.961	0.924	0.855	0.792	0.735	0.683	0.636	0.592	0.572	0.552	0.516	0.482	0.451	0.423	0.410	0.397	0.373	0.350	0.301	0.260	0.226	0.198
5	0.951	0.906	0.822	0.747	0.681	0.621	0.567	0.519	0.497	0.476	0.437	0.402	0.370	0.341	0.328	0.315	0.291	0.269	0.223	0.186	0.156	0.132
6	0.942	0.888	0.790	0.705	0.630	0.564	0.507	0.456	0.432	0.410	0.370	0.335	0.303	0.275	0.262	0.250	0.227	0.207	0.165	0.133	0.108	0.088
7	0.933	0.871	0.760	0.665	0.583	0.513	0.452	0.400	0.376	0.354	0.314	0.279	0.249	0.222	0.210	0.198	0.178	0.159	0.122	0.095	0.074	0.059
8	0.923	0.853	0.731	0.627	0.540	0.467	0.404	0.351	0.327	0.305	0.266	0.233	0.204	0.179	0.168	0.157	0.139	0.123	0.091	0.068	0.051	0.039
9	0.914	0.837	0.703	0.592	0.500	0.424	0.361	0.308	0.284	0.263	0.225	0.194	0.167	0.144	0.134	0.125	0.108	0.094	0.067	0.048	0.035	0.026
10	0.905	0.820	0.676	0.558	0.463	0.386	0.322	0.270	0.247	0.227	0.191	0.162	0.137	0.116	0.107	0.099	0.085	0.073	0.050	0.035	0.024	0.017
11	0.896	0.804	0.650	0.527	0.429	0.350	0.287	0.237	0.215	0.195	0.162	0.135	0.112	0.094	0.086	0.079	0.066	0.056	0.037	0.025	0.017	0.012
12	0.887	0.788	0.625	0.497	0.397	0.319	0.257	0.208	0.187	0.168	0.137	0.112	0.092	0.076	0.069	0.062	0.052	0.043	0.027	0.018	0.012	0.008
13	0.879	0.773	0.601	0.469	0.368	0.290	0.229	0.182	0.163	0.145	0.116	0.093	0.075	0.061	0.055	0.050	0.040	0.033	0.020	0.013	0.008	0.005
14	0.870	0.758	0.577	0.442	0.340	0.263	0.205	0.160	0.141	0.125	0.099	0.078	0.062	0.049	0.044	0.039	0.032	0.025	0.015	0.009	0.006	0.003
15	0.861	0.743	0.555	0.417	0.315	0.239	0.183	0.140	0.123	0.108	0.084	0.065	0.051	0.040	0.035	0.031	0.025	0.020	0.011	0.006	0.004	0.002
16	0.853	0.728	0.534	0.394	0.292	0.218	0.163	0.123	0.107	0.093	0.071	0.054	0.042	0.032	0.028	0.025	0.019	0.015	0.008	0.005	0.003	0.002
17	0.844	0.714	0.513	0.371	0.270	0.198	0.146	0.108	0.093	0.080	0.060	0.045	0.034	0.026	0.023	0.020	0.015	0.012	0.006	0.003	0.002	0.001
18	0.836	0.700	0.494	0.350	0.250	0.180	0.130	0.095	0.081	0.069	0.051	0.038	0.028	0.021	0.018	0.016	0.012	0.009	0.005	0.002	0.001	0.001
19	0.828	0.686	0.475	0.331	0.232	0.164	0.116	0.083	0.070	0.060	0.043	0.031	0.023	0.017	0.014	0.012	0.009	0.007	0.003	0.002	0.001	0.001
20	0.820	0.673	0.456	0.312	0.215	0.149	0.104	0.073	0.061	0.051	0.037	0.026	0.019	0.014	0.012	0.010	0.007	0.005	0.002	0.001	0.001	
21	0.811	0.660	0.439	0.294	0.199	0.135	0.093	0.064	0.053	0.044	0.031	0.022	0.015	0.011	0.009	0.008	0.006	0.004	0.002	0.001		
22	0.803	0.647	0.422	0.278	0.184	0.123	0.083	0.056	0.046	0.038	0.026	0.018	0.013	0.009	0.007	0.006	0.004	0.003	0.001	0.001		
23	0.795	0.634	0.406	0.262	0.170	0.112	0.074	0.049	0.040	0.033	0.022	0.015	0.010	0.007	0.006	0.005	0.003	0.002	0.001			
24	0.788	0.622	0.390	0.247	0.158	0.102	0.066	0.043	0.035	0.028	0.019	0.013	0.008	0.006	0.005	0.004	0.003	0.002	0.001			
25	0.780	0.610	0.375	0.233	0.146	0.092	0.059	0.038	0.030	0.024	0.016	0.010	0.007	0.005	0.004	0.003	0.002	0.001	0.001			
26	0.772	0.598	0.361	0.220	0.135	0.084	0.053	0.033	0.026	0.021	0.014	0.009	0.006	0.004	0.003	0.002	0.002	0.001				
27	0.764	0.586	0.347	0.207	0.125	0.076	0.047	0.029	0.023	0.018	0.011	0.007	0.005	0.003	0.003	0.002	0.001	0.001				
28	0.757	0.574	0.333	0.196	0.116	0.069	0.042	0.026	0.020	0.016	0.010	0.006	0.004	0.002	0.002	0.002	0.001	0.001				
29	0.749	0.563	0.321	0.185	0.107	0.063	0.037	0.022	0.017	0.014	0.008	0.005	0.003	0.002	0.002	0.001	0.001					
30	0.742	0.552	0.308	0.174	0.099	0.057	0.033	0.020	0.015	0.012	0.007	0.004	0.003	0.002	0.001	0.001	0.001					
40	0.672	0.453	0.208	0.097	0.046	0.022	0.011	0.005	0.004	0.003	0.001	0.001										
50	0.608	0.372	0.141	0.054	0.021	0.009	0.003	0.001	0.001	0.001												

Source: Robert N. Anthony, *Management Accounting: Text and Cases* (3rd ed; Homewood, Ill.: Richard D. Irwin, Inc., 1964). Used with permission.

Exhibit I

Benefit Analysis: Benefit Identification*

The benefits expected to be derived from any given investment project generally can be viewed as being both qualitative and quantitative in nature. The quantitative aspect of expected benefits refers to the volume of service which is anticipated. The qualitative aspect refers to the nature of the service which will be produced. For purposes of analysis, both of these aspects can be considered through the use of the following benefit categories:

A. Utilization
B. Service Availability
C. Nature of Expected Benefits
—degree to which patients benefit, e.g.,
Lifesaving
—full recovery
—disability
Nonlifesaving
—health restoration—full
—health restoration—partial
—fatal disease prevention
—nonfatal disease prevention
—increased patient convenience or improved operations
—number of patients who will benefit
—characteristics of patients who will benefit

Given these benefit categories or types, each proposed project must be evaluated in terms of its expected performance in respect to each category. That is, the expected benefits must be identified and measured relative to each category of benefit. Thus, for example, the type and quantity of benefits for an ambulatory care facility might be as follows:

Utilization—36%
Service Availability—service presently not available in sufficient quantity
Nature of Expected Benefits
—degree to which patients will benefit—benefits in all non-life saving areas, though approximately half of the patients are expected to benefit in regard to both categories of health restoration
—number of patients who will benefit—20,000

---

*The following material, or a variant of it, would generally be included in the Budget Officer's Budget Support and Analysis Preparation Manual but would not be provided to all staff as part of the Administrative Package.

The material is presented here as an example of a technique which can aid in the evaluation of the service/patient care benefits of alternative capital expenditures. Such evaluation is obviously needed if sound capital budget decisions are to be made.

It should be noted that the following methodology is not presented as the definitive answer to the benefit evaluation problem. Rather, it is presented as an alternative to less structured approaches and as a stimulus to the development of more accurate techniques.

—characteristics of patients who will benefit—patients of all ages will benefit, with the distribution being approximately equal

In the case of a hospital-based kidney dialysis unit, the type and quantity of benefits might be as follows:

Utilization—5%

Service Availability—service presently not available in sufficient
   quantity

Nature of Expected Results

   —degree to which patients will benefit—8 patients = full recovery

   2 patients = partial

   recovery

   —characteristics of patients who will benefit—adults (for this example, assume that all patients are adults)

f. Merger of Financial and Benefit Evaluation Data. As the final step before decision, the output of the financial and benefit evaluation steps must be merged into one or more unified measures. Unified measures should be statistics which integrate cost and benefit data into a single index which can be used for the initial rank ordering of projects.

Utilizing the methodology described in Exhibits I and II and net present value analysis, examples of the type of measures which can be developed are illustrated in the following statistics:

$$\text{Cost/Benefit Index} = \frac{\text{Net Present Value (Lifetime Benefit Value)}}{\text{Present Value of Capital Costs}}$$

$$\text{Benefit/Capital Cost Index} = \frac{\text{(Lifetime Benefit Value)}}{\text{Capital Costs}}$$

$$\text{Operating Cost Index} = \frac{\text{Annual Benefit Value}}{\text{Annual Operating Cost}}$$

These measures provide an indexing statistic which defines benefits in terms of the investment (cost) required to obtain the benefits. Of the above examples, the Cost/Benefit Index is the most comprehensive single statistic, including both capital and operating cost factors as well as the ratio of these factors to capital costs and the relationship of all financial factors to total benefits.

For projects with positive net present values and equal lifetime benefit values the larger the Cost/Benefit Index number the better the project's value, that is, a project with an index of 500 is generally more desirable than a project with an index of 60. This is the case, for, presuming benefits are held constant, the larger the numerator the better the financial aspects of the investment and the larger the final quotient. Therefore, assuming two projects with

Exhibit II

Benefit Analysis: Benefit Evaluation*

The second step in the benefit analysis process is to subjectively—but systematically—assign numerical weights or values to each category of benefit (see Exhibit I for discussion of benefit categories). The schedule of benefit weights should be determined—if the Staff Budget Committee approach discussed in the chapter is not utilized—by senior management. The weighting schedule should be reviewed annually, prior to initiation of the budget preparation process, to assure that it adequately reflects the hospital's and the community's current attitudes and priorities. A sample benefit weighting schedule is presented below:

Sample Benefit Weighting Schedule**

Benefit Category	Weight
Utilization	1 unit
Service Availability	2 units
Nature of Expected Benefit	
Lifesaving	
—full recovery	10 units
—disability	8 units
Nonlifesaving	
—health restoration—full	6 units
—health restoration—partial	5 units
—fatal disease prevention	4 units
—nonfatal disease prevention	3 units
—increase patient convenience or improved operations	1 unit

In addition to specifying the benefit weighting schedule, the relationship between the quantity of benefits and the value of weight assigned to each benefit category must be determined. This step is necessary, for in order to use the foregoing weighting schedule the weights must be expressed in terms of weighted unit per some given quantity of benefit.

---

*The following material, or a variant of it, would generally be included in the Budget Officer's, Budget Support and Analysis Preparation Manual but would not be provided to all staff as part of the Administrative Package.

The material is presented here as an example of a technique which can aid in the evaluation of the service/patient care benefits of alternative capital expenditures. Such evaluation is obviously needed if sound capital budget decisions are to be made.

It should be noted that the following methodology is not presented as the definitive answer to the benefit evaluation problem. Rather, it is presented as an alternative to less structured approaches and as a stimulus to the development of more accurate techniques.

**The above are not suggested weights. The Committee should thoroughly discuss and develop its own understanding of each benefit component so as to be able to subjectively assign weights which it feels are appropriate to local needs and values.

Thus, the hospital must determine a common denominator for each category of benefits; i.e., what percentage of utilization is equal to one unit, how many lives saved equals ten units, and so forth. A *sample* relationship schedule is presented below:

Sample Benefit-Weighting Relationship Schedule***

Benefit Category	Weight	Benefit Quantity–Weight Relationship
Utilization	1 unit	percent actually utilized
Service Availability	2 units	full value of services are presently not available in sufficient quantity; zero value if they are available
Nature of Expected Benefit		
Lifesaving		
—full recovery	8 units	10 units per each life saved
Nonlifesaving		
—health restoration		
—full	6 units	6 units per each 5,000 patients treated
—health restoration		
—partial	5 units	5 units per each 5,000 patients treated
—fatal disease		
prevention	4 units	4 units per each 5,000 patients treated
—increased patient		
convenience or improved operations	1 unit	1 unit per each 5,000 patients treated

It should be noted that the above weighting and relationship schedules are presented only as illustrations and should not be capriciously adopted. The hospital should consider the implication of several feasible schedules and independently determine the one which most appropriately reflects the community's needs and philosophies. A technique known as sensitivity analysis may be quite useful in regard to this task. In simplest terms, sensitivity analysis involves experimenting with several possible schedules and comparing the results which are obtained under each schedule. In this way, alternative schedules can be evaluated and a determination can be made as to which weighting system is the most appropriate.

Using the weighting and relationship schedules, and information about the nature of specific project benefits, the next step is to calculate the benefit value for each project under consideration. This process can be most easily explained through the use of the following examples (see Tables A and B) which rely on both the above material and the material presented in Exhibit I.

As can be seen by these examples, the total (lifetime) project benefit value is the sum of the benefit values for each benefit category multiplied by the useful life of the investment. Benefit values, by category, are determined by multiplying the benefit weight by the—according to the rela-

---

***For purposes of this sample, pediatric benefits are assumed to be weighted double; e.g., 20 units per each life saved.

tionship schedule—quantity of benefits. Thus, the benefit value calculation can be summarized as follows:

Lifetime Benefit = (Investment's Useful Life) (Annual Benefit Value)

Annual Benefit Value = the sum of: Utilization Benefit Factor, i.e.,
(percent utilization) (benefit weight)

+Service Availability Factor
+Nature of Benefit Factor, i.e., (benefit quantity by nature of benefit) (benefit weight)

The above technique provides a unique value for the annual and total useful life benefit of each investment alternative. This data can be merged, in a variety of ways, with financial data; e.g.,

$$\frac{\text{Net Present Value}}{\text{Present Value of Capital Costs}} \quad (\text{Lifetime Benefit} = \text{Cost Benefit Index Value})$$

$$\frac{\text{Lifetime Benefit Value}}{\text{Capital Costs}} = \text{Benefit/Capital Cost Index}$$

$$\frac{\text{Annual Benefit Value}}{\text{Annual Operating Costs}} = \text{Operating Cost Index}$$

to provide a set of relative indices which can be used for purposes of establishing project priority rankings.

It should be noted however, that the index values should be mechanically applied—with a rank order listing being an automatic by-product of the evaluation technique. Project rankings should be established based on management's judgment as to the total evaluation and importance of the project. The benefit indices should only serve as an input to this judgment.****

---

similar benefit values, the project with the better financial implications, i.e., the greater ratio of net cash inflows to capital costs, is, generally, the project of choice.

In the case of projects with negative net present values, the mechanics of calculating the index numbers are the same. However, due to the reversal of numerical signs (negative numbers are being calculated) the smaller the absolute index number, the more desirable (typically) is the project.

****The scope of the foregoing weighting schedule is only illustrative. For initial use, a hospital may only desire to utilize two or three benefit categories and then, as it becomes more experienced with this technique "phase in" a more lengthy and comprehensive listing. This phasing approach will simplify implementation of the benefit analysis procedure and should be considered.

Decisions

Application of the foregoing steps will produce a set of statistics which can be used to rank order alternative projects. The resulting listing does not, however, automatically dictate investment decisions for the hospital as it might for a commercial firm.

In the case of a commercial firm, unless external factors reverse the general decision rules, only projects with positive net present values would be considered as realistic investment alternatives. Unfortunately, this kind of simple decision rule is not applicable in the hospital setting.

Due to both the hospital's community resource character and its complex objective function, hospital management must consider projects with either positive or negative net present values as realistic alternatives. Moreover, because of the predominance of cost-based reimbursement, the funding decision is further compounded by the need to distinguish between projects which generate a positive net present value due to revenues and those which produce a positive value due to savings.[6]

Appendix 17-A illustrates one approach to the decision process. It should be recognized that the committee mechanism described in the appendix is just one of a variety of alternative organizational structures which can be used for making these types of decisions. The committee approach, while having certain advantages due to its interdisciplinary structure, should not be slavishly imposed. As is the case with regard to other complex organizational questions, no single correct answer exists. Each institution must structure its own solution in light of its own history, character, environment, and goals.

Capital Financing

Appendix 17-A also briefly references the role which debt (borrowing) can play in making investment decisions. Appendix 17-B addresses this issue in a bit more detail.[7] It is important to recog-

---

[6]This is necessary because, by definition, cost-based reimbursement will absorb the savings and not generate funds to meet the incremental capital costs. Therefore, these projects though having a positive net present value, have financial implications similar to projects with negative present values. If financial stability is to be provided, the hybrid nature of these projects must be identified and accounted for in the decision process.

[7]The purpose of Appendix 17-2 is to provide an introduction to capital financing alternatives. Readers interested in more information should refer to the references in the "Suggested Readings." (Continued; p. 529)

Exhibit II—Table A

Benefit Analysis Calculation

Example I

Ambulatory Care Unit

(1) *Benefit Category*	(2) *Benefit Quantity*	(3)* *Benefit Weight*	(4) *Relationship*	(5)** *Benefit Value* (Col. 2 x Col. 3)
Utilization	.36	1	percent utilized	.36
Service Availability	present service insufficient	2	sufficient; insufficient	2.00
Nature of Expected Benefit				
health care restoration—full	10,000 patients (7,500 adult; 2,500 peds)	6	5,000 pts.=6	$\dfrac{\text{Col. 2}}{\text{Col. 4}}$ Col. 3 Adult=8.25
		5.5		

health care restoration—partial	5		5,000 pts.=5	Peds=5.50
fatal disease prevention	4		5,000 pts.=4	
nonfatal disease prevention	3	2.67	10,000 patients (7,500 adult; 2,500 peds) 5,000 pts.=3	Adults=4.01
patient convenience or improved operations	1		5,000 pts.=1	Peds=2.67
TOTAL ANNUAL BENEFIT VALUE				22.79

Useful Life 30 years

Lifetime Benefit Value (22.79) (30) 683.7

---

*These weightings, once established, do not change from project to project. However, due to the benefit quantity distribution it is necessary to determine the average benefit weight. Therefore, since 10,000 patients will benefit in the first two categories, the average benefit weight is 5.5. Ten thousand patients will also benefit in the last three areas. Thus, the average benefit weight for these categories is 2.67.

**Since the adult population is 7,500 patients, the benefit value, given the relationship schedule, is equal to (1½) (average benefit weight). In the case of pediatrics, the benefit value, given the relationship schedule and the double pediatrics weighting, is equal to (½) (average benefit weight) (2).

Exhibit II—Table B

Benefit Analysis Calculation

Example II

Kidney Dialysis Unit

(1) Benefit Category	(2) Benefit Quantity	(3) Benefit Weight	(4) Relationship	(5) Benefit Value (Col. 2 x Col 3)
Utilization	.05	1	percent utilized	.05
Service Availability	present service insufficient	2	sufficient; insufficient	2.00
Nature of Expected Benefit			Col. 2 Col. 3 Col. 4	
Lifesaving —full recovery	8	10	1 life=10	80.00
—disability	2	8	1 life=8	16.00
			TOTAL ANNUAL BENEFIT VALUE	98.05
			Useful Life	6 years
			Lifetime Benefit Value (98.05) (6)	588.30

nize, however, that an in depth understanding of capital financing is beyond both the capability of a single text and the operational needs of most hospital managers.

Typically, it will be only on rare occasions, such as when large sums are needed to finance an approved renovation, expansion, or rebuilding project, that a voluntary not-for-profit hospital will need to enter the capital market.[8] Moreover, it will be even rarer that a hospital's capital market needs either require or justify its going beyond the capacity of its commercial bank.[9] In those instances, however, when a hospital must enter the capital market, management should immediately obtain the advice and assistance of an expert capital market consultant.

The capital market is a highly segmented, complex, and volatile market. Its equity component is distinct from its debt component. Morever, each is lined with potential pitfalls which can inadvertently increase either funds acquisition and/or carrying costs. Compounding the matter is the unique operating character and regulatory environment of hospitals.

Cost-based reimbursement, for example, can either positively or negatively impact a hospital's debt capacity. To the extent that bad debts and/or free service costs are not allowed as reimbursable expenses, debt capacity is limited. However, to the extent that interest costs and depreciation expenses are allowed, debt capacity—if debt repayment and depreciation schedules are synchronized—is expanded. In this latter instance, if a large proportion of a hospital's patients are covered by cost-based payers, debt capacity can easily exceed the traditional industrial guidelines, becoming a function more of the third party payer's financial condition and abilities than the condition of the hospital.

Regulatory sanctions, requiring planning agency approval of proposed projects, also impact debt capacity as well as the basic financial viability, if not legality, of a proposed investment.

Also, readers should seek out the advice of any investment banker; e.g. Goldman Sacks and Co., Blyth Eastman Dillon Health Care Funding, Inc. Smith Barney, Harris Upham & Co. Inc., Wertheim & Co., Inc. At least a general level of advice can be provided at a firm's local office.

[8] Investor owned (proprietary or for-profit) hospitals make much greater use of capital markets; obtaining their basic financing from the equity component of the market.

[9] The distinction between capital and money markets should be noted. Money markets supply short-term (working capital) funds. In contrast, capital markets are the source of long-term funds, e.g., stock, long term debt, etc. Hospitals, as discussed in Chapter 14, may make frequent use of the money market.

In view of these complexities, it is foolhardy for a hospital to attempt to either decipher or conquer the capital market on its own. The most valuable general rules which can be set out at this point are that:

—financial considerations should be included as part of the initial planning of any large scale project which might require use of the capital market for obtaining funds;

—it is generally financially sound to use debt to finance projects having revenue generated positive net present values; and

—before debt is used to finance any capital expenditure, expert advice should be obtained in order to discover not only the least cost source of capital but also to assure that the debt will not seriously impair the institution's financial position.

Conclusion

The preceding has attempted to describe in a cogent fashion the nature of the capital budgeting process. Particular emphasis has been placed upon bringing a systematic, though admittedly to some extent subjective, approach to the making of capital investment decisions.

In view of the importance of these decisions, such an approach represents perhaps only a minimal level of decision rigor. Certainly, additional research and pragmatic experimentation are needed to further refine the decision process. However, while this work is proceeding, the historical void should be filled through the implementation—on a phased basis if necessary—of budgeting processes similar to that described above and in the accompanying appendix.

Suggested Readings

American Hospital Association. *Budgeting Procedures for Hospitals.*

American Hospital Association. *Capital Financing for Hospitals.*

Cleverly, William O. *Financial Management of Health Care Facilities*, Chapter 11.

Gilbert, Robert Neal. *Capital Budgeting at Henry Ford Hospital: Analysis and Proposal.*

Griffith, John R. *Quantitative Techniques for Hospital Planning and Control*, Chapter 9.

Lindsay, J. Robert and Sametz, Arnold W. *Financial Management.*

Robinson, Roland I. *Money and Capital Markets*, Chapters 1, 9–13.

Silvers, J.B. and Prahalad, C.K. *Financial Management of Health Institutions,* Chapters 5, 6 and 7.

Topics in Health Care Financing. "Capital Financing," Fall 1978.

Topics in Health Care Financing. "Capital Projects," Winter 1975.

Van Arsdell, Paul M. "Considerations Underlying Cost of Capital." *Financial Analysts Journal,* November–December 1963.

Weston, J. Fred, and Brigham, Eugene E. *Managerial Finance, Third Edition,* Chapters 6, 7, and 8.

Appendix 17-A
Capital Budgeting*

A hospital's plant and equipment investment program can be viewed as consisting of two basic components: a long-term planning or major acquisitions component and a short-term budgeting component. The major acquisition segment of the program focuses on a new program and construction opportunities. Decisions as to which project should be undertaken should be made only after a thorough cost benefit analysis of each of the available opportunities. Financing for projects of this type is generally beyond a single year's internal capabilities. However, if these projects are to be funded either partially or totally from internal sources, then decisions as to whether or not a project is undertaken should be part of the regular annual capital budgeting process. The forms used for capital budget decision making, as well as the instructions for completing the forms and an explanation of the decision process are presented below.

Capital Budgeting: Forms and Instructions

Step 1—Initial Budget Meeting. Departmental supervisors should meet with the administrator for their department and discuss all potential capital investment expenditures for the coming fiscal year.

---

*The following material is excerpted from the budgeting procedure designed for a 300 bed community, general hospital. The organizational control relationships described in the procedure, reflect the particular organization structure of the hospital. In a different institution, the details of the process may have to be revised, e.g., more meeting and decision steps may need to be built into the procedure to properly accommodate the different organization structure. Also, in different institutions, the titles of the forms may have to be changed to reflect the particular institution's nomenclature.

Form I

Department _____

SMALL ITEM PLANT AND EQUIPMENT BUDGET REQUEST FORM

Description of Request	Quantity	Nature			Estimate of Cost		Purchase Date	Justification of Request	Decision	
		Replace.	Renova.	Addition	Total	Each			App.	Class

a. In order to avoid wasting the departmental supervisor's time in preparing detailed proposals for all potential expenditures, tentative agreement should be reached at this point as to which projects or items will be requested for the coming fiscal year.

b. Each administrator should also review with his departmental supervisors the mechanics of both the Plant and Equipment Budget Request Form and the Small Item Plant and Equipment Budget Request Form so that each departmental supervisor will know when to use each form, how to complete each form, and the nature of the supporting material which should be provided for each item listed on the Plant and Equipment Budget Request Form.

Step 2—Small Item Budget Form. Based on the tentative agreements reached in the preceeding step the departmental supervisor should complete the Small Item Plant and Equipment Budget Request Form for all expenditure requests of $500 and under (See Form I).

Example Form Entries:
—Description of Request—brief statement of the item which is being requested, e.g., electric typewriter
—Quantity—indication of the number of items requested
—Nature—indication as to whether the request is for the replacement of obsolete or worn-out equipment, renovation of obsolete or insufficient facilities, or the addition of new equipment or facilities
—Estimate of Cost—indication of unit and total purchase cost (including installation costs)
—Purchase Date Requested—indication of when the expenditure will be made. This information is needed for purposes of preparing the cash budget.
—Justification of Request—an explanation of why the item should be purchased, e.g., needed for the new secretary who is to be hired
—Decision—this column should be completed by the assistant administrator responsible for the department.

Step 3—Plant and Equipment Budget Form. Based on the tentative agreements reached in Step 1, the departmental supervisor should complete the Plant and Equipment Budget Request Form for all expenditure requests of over $500 (see Form II).

Example Form Entries:
—Description of Request—brief statement of the item, work or program which is being requested, e.g. cardiac defibulator

Form II

(DEPARTMENTAL)
PLANT AND EQUIPMENT BUDGET
REQUEST FORM

Department _____

Description of Request	Quantity	Nature			Estimate of Cost		Purchase Date	Reason for Request (brief statement)	Classi.	Priority Rank
		Replace.	Renova.	Addition	Total	Each				

—Quantity—indication of the number of items desired

—Nature—indication as to whether the request is for the replacement of obsolete or worn-out equipment, renovation of obsolete or inefficient facilities, or the addition of new equipment or facilities

—Estimate of Cost—indication of unit and total purchase cost (including installation costs)

—Purchase Date Requested—indication of when the expenditure should be made. If the expenditure will be over a number of months, the amount by month should be indicated. This information is necessary for cash budgeting purposes.

—Reason for Request—a brief statement of why the request is being made e.g., presently, one of the hospital's three defibrilators is nonoperative and cost of repair exceeds cost of replacement.

—Classification—indication of the urgency or need for the expenditure. Classification "A" should be given to those expenditures necessary for continuing or maintaining present services, including new equipment needed to meet volume growth. Classification "B" should be given to those expenditures whose principal benefit will be either a cost savings or profit within the present scope of services. Classification "C" should be given to those expenditures whose principal benefit will be an increase in quality and/or effectiveness of present services. Classification "D" should be given to those expenditures whose principal benefit will be an expansion of present services through new programs.

—Departmental Supervisors' Recommended Priority Ranking—a numerical indication of the relative importance of each of the requested items.

Step 4—Small Items: Decisions. Departmental supervisors should review both budget request forms with the assistant administrator responsible for their department.

a. The assistant administrator should examine each of the items listed on the Small Item Request Form and come to final agreement with the departmental supervisor as to whether or not the requested item should be approved and, if approved, which of the above classifications, i.e., A, B, C, or D, should be assigned to it. The decision in regard to each item should be indicated in the "Decision Column" of the Small Request Form. The approved Small Item Request Form should then be forwarded to the budget officer for inclusion in the final Plant and Equipment Budget. (It should be noted that the budgeting process for these requests is completed at this point. Therefore, care must be exercised to assure that all requests are valid and necessary).

b. The assistant administrator should examine each item listed on the Plant and Equipment Request Form and come to a final agreement with the departmental supervisor as to which items will be included in the request and the classification of each included item.

Step 5—Plant and Equipment Request: Support Documentation. Departmental supervisors should prepare supporting material for each item listed in the Plant and Equipment Budget Request Form.

a. Nature of the supporting material
    In support of each expenditure request, the departmental supervisor should prepare an expenditure proposal which indicates in detail:

—the task for which the facility or equipment is to be used;

—the necessity and importance of the task;

—the expected utilization of the facility or equipment (7 days/ week; 24 hours/day = 100% utilization);

—the extent of the current availability of the same or similar services from other sources;

—the nature of expected service/patient care benefits;

  • the degree to which patients benefit, e.g., lifesaving, health restoration, disease prevention, increased patient convenience, etc.

  • the number of patients who will benefit, and

  • the characteristics of the patients who will benefit, e.g., age, sex, etc.

—the expected life of the facility or equipment;

—the capital costs of the facility or equipment (including acquisition costs, installation costs, and major maintenance costs; and the year(s) in which these costs can be expected to be incurred);

—the operating costs of the facility or equipment—by year of operation; and

—the savings or profits (if any)—by year—which can be expected if the expenditure is made.

b. Cooperation
    In preparing the above supporting documentation, departmental supervisors should, as needed, call upon the pur-

chasing department, the budget officer, the controller's office, and administration for assistance.

Step 6—Request Package: Review. To assure that all necessary data have been provided and that there is agreement as to the items requested, departmental supervisors should review the Plant and Equipment Budget Request Form and all the required supporting documentation with the assistant administrator responsible for their department. Following this review and agreement, the request form and the supporting materials should be forwarded to the budget officer for analysis and presentation to the Plant and Equipment Budget Committee.

Capital Budgeting: Decision Process

Step 1—The budget officer should receive all departmental budget request forms and supporting materials. Additionally, he should receive from Administration, Plant and Equipment Budget Request Forms and the appropriate supporting documentation for all facility and/or equipment expenditures which Administration wishes to initiate. (The forms and the required supporting materials are identical to that previously described).

Step 2—The budget officer should analyze the information provided in the request forms and supporting documentation and prepare summary budget request forms for presentation to the Plant and Equipment Budget Committee (see Forms III, IV, V, and VI).

    a. The budget officer should review each Classification "A" request and if the request is for current operational needs, he should summarize it on the appropriate form. Those requests which do not appear to meet the Classification "A" definition should be returned to the issuing departmental supervisor for clarification or change of classification and priority.

    b. The budget officer should compute the internal rate of return for each Classification "B" item which is expected to generate a profit and summarize each of the requests on form IV-A. Net present value should be computed for each Classification "B" item which is expected to produce a savings relative to the current level of operations and summarize each of the requests on Form IV-B. Those requests which do not meet the Classification "B" definition should be returned to the proper departmental supervisor for clarification or change of classification and priority.

    c. The budget officer should compute the net present value of each Classification "C" item and summarize the costs and

Form III

SUMMARY
PLANT AND EQUIPMENT BUDGET REQUESTS
CLASSIFICATION "A" ITEMS

Description of Request	Quantity	Dept.	Total Capital Cost	Summary of Supporting Materials	Dept. Prior. Rec.	Committee Action	
						Dec.	Rk. Order

Form IV-A

SUMMARY
PLANT AND EQUIPMENT BUDGET REQUESTS
CLASSIFICATION "B" ITEMS: INTERNAL RATE OF RETURN

Description of Request	Quantity	Dept.	Capital Costs by Year	Summary of Supporting Documentation: Benefits	Dept. Prior. Rec.	Internal Rate of Return	Committee Action	
							Dec.	Rk Order

Form IV-B

SUMMARY
PLANT AND EQUIPMENT BUDGET REQUESTS
CLASSIFICATION "B" ITEMS

| Description of Request | Dept. | Quant. | Cost by Year | | Net Present Value | Summary of Supporting Documentation: Benef. | Dept. Prior Rec. | Comm. Action | |
			Capital	Oper.				Dec.	Rank Ord.

Form V

SUMMARY
PLANT AND EQUIPMENT BUDGET REQUESTS
CLASSIFICATION "C" ITEMS

Description of Request	Dept.	Quant.	Cost by Year		Net Present Value	Summary of Supporting Documentation: Benef.	Dept. Prior Rec.	Comm. Action	
			Capital	Oper.				Dec.	Rank Ord.

Form VI

SUMMARY
PLANT AND EQUIPMENT BUDGET REQUESTS
CLASSIFICATION "D" ITEMS

Description of Request	Dept.	Quant.	Cost by Year		Net Present Value	Summary of Supporting Documentation:Benef.	Dept. Prior. Rec.	Comm. Action	
			Capital	Oper.				Dec.	Rank Ord.

service and/or patient care benefits of each of the requests on the appropriate form (Form V).* Those requests which do not meet the Classification "C" definition should be returned to the proper departmental supervisor for clarification or change of classification and priority.

d. The budget officer should compute the present value of the total cost of each Classification "D" item and summarize the costs and service and/or patient care benefits of each of the requests on the appropriate form (Form VI).* Those requests which do not meet the Classification "D" definition should be returned to the proper departmental supervisor for clarification or change of classification and priority.

Step 3—Plant and Equipment Budget Committee—The summary forms should be presented to the Plant and Equipment Budget Committee (can be the Staff Budget Committee described in the chapter) for action.

a. Due to the interdepartmental nature of the Plant and Equipment Budget, a representative committee, including at least administration, nursing, the medical staff and the various general service and patient care departments should be used to review and evaluate all expenditure requests. The chairman of the committee should be appointed by the director of the hospital.

b. The Plant and Equipment Budget Committee should review all requests by classification category and recommend whether or not a request should be approved.

c. Also, the committee should rank order—in terms of priority for funding—all requests which it recommends should be approved.

---

*Note to the reader. The matter of categorizing and quantifying benefits has long been an issue of controversy. A variety of techniques ranging from a subjective approach, wherein the relative value of alternative benefits is intuitively appraised, to an objective econometric technique, wherein an attempt is made to calculate the specific dollar impact of a particular set of benefits, can be used to attempt to quantify benefits. Given the current state of the art, the econometric approach, while theoretically attractive, is encumbered with methodological and pragmatic problems which significantly impair its efficacy. Similarly, the completely subjective approach is open to criticism in that basic values are never explicitly defined or tested.

An alternative technique which attempts to recognize the deficiencies of the above approaches by adding quantified definition to subjectively established values is presented in Exhibits I and II in the chapter. It should be noted that the material illustrated in the exhibits would generally not be included as part of the forms and instructions provided in the Administrative Package. Moreover, it should be recognized that the approach presented is not the definitive answer. Rather, it is just an intermediate step toward a more effective decision process. It is presented here both as an alternative to less structured approaches and as a stimulus to the development of more accurate techniques.

1. The rank ordering of Classification "A" items should be based on a subjective evaluation of the need for each item.

2. The rank ordering of Classification "B" items should be based largely on the internal rate of return which each project will generate. That is, generally the project with the highest rate of return should be ranked first. Projects producing savings should be ranked subsequent to expenditures which will produce a profit. Generally, the project with the largest ratio of net present value to initial capital costs should be ranked first.

3. The rank ordering of Classification "C" items should be based on a subjective evaluation of the costs and benefits which will be expected from each item.

4. The rank ordering of Classification "D" items should be based on a subjective evaluation of the costs and benefits which can be expected from each item.

d. Additionally, the Committee should indicate any exceptions which it feels should be made in the general order of funding items. That is, generally, all Classification "A" items should be funded before any Classification "B" items are funded, etc. However, if the committee feels, for example, that item "D-1" should be funded prior to item "C-3", it should indicate this change in general priority.

Step 4—Committee Recommendations—The recommendations of the Plant and Equipment Budget Committee should be forwarded to the director of the hospital for consideration in determining the Plant and Equipment Budget funding decisions.

Step 5—Funding Decisions—Given the Committee's recommendations, the next issue is that of determining the total amount of funds available for plant and equipment expenditures. This determination should be made by the controller and the director of the hospital after a review of the revenue, expense, and cash budgets and the forecasted margin. Once this amount is determined, the completion of the plant and equipment budget is a relatively simple matter.

Based on the quantity of available funds, the final budget should be prepared by funding, in the appropriate order, items approved through the small item budgeting mechanism and then by funding, in the appropriate order, other approved items until the entire amount of funds is appropriated.* Thus, the general funding order, unless either the Plant and Equipment Budget Committee recommends exceptions or the director of the hospital resets the priority of specific items, would be:

Order	Classification	Item
1	A	Small Item Requests
2	A	Plant & Equipment Requests
3	B	Small Item Requests
4	B	Plant & Equipment Requests
5	C	Small Item Requests
6	C	Plant & Equipment Requests
7	D	Small Item Requests
8	D	Plant & Equipment Requests

*It should be noted that at times it may be necessary to revise the Revenue Budget or borrow in order to obtain sufficient monies to fund all necessary expenditures. The necessity of this action will depend on the size of the recommended expenditures list and the amount of funds available. Also, at times, funds may be borrowed to finance Priority "B" projects which have a profit potential and an internal rate of return greater than the interest rate.

Appendix 17-B
Capital Financing*

Except for investor owned institutions, hospitals have historically had little interaction with the private capital markets. Prior to World War II, hospital capital needs were met primarily through retained earnings and philanthropy. In the post World War II era, these traditional sources were supplemented by federal government funds provided through the Hill Burton program.

Since the mid-1960s, however, the situation has markedly changed. For a variety of economic, reimbursement, and tax reasons, philanthropy has not been able to keep up with the accelerating pace of hospital capital needs. As a result hospitals have had to look increasingly to private capital markets; i.e., borrowing (debt, since equity is not available to a non-profit hospital) as a source for needed capital.

*The material for this Appendix has been excerpted from various documents prepared by R. Neal Gilbert, Vice President, Blyth Eastman Dillon Health Care Funding Inc.; including: Capital Financing, *Topics In Health Care Financing* Vol. 5, No. 1 Fall 1978.

In entering the private capital markets, the hospital is trying to obtain funds at the most attractive possible terms. This means that the institution must not only select the optimum method of financing but also, must structure the terms and conditions of loan in a way which is most economically beneficial to it. This latter task, is a complex problem which should not be undertaken without the aid of an investment banker. With respect to the method of financing, there are several major alternatives. Each of these is discussed below.

Tax-Exempt Revenue Bonds

This financing vehicle is by far the most popular, and has gained a great deal of popularity in recent years. Forty-six states have passed enabling legislation and at least 60 percent of all long-term hospital financing is now tax exempt. Because the interest earned on these bonds is exempt from federal income taxes, investors are willing to receive from a 1½ percent to 2½ percent lower return on their investment than they would on taxable issues of similar quantity. Bonds may be issued by a state or municipal hospital authority, by a county or city, or directly by the non-profit corporation under current IRS guidelines if a beneficial interest in the facility is given to a municipality.

If the bonds are issued through an authority, title to the hospital may remain with the authority until the bonds are retired, at which time it is reconveyed to the hospital. In other cases, loan agreements lease-leasebacks or mortgage loans may be used. Bonds are usually secured by a pledge of the revenues of the hospital being financed. The credit behind them is generally not the credit of the authority or municipality, but rather the present and future financial strength of the hospital.

A hospital may issue its own tax-exempt bonds if it is an exempt charitable institution now under IRS Code, Section 501-C-3. Under this method, the hospital is required to pass title to the municipality in which the hospital is located when the bonds are retired. This is commonly referred to as the "63-20" technique, in reference to the IRS ruling establishing this financing method. This is a cumbersome, imperfect method used commonly only in those states without legislation allowing municipal issuance.

Tax-exempt revenue bonds allow for the highest ratio of financing to project cost or total assets of any method. Many facilities can finance up to 100 percent of their project costs plus financing expenses, interest during construction, and refinancing of existing debt. This is because tax-exempt credit worthiness is based more on revenue generating capability, and cash flow than on property value which is more important to investors in taxable hospital financings. In addition, this method allows for the longest maturity (30–35 years), which reduces annual debt service.

A hospital should, however, be careful to recognize that the financing expenses, including the underwriting discount, legal and printing costs, a bond reserve fund, and capitalized interest during construction, can result in the hospital borrowing more funds relative to construction costs than under some other method of financing. The processing time can also be longer because of the involvement of additional parties to the transaction, such as a public authority or municipality, the work required on the documentation, and the need for a feasibility study. A "private placement" can sometimes reduce expenses and save time but may result in a higher interest coupon rate.

Advantages*

1) Interest costs are usually 1½%–2½% lower than other methods of financing.

2) The term of the loan can be 35 years reducing annual debt service requirements.

3) Since the loan amount is determined by the ability of the facility to generate revenue, up to 100% of total project costs might be financed.

4) Bond proceeds are available before construction eliminating need for interim construction financing.

Disadvantages*

1) In some cases, title to the facility may be transferred to the authority during the life of the issue.

2) In a few states, no statutory mechanisms exist to allow hospitals to use tax-exempt financing.

3) A feasibility study executed by a recognized outside consultant firm is usually required.

4) Financing expenses, including the underwriting discount, feasibility study, bond counsel, other legal fees, and printing costs, are generally higher than in some other methods of financing.

---

*Since all segments of the capital markets are in a constant state of change, this and the other summaries should be viewed as only general guidelines.

Advantages

5) Interest payments can be capitalized during construction.

6) Tax-exempt bond issues are usually structured with "open-ended" provisions allowing for issuance of additional bonds or alternative indebtedness, provided certain levels of financial performance are maintained.

7) Existing debt can usually be refinanced.

8) Fast track construction is possible.

9) A borrower's creditworthiness can be reflected in a better rating, more flexible terms and a lower interest cost.

10) Public offering through an underwriting group taps both regional and national sources of capital among institutional and individual investors.

11) Can sometimes be privately placed.

12) Principal repayment schedule is tailored to the hospital's ability to repay. First repayment is normally scheduled for one or two years after completion of project.

Disadvantages

5) A debt service reserve fund, usually equaling one year's average principal and interest payment is generally required. The reserve fund, however, is used to pay off the last maturing bond principal and is usually reinvested in securities earning enough to pay the cost of interest on the reserve fund.

6) Bonds sold to the public require disclosure of the hospital's operating and financial history.

7) Prepayment of the bonds usually cannot be made during the first ten years: thereafter, the bonds are callable at a premium decreasing annually from about 3% to 0% in the 11th through 15th years.

Conventional Mortgages or Taxable Bonds

This health care financing alternative covers all taxable non-government guaranteed financing vehicles which utilize private institutional lenders as the source of funds. This includes mortgages, notes on either a secured or unsecured basis, term loans with commercial banks and construction loans. Institutional lenders include private and public pension funds, mutual savings banks, insurance companies, savings and loan associations, and real estate investment trusts.

This method of financing can be tailored to meet the particular financial priorities of the hospital although this flexibility is limited to the parameters of any particular lender's requirements. It is usually the speediest of all the financing techniques and can frequently be implemented in two to four months. Negotiating privately with one sophisticated lender can avoid costs and delays that can occur in methods involving governmental approval or a public offering of securities.

A disadvantage of the private placement technique is that the percentage of total project cost that can be raised through this method is generally lower than the percentage that can be raised through other financing techniques such as the government insured or guaranteed programs. This lower loan-to-value ratio dictates that a greater percentage of project cost be raised by the hospital or that the hospital be in a very strong capital position to begin with.

The hospital should be very careful in negotiating the covenants of the loan agreement. Private placements can be very restrictive with regard to pre-payment provisions and additional financing. A typical loan might be non-callable for ten years and then only at a gradually declining premium. Additional financing might only be allowed if a certain loan-to-value ratio is not exceeded.

In understanding private placements, one must keep in mind the differences between institutional lenders. Their attitudes, lending policies, and interest charges will vary dramatically depending on money market conditions, the make-up of their loan portfolio, lending criteria, interest requirements, cash flow, fiduciary responsibility and the personalities involved. What holds true for one lender may be totally inappropriate for another and what was true one time may be wrong a few months later.

These points emphasize the general need to utilize a capable investment banker in executing this method of financing. An investment banker that is thoroughly familiar with the market and is in constant contact with a large cross section of institutional lenders will be able to identify the best lenders for a particular situation. This capability will usually save the hospital time and money. In addition, an experienced investment banker will guide the hospital through the complicated negotiating process and obtain the most favorable available terms.

Advantages

1) This method often takes the shortest amount of time to implement.

2) This method of financing allows the hospital to structure a financing package most suitable to its financial priorities through negotiations with one lender.

3) The hospital does not have to conform to HEW/FHA construction standards.

4) There are no discount points required, since interest rates are freely negotiated.

5) Since the interest rate can be negotiated well before closing, the hospital can more accurately predict total costs and debt service requirements.

6) A feasibility study is frequently not required; printing expenses are reduced or avoided; and legal fees are usually less expensive than with other alternatives, particularly those involving public sale.

Disadvantages

1) The loan-to-value ratio rarely exceeds 70%. Therefore, the hospital may have to contribute a higher percentage of equity to use this method of financing.

2) The loan term may be shorter than the alternative methods of financing, 20–25 years compared with 25–30.

3) The loan covenants are usually more restrictive than in other methods.

4) The interest rate will be higher than in tax-exempt or FHA/GNMA financings.

5) Funds may be difficult to obtain when money markets are tight if the hospital is located in an unattractive area or if elements of speculation exist.

The FHA-242/GNMA Program

FHA-insured hospital mortgages were made possible in 1968 by Section 242 of Title II to the National Housing and Urban Development Act. The section authorized the Commissioner of the Federal Housing Administration (FHA) to insure mortgage loans used to finance the construction or rehabilitation of not-for-profit hospitals and the purchase of major moveable equipment for such institutions. The Act, as amended in 1970, added the eligibility for proprietary hospitals.

In 1971, marketability of the loans increased, and lower interest rates came about as a result of the lenders ability to obtain an added guarantee from the Government National Mortgage Association, a sub-agency of HUD. Under this program, an FHA approved lender, who further qualifies as a GNMA issuer, may obtain private funds to lend to hospitals, through the sale of GNMA securities. GNMA is authorized by Section 306 (g) of the National Housing Act to guarantee the timely payment of principal and interest on such securities, which are based on and backed by the mortgage loan issued by FHA.

Hospitals utilizing the FHA-242/GNMA program may borrow up to 90 percent of the replacement value of the facility for a term of up to 25 years plus the period of construction. For hospitals with sufficient equity in the form of existing property, plant, and equipment, the financing program may be used to finance 100 percent of eligible project costs.

The process by which hospitals obtain an FHA commitment is to file a loan application with the Department of Health, Education and Welfare (HEW). Under an agreement between HEW and FHA, HEW has the responsibility for evaluating and passing on its project approval to FHA. The evaluation process is conducted in three principal areas: financial feasibility, architectural and engineering conformance to federal guidelines and service program need. In most instances, an independent feasibility study supports the basic application documentation. Notwithstanding a favorable evaluation by HEW, the project application is then analyzed by the multi-family mortgage credit section of FHA for conformance with numerous other financing guidelines. Furthermore, all hospitals must have project approvals from local HSA's and federally recognized Certificates of Need.

Advantages

1) Load-to-replacement value ratio can be as high as 90%.

2) The value of the land, existing buildings, and major moveable equipment may satisfy hospital's equity requirement.

3) Most preparation and application costs can be included in eligible costs.

4) The United States Government's full faith and credit guarantee allows the hospital to secure an attractive interest rate.

5) The GNMA Construction Loan Certificate enables the hospital to obtain both construction and permanent financing in a single package at the same interest rate.

6) If the hospital is undergoing an expansion or modernization program, eligible debt can include refinancing of existing debt.

7) The term of the loan can be as much as 25 years after completion of construction.

8) Prepayment of 15% of the original principal amount is permitted in a calender year without penalty. In addition, the loan can be structured to allow for prepayment in excess of this amount at any time for a negotiated penalty.

9) FHA/GNMA financing is extremely compatible with other government programs.

Disadvantages

1) Processing of the FHA application can be time-consuming.

2) Construction must conform to FHA/HEW standards.

3) Construction labor costs can be higher than other methods of financing because of strict government regulations.

4) If the FHA cupon rate is below current money market rates, the hospital must pay front-end discount points to bring the yield to the investor up to market levels.

5) The hospital must pay an annual mortgage insurance premium of ½ of 1% of the unamortized principal amount.

6) The hospital must pay front-end inspection and filing fees totaling .8 of 1% of the principal amount.

FHA-242/GNMA Insured and Guaranteed Tax-Exempt Revenue Bonds

A recent breakthrough in hospital finance has been achieved through the development of a unique financing program which combines the advantages of the FHA-242/GNMA program with those of tax-exempt revenue bonds.*

The essence of the program is the issuance of hospital tax-exempt revenue bonds which are 100 percent collateralized by Government National Mortgage Association securities, which in turn are backed by the full faith and credit of the United States government.

These combined financing programs significantly reduce the interest rate for borrowed funds, and result in a decrease in debt service costs and cash requirements. These cost savings will be passed on to third party payors and ultimately to the health care consumer.

The hospital's investment banker obtains an FHA-242 mortgage insurance in the ordinary manner, issues GNMA securities, structures and places the tax-exempt bond issue for the proposed capital project. The proceeds from the sale of the bond issue are deposited with a Trustee to be used to purchase the GNMA guaranteed securities that are generated by and based on the FHA insured mortgage. The Bonds issued are equal in amount to the FHA insured mortgage principal and collateralized by a pledge of the purchased GNMA securities and payments thereon. The pledge of the purchased GNMA securities as collateral provides security sufficient to allow the tax-exempt bonds to receive at least an AA rating. As the interest rate on the GNMA securities and underlying hospital mortgage is set at a level sufficient to pay the debt service on the resulting tax-exempt bonds, there is a substantial decrease in the hospital's debt service in comparison to the debt service associated with other capital financing alternatives.

Upon FHA's initial approval of the project, the Hospital Finance Authority is notified of a potential bond issue to effect a combination financing, its size and anticipated sale date. The investment banker works with both bond counsel and FHA/GNMA counsel to prepare the necessary loan documentation such that upon final FHA approval of the mortgage loan, the bond sale occurs simultaneously with the FHA loan closing.

---

*In April 1979 the Department of Housing and Urban Development issued an opinion that this financial mechanism could no longer be used for hospital financings. This decision by the Department is currently (May 1979) being appealed in the courts.

The bond issue size is equal in amount to the principal of the GNMA securities to be issued and the underlying FHA insured mortgage. The proceeds of the bond issue are deposited with a Trustee for the benefit of the bondholders, and used to purchase the GNMA securities in the Authority's name, as they are generated throughout the construction period. The interest rate on the FHA insured mortgage and GNMA securities is set to meet principal and interest payments on the tax-exempt bonds when due. As the interest rates on the mortgage and GNMA securities must be set prior to loan closing the hospital's investment banker negotiates privately with potential bond investors to obtain a fixed interest rate commitment for the bond issue purchase, to be executed at FHA loan closing.

During the construction period when the Trustee is accumulating the GNMA securities, the balance of the bond proceeds are invested in qualified securities acceptable to the bondholders and whose maturities and interest payments thereon will be sufficient to provide funds to purchase the GNMA securities and to meet the debt service on the outstanding bonds.

The tax-exempt bond issue is structured with a term of 25 years plus the construction period with no principal repayment during construction and with maturities such that the monthly GNMA payments to the Authority accumulate to pay the bonds debt service when due.

Farmers Home Administration (FMHA) Guarantee and Direct Loan Programs for Hospitals

The Rural Development Act of 1972 authorized Farmers Home Administration (FMHA) to fund essential community facilities including hospitals, clinics, and other health related facilities. Credit is provided for the construction or renovation of these health facilities through two of the FMHA programs: the Community Facilities Program and the Business and Industrial Loan Program. Both programs also provide funds to non-health related community facilities and have policies stating which types of facilities have priority over others for receipt of credit assistance.

Each program is allocated a certain amount of credit yearly, on a national level which is then distributed to the states and eligible territories based on population and income figures. Within these geographic areas, each program can extend credit only up to its budgeted amount each year with priority given to those individual applicants whose projects fall within the highest priority FMHA categories of project types. Historically, the demand for assistance under both these programs has exceeded the yearly budget allocations resulting in many lower priority projects being turned down thus not being constructed at all or being forced to rely on conventional sources of funds.

To be eligible for assistance under either program, a proposed health care project must meet certain standard criteria and provide certain assurances including:

a) Compliance with the State Medical Facilities Plan
b) Possession of a Certificate of Need
c) Demonstration of financial ability to repay loan
d) Compliance with state and local building and zoning ordinances
e) Possession of clear title to the project's assets
f) Provision of non-discrimination and equal employment opportunity assurances

The Business and Industrial Loan Program (B&I)

Assistance under the B&I Program is available to any legal entity, public or private, for profit or non-profit that proposes to finance a project that will improve the economic or environmental climate of a rural area, with priority given to projects which save existing jobs or create the highest number of new permanent employment opportunities. To be eligible for assistance, the proposed project must be in any area outside the boundary of a city of 50,000 or more population or outside a city's adjacent areas with population density exceeding 100 persons per square mile. Priority is given to those projects in areas of population of 25,000 or less.

The assistance provided is in the form of a FMHA loan guarantee, where the loan is arranged with, made, and serviced by a private lender who is indemnified by FMHA for a certain percentage of his losses should a default occur. FMHA can provide a guarantee of up to 90 percent of the principal and interest on the loan to the private lender. In return for this guarantee the applicant must pay FMHA a fee equal to 1 percent of the guaranteed principal amount at loan closing.

The benefit of the FMHA guarantee to the lender is not primarily to strengthen the financial credit of a proposed project to give it access to private lenders, but to provide the lender with a federal government guarantee so that he can provide funds to certain project types in excess of that amount allowed for these projects without the guarantee. As the projects receiving the FMHA guarantee must be good credit risks to qualify for assistance, receipt of the guarantee plus the payment of the 1 percent fee by the applicant will generally result in financing whose cost is not appreciably lower than that normally associated with conventional sources.

Fiscal year 1978 funding for the B&I Program is $1 billion on a national level.

The Community Facilities Loan Program (CFL Program)

Credit assistance under the CFL Program is available to all political subdivisions of a state and other organizations operated on a non-profit basis such as districts, authorities, corporations, associations, and cooperatives. The purpose of the program is to provide funds for the construction and equipping of essential facilities to serve the community where located which cannot obtain commercial credit on "reasonable terms or at reasonable rates." In determining that commercial credit is not available on these terms FMHA will examine only private market sources not the terms available under other government programs for hospital financing such as FHA-242 insured mortgages. In determining the "reasonableness" of private market terms FMHA will consider front-end costs as well as interest rate and the project's ability to pay debt service under those conditions.

In addition to the nonavailability of credit criteria, eligibility for the CFL Program is subject to the following conditions:

1. The proposed project must be located in a rural area of under 10,000 population with priority given to those projects in areas of less than 5,000 population.
2. Applicant must show legal authority to construct, operate and maintain the proposed facility.
3. Private non-profit sponsors must show significant community ties as evidenced by community control of the governing board or substantial public funding via taxes or philanthrophy.

If an applicant and proposed project is found eligible for direct FMHA loan assistance, there are a number of requirements that must be met prior to loan closing and during and after construction.

A Note of Caution

In addition to the foregoing, some of the financing alternatives can be combined, in some cases resulting in an optimal financing package. The financing techniques vary in time requirements, processing procedures, costs flexibility, interest rates and impact on cash flow. Each alternative requires a professional financial expertise to insure proper execution and each has advantages and disadvantages that must be carefully evaluated before one approach is selected.

Chapter 18

Management Reporting

An outstanding feature of a hospital budget system should now be apparent: effective budgeting requires group participation by personnel from responsibility centers upward to the administrative offices. That participation should not be one of a token partnership, but an active one where the employee involved feels input from his level is important in planning and in accomplishing objectives.

Budgeting should be a living process with a reasonable degree of flexibility, fluidity, and mobility to meet changing conditions and unforeseen exigencies. Changing conditions could occur within a budget period or, more likely, within the time span leading to the projected planning horizon.

If the position is taken that budgeting is a dynamic rather than a static process, one must be prepared to adjust to changes in demand for services, changes in the costs of services or supplies, and changes in a variety of other conditions which force adjustments in budgetary projections.

The next logical thought is: If a hospital's manager and its governing board are to retain their managerial perspective and administrative balance by keeping the budget process adaptable to change and flexible in response to changing needs, they must be kept informed.

Plans are good only as road maps (as earlier suggested). Operations people must read the signposts and change routes when necessary to reach objectives, if the first route or plan proves unworkable or ineffective. Information about the flow of operations must be fed constantly into the system, so that, in a sense, there is a continuous register of the blood pressure, temperature, and other vital systemic signs.

(The authors digress a moment to make an important point by analogy: Think of a hospital in terms of a commercial venture. Most administrators realize what a precarious situation the A & P supermarket chain is in when it attempts to operate on a net profit of one or two percent. Executives in that kind of operation, as recent history demonstrated, are walking forever on the brink of disaster. However, they do have some capability to adjust prices and to change marketing emphasis within a competitive framework in an attempt to retain profitability. Hospitals also often operate on less than a two percent margin, but have a very limited maneuverability in changing operating conditions to avoid deficits or even disaster. This digression, it must be evident, was made to emphasize the great need of keeping "on top of things" in order to maintain the solvency of a hospital. That means accurate, relevant information must be available when needed.)

Information Flow

If management is to have access to relevant, accurate information, it must plan a flow of information on the basis of daily, monthly and, possibly, quarterly inputs so that comparisons with planned results as well as with previous periods can be charted and trends can be projected. This flow of information can come up the organization's "escalator stairway" by the same route as did the original planning information. Later in this chapter this stairway concept will be considered not only in the sense of information flowing upward, but also in the context of the downward flow of performance data.

Ideally, the budget officer, through the hospital's chief financial officer, should direct the financial and performance reporting system. This system should provide for the exchange of actual performance and corrective action information between persons in charge of the various cost centers, departments, divisions, and programs of the hospital. Reports of financial and work performance will enable managers at the various levels to measure the performance of their responsibility centers in terms of the objectives set for the budget period. Since each person in charge of a responsibility center or group of responsibility centers participates in the planning and budgeting process, each manager should expect, in turn, to receive reports which can be used to monitor and to evaluate performance.

To return to the information stairway concept, data are input at the various organizational levels (cost centers, departments, divi-

Figure 18-1

Organizational Information Stairway

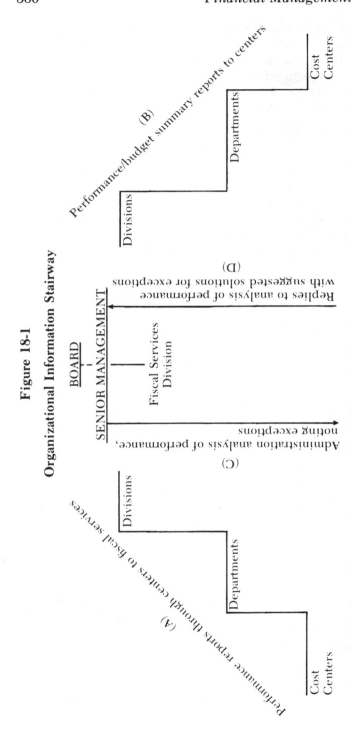

Legend: (A) indicates the upward movement of monthly reports of manhours registered, work units performed, and patients served from the various centers and divisions to the fiscal services office. (The fiscal office collects data from all necessary sources and prepares summary reports of hospital performance as related to budget projections. Complete summaries are sent to senior management.) (B) indicates movement of departmental performance/budget projection summaries from the fiscal services office to the various departments or centers. (C) marks the movement of memoranda on analyses of performance/budget projections with notations on exceptions from the senior administrator to divisional offices and down to all centers. (D) marks the movement of replies as memoranda of (C) with suggested remedies for the exceptions.

sions) and moved through the organizational hierarchy to the fiscal services division. The fiscal services office collects the responsibility center data inputs, adds financial data, collates it, and prepares reports which portray actual performance. These reports should, at a minimum, compare actual performance with that anticipated in the budget projections, usually on a monthly or quarterly basis, and summarize performance to date with budget projection to date for the budget year.

To complete the up and down of the information flow concept, the fiscal services division must prepare reports which interpret the operations/budget information for the responsibility center managers and send the reports down to them so they can evaluate performance in budget terms. This concept is shown in Figure 18-1.

A word of warning must be repeated. The authors realize that it is impossible to design a budget system which will fit the needs of every hospital in every detail. However, the basic principles and objectives of a performance reporting system can be identified and can serve as general guidelines. In the pages which follow several examples of reports will be given which may not fit the particular needs of some institutions precisely. Nevertheless, it is believed that the principles being described can be adapted to most situations.

In order to get the reporting mechanism into proper perspective, it should be remembered the discussion will be focused on expense and capital budgets principally, and on the revenue budget to a lesser degree.[1]

Statistical Reports

As stated earlier, the fiscal services division is responsible for collecting data input, for generating financial statistics, and for obtaining any other information needed to compile reports for the comparison of the hospital's performance to the budget projections. This information can come from many sources so that the fiscal services division can fulfill its clearinghouse function of collecting data and preparing budget reports for management to interpret and act upon.

A brief examination of the reporting activities of a nursing de-

---

[1]Revenue is beyond the control of line management because prices or fees are set by senior management. Volume of services rendered also is largely beyond the control of line management. Therefore, it is unreasonable either to expect or hold line management accountable for revenue performance. Since they should not be held accountable, it is generally not necessary to report revenue to line management.

partment may illustrate how one department might feed information into the system. The fiscal services division would then assimilate these data for reports to the various levels of management.

Nursing. The nursing department is the largest in terms of personnel in the hospital. Furthermore, all inpatients are statistics in the various units of the department. Two types of information about nursing which need to be gathered are patient population and nurse staffing. Most hospitals collect patient information in a midnight census. This is a convenient method and time for determining what beds are occupied and by whom. This census can be used for daily room charge billings and for calculating official occupancy rates. The data on a patient's status at midnight on any given day should include, as a minimum: room number; bed number (if not a private room); and name, age, and sex of the patient. The percentage of the total beds which are occupied will give the occupancy rate.

The authors do not wish to make a point as to how the information should be collected. This could be done by either manual or automated methods. The basic information can be assembled on a worksheet. For example, a nursing unit might be considered a responsibility center; the total inpatient nursing department might be a cost center. For an example we have selected a single nursing unit, Second Floor North, a twenty-bed surgical nursing unit. A worksheet for the midnight census of June 14, 1976 for the responsibility center known as Second Floor North (2N) could contain the necessary patient statistics as shown in Figure 18-2.

If the total inpatient nursing department is considered a cost center, it seems likely the work sheets of all the inpatient nursing units for June 14, 1976 would be summarized for nursing administration in a form similar to that shown in Figure 18-3. It will be noted that this sheet gives occupancy and occupancy percentages for each unit and for the total hospital for that day.

Another element which is useful in performance evaluation is a work measurement statistic. One of the most common measurements used in nursing departments is the ratio of hours of nursing per patient day. A worksheet for 2N for June 14, 1976 might show the roster of the nursing staff of that unit for three shifts as described in Figure 18-4. From this roster worksheet the total nursing hours can be divided by the number of patients to determine the nursing hours/patient ratio. (Note that in the example no recording was made of the time worked by the supervisor, clinical nursing specialist, or by therapists giving direct care. A hospital designing

Figure 18-2

Midnight Census Worksheet

Unit **2N**   Date_____ June 14, 1976

Room	Bed	Patient	Sex	Age
2N1	A	Aaron Unger	M	32
	B	D. C. Anders	M	59
2N2	A			
	B			
2N3	A	D. Dillon	F	26
	B	Alissa Havens	F	29
2N4	A	G. Bisbee III	M	62
	B	Bernard Dosson	M	66
2N5	A	Gene Sibery	M	45
	B			
2N6	A	Amy Friedman	F	65
	B			
2N7	A	T. Dillon	M	37
	B	Tim Tuller	M	32
2N8	A	D. Dodak	F	18
	B	Pamela Smith	F	23
2N9	A	John Newman	M	47
	B	Brian Blitz	M	55
2N10	A	K. Bisbee	F	42
	B	Gina Luneckas	F	22

Bed Complement	20
Patients	16
Occupancy rate	80%
Patients 65 or older	2

Figure 18-3

Midnight Census, Summary Sheet

			June 14, 1976
Unit	Beds	Occupied	Percentage
2N	20	16	80%
2S	20	12	60
2E	20	18	90
2W	20	14	70
3N	20	16	80
3S	20	14	70
3E	20	12	60
3W	20	20	100
4N	20	20	100
4S	20	18	90
4E	20	15	75
4W	20	20	100
ICU	10	5	50
CCU	5	2	40
OB	15	5	33.3
PED	10	5	50
Long-term	20	18	90
	300	230	
Nursery	10	6	60%

Average occupancy, excluding nursery 76.7%

a work measurement formula might wish to prorate some of the work statistics to units served by these special staff members or might wish to charge this personnel to nursing administration.)

Still another possibility to be considered by those who wish to inject an element of quality of care into the work measurement statistic would be to weight the work of the nursing staff. An example is given in Figure 18-5. In this example the basis of weighting was the relationship of salary rates to position, taking the staff nurse's rate as 1.00. Under this rating scale, the head nurse was weighted as 1.25 times the hours she worked; staff nurse 1.00; licensed practical nurse 0.75; and aide or orderly 0.50. Other values for weighting could be used for assessing quality of care. According to a weighting plan, as can be seen, two rosters of the same number of nursing employees with different distributions of professional training could show quite different values on a quality of nursing scale.

Figure 18-4

Worksheet

Nursing Staff Schedule

Unit 2N   Date June 14, 1976

Position	Morning	Hours worked	Afternoon	Hours worked	Evening	Hours worked
Head nurse	Mackis Berman	8				
RN	E. Killingsworth	8	D. Cohn	8	G.L. Warden	8
LPN	S. Holloway	8	R. Snyder	8		
Aide	E. Tuller	8	G.S. Eide	8	R. Klein	8
	Hours per shift	32		24		16

Total hours, all shifts	72
Total patients on census	16
Average hours per patient	4.5

In the examples given of data collection in the nursing department, statistics have been gathered daily, at the unit level, on patient census and nursing work hours. Generally, these data would be transmitted to nursing administration where they would be summarized each month. A monthly report would be sent through the divisional office to the fiscal office for the final compilation of the monthly hospital performance/budget projection reports for four levels of management. An example of a nursing department monthly census and work hours summary prepared for the fiscal office is given in Figure 18-6.

Other responsibility and cost centers. All departments will not have the same data to collect although they will be similar, for staffing and work units will be the basic considerations. Radiology and clinical laboratory both must consider the ratio of weighted work units to staffing. They also are concerned with work scheduling to meet service demands. Physical therapy may have a weighted treatment modal system as a work measurement; dietary may report in number of meals served, the laundry in pounds of linen washed—whatever the unit of measurement, a performance report finally reaches the senior administrator's desk against which he can match the projections for the budget period.

Figure 18-5

Worksheet

Nursing Staff Schedule Weighted for Quality of Care

Unit 2N		Date June 14, 1976

Morning shift

1 Head nurse	8h. x 1.25	10
1 RN	8h. x 1.00	8
1 LPN	8h. x .75	6
1 Aide	8h. x .50	4

Afternoon shift

Head nurse	x 1.25	
1 RN	8h. x 1.00	8
1 LPN	8h. x .75	6
1 Aide	8h. x .50	4

Night shift

Head nurse	x 1.25	
1 RN	8h. x 1.00	8
LPN	x .75	
1 Aide	8h. x .50	4

	Weighted hours values	58

Total weighted hour values   58

Total patients on census   16

Average weighted hour values per patient   3.625

In a responsibility center, as shown in Figure 18-7, the principal items to be covered would be:

—Personnel costs
—Work units performed (where applicable)
—Occupancy rates (where applicable)
—Revenue (where applicable)[2]
—Capital expenditures (where applicable)[3]
—Other expenditures (supplies, etc.)

---

[2]Although revenue is beyond the control of line management, revenue figures can be used comparatively with expenses to determine operation realities.

[3]Depending on the level of activity, capital expenditures may need a separate report.

Figure 18-6

Nursing Department Monthly Census and Work Hours Summary

June, 1976 (30 days)

Unit	Beds per Unit	Mo. Bed Complement (beds x days)	Patient Days per Unit for Month	Occupancy % per Unit	Nursing Hours for Month	Average Nursing Hours per Patient Day
2N	20	600	480	80%	2,160	4.5
2S	20	600	360	60	1,800	5.0
2E	20	600	540	90	2,160	4.0
2W	20	600	438	73	1,971	4.5
3N	20	600	420	70	2,016	4.8
3S	20	600	510	85	2,142	4.2
3E	20	600	402	67	2,010	5.0
3W	20	600	570	95	2,166	3.8
4N	20	600	402	67	2,010	5.0
4S	20	600	492	82	2,214	4.5
4E	20	600	450	75	2,025	4.5
4W	20	600	420	70	1,932	4.6
ICU	10	300	180	60	1,080	6.0
CCU	5	150	75	50	600	8.0
OB	15	450	225	50	900	4.0
PED	20	600	288	48	1,152	4.0
Long-term	20	600	540	90	1,890	3.5
	310	9,300	6,792		30,228	

Percentage Occupancy = $\dfrac{6{,}792}{9{,}300}$ = 73.03%

Average Nursing hours per patient day = $\dfrac{30{,}228}{6{,}792}$ = 4.45 h.p.p.d.

Figure 18-7

Monthly Budget Report, June 1976

Nursing Unit 2N				
	Month		*Year to Date*	
Item	Budget	Actual	Budget	Actual
Personnel costs	$9,500.00	$10,200.40*	$60,000.00	$62,000.20
Work units per patient day	4 hours	4.5 hours*	4 hours	4.2 hours*
Occupancy rate	83%	80%	82%	81%
Supplies	$4,000.00	$3,920.00	$24,000.00	$22,400.00*

*A five percent variance figure is used to illustrate the principle of exceptions—an automatic signal that administration should investigate the deviation from the budget projection. Any percentage or degree of deviation can be used, but it should be agreed upon by administration and line managers on a mutual basis at the beginning of the budget period.

Financial and Performance Reports

The point was made in the information flow illustration that information moves two ways. First, reports are sent "up" to the fiscal services division. In addition to the data from cost centers, the fiscal services division collects data from other sources as needed to compile performance reports. Second, the fiscal services division sends performance reports, designed for the pertinent level of operation, back to management. This series of reports allows each level of management to review performance against budget projections.

A performance report for a responsibility center called nursing unit (2N) is shown in Figure 18-7. The operations items can be compared with budget projections. The format of the report and the manner in which it is compiled will vary among hospitals. The reports, however designed, should show deviations (exceptions) from the performances projected in the budget. The exceptions should be studied by the manager and his superior in order to review the factors affecting operations: workload/revenue ratios; salary adjustments; unforeseen expense; and even unrealistic projections.

Departmental or multiple cost center supervisors should also receive summary reports each month. These reports should compare actual expenses and work performance for the month and for

Figure 18-8

Departmental Monthly Expense Report

Center_____			Month_____	
Unit		*Month*	*Budget year to date*	
	Actual	Budget	Actual	Budget
2N	$	$	$	$
2S				
2E				
2W				
3N				
3S				
3E				
3W				
4N				
4S				
4E				
4W				
ICU				
CCU				
OB				
PED				
L-T				
Total				

the budget year to date with budget projections for all the cost centers for which the manager is accountable. An example is shown in Figure 18-8.

In the same manner, divisional and succeeding levels of management should receive monthly summary reports of expenses and performances for all departments/cost centers reporting to them. An example of a program level report, one for the Patients' Services Program, is given in Figure 18-9.

Finally, a monthly summary report which compares actual expenses and work performance for the whole hospital with budget projections should be prepared by the fiscal services division for senior management. An example is given in Figure 18-10.

In addition, the fiscal services division should be asked to prepare a variance report for the senior administrator. This report should identify any significant variances or exceptions from budget projections. This itemized list can be a valuable worksheet on which to focus suggestions for solutions to exceptions to the budget. See Figure 18-11.

Suggested solutions to exceptions to budget projections should be sought from line management. This statement is posited on the

Figure 18-9

Expense Summary Report

Patient Service Program*

	Month			*Year to Date*		
Centers	Actual	Budget	Variance	Actual	Budget	Variance
Nursing						
Pharmacy						
P.T.						
Inhalation therapy						
Medical records						
Medical secretaries						

*This report is designed for the associate administrator or other head of a hospital division.

Source: Adapted from Berman and Bash, "Operational Budgeting Systems," and used with permission.

same thinking that concluded that line management involvement was basic to budget planning. The line manager is at the point of performance in the operation of a health facility. He should have excellent insight into the problems and needs to be faced in effecting good management and in meeting budget projections. Consequently, each manager should be required to file a report on each significant budget exception in his area of responsibility. The form can be quite simple: identification of the unit and the exception; and statement of the proposed solution of the exception. An example is given in Figure 18-12.

The method of discussion of exceptions and proposed solutions, and the manner in which steps are taken to correct the exceptions, will vary from hospital to hospital and from exception to exception. Generally stated, communication will take place at the several levels of management as necessary. Input should be possible at any level from the lowest to the highest whenever any of the management personnel can contribute to the solution of a problem.

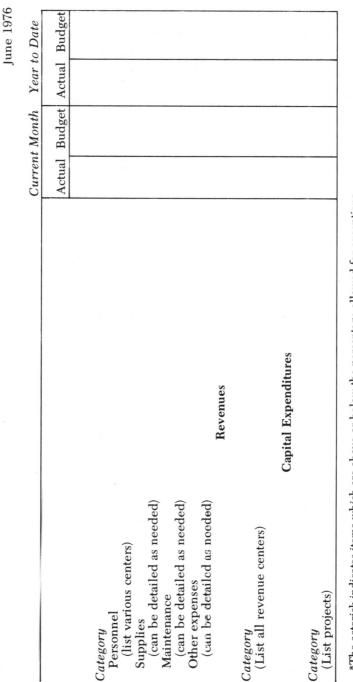

Figure 18-10
Summary Budget Report
Expenditures

June 1976

	Current Month		Year to Date	
	Actual	Budget	Actual	Budget

Category
Personnel
 (list various centers)
Supplies
 (can be detailed as needed)
Maintenance
 (can be detailed as needed)
Other expenses
 (can be detailed as needed)

Revenues

Category
(List all revenue centers)

Capital Expenditures

Category
(List projects)

*The asterisk indicates items which are above or below the percentage allowed for exceptions.

Figure 18-11

Expense Summary Report of Significant Budget Variances*

	Month		*Year to Date*	
Cost Centers	Actual	Budget	Actual	Budget

*This report is designed for the chief administrative officer of the hospital.

Source: Adapted from Berman and Bash. "Operational Budgeting System," with permission.

Figure 18-12

Budget Variance Report

RC Supervisor's Follow-Up

Month_____ Year_____

RC_____

    Variances:

    Cause:

    Solution:

Source: adapted from Berman and Bash, "Operational Budgeting Systems," with permission.

It should be recognized, however, that merely because an exception is identified, corrective action may not be either necessary or appropriate. The budget should be examined for acceptability *prior* to taking corrective action. Situations where signals of exceptions might call for budget changes as opposed to corrective action are:

—Change of environment might call for budget revision.
—The assumptions on which the dollar budget was developed may not have been valid.
—Furthermore, year to date figures should be looked at warily so new monthly budget needs are not penalized to make up for previous exceptions. Also, management should keep in tune with external indicators to ensure that there is a realistic climate for budget consideration. Those external indicators should include complaints of patients' families and of nurses, findings of the utilization review committee and other committees, as well as all indications of community health care needs.

The art of administration becomes a necessary element in budget/performance reconciliation. Assuming that budget construction has been done with realistic guidelines, the problem of coping with exceptions and deviations is not insurmountable if it is accomplishable at regular intervals.

Annual Reports

Annual summary reports will evolve from the monthly, quarterly, and semiannual reports. The annual reports will show performance expressed in actual expenses, revenues, capital spending, and work output correlated with projected figures. These reports along with the balance sheet of assets and liabilities are the basic data on which management policy decisions—financial and otherwise—can be made.

Public Accountability

A practice which is becoming more common each year is for the hospital to make an annual public accounting to its community. These reports are similar to those made by commercial corporations to their stockholders. These documents tell what the financial condition of the hospital is: what the flow of revenues and expenses has been; and what changes have occurred in the capital account. This annual report gives the hospital an excellent opportunity to tell its community what it has done to supply good health

Figure 18-13

Financial Results

	June, 1975	June, 1974
Salaries & Wages	$ 6,996,076	$ 5,829,470
Contractual Services	1,426,951	1,220,938
Employee Health & Welfare	845,977	614,902
Specialty Supplies	894,232	765,749
General Supplies	1,095,024	844,472
Depreciation	541,225	512,377
Other Expenses	478,820	418,998
Funds for Improvement of Patient Services	753,775	730,922
Total Expenses	$13,032,080	$10,937,828

	June, 1975	June, 1974
Inpatient Income	$12,056,388	$10,460,556
Outpatient Income	1,594,750	1,267,974
Gross Income	13,651,138	11,728,530
Deductions (Non-paid Services)	666,952	856,282
Net Patient Revenue	12,984,186	10,872,248
Non-Operating Revenue	47,894	65,580
Total Income	$13,032,080	$10,937,828

Source: St. Mary's Hospital (Decatur, Ill.) 1975 Report, used with permission.

care to persons in its service area. Some hospitals develop a narrative style which adds a human interest element to the story. The specialized treatment centers are described, educational divisions are photographed, personnel and their contributions to good care are talked about, and the medical staff is listed by name and specialty. Quite often statistics are listed which are believed to be of interest to the public, such as: number of patients admitted and discharged; surgery performed; therapy treatments given; laboratory tests performed; and activities of volunteer groups. Babies born, average census, and average length of stay are statistics also commonly quoted as are the number of anesthetics administered, the meals served, the prescriptions filled, the x-rays taken, the pounds of laundry processed, the social service cases handled, and the EEGs and ECGs performed. Some hospitals show a distribution of patients by sex, age, point of origin, or classification of payment. Others show how the patient dollar is spent: how many cents for nursing, housekeeping, dietary, ancillary services, administration, maintenance, etc. See Figures 18-13, 14, 15.

Figure 18-14

Statistics from St. Mary's Hospital for 1974 and 1975

	1974	1975
Admissions	17,007	16,856
Discharges (adults and peds.)	16,902	16,932
Births	1,511	1,458
Newborns discharged	1,504	1,480
Average daily census	333.1	338.1
Average length of stay, days	7.2	7.3
Percentage occupancy	81.3	82.5
Patient days (adults and peds.)	121,592	123,419
Patient days (newborn)	6,356	6,131
Anesthetics	7,435	7,538
Central Supply requisitions	223,783	235,260
Emergency Room visits	28,386	32,555
Laboratory tests	533,960	599,861
EEG examinations	1,724	1,849
ECG examinations	8,679	9,178
Meals served	523,582	525,504
Surgical procedures	7,585	7,988
Pharmacy prescriptions	182,885	203,456
Physical Therapy treatments	16,567	18,635
Respiratory Therapy hours	74,400	96,770
X-ray procedures	55,357	58,305
Social Service cases	771	1,404
Laundry pounds processed	1,676,261	1,718,560

Source: St. Mary's Hospital, Decatur, Illinois. Used with permission.

These annual reports to the public tend to humanize the hospital image, particularly those of the larger institutions. The physicians, nurses, and other staff members who are described tend to become warm human beings rather than figures in starched white uniforms. Even the balance sheet shows how closely expenditures for giving good care come to consuming all the hospital's revenues.

Some hospitals tell their story in well-designed brochures similar to corporation reports to stockholders. These can be mailed to friends and employees of the hospital, can be used to inform prospective donors. The story also can be told by buying advertising space in the local newspaper in the same way any public agency does which must make a formal report of its activities to the community. Whatever means is used, the objective should be to tell as much as possible to as wide a segment of the public as can be reached about what the hospital is doing to serve its community and how it is spending its money to do the job.

Figure 18-15

Patient Dollar Distribution, St. Mary's Hospital, 1975

General Administration	$ .13
Nursing Care	.25
Other Medical Services	.37
Dietary	.07
Patient Record Administration	.05
Plant, Maintenance, Repair	.07
Laundry, Linen	.02
Housekeeping	.04
	$1.00

Source: St. Mary's Hospital, Decatur, Illinois. Used with permission.

As a conclusion to this chapter, it would seem fair to say that a program of good planning and budgeting is one of the principal tools of the financial management of hospitals. In like manner, accurate, timely, and two-way reporting is one of the important elements of an effective, comprehensive planning and budgeting system. Given the general guidelines described in this chapter, the authors believe it is possible for a hospital financial team to design a performance reporting system that will fit the particular need of its institutions.

Information Systems and Reporting

Up to this point in the chapter, the discussion of management reporting has been from the standpoint of the information to be generated and the flow of that information within the hierarchy. It was stated that individual hospitals have different needs for information and have different facilities and capabilities for collecting and disseminating it. At one end of that facilities spectrum could be a primitive, manual method using simply a pencil and paper, at the other a sophisticated computer system.

According to a study by the Hospital Financial Management Association, *The State of Information Processing in the Health Industry* (1976), over 90 percent of the institutions responding to a questionnaire were using electronic data processing (EDP) for at least one application. Of the institutions' EDP applications, 60 percent had in-house facilities (with the trend to mini-computers), and the other 40 percent contracted for some kind of outside services. The functions most used were payroll accounting (88.9 percent), accounts receivable, inpatient billing, and outpatient billing, in that order.

Computerized information systems for health care facilities can be classified into two general categories. They are the Administrative Information System (AIS) which is the widest application of the art, and Clinical Information System (CIS) the nomenclature used by Charles J. Austin and others. (CIS is sometimes called Medical Information System (MIS), the title used in the El Camino Hospital project in Mountainview, California, and by others.)

AIS collects and uses data from and for:

- Admissions, discharges, census
- Facilities utilization and scheduling
- Accounting
- Materials handling
- Payroll
- Personnel
- Budgeting
- Financial planning and modeling

The CIS and MIS systems, as the titles indicate, are focused on the clinical care of patients and are likely to include information from or for:

- Medical records
- Physicians' orders
- Clinical laboratory
- Radiology
- EKG and EEG
- Pharmacy

The Administrative Information System

The Administrative Information System is easier to implement and operate because the data handled are more likely to be factual rather than judgmental, fewer employees are involved, and training is less difficult because of the predominantly factual aspects.

Admissions, discharges, preadmission appointments, and bed census information, when put into a computer system and programmed to give desired summaries in printouts, can be of great value in the management reporting process.

Facilities utilization and scheduling input can be very useful not only for efficient operation, but also as basic information for planning and budgeting.

Accounting is a key source of information for the management reporting process. Accounting can include not only general ledger accounting, accounts receivable and payable, patient billings, but also budget monitoring, cost analysis, allocation of costs of non-revenue departments to revenue cost centers, third party billings and reports, and generation of varied financial information as an input to the reporting system.

Materials handling can include purchasing (and relate it to the monies available under the budget), inventory control (which strangely enough seems to be a weak point in many hospitals), and inventory value adjustments.

Payroll management was one of the first computer applications in hospitals and came into being via bookkeeping machines and other mechanical devices. Most hospitals have some kind of EDP payroll application. Of that number, many have contracted with outside sources. Payroll information can be coupled with personnel data to furnish basic material for cost projections and management planning.

Personnel data systems can generate information about the staff which can be useful for reporting and planning. These data can summarize turnover and absenteeism, employee characteristics, employment trends, and departmental incidents to help with cost projections and departmental planning. Some hospitals have used employee profiles developed on computers to indicate abilities and capabilities in addition to those necessary for the job assigned. In case of emergency, the employee may be shifted to cover possible staff shortages. This can be an important factor in planning for emergencies.

Budgeting is of central importance in any kind of hospital informational system, manual or computerized. In any effective system, information on costs, revenues, personnel, utilization, scheduling, purchasing and inventories, construction, planning, and institutional needs and activities is channeled to the administration and the budget officer.

Financial planning and modeling can be done effectively only on valid information. The computer, properly programmed, can supply the means of information output, assimilation, and plan or model design far superior to any manual operation.

Clinical Information System (CIS) (MIS)

The clinical system collects data about the physician's orders, the nurse's notes, any nursing plan, medications, therapies, laboratory services, radiology, EKG, EEG, and the use of special units such as the emergency room, the delivery room, the operating rooms, the intensive care unit, cardiac care, outpatient clinic, and other special services for patients.

As stated before, a CIS program is much more difficult to implement because of judgmental elements affecting the information put into the system and because of the greater number of persons involved. However, information can be generated in the CIS which would be useful in financial planning. This information could be composed of data on facilities and equipment use and scheduling, on quality of care indices, profiles of ancillary services, drug distribution and pharmacy costs, and any other needed information which could be programmed.

Many variations of information systems are evolving. Hopefully, they are being tailored to the needs of the individual institution, rather than being purchased as a packaged deal from a commercial supplier. In differing degrees, departments or sectors in information systems are being integrated or designed in parallel or tandem so that necessary information can be retrieved at different levels. All this is working toward a total hospital information system (THIS). A group at Yale has designed a regional information system. This regional effort, however, must be based on uniformity of reporting and recording of information, if there is to be a workable exchange of data.

The human element seems to be the weakest point. First, there is a lack of knowledge at the administrative level about what information is important to put into the system, and how to implement the system. (The so-called information explosion of the past generation was cursed before computers became so common. Then, we complained about all the unnecessary paper work we had to do. With computers, we marveled at how much information we could put into the monster. Now, we are beginning to realize that we have to be selective: what do we *need* to know?)

The second human element is the persons who are responsible for input and output. After the system has been designed in a suitable manner for processing the desired kind of information, how can the physicians, nurses, and others on the staff be trained to use the system and be convinced it's worth all the effort. Without the full and proper participation by these key people, the system doesn't operate up to potential.

The final word is, of course, that financial officers, administrators, and planners should use whatever information is available to the best possible advantage in the reporting process.

Hospital Administrative Services

More than 2,800 hospitals—running the whole gamut of bed size, kinds of services offered, and teaching activity—use the Hospital Administrative Services of the American Hospital Association as an adjunct to any internal reporting system or other statistical collection from hospital records. The HAS data bank offers profiles of departmental costs and revenues, employe productivity, utilization of services and units of care, and man hours per patient day or service modality.

Hospitals which subscribe to the HAS have the ability to know not only their own performance, but also their performance relative to that of other institutions of like size, and to others in all of the nine census regions of the country. Monthly, quarterly, and six month national data reports not only enable financial officers to compare the hospital's productivity, costs and revenues, and utilization of inhospital departments, outpatient clinics, and extended care units to other institutions, but also to chart the trends in these activities. HAS was designed to be a tool for financial managers and administrators. In 1979, HAS introduced a new product, Monitrend, designed to make comparative management data increasingly useful to the operating administrator.

Suggested Readings

American Hospital Association. *Budgeting Procedures for Hospitals.*

Andrews C.T. "Financial and Statistical Reports for Administrative Decision-Making in Hospitals."

Ambrose, Donald M. "A Sensor and Monitor for a Manpower Control System."

Austin, Charles J. *Information Systems for Hospital Administration.* Ann Arbor: Health Administration Press, 1979.

Austin, Charles J. and Greene, Barry R. "Hospital Information Systems: A Current Perspective." *Inquiry*, XV:2.

Berman, Howard J. and Bash, Paul L. "Operational Budgeting Systems: Hackley Hospital, Muskegon, Michigan."

Falcon, William D., ed. *Reporting Financial Data to Management.*

Part V
The Future

Chapter 19

Future Trends in Hospital Financing

In this fourth edition of *The Financial Management of Hospitals*, the material presented in earlier editions has been revised and updated to reflect changes taking place during the eight years since the first publication. However, the discussion of expected trends in health care delivery and the implications for financial management have remained largely applicable today and for the near future.

Eight years ago the authors said certain ideas or beliefs were accepted as foregone conclusions by the American people because they had been repeated and heard so often. Many of those fixed beliefs are still prevalent today.

Consider some of those fixed ideas and beliefs mentioned in the previous editions of this book:

Inflation will continue and will be almost impossible to control. Labor unions, now that they are organized both by industry and on a nationwide basis, have such tremendous power that they can demand and they will receive. We hear talk of plumbers, electricians, carpenters and other skilled workers making fabulous incomes in a few years ($50,000–$100,000 a year, depending on how expansionary the imagination), greater than many highly educated professional people. If this becomes true, it will skew all the economists' curves and put the unorganized breadwinner, the retired person, and the unskilled in a precarious position. The possible course of inflation demands a lot of thought as does the possibility that it cannot be limitless without chaos.

The social welfare load will continue to rise in dollars and numbers of recipients until Americans will begin to ask each other who is left to pay the bills. Truly, social welfare expenditures—federal, state, and local—have zoomed upward so rapidly that total welfare expenditures now approximate 15 percent of the Gross National Product. Health expenditures make up a large portion of the social welfare costs. Much of the hospital expense for the medically indigent is paid through Medicaid. In turn, Medicaid rates of payment, to all practical purposes, are negotiated rates. If hospital expenses rise beyond the ability of the federal government to pay at cost reimbursement rates from Medicaid monies, will the Congress vote additional funds or will the hospitals be asked to accept negotiated rates which may for the most part be below economic costs?

Hospital prices will continue to rise unchecked. Twenty years ago when those persons who tried to project the cost of hospital care said it would not be long before the average daily cost of general hospital care would be $100, it seemed impossible. Now that that impossibility is a fact, can we supinely accept some of the present predictions of $300, $500, or $1,000 a day average cost for hospital care within the next decade?

Blue Cross benefits will continue to increase. The Blue Cross premium more and more is something the employer pays. Blue Cross benefits, therefore, have become bargaining points in more and more union contract negotiations. The employee, through this growing change, has become farther and farther removed from the realities of the cost of his Blue Cross or other insurance coverage. He has asked for greater benefits each contract period: prescription drugs, dental care, and other special benefits. This will keep increasing within our present system.

Blue Cross can keep increasing rates. As benefits and hospital costs increase, so must Blue Cross premiums. Every year or so, it seems, the Blue plans ask their state regulatory bodies for permission to raise premium rates. Their books justify the requests in most cases, but the following question should be asked: Will the well ever run dry for Blue Cross?

Drugs perform miracles, doctors are omniscient. This is the age of pills—miracle pills that kill infections, relieve tensions, brighten the day and obliterate depressions, and do other marvelous things not related to hospital financial management. The sulfa drugs, penicillin and some other antibiotics truly are the greatest miracle drugs since the use of quinine was discovered for the treatment of malaria, but we as a people sometimes like to believe in total miracle medicine. We want all our drugs to work miracles (if only for today until another miracle replacement appears tomorrow) and we want to think of our physicians as omniscient savants who can assure us good health no matter how we misuse our bodies. With miracle drugs and with supermen as physicians, our worries about a comprehensive health care system would seem to be a formality if we could just lick the problem of logistics.

The fee-for-service concept for physicians is inviolable. The medical profession in this country traditionally has believed in a fee-for-service method of payment. This is one reason the A.M.A. was horrified with the capitation payment system for general practitioners and the salary plan for specialists instituted under the National Health Service in England. Fee-for-service has been a stumbling block under Blue Shield, and a source of national scandal about the enormous totals of fees a minority of physicians collected under Medicare and Medicaid.[1] The fee-for-service concept may be becoming worn out. Certainly it will be re-evaluated.

Only peer review of a physician's work should be allowed. Only a doctor can accurately judge or criticize another doctor's work is the position commonly taken by the medical profession in regard to quality control of professional services. This also might imply that only doctors should impose penalties on fellow doctors, unless, of course, a legal matter is involved. Peer review has been a principle many other professionals have used to protect their professions on the assumption the general public does not have the expertise to criticize competently. Peer review organized on a multi-hospital or on a regional scale seems to be shaping up slowly under the Medical Foundations and Professional Standards Review Organizations.

The computer answers all questions. This has been not only the age of the pill, but also of the computer. To the computer and its lightning calculations we have attributed infallibility limited only by the ability of fallible man to program it correctly. Computers have been adapted to medical diagnostic work as well as record-keeping and a thousand other uses in health care. Some persons think that some day they will be able to turn themselves over to a

---

[1]*Medicare and Medicaid: Problems, Issues, and Alternatives.* Report of the staff to the Committee on Finance, U.S. Senate, Russell B. Long, Chairman. Feburary 9, 1970, pp. 163 ff.

computer on a health production line and be diagnosed, treated, and cured of their illnesses in a twinkling of those computer lights. It seems like one step this side of the millenium, if you are a believer—either in the computer, or in the Great Day.

National Health Care

In the United States we have reached the point of saying that adequate health care is a *right* of every person. We haven't defined "adequate" very well, but we mean at the very least that a person who becomes ill should be able to get necessary health care without too much trouble or too long a wait for service. In other words, health service should be available within the range of the patient's mode of transportation, within his ability to pay or not, and within the time needs for proper treatment.

It is a worthy goal to wish to provide the "adequate" care so inadequately defined above. Many persons would like to set the sights higher than merely providing palliative care of illness. They would try to remove or temper causes of disease and illness whether they were systemic, psychological, environmental, social, hereditary, or epidemic. These higher goals are commendable and should be considered carefully in any long-range planning. The attainment of these long-range goals implies such a tremendous change in American life and culture that they can be brought about only with careful planning and common consent. They really demand a social revolution.

As stated before, it is an axiom that adequate health care is the right of every American. Related to the growth of the feeling that adequate health care is a *right* (rather than a privilege) has been political activity to bring about better health protection. Political discussion of health care has been taking place in this country since the days of Theodore Roosevelt early in this century. You probably could find that the social concept of health care for all ricocheted off Chancellor von Bismarck of nineteenth century Germany from some Greek philosopher in the era before Christ.

The problem is not in setting the goal of adequate health care for every person, but in attaining the goal. Americans have a great weakness in believing that if they have money to pay for a thing or a service, nothing should prevent them from having it. The United States has been said to be the wealthiest, most powerful nation on earth. Americans spend twice as large a percentage of their GNP on health care as most other Western nations, have developed medical technology and skills to a high degree, and have spent more lavishly on gleaming hospitals and sophisticated equipment—but have not learned to deliver effective health care to all citizens as well as some of the European nations spending at half the American rate.

Labor, business, health professions, and politicians have all presented ideas to Congress for structuring a health care system. The ideas have ranged from provision for a completely open system under which every health service would be provided to every American without cost at time of delivery of service to more restrictive plans covering special groups or catastrophic illnesses. Discussions have covered the many facets of health care and the ways various plans would be implemented.

Some who want the open system favor implementing it totally in one swoop. They would have an appointed day and open the gates for all with real or imagined illnesses to come in for treatment. Others shudder at this swoop approach and point to the Medicaid and Medicare experience which demonstrated the inability of statistical and actuarial minds to anticipate the flood of demand for care that developed after the plans went into effect. Adequate and satisfactory health care did not necessarily follow merely because it was made available by law.

Patently, if a comprehensive, open system were implemented totally on an appointed day in the near future there would not be enough trained health manpower and proper facilities available in every situation to meet the demand for care.

Some proponents of the open system argue that a comprehensive plan should be implemented in segments in order to absorb the anticipated increase in demand efficiently. It has been suggested that, since Medicare covers the population aged 65 and over and certain other disabled persons, the next group with high priority would be children and young persons under 25 years of age who are just getting started in adult life. After the care of this group has been absorbed and consolidated in an open system then the remainder of the population could be admitted in one or two segments.

Another approach for segmental implementation is illustrated by the care for patients needing renal dialysis provided under the SSA (Medicare) Amendments of 1972. Certain things may be learned by this diagnostic approach under Medicare. It is possible that a series of renal dialysis centers will be operated under strict criteria in an effort to prevent unnecessary expansion of services in areas adequately covered, and, conversely, to ensure that services are available in all areas where needed. Again, this thinking is based on giving proper attention to efficient delivery of health care.

Some planners predict the use of a pluralistic system as opposed to the monolithic open system. Those favoring a pluralistic approach are not denying that a uniform system might eventually result from multiple approaches.

Naturally the ideal system would be one which delivered the best possible health care within fiscally supportable resources of manpower and facilities—no matter which approach was used.

The elements of pluralism most often mentioned are variations in insurance coverage or in modes of treatment. Compulsory full insurance coverage is often suggested, or compulsory insurance for catastrophic illness as an alternative. Several plans might be tried in the country concurrently: HMOs might be developed in one area, hospital-connected ambulatory centers in another, visiting nurse service might be raised to new levels, satellite organizations and regional planning might be used in pilot projects. Several approaches might be offered as options to the same group. (The choice between health insurance fully paid by the employer and a wider HMO coverage with the employee paying any additional premium has been used successfully already.)

The sheer magnitude of implementing a national comprehensive health care coverage in a country as big and as diversified as the United States suggests that gradualism and pluralism are both quite likely to be elements in the approach.

An Unmanageable Situation

A seemingly unsurmountable obstacle to national comprehensive health care is the lack of organization or direction of the participants. There is no health care system, many say, only a "nonsystem." We are said to be riding in a speeding automobile without brakes and with defective steering gear. We have many independent, unmanageable providers. Too many critical events happen without planning, or without being subject to a superintendent, if there is a plan.

Physicians' strong, united front to defend their fee-for-service practices was mentioned previously. They would resist as fiercely any effort to set up a plan for distributing physicians so that rural areas, inner cities, and other areas lacking doctors could be covered. Physicians will continue to fight rear guard action against utilization review to limit hospital stays. They prefer any review to be done by colleagues on their own medical staff rather than by physicians connected with PSROs or other agencies. To be reviewed by a computer is unconscionable.

Many hospitals are still in a status struggle, each likely to be looking at its neighbor to see if the other hospital is adding a new piece of sophisticated equipment or forming a new team for some highly specialized procedure. Hospitals are plagued by the imbalance in bed supply: some have too many beds and some have too few. Unfortunately the oversupplied areas usually are not located so that they can help the undersupplied. Hospitals are becoming more expensive to operate each year, and the flexibility of operation needed to reduce or contain costs is quickly disappearing. There needs to be a lever which can be grasped to bring a runaway situation under control.

Paraprofessionals and technicians are increasing in and out of hospitals with great rapidity. Paraprofessionals are organizing and pressing forward their claims to professionalism and all that implies in higher fees and more fractionated activities. The growth in number of paraprofessionals and technicians may have been one contributing factor in the increase of employee-patient ratio in hospitals. Personnel in hospitals in the past decade have increased from about two (FTE) employees per patient to over three (FTE) employees per patient. It is fair to ask if, because of this increase in number of employees, quality of care has increased, or if lives have been saved.

Patients have a responsibility in any system designed to deliver comprehensive health care. The patient should ask himself if he is being reasonable in the service he requests. He should be concerned with the zooming costs of health care even if his employer pays his hospital and medical insurance. Even though health insurance is a fringe benefit, every worker pays indirectly by receiving a lower pay rate or by paying more for products he buys. For example, at a 1975 institute a speaker stated that the health benefits package for General Motors employees and retirees costs $135.00 for every GM car manufactured. The dollar costs of health benefits has undoubtedly risen since then.

It would seem likely that certain conditions would naturally accompany the development of a national health plan. All indications are for: more control over utilization of health services; more control over providers of care, including physicians, hospitals, and other health care agencies; more control over the expansion of facilities and over patient referral systems; and more control over costs.

Utilization Controls

Control over utilization of health care facilities may be evidenced in several ways:

(1) Utilization review may partially ignore the old belief that only peer review is acceptable, that only physicians should judge the work of fellow physicians. It is conceivable that a national system similar to the inspection visitations of representatives of the Joint Commission on Accreditation of Hospitals (JCAH) would be used to review hospital utilization. Conjointly with the JCAH-type inspection, a computerized system such as the Professional Activity Study (PAS) could be used to monitor the medical records for possible overutilization of the hospital. As previously suggested, regional organizations such as Professional Standards Review Organizations (PSROs) are becoming more active.

(2) Utilization might be influenced and lessened somewhat by limiting malpractice liability. Physicians presently may be tempted to overutilize; to overorder on laboratory tests, x-rays, and other paramedical services; to hospitalize quicker than necessary; to request consultations more routinely than necessary for quality care. Some physicians may feel through this overutilization there is an added margin of safety against malpractice suits and judgments. If malpractice liability were limited, physicians might not feel it necessary to order as high a level of services as at present as a defense against malpractice suits.

Cost Controls

All the proposed plans for comprehensive health care have built-in implications of cost controls because of the tremendous operating expenses any national plan will entail. Cost controls without loss of quality of care will be the necessary goal. Costs must be controlled if the ideal of adequate health care for all citizens is to be realized within the limits of what the public is able and willing to pay.

Health care is the most important public problem in the minds of health professionals, and costs may seem secondary. However, when one considers the interests of others and the demands these interests make on public and private monies, then one can see the tremendous importance of containing health costs in order to attain health goals. Other citizens are deeply interested in wiping out poverty, in educating every American child to his potential, in curbing environmental pollution, in keeping the defenses high, in rebuilding the decaying cities, in preserving the natural resources, in enlarging the highway system, in equalizing rights, in promoting the arts, and in bringing peace into the world and safety in our streets. Health care must compete with every one of those interests and hundreds of other demands which could be added. Costs must be kept within reason if we are going to be able to buy as much health care as we need.

The hospital must operate more efficiently whether or not it retains its autonomy. In fact, it must be more efficient even if it: remains a 200 bed community hospital under the direction of its local board of trustees; becomes a part of a regional authority; or if it comes under the umbrella of the federal government. If every citizen is to be able to receive adequate and necessary care, the hospital must determine that the care, in fact, is necessary, that it is of good quality, and that the cost is within realistic limits.

Three possible ways costs can be kept realistic are to: (1) set hospital charges on a projective basis with incentives for reducing costs rather than having reimbursements based on present "costs;" (2) put some real teeth in areawide planning and make it work; and (3) regionalize facilities on the foundations laid by good area planning.

Projective Rates and Incentives

One of the controls being applied to hospitals by third parties, particularly Blue Cross and the federal government, is the use of projective rates with a built-in incentive as a means of figuring reimbursements. The general plan is to project costs for a fiscal year based on detailed budgeting and subject to negotiations between the hospital and the third party. Once a rate based on projected costs is adopted, an incentive can be introduced. This incentive can be as follows (or something similar): If the hospital could operate during the fiscal year at lower than the projected cost, there would be an agreement about dividing the difference between projected and actual costs between the hospital and the third party. This division of the difference, in substance, would amount to a plus factor.[2]

---

[2] See "What Experiments in Prospective Reimbursements Are Teaching Providers, Agencies, Third Parties" by Glenn J. Martin, *Hospital Financial Management*, November 1970, pp. 3–7.

The projective rate plan (or the prospective reimbursement concept) has run into some difficulties where its acceptance has been resisted. Furthermore, critics of the idea argue that such a small part of the cost of running a hospital is subject to budget trimming that any savings would be of little consequence. However, in spite of resistance, there will continue to be experiments conducted in this plan of paying hospitals.

Areawide Planning

Areawide planning for health care is being recommended by the American Hospital Association, legislated by Congress, and supported by many individuals prominent in the health industry as a necessary factor in any comprehensive health scheme.[3]

Regionalization and Shared Services

One of the final goals of areawide planning is expressed in the concept of regionalization. This concept is graphically presented as a web with the full service hospital at the center surrounded at varying distances by satellite hospitals with more limited services available and by neighborhood or rural health centers. All these facilities are interconnected to allow for patients to move from the periphery toward the center, or in the reverse, according to the needs for care and facilities.

The regional hospital at the center could be a university medical center or a teaching hospital with most all of the medical specialties represented and with all the principal health care facilities and services available for the care of patients. Usually, primary care would be supplied at the periphery in one of the neighborhood or rural centers. If more extensive treatment were needed the patient could be referred to the satellite or to the central (regional) hospital. In reverse, the patient could be referred from the center hospital outward through the centers if less intensive but continued care were required after discharge from the central hospital. Beyond the regional or central hospital might be a hospital with a statewide catchment area.

A variation from the web format might be a hierarchical tree method in which facilities would be rated for care capabilities.

---

[3]Great expectations have resulted from the passing of National Health Planning and Resources Development Act of 1974 (P.L. 93–641) which calls for new dimensions in health planning. The full effect has not been realized.

Patients would move up the tree of rating for facilities as need for more sophisticated care increased.

No matter what configuration is used for regionalization, three key structured characteristics might be considered: (1) ownership; (2) administration; and (3) financial management.

If the present health care system were to adopt a regionalization plan, this would mean voluntarism and individual ownership of facilities would be put to a severe test. The medium-sized and small hospitals would have to agree to a secondary position. With a university medical center or another large teaching hospital at the regional hub, this might mean a state-owned hospital was dominant over a group of community-owned voluntary hospitals and health centers. The situation might require a super-body, an area council representing all facilities, to make policy decisions, and to make the hard decisions on ratings and on referral policies.

To administer a network of health facilities working cooperatively on a regional basis might require some new thinking. Much would depend on ownership. If a central hospital owned satellites and/or neighborhood or rural health centers, the management probably would be centered in the parent organization. If each facility were a discrete entity, the other extreme might be expected: decentralized management. For administration of a region with decentralized management, there again would be a role for a super-body to synchronize activities.

For the financial manager, regionalization could be either a blessing or a burden. The facilities in a region or an area, working with the area planning council, could pool depreciation funds, for example. A pooling of funds could make assets available to member facilities, when needed, at the lowest possible costs. Certain services can be shared by member facilities within a region to the financial benefit of all. If the financial manager makes a determined effort he can find many financial benefits. Conversely, if he does not watch carefully, he may miss opportunities to benefit.

Self Control

Recently in a meeting in Stockholm called to consider the problems of the delivery of health care and attended by leaders in the field from Western European countries and the United Kingdom, Dr. DeGroot of the Nationaal Ziekenhuisinstituut of the Netherlands made a plea for "self-care." He was not referring to the self care of ambulatory inpatients which we think of as a part of Progressive Patient Care. He was asking that emphasis be put on educating the populace in taking better care of their bodies as an initiatory step in care to precede and possibly to some degree obviate what we call "primary care."

With all due credit to Dr. DeGroot, the authors of this volume suggest that "self-control" might be a better way of expressing a realistic need if the comprehensive health care system talked about is to become workable. However, realistically or cynically— whatever way you care to characterize the attitude—self-control will be difficult to make effective.

By self-control and its effect on health care, we mean if drunks did not drive automobiles, there would be a dramatic decrease in highway fatalities and in the workloads in hospital trauma centers and emergency rooms. If the smoking of cigarettes and other forms of tobacco could be cut drastically, we are told that lung cancer and heart diseases would be greatly reduced. In addition to our bad habits, most of us eat too much and exercise too little. Self-control might reduce the load of medical and hospital care and lengthen the life span.

Cynicism creeps in also when someone mentions health education. The schools, the government, the insurance companies and many other organized agencies have been telling the dangers of alcohol, tobacco, V.D., and drugs. In spite of all the publicity there are still too many who drink and drive and kill and maim. The sale of cigarettes continues to rise without benefit of television or radio advertising and in spite of the countercampaign of advertising which displays the horrible consequences of smoking with graphic and artistic talent. The specters of lung cancer, emphysema, and heart disease are not enough to check the dependence on nicotine even among alert and sophisticated youth. Disappointingly, the same alert, sophisticated youth with freedom in sexual conduct are spreading venereal diseases at epidemic rates. A generation ago physicians thought the day had come when V.D. could be obliterated from civilized countries. They knew they would no longer have to depend on Erlich's magic bullet, salvarsan and its refinements, to treat syphilis or on protargol, potassium permanganate, and other prolonged treatments for gonorrhea, because penicillin had been discovered. Since then the medical armamentarium has been increased, treatments have been shortened and made less painful. In spite of all this, venereal diseases continue to spread. Action on the part of persons exposed to V.D. or suspicious of a lesion or discharge, or, in fact, of any abnormal body sign could help control V.D. The overt results of V.D. are chilling to think about (blindness, sterility, even insanity) but the covert effects are more subtle and hidden but add up to sickness, lost work, and costly health care. New tests for gonorrhea no more bothersome to administer or read than a test for TB may overcome the reluctance of many women to ask voluntarily to be checked. Health departments, clinics, and family physicians are all interested in detecting and treating V.D. with privacy to the patient.

Drug misuse is as senseless as drunk driving, excessive smoking, or untreated V.D. Drug misuse can be legal. Today probably the largest category of drugs prescribed by the physicians is that of tranquilizers and barbiturates. A sleeping pill seems harmless now and then, a tranquilizer may seem to help relieve the little pressures of life. Somewhat opposite to the sedatives are the amphetamines which were originally used for crash dieting and weight reduction. Later these pills were used as energizers by soldiers, athletes, race horses—and now by ordinary mortals. So we have become a drug culture quite legally: to sleep, to reduce, to sedate and tranquilize, to pep up, and to overcome depression. We have come to depend more and more on legal drugs to buoy us up and to help us endure the pressures of a highly protective society. We have done this at the expense of our health in many cases. The authors suggest a sane attitude toward the use of legal drugs by physicians and patients might be an effective control in preventing some of the illness and costly health care.

Illegal drug use is another problem for which there seem to be no simple answers. Some of the same sedatives and the same energizers being prescribed legally are also being sold illegally to youngsters and oldsters as well. The dosage used for a kick or a thrill unfortunately often dangerously exceeds that recommended by the pharmacopeia for medical use. As we all know too well, illegal drug usage has spread from "uppers" and "downers," and marihuana and LSD to narcotics (hard drugs), worst of all to heroin. To throw off the hard drug habit evidently makes almost impossible demands on self-control, but it could be worthwhile in a life and death gamble.

Cynical and moralizing as the authors appear, they see a possible glimmer of hope for self-control. A century which is just three-quarters over has witnessed many miraculous advances in preventive health care. There has been the eradication, disappearance, or potential control of polio, tuberculosis, malaria, smallpox, pneumonia, scarlet fever, yellow fever, diphtheria, typhus, syphilis and gonorrhea. Possibly human beings can now use self-control as a preventive measure to reduce sickness and death and make the most of medicine's advances.

Summary

This chapter contains a large amount of conjecture, and hopefully some stimuli for thoughts about the future of hospital financial management.

Some of the factors mentioned seem to the authors to have high probability of happening. This wave of the future will probably bring:

—Projective rates for hospitals with built-in incentives as ongoing
—Areawide planning effectively administer
—Pooled depreciation by areas
—Greater shared services
—Less fee-for-service for physicians and more capitation and salary reimbursement
—Tighter controls on utilization
—A comprehensive health care system
—A growth in prepaid group practices

The wave of the future is going to bring exciting times to every health care decision maker and particularly to the hospital financial manager.

Glossary

Accelerated Depreciation—Depreciation methods that write-off the cost of an asset at a faster rate than the write-off under the straight-line method. The two principal methods of accelerated depreciation are: (1) sum-of-years digits and (2) double declining balance.

Accounting—The art of recording, classifying and summarizing in a significant manner and in terms of money transactions which are, at least in part, of a financial character—and interpreting the results thereof.

Accounting Costs—All tangible costs which can be measured in terms of release of value.

Accounts Receivable—Amounts due from patients for services rendered to them.

Accrual-Basis Accounting—An accounting system wherein revenue is recorded in the accounting period in which it is earned, whether or not cash has been received; and expenses are recorded in the accounting period in which they are used or consumed in producing revenue, whether or not cash is disbursed in the payment of those expenses.

Accruals—Continually recurring short-term liabilities. Examples are accrued wages, accrued taxes, and accrued interest.

Accrued Interest—Interest earned on a bond issue from the dated date to the date of delivery. Accrued interest is credited to the issuer at delivery.

Aging Schedule—A report showing how long accounts receivable have been outstanding. It gives the percent of receivables not past due and the percent past due by, for example, one month, two months, or other periods.

Algebraic Method—A cost finding technique involving the simultaneous distribution of general service cost center costs to both general service and final cost centers.

Amortize—To liquidate on an installment basis; an amortized loan is one in which the principal amount of the loan is repaid in installments during the life of the loan.

Asked Price—The price at which bonds are offered to potential buyers.

Assignment—A relatively inexpensive way of liquidating a failing firm that does not involve going through the courts.

Authority—A municipal or state entity formed through a special legislative act to perform the specific function of distribution of bonds.

Bad Debts—An account which is charged off due to the fact that it is unpaid, although the patient has the ability to pay.

Balloon Payment—When a debt is not fully amortized, the final payment is larger than the preceding payments and is called a "balloon" payment.

Bank Line—The funds that a bank keeps available to a borrower, which can use some or all of its line at any time.

Bankruptcy—A legal procedure for formally liquidating a business carried out under the jurisdiction of courts of law.

Basis Point—One basis point is equal to one one-hundredth of one percent or .01 percent.

Benefits—A payment or service provided under an insurance policy or prepayment plan. In the case of Blue Cross, the payments are made directly to the hospital on behalf of all patients who are covered. Commercial insurers either make payments to the hospital or the patient.

Best Efforts Underwriting—A relationship where the underwriter acts as agent for the issuer and there is no commitment to purchase any of the bonds. If the underwriter has given a Firm Commitment, he is acting as principal and has agreed to buy the entire issue.

Bid—The price buyers offer to pay for bonds; the price at which sellers may dispose of them.

Bond—A long-term debt instrument.

Bond Discount (or Debt Discount)—Amount by which the selling (or purchase) price is less than the face value of a bond or other form of indebtedness.

Bond Premium (or Debt Premium)—Amount by which the selling (or purchase) price exceeds the face value of a bond or other form of indebtedness.

Book Value—The value of an asset as shown in the accounting records of a firm.

Capital Asset—An asset with a life of more than one year that is not bought and sold in the ordinary course of business.

Capital Budgeting—The process of planning expenditures on assets whose returns are expected to extend beyond one year.

Capital Rationing—A situation where a constraint is placed on the total size of the capital investment during a particular period.

Capital Structure—The permanent long-term financing of the firm. Capital structure is distinguished from *financial structure*, which includes short-term debt plus all reserve accounts.

Capitalization—The capital of a hospital includes the long-term debt (including current portion of long-term debt and capital equipment leases), capitalized leases, and both restricted and unrestricted fund balances. Pro-forma capitalization reflects these categories after giving effect to proposal financing.

Capitalization Rate—A discount rate used to find the present value of a series of future cash receipts; sometimes called *discount rate*.

Cash Budget—A schedule showing cash flows (receipts, disbursements, and net cash) for a firm over a specified period.

Cash Cycle—The length of time between the purchase of raw materials and the receipt of the cash which is generated due to the sale of the final product.

Cash Inflows—Revenues actually received by the hospital.

Cash Outflows—Expenses actually paid by the hospital.

Certificate of Need (CON)—A confirmation, usually legal in nature, by an approved agency that a proposal for establishing a program or constructing a facility meets an estimated unmet need in a defined service area.

Chart of Accounts—A listing of accounts and titles, with numerical symbols, employed in a compilation of financial data concerning the assets, liabilities, capital, revenues, and expenses of an enterprise.

Chattel Mortgage—A mortgage on personal property (not real estate). A mortgage on equipment would be a chattel mortgage.

Collateral—Assets that are used to secure a loan.

Commercial Paper—Unsecured, short-term promissory notes of large firms, usually issued in denominations of $1 million or more. The rate of interest on commercial paper is typically somewhat below the prime rate of interest.

Compensating Balances—Cash deposits required by a bank as partial compensation for lending and other services which it provides to a hospital.

Compound Interest—An interest rate that is applicable when interest in succeeding periods is earned not only on the initial principal, but also on the accumulated interest of prior periods. Compound interest is contrasted to *simple interest*, in which returns are not earned on interest received.

Compounding—The arithmetic process of determining the final value of a payment or series of payments when compound interest is applied.

Conditional Sales Contract—A method of financing new equipment by paying it off in installments over a one- to five-year period. The seller retains title to the equipment until payment has been completed.

Continuous Compounding (Discounting)—As opposed to discrete compounding, interest is added continuously rather than at discrete points in time.

Cost—The monetary valuation applied to an asset or service that has been obtained by an expenditure of cash or by a commitment to make a future expenditure.

Cost-Based Reimbursement—The reimbursement approach generally used by third party payers. Under this approach, the third party pays the hospital for the care received by covered patients at cost; with the expense elements included and excluded from cost determined by the third party.

Cost Finding—The process of apportioning or allocating the costs of the non-revenue-producing cost centers to each other and to the revenue-producing cost centers on the basis of the statistical data that measures the amount of service rendered by each center to the other centers.

Cost of Capital—The discount rate that should be used in the capital budgeting process.

Cost-Plus Contract—A type of agreement widely used in construction, in which the owner agrees to pay for all costs incurred by the contractor in executing the plans and specifications, "plus" an additional amount (fixed sum, percentage or other arrangement) as fee or profit.

Coupon Rate—The stated annual rate of interest which the borrower promised to pay to the bond holder.

Current Yield—The percent relation of the annual interest received to the price of the bond.

Debenture—A long-term debt instrument that is not secured by a mortgage on specific property.

Default—The failure to fulfill a contract. Generally, default refers to the failure to pay interest or principal on debt obligations.

Depreciation—The annual estimated cost of expired services of fixed assets.

Direct Distribution—A cost finding technique involving the distribution of general service cost center costs directly to final cost centers.

Discounting—The process of finding the present value of a series of future cash flows. Discounting is the reverse of compounding.

Discounting of Accounts Receivable—Short-term financing where accounts receivable are used to secure the loan. The lender *does not* buy the accounts receivable, but simply uses them as collateral for the loan. Also called "pledging of accounts receivable."

Double Distribution—A cost finding technique involving the distribution of general service cost center costs first to the appropriate general service centers and then to final cost centers.

Economic Cost—The full cost of operations. It includes both tangible and intangible costs.

Economical Ordering Quantity (EOQ)—The optimum (least cost) quantity of merchandise which should be purchased in any single order.

Endowment Fund—The account group used to record transactions arising from funds which have been given to the hospital and for which a moral and legal responsibility exists to comply with the terms of the endowment.

Equity—The net worth of an enterprise.

Expected Return—The rate of return a firm expects to realize from an investment. The expected return is the mean value of the probability distribution of possible returns.

Expenses—Costs that have been used or consumed in carrying on some activity and from which no measurable benefit will extend beyond the present. In the broadest sense, expense includes all expired costs.

Factoring—A method financing accounts receivable under which a firm sells its accounts receivable (generally without recourse) to a financial institution (the "factor").

Federal National Mortgage Association (FNMA) (Fannie Mae)—A federal agency which purchases FHA insured mortgages, to assure a wider secondary market for such securities.

Financial Structure—The entire right-hand side of the balance sheet—the way in which a firm is financed.

Fixed Assets—Assets of a relatively permanent nature held for continuous use in hospital operations and not intended to be converted into cash through sale.

Fixed Charges—Costs that do not vary with the level of output.

Fund Accounting—A system of accounting wherein the hospital's resources, obligations, and capital balances are segregated into the accounts into logical groups according to legal restrictions and administrative requirements. Each account group, or fund, constitutes a subordinate accounting entity, created and maintained for a particular purpose.

Funded Debt—Long-term debt.

General Fund—The account group used to record transactions arising out of the general operations and the regular day-to-day operations of the hospital.

General Obligation—A bond secured by pledge of the issuer's full faith, credit and taxing power.

Goodwill—Intangible assets of a firm established by the excess of the price paid for the going concern over its book value.

Government National Mortgage Association (GNMA) (Ginnie Mae)—A federal agency which issues its own securities on the open market, which are backed by the yields on federally insured mortgages.

Indenture—A formal agreement between the issuer of a bond and the bond holders.

Insolvency—The inability to meet mature or due obligations.

Internal Control—The plan of organizaticn of all the coordinate methods and measures adopted within a business to safeguard its assets, check the accuracy and reliability of its accounting data, promote operating efficiency, and encourage a change to prescribe managerial policies.

Internal Rate of Return (IRR)—The rate of return on an asset investment. The internal rate of return is calculated by finding the discount rate that equates the present value of future cash flows to the cost of the investment.

Investment Banker—Also known as ar underwriter, is the middle-man between this issuer and the public market. The investment banker usually functions as principal rather than agent and initially purchases all of the bonds from the issuer.

Line of Credit—An arrangment whereby a financial institution commits itself to lend up to a specified maximum amount of funds during a specified period.

Liquid—Refers to the ability to rapidly sell marketable securities without a loss in principal.

Liquidity—Refers to a firm's cash position and its ability to meet maturing obligations.

Lock-box Plan—A procedure used to speed up collections and to reduce float.

Marginal Cost—The cost of an additional unit. The *marginal cost of capital* is the cost of an additional dollar of new funds.

Marketable Security—Short-term financial instruments which can be readily bought or sold without a loss in principal. Often used as a short-term investment alternative for temporary surplus cash balances.

Money Market—Financial markets in which funds are borrowed or loaned for short periods. (The money market is distinguished from the capital market, which is the market for long-term funds.)

Mortgage—A pledge of designated property as security for a loan.

Municipal Bond—A bond issued by a state or a political subdivision, such as a county, city or village. The term also refers to bonds issued by state agencies and authorities. Generally, interest paid on municipal bonds is exempt from federal income taxes. The term municipal bond is usually synonymous with "tax-exempt bond."

Negotiated Underwriting—A private sale of the bonds by the issuer as contrasted to the advertisement for public bids. Most hospital bond underwritings are negotiated due to special marketing considerations.

Net Worth—The capital and surplus of a firm.

Objective Probability Distributions—Probability distributions determined by statistical procedures.

Opportunity Cost—The rate of return on the best *alternative* investment that is available. It is the highest return that will *not* be earned if the funds are invested in a particular project.

Overstocked—A condition wherein inventory stocks exceed demand.

Par Value—The face amount of the bond. The amount of money due at maturity—usually $1,000.

Plant Fund—Account group used to record the transactions involving the hospital's investment in land, buildings, and equipment.

Pledging of Accounts Receivable—Short-term borrowing from financial institutions where the loan is secured by accounts receivable. The lender may physically take the accounts receivable but typically has recourse to the borrower; also called *discounting of accounts receivable*.

Points—The same as "percentage." In the case of a bond, a point means $10 since a bond is quoted as a percentage of $1,000.

A bond or bond issue which is discounted two points is quoted at 98 percent of its par value.

Prepayment Provisions—The provision in the bond or mortgage indenture which specifies at what time and on what terms repayment of principal amount may be made prior to maturity.

Present Value (PV)—The value today of a future payment, or stream of payments, discounted at the appropriate discount rate.

Prime Rate—The rate of interest commercial banks charge very large, strong corporations.

Private Placement—The placement of an issue in the private (i.e., nonpublic) money markets. This private market is composed of different types of financial institutions (banks, life insurance companies, pension funds, REITs, etc.).

Prospectus—Commonly, a written document conforming to state and federal regulations containing disclosures about a business entity which is seeking additional debt or equity financing, together with information about the terms and purposes of the financing.

Rate of Return—The internal rate of return on an investment.

Recourse Arrangement—A term used in connection with accounts receivable financing. If a firm sells its accounts receivable to a financial institution under a recourse agreement then, if the account receivable cannot be collected, the selling firm must repurchase the account from the financial institution.

Redemption Provision—A provision allowing the issuer, at its option, to call the bonds at fixed price after a certain date.

Refunding—New securities are sold by the issuer and the proceeds used to retire outstanding securities. The object may be to save interest cost, extend the maturity of the debt or to relax certain existing restrictive covenants.

Registered Bonds—Bonds which are registered with the bond trustee which designate ownership. Transfer of ownership of the bonds must be registered with the bond trustee in order that new bond holders continue to receive principal and interest.

Regression Analysis—A statistical procedure for predicting the value of one variable (dependent variable) on the basis of knowledge about one or more other variables (independent variables).

Relative Value Units—Index number assigned to various procedures based upon the relative amount of labor, supplies, and capital needed to perform the procedure.

Responsibility Accounting—An accounting system which accumulates and communicates historical and projected monetary and statistical data relating to revenues and controllable expenses, classified according to the organizational units producing the revenues and responsible for incurring the expenses.

Revenue Bond—A bond payable solely from the revenue generated from the operation of the project being financed. In the case of hospital revenue bond financing, the bonds are typically payable from the gross receipts of the hospital.

Salvage Value—The value of a capital asset at the end of a specified period. It is the current market price of an asset being considered for replacement in a capital budgeting problem.

Self-Responsible Patient—A patient who pays either all or part of his hospital bill from his own funds as opposed to third party funds.

Serial Bonds—Not a distinct class of bonds but rather an issue of bonds with different maturities, as distinguished from an issue where all of the bonds have identical maturities (term bonds). Serial bonds are usually retired either in equal annual amounts or on a level debt service basis.

Series Bonds—Secured by the same assets or revenue, but issued at intervals with different dates. They may or may not mature at the same time.

"63-20" Financing—A type of tax-exempt hospital financing requiring a special ruling from the Internal Revenue Service based upon a 1963 Ruling (#20). The bonds are issued by the hospital and when fully retired, title is tendered to a municipality or other public body.

Step Down—A cost finding technique involving a single distribution of general service cost centers to both general service and final cost centers.

Stock-out—A condition wherein demand exists for inventory items but none are available.

Subjective Probability Distributions—Probability distributions determined through subjective procedures without the use of objective data.

Subordinated Debenture—A bond having a claim of assets only after the senior debt has been paid off in the event of liquidation.

Tangible Assets—Physical assets as opposed to such intangible assets as goodwill and the stated value of patients.

Tax-Exempt Bond—A bond upon which the interest is exempt from federal income taxes.

Term Loan—A loan generally obtained from a bank or insurance company with a maturity greater than one year. Term loans are generally amortized.

Third Party Payers—An agency such as Blue Cross or Medicare program which contracts with hospitals and patients to pay for the care of covered patients.

Trade Credit—Interfirm debt arising through credit sales and recorded as an account payable by the buyer.

Underwriter—Generally, one or more investment bankers, who, for a fee, undertake to market a debt or equity security issue for the issuing entity or, in the case of a secondary offering, for the selling shareholders.

Working Capital—Refers to a firm's investment in short-term assets—cash, short-term securities, accounts receivable, and inventories. *Gross working capital* is defined as a firm's total current assets. *Net working capital* is defined as current assets minus current liabilities.

Wraparound Mortgage—A mortgage loan in which the lender takes a junior lien position, but undertakes to make the payments on the prior lien, usually without assuming any legal obligation to pay it. This device is used to leverage an additional loan by charging a higher rate of interest on both old and new balances, while paying only the lower prior rate.

Yield—The rate of return on an investment—the internal rate of return.

Sources

Segments of the glossary were adapted from the following sources:

Hay, Leon E. *Budgeting and Cost Analysis for Hospital Management.*

Lindsay, J. Robert and Sametz, Arnold W. *Financial Management: An Analytic Approach.*

Moyer, C.A. and Mautz, R.K. *Intermediate Accounting: A Functional Approach.*

Seawell, L. Vann. *Hospital Accounting and Financial Managment.*

Seawell, L. Vann. *Principles of Hospital Accounting.*

Taylor, Philip J. and Nelson, Benjamin O. *Management Accounting for Hospitals.*

Topics in Health Care Financing, Fall 1978.

Weston, J. Fred and Brigham, Eugene F. *Managerial Finance.*

Bibliography, Part A

Aday, Lu Ann and Andersen, Ronald. *Development of Indices of Access to Medical Care.* Ann Arbor: Health Administration Press, 1974.

American Hospital Association. *Budgeting Procedures for Hospitals.* Chicago: The Association, 1971.

American Hospital Association. *Chart of Accounts for Hospitals.* Chicago: The Association, 1966.

American Hospital Association. *Cost Finding and Rate Setting for Hospitals.* Chicago: The Association, 1968.

American Hospital Association. *Internal Control and Internal Auditing for Hospitals.* Chicago: The Association, 1969.

American Hospital Association. "Principles of Payment for Hospital Care." Chicago: The Association, 1963.

American Hospital Association. *Report of a Special Committee on the Provision of Health Services.* Chicago: The Association, 1970.

American Hospital Association. *Report of the Task Force on Principles of Payment for Hospital Care.* Chicago: The Association, 1963.

American Hospital Association. *Statement on the Financial Requirements of Health Care Institutions and Services.* Chicago: The Association, 1969.

American Hospital Association. *Uniform Hospital Definitions.* Chicago: The Association, 1960.

Andersen, Ronald and Anderson, Odin W. *A Decade of Health Services.* Chicago: The University of Chicago Press, 1967.

Anderson, Odin W. *Blue Cross Since 1929: Accountability and Public Trust.* Cambridge, Mass.: Ballinger, 1975.

Anderson, Odin W. *The Uneasy Equilibrium.* New Haven: College & University Press, 1968.

Association of University Programs in Health Administration. *Financial Management of Health Care Organizations: A Referenced Outline and Annotated Bibliography.* Washington, D.C.: The Association, 1978.

Austin, Charles J. *The Politics of National Health Insurance.* San Antonio: Trinity University Press, 1975.

Austin, Charles J. *Information Systems for Hospital Administration.* Ann Arbor: Health Administration Press, 1979.

Austin, Charles J. and Greene, Barry R. "Hospital Information Systems: A Current Perspective." *Inquiry,* Vol. XV, No. 2, pp. 95–112.

Ball, Robert M. *Social Security: Today and Tomorrow.* New York: Columbia University Press, 1978.

Barnes, E.H. *Barnes on Credit and Collection.* Englewood Cliffs, N.J.: Prentice-Hall, 1961.

Bartizal, John R. *Budget Principles and Procedures.* Englewood Cliffs, N.J.: Prentice-Hall, 1940.

Baumol, William J. "The Transactions Demand for Cash: An Inventory Theoretic Approach." *Quarterly Journal of Economics,* November, 1952.

Beranek, William. *Analysis for Financial Decision.* Homewood, Ill.: Irwin, 1963.

Beranek, William. *Working Capital Managment.* Belmont, Calif.: Wadsworth, 1966.

Berg, Gordon H. and Tucker, John M. "Techniques for Arranging Hospital Financing." *Financial Management,* Spring 1972, pp. 48–57.

Berki, Sylvester E. *Hospital Economics.* Lexington, Mass.: Heath, 1972.

The Boston Consulting Group, Inc. *Reimbursing Hospitals on Inclusive Rates.* Rockville, Md.: The National Center for Health Services Research and Development, Department of Health, Education and Welfare, 1971.

Boulis, Paul S. and Funk, Denise A. *Patient Care Coordinator Program.* Chicago: Blue Cross Association, 1974.

Bower, James B.; Connors, Edward J.; Mosher, John E.; Rowley, Clyde S., Jr. *Hospital Income Flow: A Study of the Effects of Source of Pay on Hospital Income.* Madison, Wisc.: Mimir Publishers, Inc. for The University of Wisconsin Graduate School of Business, 1970.

Bower, James B. and Schlosser, Robert E. "Internal Control—Its True Nature." *The Accounting Review,* Vol. 40, No. 2, April 1965.

Brook, Robert H. *Quality of Care Assessment: A Comparison of Five Methods of Peer Review.* Washington, D.C.: Department of Health, Education, and Welfare, Pub. No. HRA–74–3100, 1973.

Brookings Institution. *Setting National Priorities: the 1974 Budget.* Washington, D.C.: The Institution, 1974.

Brown, Ray E. *Judgment in Administration.* Hightstown, N.J.: McGraw-Hill, 1966.

Bulloch, James. "Responsibility Accounting—A Results Oriented Appraisal System." *Management of Personnel Quarterly,* Winter, 1964, pp. 25–31.

Bureau of Public Health Economics and Department of Economics, The University of Michigan. *The Economics of Health and Medical Care.* Ann Arbor: The Bureau, 1964.

Calman, R.F. *Linear Programming and Cash Management: Cash ALPHA.* Cambridge, Mass.: The MIT Press, 1968.

Carter, Eugene and DeKoff, Newton. "Health Insurance for the Aged: Number of Hospital and Extended Care Facility Admissions by State." *Research and Statistics Notes,* October 15, 1940.

Caruana, Russell A. *A Guide to Organizing the Hospital's Fiscal Services Division.* Chicago: Hospital Financial Management Association, 1974.

Citizens Research Council of Michigan. *A Report to the Michigan Task Force on Medicaid and Health Care Costs.* Detroit: The Council, 1978.

Cleverly, William O. *Financial Management of Health Care Facilities.* Germantown, Md.: Aspen Systems, 1975.

The Committee for National Health Insurance. *Facts of Life: Health and Health Insurance.* Washington, D.C.: The Committee, 1969.

Committee on Finance, United States Senate. *Medicare and Medicaid: Problems, Issues, and Alternatives.* Washington, D.C.: U.S. Printing Office, 1970.

Corning, Peter A. *The Evolution of Medicare.* Washington, D.C.: Social Security Administration Research Report No. 29, 1969.

Cunningham, Robert M., Jr. *Governing Hospitals: Trustees and the New Accountabilities.* Chicago: American Hospital Association, 1976.

Detwiller, L.F. *The Consequences of Health Care Through Government: A Study of the Social and Financial Effects of Canada's Health Care Programs.* Sydney, Australia: Office of Health Care Finance, 1972.

Dewing, Arthur S. *The Financial Policy of Corporations.* New York: The Ronald Press, 1953.

Dominion Bureau of Statistics. "Canadian Schedule of Unit Values for Clinical Laboratory Procedures." Ottawa: The Bureau, 1971.

Dominion Bureau of Statistics. "Canadian Schedule of Unit Values for Physiotherapy and Occupational Therapy." Ottawa: The Bureau, 1971.

Donabedian, Avedis. *Aspects of Medical Care Administration.* Cambridge, Mass.: Harvard University Press, 1973.

Durbin, Richard L. and Springall, W. Herbert. *Organization and Administration of Health Care.* Saint Louis: Mosby, 1969.

Earhart, Charles H. "An Analysis and Development of Standards for Selected Financial Ratios in Voluntary Non-Profit General Hospitals." University of Iowa master's thesis, 1971.

Ehrenreich, Barbara and Ehrenreich, John. *The American Health Empire: Power, Profits, Politics.* New York: Random House, 1970.

Eilers, Robert D. "Postpayment Medical Expense Coverage." *Blue Cross Reports,* September, 1969.

Falcon, William D., ed. *Reporting Financial Data to Management.* New York: American Management Association, 1965.

Feldstein, Martin. *The Rising Cost of Hospital Care.* Washington, D.C.: Information Resources Press, 1971.

Ferber, Bernard C. and Lichterman, Michael S. "Principal Sources of Payment for Patients Discharged from Chicago Area Short-term General Hospitals." Chicago Hospital Council, 1977.

Flook, E. Evelyn and Sanazaro, Paul J., eds. *Health Services Research and R&D in Perspective.* Ann Arbor: Health Administration Press, 1973.

Foyle, William B. "Merge the Plant and General Funds—Why Not?" *Hospital Accounting,* Vol. 19, No.6, June, 1965, pp. 2–5.

Friedman, Emily and Wendorf, Carl. "Medicaid." *Hospitals*, August 16, 1977; September 1, 1977; September 16, 1977; October 1, 1977; November 1, 1977.

Funk, Denise A. *Health Data Systems: An Informational Manual.* Chicago: Blue Cross Association, 1973.

Gibson, Geoffrey; Bugbee, George; and Anderson, Odin W. *Emergency Medical Services in the Chicago Area.* Chicago: University of Chicago Center for Health Administration Studies, 1970.

Ginzberg, Eli. *The Limits of Health Reform: The Search for Realism.* New York: Basic Books, Inc., 1977.

Griffith, John R. *Measuring Hospital Performance.* Chicago: Blue Cross Association, 1978.

Griffith, John W. *Quantitative Techniques for Hospital Planning and Control.* Lexington, Mass.: Heath, 1972.

Griffith, John R.; Hancock, Walton M.; Munson, Fred C., eds. *Cost Control in Hospitals.* Ann Arbor: Health Administration Press, 1976.

Hauser, Richard. "How to Build and Use a Flexible Budget." *Financial Management*, August, 1974.

Health Insurance Institute. *Source Book of Health Insurance Data.* New York: The Institute. 1976–1977.

Heaney, Charles T. and Riedel, Donald C. "From Indemnity to Full Coverage: Changes in Hospital Utilization." *Blue Cross Reports*, October, 1970.

Heckert, J.B. and Willson, J.D. *Controllership.* New York: Ronald, 1963.

Herkhimer, Allen G. *Understanding Hospital Financial Management.* Germantown, Md.: Aspen Systems, 1978.

Hess, Irene; Riedel, Donald C.; Fitzpatrick, Thomas B. *Probability Sampling of Hospitals and Patients: Second Edition.* Ann Arbor: Health Administration Press, 1976.

Hillier, Frederick E. and Lieberman, Gerald J. *Introduction to Operations Research*, Second Edition. San Francisco: Holden-Day, 1974.

Hodge, Melville H. *Medical Information System: A Resource for Hospitals.* Germantown, Md.: Aspen Systems Corp., 1977.

Holahan, John. *Financing Health Care for the Poor: The Medicaid Experience.* Lexington, Mass.: D.C. Heath & Co., 1975.

Holahan, John. *Physician Supply, Peer Review and Use of Health Services in Medicaid.* Washington, D.C.: The Urban Institute, 1976.

Holahan, John; Scanlon, William; and Spitz, Bruce. *Restructuring Federal Medicaid Controls and Incentives.* Washington, D.C.: The Urban Institute, 1977.

Holahan, John; Spitz, Bruce; Pollak, William; and Feder, Judith. *Altering Medicaid Reimbursement Methods.* Washington, D.C.: The Urban Institute, 1977.

Holahan, John and Stuart, Bruce. *Controlling Medicaid Utilization Patterns.* Washington, D.C.: The Urban Institute, 1977.

Hopp, Michael. "Purchasing and Accounting Information System." Ann Arbor: Community Systems Foundation, 1966.

Hospital Financial Management Association. *Managing the Patient Account*. Chicago: The Association, 1970.

Hospital Financial Management Association. *Planning the Hospital's Financial Operations*. Chicago: The Association, 1972.

Hospital Financial Management Association. *Safeguarding the Hospital's Assets*. Chicago: The Association, 1971.

Hospital Financial Management Association. *The State of Information Processing in the Health Care Industry*. Chicago: The Association, 1976.

Hospital Planning Council of Metropolitan Chicago. "Capital Financing of Voluntary Hospitals: The Role of Contributions." Chicago: The Council, 1971.

Hospital Planning Council of Metropolitan Chicago. "Capital Financing of Voluntary Hospitals: The Role of Debt Funds." Chicago: The Council, 1971.

Hospital Planning Council of Metropolitan Chicago. "Capital Financing of Voluntary Hospitals: The Role of Government Assistance." Chicago: The Council, 1971.

Hospital Planning Council of Metropolitan Chicago: ' Capital Financing of Voluntary Hospitals: The Role of Internal Funds." Chicago: The Council, 1971.

Indiana University Graduate School of Business. *Third Party Reimbursement for Hospitals*. Bloomington, Ind.: The School, 1965.

Kaiser Foundation Medical Care Program. "Kaiser Foundation Medical Care Program." Oakland, Calif.: The Foundation, 1970.

Kennedy, Edward M. *In Critical Condition: The Crisis in America's Health Care*. New York: Simon and Schuster, 1972.

Knight, W.D. "Working Capital Management—Satisfactory Versus Optimization." *Financial Management*, Spring, 1972, pp. 33–40.

Kovner, Anthony R. and Neuhauser, Duncan, eds. *Health Services Management*. Ann Arbor: Health Administration Press, 1978.

Krizay, John and Wilson, Andrew A. *The Patient as Consumer: Health Care Financing in the United States*. Lexington, Mass.: Heath, 1974.

Law, Sylvia A. *Blue Cross: What Went Wrong?* New Haven: Yale University Press, 1974.

Lerner, Monroe and Anderson, Odin W. *Health Progress in the United States: 1900–1960*. Chicago: The University of Chicago Press, 1963.

Lindsay, Franklin A. *New Techniques for Management Decision-Making*. Hightstown, N.J.: McGraw-Hill, 1963.

Lindsay, Robert and Sametz, Arnold W. *Financial Management: An Analytical Approach*. Homewood, Ill.: Irwin, 1967.

Lippold, Ronald C. *Hospital Credit Training Manual*. Saint Louis: The Catholic Hospital Association, 1970.

Lipson, Stephen H. "Antitrust Implications of Voluntary Rate Review." *Hospital and Health Services*, Winter 1979, pp 93–101.

Lipson, Stephen H. *Development of the Virginia Hospital Rate Review Program*. Richmond: Virginia Hospital Research & Education Foundation, 1976.

Lipson, Stephen H. and Hensel, Mary D. *Hospital Manpower Budget Preparation Manual*. Ann Arbor: Health Administration Press, 1975.

Loebs, Stephen F. "Medicaid: A Survey of Indicators and Issues." *Hospitals and Health Services Administration*, Fall 1977, pp. 63–90.

Loebs, Stephen F. *Variations Among States in Selected Optional Decisions in the Medicaid Program*. A University of Michigan doctoral dissertation. Ann Arbor: University Microfilms, 1974.

McNerney, Walter et al. *Hospital and Medical Economics*, 2 vol. Chicago: Hospital Research and Educational Trust, 1962.

MacStravic, Robin E. *Determining Health Needs*. Ann Arbor: Health Administration Press, 1978.

Magee, John R. and Boodman, D.M. *Production Planning and Inventory Control*. Hightstown, N.J.: McGraw-Hill, 1967.

Manitoba Hospital Association. *Hospital Management and Accounting Manual for Automated Systems*. Winnipeg: The Association, 1969.

Manney, James D. *Aging in American Society*. Ann Arbor: The Institute of Gerontology, 1975.

Mannix, John R. "Blue Cross Reimbursement for Hospitals." Paper presented at Hospital Summer Management Course, Center for Continuing Education, The University of Michigan, 1969.

Markstein, David L. "How to Make Short-Term Cash Work at Full-Time Rates." *Modern Hospital*, Vol. 114, No. 1, January 1970, pp. 63, 64, 134.

Markstein, David L. "The Pros and Cons of Credit Cards for the Hospital Field." *Modern Hospital*, June 1970, pp. 70,72,78.

Martin, Glenn J. "What Experiments in Prospective Reimbursement are Teaching Providers, Agencies, Third Parties." *Hospital Financial Management*, Vol. 24, No. 10, November 1970, pp. 3–7.

Martin, Lawrence E. "Reimbursements by All Inclusive Rates." *HSRD Briefs*. National Center for Health Services Research and Development, Dept. HEW, 5600 Fishers Lane, Rockville, Md. Summer 1970.

Melkonian, Donna J. and Raichel, Theodore M. *Provider Review Manual (Plan Utilization Review Program)*. Chicago: Blue Cross Association, 1974.

Michigan Task Force on Medicaid and Health Care Costs. *Report of the Michigan Task Force on Medicaid and Health Care Costs*. Ann Arbor: The Task Force, January 1979.

Miller, Merton H. and Orr, Daniel. "An Application of Control Limit Models to the Management of Corporate Cash Balances" in *Proceedings of the Conference on Financial Research and Its Implications for Management, Stanford University*. Robichek, Alexander A., ed. New York: Wiley, 1967.

Miller, Merton H. and Orr, Daniel. "Model for the Demand for Money by Firms." *Quarterly Journal of Economics*, August, 1966, pp. 413–435.

Moyer, C.A. and Mautz, R.K. *Intermediate Accounting: A Functional Approach*. New York: Wiley, 1962.

Mueller, William J., and Soder, Earl. "Rate Setting." *Hospital Accounting*, Vol. 18, No. 12, December 1964.

Murphy, Thomas. "The Hospital Treasurer and Controller: Duties and Responsibilities." *Hospital Financial Managment*, Vol. 24, No. 4, April 1970, pp. 11–14.

Myers, Robert J. *Medicare*. Homewood, Ill.: Irwin, 1970.

National Center for Health Services Research and Development. *Administrative Cost Determination Manual for Hospital Outpatient Accounting*. Rockville, Md.: 1972.

National Center for Health Services Research. "Demonstration and Evaluation of a Total Hospital Information System," DHEW Publication No. (HRA) 77-3188, July 1977.

Novick, David. *Program Budgeting: Program Analysis and the Federal Budget, Second Edition*. Cambridge, Mass.: Harvard University Press, 1967.

Odiorne, George. *Planning the Hospital's Financial Operations*. Chicago: The Hospital Financial Management Association, 1972.

O'Donoghue, Patrick. *Evidence About the Effects of Health Care Regulation*. Denver: Spectrum Research, 1974.

Orgler, Yair E. *Cash Management and Models*. Belmont, Calif.: Wadsworth, 1970.

Perlman, Mark; Adams, Jeffrey; Wolfe, Harvey; Shuman, Larry. *Methods for Distributing the Costs on Non-Revenue Producing Centers*. Ann Arbor: University Microfilms Hospital Abstract 10600AC, 1972.

Provost, George P. and Heller, William M. "How Break-Even Pricing of Drugs Works." *Modern Hospital*, Vol. 94, No.5, May 1960, pp. 122–126.

Pyhrr, Peter A. *Zero Base Budgeting*. New York: Wiley, 1973.

Quirin, G. David. *The Capital Expenditure Decision*. Homewood, Ill.: Irwin, 1967.

Raitz, Robert E. "The Effect of Using an Economic Order Quantity Formula and Exponential Smoothing to Reduce Hospital Purchasing Costs." Master's thesis, the University of Minnesota, 1964.

Reed, Louis S. and Carr, Willine. *The Benefit Structure of Private Health Insurance, 1968*. Washington, D.C.: Social Security Administration, Office of Research and Statistics, Research Report No. 32, 1970.

Reed, Louis S. and Dwyer, Maureen. *Health Insurance Plans Other than Blue Cross or Blue Shield Plans or Insurance Companies*. Washington, D.C.: Social Security Administration, Office of Research and Statistics, Research Report No. 35, 1971.

Rice, Thomas R. "The Development of a Double Weighting Charge Structure for Physical Therapy." Master's thesis, Duke University, 1970.

Riedel, Donald C.; Walden, Daniel C.; Singsen, Antone G.; Meyers, Samuel; Krantz, Goldie; Henderson, Marie. *Federal Employees Health Benefits Program Utilization Study*. Washington, D.C.: Department HEW, 1975.

Roemer, Milton I.; Dubois, Donald M.; Rich, Shirley W., eds. *Health Insurance Plans: Studies in Organizational Diversity*. Los Angeles, Calif.: University of California, 1970.

Rorem, C. Rufus. *Origins of Blue Cross*. Privately published, 1971.

Salling, Raymond C. "Can Your Inventory Control Be Scientific?" *Modern Hospital*, October 1964, pp. 34, 36.

Schein, Edgar H. *Organizational Psychology*. Englewood Cliffs, N.J.: Prentice-Hall, 1972.

Seawell, L. Vann. *Hospital Accounting and Financial Management*. Berwyn, Ill.: Physicians Record Co., 1964.

Seawell, L. Vann. *Introduction to Hospital Accounting*. Chicago: Hospital Financial Management Association, 1971.

Seawell, L. Vann. *Hospital Financial Accounting: Theory and Practice*. Chicago: Hospital Financial Management Association, 1975.

Seawell, L. Vann. *Principles of Hospital Accounting*. Berwyn, Ill.: Physicians Record Co., 1960.

Shelton, Robert M. "The Hospital Financial Manager Today." *Hospital Financial Management*, Vol. 24, No. 4, April 1970, pp. 4–6, 40, 41.

Silvers, J.B. and Prahalad, C.K. *Financial Management of Health Institutions*. New York: Spectrum Publications, 1974.

Skolnik, Alfred M. and Dales, Sophie R. "Social Welfare Expenditures in Fiscal Year 1970." *Research and Statistics Notes*, November 30, 1970.

Smalley, Harold E. and Freeman, John R. *Hospital Industrial Engineering*. New York: Reinhold, 1966.

Social Security Administration. *Medicare, 1972: Enrollment*. Washington, D.C.: Government Printing Office, 1975.

Social Security Administration. *Medicare, the First Nine Months*. Washington D.C.: Government Printing Office, 1967.

Social Security Administration. *Medicare, 1972: Reimbursement by State and County*. Washington, D.C.: Government Printing Office, 1975.

Somers, Anne R. and Somers, Herman M. *Health and Health Care: Policies in Perspective*. Germantown, Md: Aspen Systems Corp., 1977.

Somers, Herman M. and Somers, Anne R. *Doctors, Patients and Health Insurance*. New York: Doubleday Anchor Books, 1962.

Somers, Herman M. and Somers, Anne R. "Major Issues in National Health Insurance." *Milbank Memorial Fund Quarterly*, Vol. L, No. 2. Part I, pp. 177–210.

Somers, Herman M. and Somers, Anne R. *Medicare and the Hospitals*. Washington, D.C.: The Brookings Institution, 1968.

Spiegel, Allen D. and Podair, Simon, eds. *Medicaid: Lessons for National Health Insurance*. Rockville, Md.: Aspen, 1975.

Stevens, Robert and Stevens, Rosemary. *Welfare Medicine in America: A Case Study of Medicaid*. New York: The Free Press, 1974.

Stone, Bernell K. "The Use of Forecasts and Smoothing in Control-Limit Models for Cash Management." *Financial Management*, Spring, 1972.

Stuart, Bruce C. and Bair, Lee A. *Health Care and Income: The Distributional Impacts of Medicaid and Medicare Nationally and in the State of Michigan*. Lansing, Mich.: State of Michigan Department of Social Services, 1971.

Stuart, Bruce C. and Spitz, Bruce. *Rising Medical Costs in Michigan*. Lansing, Mich.: State of Michigan Department of Social Services, 1973.

Sutermeister, Robert A. *People and Productivity.* Hightstown, N.J.: McGraw-Hill, 1969.

Symonds, Curtis W. *Basic Financial Management.* New York: American Management Association, 1969.

Tonkin, G.W. "The Controller's Role on the Management Team." *Hospital Financial Management,* Vol. 24, No. 4, April 1970, pp. 7–9.

Tunley, Roul. *The American Health Scandal.* New York: Dell, 1966.

U.S. Department of Health, Education and Welfare. *Recommendations of the Task Force on Medicaid and Related Programs, November, 1969.* Washington D.C.: Government Printing Office, 1969.

U.S. Department of Health, Education and Welfare, *Health: United States, 1978.* Washington, D.C.: Government Printing Office, 1978. DHEW Publication No. (PHS) 78-1232.

Van Arsdell, Paul M. *Corporation Finance: Policy, Planning, Administration.* New York: Ronald, 1968.

Van Horne, James C. *Financial Management and Policy, Part II.* Englewood Cliffs, N.J.: Prentice-Hall, 1969.

Wacht, Richard F. "Toward Rationality in the Allocation of Hospital Resources." *Financial Management,* Spring 1972, pp. 66–71.

Waldman, Saul and Peel, Evelyn. "National Health Insurance: A Comparison of Five Proposals." *The Journal of the American Osteopathic Association.* Vol. 70, December 1970, pp. 382–395.

Walls, Edward L., Jr. "Hospital Dependency of Long-Term Debt." *Financial Management,* Spring 1972, pp. 42–47.

Warner, D. Michael and Holloway, Don C. *Decision Making and Control for Health Administration.* Ann Arbor: Health Administration Press, 1978.

Wath, Jacquelyn J. "Health Insurance for the Aged: Participating Health Facilities, July 1970." *Health Insurance Statistics,* January 15, 1971.

Weeks, Lewis E. and Berman, Howard J., eds. *Economics in Health Care.* Germantown, Md.: Aspen Systems Corp., 1977.

Weeks, Lewis E.; Berman, Howard J.; and Bisbee, Gerald E., Jr., eds. *Financing of Health Care.* Ann Arbor: Health Administration Press, 1979.

Weston, J. Fred and Brigham, Eugene F. *Managerial Finance, Third Edition.* New York: Holt, Rinehart and Winston, 1969.

Wheelwright, Steven C. and Makridakis, Spyos G. *Forecasting Methods for Management.* New York: Wiley, 1973.

Williams, John Daniel and Rakich, Jonathan S. "Investment Evaluation in Hospitals." *Financial Management,* Summer 1973.

Williams, William J. "A Report on Insurance and Prepayment for Medical Care." A master's thesis Xavier University, Cincinnati. Ann Arbor: University Microfilms Hospital Abstract IN 2026. 1964.

Wilson, Florence A. and Neuhauser, Duncan. *Health Services in the United States.* Cambridge, Mass.: Ballinger, 1974.

Wren, George R. *Modern Health Administration.* Athens, Ga.: University of Georgia Press, 1974.

Young, D,E. "Effective Presentation of Reports: Information for Understanding," in *Reporting Financial Data to Management.* New York: American Management Association, 1965.

Bibliography, Part B[1]

(Classified as: Accounting, Administration, Health Services, Insurance and Prepayment, Outpatient Services, and Utilization Review.)

ACCOUNTING

Adair, Jerry D.
A Feasability Study of an All-Inclusive Rate Structure for Today's Hospitals
Duke University, Durham, N.C., 1970, 52 pp.
Available from University Microfilms.

An evaluation of the inclusive rate system and a comparison with the itemized charge system. Discussion of variations of the inclusive rate includes the straight line charge, modified straight line, and straight line with special charges. Equitability and the "share-the-hazard" principle are also examined. Disadvantages of itemized charge system are listed as excessive bookkeeping, non-use of services because of expense, and the surprise element in patient's bill. Advantages of inclusive rates given are their predictable nature, ease of rate changing, patient and third party acceptance. Data from four hospitals were collected, to "determine whether an average charge per patient day is generally a valid measure to represent the total charge to all patients . . . " Variations in charges result from different clinical services within systems rather than from the systems as a whole, therefore, if the inclusive rate is used it should be based on clinical service.
Hospital Abstract AC2–5830.

---

[1]The abstracts printed in Bibliography Part B are republished from *Abstracts of Hospital Management Studies* with permission. The full text of each abstracted document is available as indicated. Those marked "Available from University Microfilms" can be ordered from University Microfilms, 300 N. Zeeb Road, Ann Arbor, Michigan 48106 by the Hospital Abstract Number.

Andrews, Charles T.
Financial and Statistical Reports for Administrative Decision-Making in Hospitals
Indiana University, Bloomington, Ind., 1968, 261 pp.
Available from University Microfilms

The purpose of this study was to investigate the information needs of hospital administrators for decision-making and to then develop model financial and statistical reports which would best meet these information needs. In order to develop the model reports it was necessary to determine the content of specific reports, how frequently the information was needed, and the best format for presenting the information.

Interviews were conducted separately with selected hospital administrators and financial officers to obtain data as to areas of administrative decision-making, the information required, the frequency of which the information was needed, and the current reporting practices in the hospital represented. The interviews with the financial officers were to determine their awareness of the administrators' information needs. Basically the same questions were used for these interviews. The results of the interviews indicated there was not uniformity in current financial reporting practices as to frequency, content or format.

Based upon the results of the research, model financial and statistical reports were developed. The objectives of the model reports were to assist the administrator by pointing up areas needing his attention, and to provide an accurate portrayal of facts through interpretation and analysis by the financial officer.
Hospital Abstract ACO–5406.

Arafa, Said M.
Accounting Information for Planning and Control Models: The Case of PERT and Critical Path Method
University of California, Berkeley, Calif., 1970, 323 pp.
Available from University Microfilms

The purpose of this study is to demonstrate with reference to an empirical situation and within a conceptual framework how accounting can serve as the primary formal information system for the purpose of a given decision model, and how accounting information can be extended to meet the information requirements of the model. Data for this study were secured through a thorough case study of a large construction company which undertakes large industrial and heavy construction projects and which has a relatively long experience with the application of the model examined

in this study, the PERT-CFU model. Improvements in accounting information provided for central feedback purposes are recommended through a suggested system of variance analysis that integrates unit cost control with activity-progress control needed for the model. The proposed system is extended to provide useful information for updating cost estimates at completion.
Hospital Abstract AC1–6292.

Barten, Frederick J.
A Comparison Utilizing Two Cost Finding Systems of Inpatient Reimbursement Under Current Formulas and Universally Applied RCC
Program in Hospital Administration, The University of Michigan, Ann Arbor, Mich., 1968, 70 pp.
Available from University Microfilms

A study which attempts to measure the impact of arbitrary rate setting practices when these rates are used for reimbursement calculations under RCC formula. Actual charges and reimbursement charges of the 287 bed Annapolis Hospital in Wayne, Michigan were compared to those which would have been received under a system of charges, systematically related to departmental costs under two different schemes of cost finding. The results of the analysis indicate that although the total revenue of the hospital would change only slightly, the RCC formula is open to manipulation by means of the arbitrary charges which are set. In addition, the amounts paid by Blue Cross, Medicare, and other third party payers vary from three to 10%. The kind of cost allocation system used does influence the results. A fully automated simultaneous equation solution gives different results from the stepdown approximation used by the cost allocation program of the Hospital Administrative Services Corporation.
Hospital Abstract AC1033

Bash, Paul L.
Can Capital Budgeting Work in Hospitals?
Hospital Administration, Vol.16, No. 2, Spring 1971, pp. 59–64.

Author discusses some of the important considerations hospitals must face if capital budgeting techniques are to be used in making investment decisions. It is suggested a first step is to spell out the goals of the organization and that capital budgeting will work only if the hospital can tolerate having its true goals brought into open discussion. Other considerations discussed include measuring non-monetary benefits, evaluation of existing programs, and resolving inter-hospital competition. It is concluded any hospital

with cost finding, budgeting and forecasting capability can master capital budgeting, but the two major questions which need resolution are: "Can the hospital organization stand the strain?" and "Can planning agencies provide appropriate support?".
Hospital Abstract AC1–6920.

Bauer, Katharine G.
Improving Information for Hospital Rate Setting
Harvard Center for Community Health and Medical Care, Boston, 1976, 272 pp.

Based on the findings of a series of working papers on the use of data in hospital ratesetting, recommendations are offered for Federal and State officials charged with developing guidelines or regulations concerning information for hospital ratesetting. Following a summary of the project and of its conclusions, the range of information that Blue Cross and State ratesetting programs employ is reviewed, and additional kinds of data that appear to be required are discussed. The nature of data available for monitoring the effects of ratesetting programs is examined, in regard to achieving the cost containment and related objectives of the programs and to possible counterproductive responses the programs might set in motion. Difficulties to be anticipated in transitions to new accounting and reporting systems are noted, and steps that might be taken to ease the changeover are suggested. Shortcomings in the quality of data available to rate setters are pointed out, and the potential for uniform reporting and accounting, together with more extensive auditing, to address these shortcomings is discussed. The need to eliminate duplicate reporting of data from hospitals is stressed, and approaches to doing so are suggested.
Hospital Abstract 17761 AC

Bauer, Katharine G.
Uniform Reporting for Hospital Rate Reviews. Criteria to Guide Development and Proceedings of a 1975 Conference
Harvard Center for Community Health and Medical Care, Boston, 1975 88 pp.

Criteria for use in developing uniform reporting systems for hospital rate review are offered, and the proceedings of a conference on uniform reporting for hospital rate review held in Washington, D.C., in summer of 1975 are documented. The criteria, which focus on the reporting of revenue, costs, and statistics to provide comparability in cost/budget reports, are based on interviews with executives in rate-setting bodies and hospital associations in five

States, and on observations of data problems in case studies of 11 hospital rate-setting programs. They are grouped in three sections: those that might govern the design of uniform reports, those that concern the analyses derived from the reports, and those that concern implementation of new reporting systems. The 1975 conference involved 16 participants representative of rate-setting bodies, hospital associations, and other groups with experience in reporting systems. The papers cover the following subjects: proposed criteria for reporting systems; the American Hospital Association's 1975 chart of accounts; a matrix reporting system under development in New York; California's phased-in process for uniform reporting and budgeting; the feasibility of a complex reporting system for primary level hospitals; matching cost and revenue to detailed functional reporting centers; using length-of-stay norms in rate setting; information payment by case; and ways to account for case mix and complexity.
Hospital Abstract 18427 AC

Beck, Richard H.
A Guideline for Financial Ratio Analysis of Publicly Owned Nursing Home and Extended Care Facility Corporations
Graduate Program in Hospital and Health Administration, University of Iowa, Iowa City, Iowa, 1971, 136 pp.
Available from University Microfilms

Paper discusses the need for responsible financial management of publicly owned nursing homes and extended care facilities. Suggestions are made for establishing a framework for a system of financial ratio analysis, using 12 ratios considered applicable to the nursing home industry. Twenty corporations are described and their individual ratios enumerated on the basis of balance sheets and income statements for fiscal 1970. Tables show liquidity, activity, leverage and profitability ratios for all 20 corporations.
Hospital Abstract AC1–7016

Bennett, Max D.
An Evaluation of Hospital Charges for Patients Discharged with the Same Primary Diagnosis
University of Michigan, Ann Arbor, Mich., 1968, 42 pp.
Available from University Microfilms

This study, conducted at the Johns Hopkins Hospital, analyzes the statistical distribution of hospital charges associated with the care of patients discharged with one of nine selected primary diagnoses. The objective of the study was to determine the feasibility of using costs by diagnosis for purposes of budgeting and reimbursement. Charge data were used as an approximation of cost.

The coefficient of variation was used to analyze the distributions about the mean cost in the nine diagnostic categories. An analysis of the coefficient found all nine diagnoses were of medium or high variation. The coefficients ranged from 41% to 68%.
Hospital Abstract AC2011

Berman, Howard J.
Debt: How Much is Too Much?
Hospital Financial Management, Vol. 23, No. 9 November 1969, pp. 12–13.

Description of a quantitative technique (probabilistic cash forecasting) for determining debt capacity. The author describes and illustrates with an example how a hospital can determine the amount of debt which it can safely hold.
Hospital Abstract AC0032

Berman, Howard J.
Financial Management: Necessity or Nicety?
Hospital Administration, Vol. 15, No. 3, Summer 1970, pp. 84–90

A review article with references on the value and importance of financial management tools and techniques in hospital operations. The usefulness of financial management tools in controlling internal operations, operating financial systems, and making capital investment decisions is explained. Also, references to appropriate research are provided. The author concludes that competent financial management is necessary for efficient and effective hospital operations.
Hospital Abstract ACO–5834

Berman, Howard J.
Ratio Analysis: A Technique for Financial Management in Hospitals
University of Michigan, Ann Arbor, Mich., 1968, 49 pp.
Available from University Microfilms

Study develops ratio values for hospitals to use in estimating financial efficiency which are based on a normal financial plan (presented in traditional corporate finance format as opposed to fund accounting style which AHA suggests) and explains what the ratios mean and how they can be used. Ratio analysis—its limitations and potential value—is discussed. The ratios developed include: 1) Guides to Capital Distribution—cash and near cash to total assets; current assets to total assets; and fixed assets to total

assets. 2) Guides to Liquidity—current ratio; and acid test ratio; 3) Guide to Protective Margins—current liabilities to total assets. A comparison of actual ratios to normal values shows an estimated relative financial efficiency of a particular hospital. Study devises a normal financial plan for 100 bed hospital with average length of stay of seven days. Assumptions are made as to operating parameters such as percent of wages and salaries to total expenses, purchase discounts, supply and materials ordering and payment schedules, etc. Plan can be adapted to different size hospitals if operating parameters are the same. Study also includes discussion of hospital debt capacity. Appendices include working papers which explain how each of figures in normal financial plan presented were derived.
Hospital Abstract AC1051

Berman, Howard J. and Bash, Paul L.
Capital Investment Decisions
Bureau of Hospital Administration, The University of Michigan, Ann Arbor, Mich., 1971, 98 pp.
Available from University Microfilms

This report, designed to provide a practical procedure for evaluating and selecting capital investment opportunities, is comprised of two sections, each intended as a separate manual. Section 1 is the Project Application Manual. It includes a description of the structure of the capital investment process, forms to be used in submitting projects to the Planning Association and an explanation of data needed to complete the forms. Section 2 is the Investment Decision Manual and provides a detailed explanation of the mechanics of evaluating and rank-ordering proposed investments.
Hospital Abstract AC3–6960

Berman, Howard J. and Bash, Paul L.
Operational Budgeting Systems: Hackley Hospital, Muskegon, Michigan
Bureau of Hospital Administration, The University of Michigan, Ann Arbor, Mich., 1970, 151 pp.
Available from University Microfilms

A report on the budgeting practices and procedures of a 400 bed voluntary, nonprofit hospital. Authors examine the present budgeting procedures and present recommendations as to how the existing system can be improved in order to provide a budgeting process which is both compatible with and facilitates managment by objectives and responsibility accounting. In those areas where

current budgets do not exist; e.g., plant and equipment and cash, detailed, step-by-step guidelines for the preparation of operational budgets are provided. Also, a detailed procedure for projecting service volume by cost center is included. Additionally, a chapter is devoted to expense budget reporting and the techniques for adjusting actual performance to budgeted expectations in order to produce an effective responsibility accounting system. Sample forms, reporting formats and worksheets are included.
Hospital Abstract AC1–6152

Blume, Frederick R.
Hospital Debt Management and Cost Reimbursement
Topics in Health Care Financing, 3:1, 1976, pp. 69–81.

Article discusses some of the important factors relating to hospital debt management and the problems imposed by present cost reimbursement regulations: alternative sources for capital; competition in money markets; and structuring a debt issue. It is concluded if hospitals want to retain access to private capital markets, they must have a thorough understanding of the impact of cost reimbursement that ignores replacement cost depreciation, the operating cost of bad debts and charity care and necessity of generating a return on equity capital.
Hospital Abstract 17067 AC

Brown, Jonathan B.; Rowland, Diane; Sweetland, Margaret
Exchange of Information Between Hospital Rate Setting and Certificate of Need Agencies: Selected State Experiences
Harvard Center for Community Health Medical Care, Boston, 1976, 85 pp.

The exchange of information between and within the organizations that share regulatory authority over medical care institutions in New York, Arizona, and Connecticut is discussed. New York provides several examples of information sharing between certificate of need and rate setting bodies. The most successful linkages are said to be the financial feasibility analyses that accompany each certificate of need review and the architectural cost monitoring that accompanies the process of planning and construction. One lesson that emerges from the New York experience is the impact on information sharing of a regulatory structure administered in one agency led by one decisionmaker. The integration of rate review and regulatory functions in Arizona is said to offer several advantages: good communication between rate review and certificate of need analysts, as well as with licensing and certifica-

tion reviewers; full access by analysts at the State and area levels to each others' files; the need for only one filing package from applicants for certificate of need and rate review for use by both State and local agencies; and more informed decisionmaking. The Arizona system is handicapped by the fact that rate recommendations are not enforceable and by inadequate numbers of staff analysts. Connecticut's Commission on Hospitals and Health Care is said to provide a vehicle for close coordination of rate review and facility proposal review. However, the opportunity for closely aligned information activities has not been fully utilized due to both internal and external constraints.
Hospital Abstract 17773 AC

Cannedy, Lloyd L.
An Inquiry into the Utilization of Money-Market Investments by Non-Federal General Hospitals in the United States Exceeding 500 Beds
University of Alabama, Birmingham, Ala., 1968, 114pp.
Available from University Microfilms

An inquiry of utilization for investments by hospitals of nine representative types of short-term securities over three time periods was sent to 169 non-federal general hospitals exceeding 500 beds. The 96 hospitals responding were categorized by type of control, and location in seven geographical districts. Money-market operations are discussed.

U.S. Treasury bills were utilized most often; bankers' acceptance least. Religiously-controlled institutions and institutions in the midwest generally dominated in utilization. No dependence was found between nonutilization and either type of control or location.
Hospital Abstract AC0022

Canter, Eric W.
Business Office: Outpatient Charge Processing Analysis
National Cooperative Services Center for Hospital Management Engineering, Chicago, Ill., 1975, 22pp.

The objective of this study analyzed the errors, time required, and process involved with outpatient billing. A random work sampling of 20 patient visits per department was performed, although no discussion of sampling techniques is provided. Supplemented by interviews, charts and flow charts were created to indicate type of error by day of week, and time involved with error detection/ correction. Exhibits, in addition to data charts and process flows, include the Data Collection Form and the Patient Visit Worksheet. Findings pertaining to billing errors reflected that failure to check requested tests or making incorrect tests were the highest occurrence of errors. In addition the author discovered that weekends had a high incidence of errors, with Sunday the highest. Regarding the process itself, it was determined that approximately 35 hours per day are spent in editing charge mistakes. Cost calculations for this time are also shown. Recommendations provided for the elimination of certain charge documents, and alteration of the process flow. Both procedural steps and flow charts of proposals are provided.

Hospital Abstract 13440 AC

Catholic Hospital Association
  Guides to Hospital Administrative Planning and Control Through Accounting
The Association, Saint Louis, 62 pp.
Available from University Microfilms

A manual for administrators which presents the uses of accounting and statistical data in specific, but nontechnical terms. Adoption of uniform principles, such as accrual accounting, internal controls, and fund account-coordination and control, are discussed. In particular, cash, payroll, and capital expenditures budgeting are treated. Reports recommended by administrator, how they should be interpreted by him, and what uses he can make of them are discussed in considerable detail. Strict consistency in methods and usage of accounting data is suggested.

Hospital Abstract 1

Choate, G.M.
  Financial Ratio Analysis
Hospital Progress, January 1974, pp. 49–57, 67

Financial ratio analysis enables hospital administrators to rapidly and comprehensively digest routine financial statements in a minimum amount of time with a maximum acquisition of useful information. Part 1 explains how routine financial statements need to be modified in order to facilitate useful ratio analysis. Part 2 defines and explains the ratios themselves. Part 3 outlines how to use financial ratios and demonstrates their use by comparing actual ratio data from the industry sample, and Part 4 discusses the frequency with which ratio analysis should be employed.

Hospital Abstract 12219 AC

Cleverley, William O.
An Input-Output Model for Hospital Costing
Bulletin of the Operations Research Society of America, Vol. 22, No. 1, Spring 1974.

The basic objective of this paper will be to apply input-output methodology as an alternative cost finding system in a hospital. Simple regression analysis will be used to develop estimates of the technological coefficients. Cost functions for the defined final product centers will be developed that will separate costs into their variable and fixed components and account for the effects of interdepartmental transfers of service. These two features are not present in existing cost finding systems. Differences between the two cost systems will be analyzed with special emphasis on potential pricing decisions.
Hospital Abstract 13221 AC

Cleverly, William O.
One Step Further: The Multi-Variable Flexible Budget System
Hospital Financial Management, 30:4, 1976, pp. 34–44.

Describes a method for developing a multi-variable, flexible budget system using existing data of a nursing cost center for budgeting RN, ancillary and total hours to illustrate how a system can be developed and what level of improved accuracy might be expected.
Hospital Abstract 19039 AC

Colner, Alan N.
The Impact of State Government Rate Setting on Hospital Management
Health Care Management Review, 2:1, 1977, pp. 37–49

Article describes the experiences of three of the nine states which currently have commissions with statutory responsibility to review and approve their hospitals' budgets and/or rates: Maryland, New Jersey and Massachusetts. The rate-setting system in these states oversees a hospital budget or rates on a prospective basis, but in politics, legislation, regulations and prospects for the future, complexion of rate-setting varies considerably among these three states. Implications of rate-setting programs on internal hospital management, and the need for coordination of rate-setting, planning and certificate-of-need are discussed. Article finds when decisions are not coordinated, planners may approve capital costs of a project while rate-setters may disallow operating costs to run it or interest costs to repay the debt.
Hospital Abstract 18085 AC

Comptroller General of the United States
Need to More Consistently Reimburse Health Facilities Under Medicare and Medicaid. Report to the Congress, 1974, 50 pp.
Available from Government Accounting Office, Publications Section, 441 G Street, N.W., Washington, D.C. 20548.

The findings of a General Accounting Office review of Medicare and Medicaid reimbursements to proprietary hospitals and skilled nursing care facilities are presented in a report by the Comptroller General to Congress. Three Medicare intermediaries, 5 subcontract intermediaries, 4 State Medicaid agencies, 11 proprietary hospitals, and 19 proprietary skilled nursing facilities were investigated to determine whether, as of 1974, Medicare and Medicaid payments to hospitals and Medicare payments to nursing facilities were being made on a uniform and equitable basis by the various agencies, contractors, and subcontractors. In addition, Medicare and Medicaid audits for 27 California hospitals were reviewed to further assess the situation. The study found that intermediaries using the same published Social Security Administration (SSA) guidelines made different interpretations about whether and how much of certain costs were allowable or reimbursable by Medicare. In some cases, the inconsistent treatment resulted in overpayments for several years. SSA regulation and guideline terms were found to be inadequately defined. Although progress was noted in exchanging Medicare and Medicaid audit findings, there was no apparent systematic exchange of audit information in about 20 States and jurisdictions. These and other findings are discussed at length, and recommendations are offered.
Hospital Abstract 17758 AC

Cosner, John S.
Capital Financing for Hospitals: Lease Versus Buy
The University of Michigan, Ann Arbor, Mich., 1972, 53 pp.
Available from University Microfilms

Study is a comparative analysis of purchasing and leasing as alternative methods by which a hospital might procure assets. The methodology developed for the analysis follows these procedures: conversion of all monetary values to net present value; make equivalent the features of the alternative proposals; comparison of cash flows at new present value; and optimization of each alternative. Application of this methodology is illustrated using McPherson Community Health Center in Howell, Michigan as a case study. The hospital was in a severe cash bind and needed to acquire a blood-gas PH machine costing $6,335. Alternatives the hospital had were to lease for either a three or five year period or borrow funds and purchase the equipment. Evaluation of each alternative is presented, using the proposed methodology. Findings indicate borrowing is the most favorable option for the hospital from a financial viewpoint, while the extended five year lease would be the most favorable for the third party payers. It is concluded that when third party reimbursements are not directly based on costs the net present value of required expenditures provides the best basis for comparing alternatives. If reimbursement is based on costs the hospital prefers the alternative which results in the greatest net cash flow while third party payers (and all consumers) prefer the alternative resulting in lowest net present value of reimbursements. Study also concludes divorcing of reimbursements from costs is the best method for achieving economic rationality and payment mechanisms such as prospective reimbursements or capitation make the optimization point the same for both the hospital and the consumer.

Hospital Abstract AC3–7838

Dittman, David A.; Ofer, Aharon R.
The Effect of Cost Reimbursement on Capital Budgeting Decision Models
Topics in Health Care Financing, 3:1, 1976, pp. 35–50.

Article illustrates effect cost base reimbursement has on four basic capital budgeting models: accounting rate of return; payback; internal rate of return; and net present value. The usefulness of the various models is discussed. It is concluded that the time ajusted rate of return techniques of internal rate of return and net present values are superior since they take into account size and timing of the cash inflow. When used to choose between alternative investment projects, it allows the manager to ration his capital so the organization earns the highest compound rate on its investment and thus insures the best possibility of the organization's economic arrival.

Hospital Abstract 17069 AC

Dittman, David A.; Ofer, Aharon
The Impact of Reimbursement on Hospital Cash Flow
Topics in Health Care Financing, 3:1, 1976, pp. 27–31

Article illustrates the effect third party reimbursement has on the investment decision process of health care institutions. Two examples are outlined: the hospital makes a cost saving invest-

ment in labor-saving equipment; and the hospital purchases revenue generating equipment. In both instances it is shown that cost based reimbursement affects the net cash flow realized. While a cost savings investment reduces total operating cost, it also reduces the cost based used in calculating the amount of reimbursement and thus reduces revenue generated. Similarly since for part of services provided the hospital will get compensated on the basis of the cost of providing the service rather on the basis of price charged for the service, the revenue generated by a given treatment will not equal quantity provided times price charged.
Hospital Abstract 17070 AC

Dowling, William L. (ed.)
Prospective Rate Setting
Topics in Health Care Financing, 3:2, 1976, 167 pp.

This issue of *Topics in Health Care Financing* is concerned exclusively with prospective rate setting (PR), presenting seven papers which explore what is being done to provide administrators and financial managers with up-to-date information about the nature of PR and how it might affect their institutions. The first paper describes goals of PR systems and the various ways systems are designed, organized and sponsored. The next two papers describe the PR systems used in Rhode Island and Washington State. In Rhode Island, budgets are negotiated on a one-to-one basis between Blue Cross and each hospital, but within a statewide "maxi-cap"—an aggregate cost-increase ceiling. In Washington, rates are set by a state commission, and each hospital's budget is judged in comparison to budgets of its peers. The fourth paper summarizes findings from five SSA sponsored evaluations of PR systems which indicate PR programs were moderately successful in lessening the pace of hospital cost inflation. The fifth paper describes administrative responses to the Michigan Blue Cross PR program, a system which establishes a total budget within which hospitals must operate for the coming year rather than setting per diem or per specific service rates. The sixth paper outlines what managers should be doing to prepare their institutions for PR and what changes can be expected in accounting and financial management practice. The last paper discussed data requirements for rate setting and planning and current inadequacies of data provided to rate setting agencies.
Hospital Abstract 18086 AC

Earhart, Charles H.
   An Analysis and Development of Standards for Selected Financial Ratios in Voluntary Non-Profit General Hospitals

Program in Hospital and Health Administration, University of Iowa, Iowa City, Iowa,1971, 99 pp.

Study examines nine financial ratios relevant to hospital financial management in a sample of U.S. short-term voluntary hospitals representing nine geographic regions and six size categories. The nine ratios analyzed include: operating assets to operating liabilities; quick assets to operating liabilities; current debt to net worth; total debt to net worth; net revenue from operations to accounts receivable; net profit to total assets; net revenue from operations to net worth; and net revenue from operations to working capital. Standards are developed for the nine ratios from data gathered from letters mailed to administrators requesting the latest annual report including a balance sheet and income statement. These standards are shown for median, upper quartile and lower quartile for each of the 54 hospital size-region combinations. It is concluded the response rate (49.27 per cent) indicates considerable interest in financial ratio standards and standards should be determined for more ratios than those used in the study and for other ownership types of hospitals. Study also concludes there is a need for more uniform hospital accounting terminology and accounting methods.
Hospital Abstract ACO–6485

Economic Stabilization Program
   Acute Care Hospitals: Planning and Executing Capital Projects Under Cost Controls

Government Printing Office, Washington D.C., 1974, Stock Number 4114–00032, 26 pp.

The purpose of this document is to facilitate the planning and implementation of capital expenditure projects while meeting the cost control objectives of planning agencies, hospitals and programs, such as Phase IV. Principal topics include preliminary program planning, initial construction cost estimates, the review of capital needs, feasibility study, financing requirements, Phase IV requirements, planning agency approval, project development and start-up, and the postcompletion audit.
Hospital Abstract 12346 AC

Elnicki, Richard A.
Accelerated Depreciation: Best for "Growth" Hospitals
Hospital Financial Management, Vol. 23, No. 3, March 1969, pp. 7–10

Recommendation of sum-of-the-years'-digits depreciation (SYD) over straight line depreciation (SL) in Medicare reimbursement calculations for growth hospitals which are able to recover costs and reinvest depreciation funds. Artificial data supply an example comparing continuous investment policy under either method over an eight-year period, covering the cycles of original reinvestment depreciation and reinvestment-only. The SYD method generated 35 percent more in depreciable assets than SL.
Hospital Abstract AC1049

Elnicki, Richard A.
A Theory of Hospital Financial Analysis
Health Services Research, Vol. 4, No. 1, pp. 14–41

The problem of determining the financial status of a group of hospitals was posed by the Connecticut Regional Medical Program in 1967 with the question: Are Connecticut's general hospitals financially healthy? The economist assigned to explore the question here describes the economic concepts and the methodology from which models applicable to voluntary hospitals were developed, utilizing the accepted modes of analysis and standards of for-profit business. The basic index of financial health investigated is self-sufficiency, with plant liquidation, revenue control and the role of private payers, and cost control studied as factors affecting the financial status of hospitals.
Hospital Abstract AC0024

Feldstein, Paul J.
An Empirical Investigation of the Marginal Cost of Hospital Services
Doctoral dissertation, University of Chicago, 1961, 77 pp.

Report from a doctoral dissertation of a study at Methodist Hospital of Gary, Indiana, from January 1956 to December 1958 examines short-run marginal costs in separate hospital departments on monthly basis. Independent variables used to estimate costs were adult patient-days, staff days off with pay, and changes or substitution in techniques or production. Cost estimates were statistically computed by a multiple regression analysis; the results for each department were expressed in "marginal costs per patient day." Functions for these are given, with supporting data. It was found that marginal cost of an additional patient-day is small, i.e. changes in short-run costs resulting from changes in hospital's occupancy rate were small. Other uses for this method of cost estimation, and summary of factors affecting hospital costs given. Hospital Abstract AC10, No. 56

Foyle, William R.
Evaluation of Methods of Cost Analysis
Unpublished, 18 pp.
Available from University Microfilms

The author evaluates five cost methods available to hospitals for cost determinations. The evaluations were based on results of cost analyses made in each of two years in three hospitals. Comparisons are expressed in ratios for the revenue department of general hospitals. A comprehensive discussion of the problems of reciprocal distribution and the methods used to recognize reciprocity of services is included. In addition, the material includes a discussion of the practicality of using simultaneous equations in distributing service departments in hospital cost analyses.
Hospital Abstract AC1001

Gilbert, R. Neal
The Bond Rating: A Major Ingredient to Hospital Capital Financing
Eastdil Health Care Funding, Inc., New York, 1977, 7 pp.

The bond rating of a hospital is critical to its ability to attract investors and secure loans. A bond rating, simply put, is a hospital's credit rating, which is expressed on an A-B-C scale by a credit rating service such as Standard and Poor's, Moody's or Fitch's. The highest rating, meaning the most secure investment, is given as Aaa by Moody's and AAA by Standard and Poor's. Upper medium risk is rated at A, which is the rating most commonly given to hospitals. This article outlines how hospitals can obtain a good bond rating, by going over which of the hospital's financing records, resources, personnel profiles, statistics, budget information, etc., should be presented during the credit ratings process, by describing the necessary planning, and by detailing the work of the staff of the rating agency. Explanations of Moody's and Standard and Poor's ratings scales are included with this article as Exhibits I and II.
Hospital Abstract 18124 AC

Gilbert, R. Neal
The Certificate of Need: A Major Ingredient to Capital Financing
Eastdil Health Care Funding, Inc., New York, 1977, 7 pp.

This article describes the process by which a hospital obtains a certificate of need, the most critical element in the financing pro-

cess. Title XVI of the National Health Planning and Resources Development Act of 1974 provides funds to establish a nationwide network of Health Systems Agencies. A Health Systems Agency (HSA) is a private non-profit corporation or public entity designated by the state's governor to oversee and coordinate health planning and development at the local level. At the state level, development is coordinated by the State Health Planning and Development Agency (SHPDA), under whose jurisdication comes the State Certificate of Need Program. This program applies to new institutional health services proposed within the state. No arrangement or commitment for financing a new institutional health service may be made unless a certificate of need for such a commitment has been granted. To obtain one, a Letter of Intent must be submitted to both the HSA and the SHPDA to begin the process. The review can take no longer than 90 days, during which the cost and feasibility of the proposed project as well as the past financial history of the hospital are scrutinized.
Hospital Abstract 18123 AC

Gilbert, R. Neal
Hospital Capital Budgeting Principles and Techniques

Hospital Progress, Vol. 56, No. 6, June 1975, pp 56–59

Article reviews the principles of capital allocation and describes 12 characteristics of an ideal capital budgeting system. Author discusses four steps in the development of the ideal system: preparing an operating budget; setting the scope of the capital budget; fixing responsibility for capital planning; and generating a budget calendar, manual, and package.
Hospital Abstract 14486 AC

Gilbert, R. Neal
Hospital Capital Budgeting System Development

Coopers and Lybrand, Philadelphia, Pa., 1975. 23 pp.

The main objective of this article is to develop a mechanism which would help to insure that the capital resources of the health care institution are allocated in the most efficient and effective manner possible consistent with the delivery of high quality health care. The author approaches the issue of capital budgeting by grouping hospital capital expenditures into three broad categories: large, intermediate, and small.
Hospital Abstract 13659 AC

Gilbert, R. Neal
The Hospital Capital Financing Crisis
Coopers and Lybrand, Philadelphia, Pa., 1974, 26 pp.

Paper examines capital financing situation in the hospital industry and the part cost-based reimbursement contributes to the problem of obtaining sufficient capital. Analysis of data pertaining to sources of financing capital and construction costs indicates since enactment of Medicare, the relative amounts of philanthropic sources of capital have experienced major decreases, government sources continue to decrease and patient care revenue is the primary source of funds for capital financing. Thus hospitals depend on third parties as their major source of revenue. Analysis indicates use of historical cost depreciation methods, even on an accelerated basis is inadequate, with inflation compounding the problem. A methodology whereby third parties can provide adequate capital funds for participating hospitals is suggested. Paper proposes reflecting depreciation on a price-level basis whereby original asset cost is adjusted through use of price indices such as Consumer Price Index and Implicit Price Deflator. The objective is to recover current dollars equivalent to present value of facilities and equipment. Paper also outlines strategies whereby health care administrators can temporarily ease capital financing problems.
Hospital Abstract 13656 AC

Gilbert, R. Neal
The Principles of Capital Budgeting for Hospitals
Coopers and Lybrand, Philadelphia, Pa., 1974, 12 pp.

Paper develops principles for efficient and effective allocation of capital resources in hospitals. Essential elements of an ideal hospital capital budgeting system are outlined and discussed: cost containment; planning; coordination; control; assessment of future financial support requirements; communication; and acceptability. In developing a hospital capital budgeting system paper discusses following necessary procedures: implementation of an operating budget; determination of scope of capital activities subject to annual budgeting process; fixing responsibility for capital planning; preparation of a budget calendar which puts capital budgeting process on a fixed time horizon; development of a budget manual outlining responsibilities of each participant; and preparation of a budget package which contains budget calendar and manual and all necessary forms, data and statistics for making accurate forecasts of capital activity.
Hospital Abstract 13658 AC

Gilbert, Robert N.
Capital Budgeting at Henry Ford Hospital: Analysis and Proposal
University of Michigan, Ann Arbor, Mich., 1974, 76 pp.
Available from University Microfilms

The objective of this study is to develop a mechanism which will help to ensure that the capital resources of Henry Ford Hospital are allocated in the most efficient and effective manner possible consistent with the delivery of high quality health care. Although the author finds a relatively sophisticated capital budgeting process in use at Ford Hospital, he notes certain weaknesses. With the strengths and weaknesses of the present capital budgeting system in mind, the author designs a new system which incorporates aspects of the current system and consists of four stages. In the first stage, the description process, detailed quantitative and qualitative data are entered on revised capital planning forms. This is meant to facilitate later evaluation and summary. The verification process is a second stage aimed at improving the reliability of the information provided in the capital planning forms. The third stage, the evaluation process, uses input from the clinical staff to augment cost-benefit analysis. The decision process is the final stage of the system and more formal decision-making protocols are specified.

This system gives department heads significant authority in allocating capital funds for small capital expenditures. Expenditures in the intermediate range go through a more sophisticated budgeting process, while large capital expenditures are subject to extensive review and analysis proportionate to their size.
Hospital Abstract 12307 AC

Gottschalk, Carl A.
An All-Inclusive Daily Rate
Hospital Forum, Vol. xiii, No. 3, June 1970, pp. 8–10, 20

Describes the West Valley Community Hospital, Encino, California method of determining daily charge to patients under an all-inclusive rate. Results, after three years, show admissions increased, average length-of-stay and paperwork decreased, less patient shock at hospital bill size, since they know the charges in advance.
Hospital Abstract AC2–5904

Grooms, Ferris L.
**An Analysis of the Impact of Medicare on Hospital Financial Reporting
Practices**
Texas Tech University, Lubbock, Texas, 1971
Available from University Microfilms

The author concluded that Medicare has imposed sophisticated accounting and reporting practices upon hospitals, which are generally resolved within the framework of accepted accounting principles.
Hospital Abstract 08776 AC

Gulinson, Sheldon K.
A Study of the Direct Cost to the Hospital of Processing Duplicate Coverage Third Party Claims
Duke University, Durham, N.C., 1969, 21 pp.
Available from University Microfilms

A study to determine the problem posed by processing duplicate coverage third party claims at Wilson Memorial Hospital, a 254-bed community general hospital. The volume, cost of processing, and the negative costs of holding interest-free money by the hospital were studied. The author concludes that the policy of not charging a patient directly for processing additional third party claims should be continued because (1) the cost is insignificant, (2) the magnitude of establishing a charging system is not justified and (3) negative public relations would outweigh any benefits.
Hospital Abstract AC3016

Hellinger, Fred J.
Prospective Reimbursement Through Budget Review: New Jersey, Rhode Island, and Western Pennsylvania
Inquiry, 13:3, 1976, pp. 309–320

Analyzing prospective reimbursement programs through budget reviews in three states, the author finds that the programs are ineffective in controlling hospital cost escalation. Budget reviews of individual hospitals are cumbersome operations. The development of cost and productivity screens may or may not be effective in eliminating the need for individual review.
Hospital Abstract 19056 AC

Heuerman, James N.
A Study of the Primary Sources of Payment and Related Payment Cycles at Evanston Hospital
University of Minnesota, Minneapolis, Minn., 1971, 72 pp.
Available from Univeristy Microfilms

Study investigated primary sources of income of Evanston Hospital in Illinois to determine effective means of improving cash flow. Four primary payers are identified: Blue Cross; Medicare; commercial insurance companies; and self-pay. Payment cycles which include number of days from discharge to billing of primary

payer, number of days between billing and posting of final payment and number of days from admission to receipt of confirmation of benefits from third party payers are computed for each of the primary payers. Study found the four primary payers accounted for 96 percent of hospital income, of which self-payers accounted for 17 percent. Significant differences were found between the primary payers in all three phases of the payment cycle. Of all payers, Medicare had the best performance for total payment cycle and for time between discharge and payment. Data indicated time between discharge and billing was shortest for self-pay because there was no confirmation of benefits needed. Commercial insurance was found to have the best record for confirmation of benefits. Comparison of findings with four income studies conducted primarily in smaller rural hospitals indicate payment performance of Medicare and self-pay at Evanston Hospital appears to be considerably lower.
Hospital Abstract 07845 AC

Holder, William W.
The Impact of Selected Third Party Reimbursement Policies on Capital Expenditure Decisions for General Hospitals
University of Oklahoma, Norman, Okla., 1974, 184 pp.
Available from University Microfilms

This study was concerned with the effects the advent of Medicare and Medicaid have had upon the capital expenditure decisions of short-term, general, non-federal, not-for-profit hospitals in the state of Oklahoma. The purpose of the study was to ascertain whether or not sample hospitals have responded, and if so in what way, to the presence of the Medicare rules and regulations. A closely related problem resolved involved the sophistication of hospital administration in evaluating economic aspects of proposed capital expenditures. In this manner both the effects of the advent of Medicare and Medicaid could be isolated as well as determining the responsive ability of hospital administrations to various programs of incentives. It was determined that hospital administrations have significantly altered the methods of capital expenditure planning and evaluation in response to Medicare and Medicaid. In general, hospitals now plan for longer periods of time and in much greater detail than in 1966.
Hospital Abstract 13882 AC

Hospital Survey Committee
Debt Financing Alternatives for Hospital Construction
The Committee, Philadelphia, Pa., 1973, 48 pp.

Report is a systematic study of hospital financial planning. Rapid inflation in construction costs over the past several years has created a financial crisis in many hospitals. Study explains the implications of this crisis and offers several alternative means of debt financing as a means of ameliorating the situation. Report considers the hospital's ability to repay debt; major interrelating factors affecting cash flow; hospital debt limitations; and cost comparisons of major types of financing in its analysis.
Hospital Abstract 12742 AC

Jaeger, John W., Jr. and Hardwick, C. Patrick
Negotiated Budget Incentive Pilot Program
Blue Cross of Western Pennsylvania, Pittsburgh, Pa. Research Series No. 7, 1971, 35 pp.

Report describes a pilot program conducted in one hospital which evaluated the effectiveness and practicality of using an individually approved and negotiated budget as a basis for hospital reimbursement by Blue Cross throughout Western Pennsylvania. Methodology involved a comparison of the hospital's 1969 total and departmental expenditures with a control group of four similar hospitals. Secondly, an evaluation was made of the hospital's budgeting techniques and management practices as well as an analysis of economic factors which may affect future expenses. After the process of comparison and evaluation, appropriate budget adjustments were discussed with the administrator and the approved budget was negotiated and used as a target for computation of reimbursement and subsequent incentive or penalty payments. Report includes cost data for each department of the study hospital and the control group. No actual transfer of funds, based on this study, occurred but the administrator used the budgeting process as a management tool in discussing major variances with department heads. Two major findings of the study are: there is greater educational value in this method of budgeting and negotiating hospital expenditures for both third-party and hospital management than under the present method; and any application of this type of program to several hospitals would involve serious problems in time, expense and administrative effort.
Hospital Abstract AC1–6950

Johnson, Richard W.
Capital Budgeting for a Group Practice
Medical Group Management, Vol. 22, No. 1, Nov.-Dec. 1974, pp. 10–14

A step-by-step explanation of capital budgeting decision making for a group practice is presented in this article. The concepts of

present values (a tool for drawing cash flows from the future to the present), depreciation, and the effects of taxes on additional expenses are discussed first. Next a demonstration of a method of capital budgeting for an echocardiograph set and its associated equipment is worked through. The various steps include: estimation of income; estimation of additional expenses; the effects of depreciation; establishment of after-tax cash flow; and estimation of present value of after-tax proceeds. This is followed by a comparison of leasing versus buying. The major point here is that while leasing is often more expensive than buying, the entire lease payment is tax deductible and a purchase is not.
Hospital Abstract 13530 AC

Kaitz, Edward M.
Pricing Policy and Cost Behavior in the Hospital Industry
Frederick A. Praeger, New York, N.Y., 1968, 205 pp.

A study to establish and evaluate the relationship between the financial and accounting techniques used by the third party payment system and the price determination, cost control, and capital-budgeting decisions within the individual hospital. The study included an analysis of the operating characteristics of the hospital industry, a review of the legislative and financial background of the third party payment system, and an analysis of the decision-making process with a sample population of rural, suburban, and urban hospitals in the Commonwealth of Massachusetts. It was concluded that the industry's growth has been characterized by a steady dilution of resources, and that the third-party system has provided the motivation for the inefficient allocation of resources in the hospital industry. The conclusions led to the recommendation that the present Blue Cross hospital "partnership" be dissolved. It is also recommended that Medicare and Medicaid find some alternative to their cost-based reimbursement system.
Hospital Abstract AC2012

Kovner, Anthony R. and Lusk, Edward J.
Effective Hospital Budgeting
Hospital Administration, Vol. 18, No. 4, Fall 1973, pp. 44–64.

Article discusses reasons why hospitals have not effectively used capital budgeting, recommends how investment proposals may be more effectively evaluated and outlines methods for implementing these recommendations. Recommendations are based on a study of three large urban non-profit hospitals which indicated top management failed to isolate relevant investment costs or specify benefits to be derived from investments. Article specifies four requirements for more effective operational budgeting: responsibility accounting; subdivision of hospital into performance centers; incentive to control costs; and development of performance standards to evaluate hospital output. It is suggested several preconditions are necessary—provision of cost reduction incentives by reimbursement agencies and incorporation of several critical intrahospital organizational changes. Article suggests major institutional constraints may inhibit efforts to establish preconditions necessary for implementing suggested system changes. Hospital Abstract 11795 AC

Krembs, James W.
  A Cash Forecasting System
Xavier University, Cincinnati, Ohio, 1973, 59 pp.
Available from University Microfilms

The object of this study is to provide hospital administration with a statistical method for forecasting cash flows. Two phases of prediction are discussed: predicting cash income on a six month and a 12 month basis; predicting cash expenditures, both wage and non-wage. Traditional methods for figuring debt retirement, working capital differential, receipts and disbursements and monthly cash needs are described and evaluated. Finally, the author presents the results of applying the cash forecasting system in Aultman Hospital, Canton, Ohio. The study is concluded by an optimistic evaluation of the cash forecasting system given the mechanical difficulties encountered in categorizing the data. Hospital Abstract 11332 AC

Laffey, William J.; Lappen, Stan
  Tax-Exempt Hospital Financing: Revenue Bonds
Health Care Management Review, 1:4, 1976, pp. 19–30

This article discusses the use of tax-exempt revenue bonds as a method of hospital financing, their advantages, costs and risks. Factors affecting the net interest cost of such bonds were identified and are described as 11 variables which can be correlated to such cost. These variables are: size of hospital, its occupancy rate, net revenue, population base, state or local affiliation, and percentage of third-party cost-based reimbursement; the size of the bond issue, whether it is insured, whether it would add to the hospital's revenue generating capacity, whether there will be an excess over debt-service payable, and whether a percentage of the issue will be devoted to a contingency fund. Correlations indicate

that hospitals planning to issue such bonds can influence the net interest cost by instituting in advance measures which will reduce risks and insure adequate cash flow. analysis shows that key factors are the debt-service coverage ratio and size of service area.
Hospital Abstract 17561 AC

Lash, Myles P.
The Development of an Expense Budgeting Procedure
Program in Hospital Administration, The University of Michigan, Ann Arbor, Mich., 1970, 68 pp.
Available from University Microfilms

Report describes procedures undertaken tc develop an expense budgeting program for Annapolis Hospital which will project the volume and cost of services to be rendered during a future operating period. Regression analysis calculations used for projection of volume of patient days for all nursing units are described in detail. This figure is then related to the production volume estimates of each cost center. The hospital departments are categorized into one of three different cost centers: one where there is a direct relationship between number of patient days and service provided by the department; one where the relationship between the number of patient days and service rendered is direct and the use of relative value scales is necessary, e.g., radiology and laboratory; and where there is only an indirect relationship between patient days and output, e.g., housekeeping. Procedures for determining the volume of activity for each of the three categories of department are described. The final procedures in expense budgeting involve determination of personnel and supplies expense budget and equations used for these calculations are explained.
Hospital Abstract AC1–6955

Lave, Judith R. and Lave, Lester B.
Hospital Cost Functions: Estimating Cost Functions for Multi-Product Firms
Carnegie-Mellon University School of Industrial Administration. Pittsburgh, Pa., 1969, 38 pp.

Describes a method of estimating the cost function of hospitals which takes into account the multi-product nature of the output (education, research, patient care and community services). Using data consisting of time series on many firms, two procedures were developed which authors believe can be applied to other multi-product and multi-service industries as well as to hospitals. Estimation techniques are explained in detail and the results of test-

ing several hypotheses discussed. Results of initial analysis were found to be similar to those reported in the literature for other techniques. Conclusion of researchers was that the proposed method of estimating hospital costs shows promise. Future research should concentrate on determining absolute levels of cost, rather than on explaining changes in cost.
Hospital Abstracts AC1-7051

Leaman, Elmer L.
Tax-Free Revenue Bonds: An Alternative to Capital Financing in Voluntary Non-Profit General Hospitals in Pennsylvania
University of Alabama, Birmingham, Ala., 1972
Available from University Microfilms

Thesis documented capital needs and capital financing trends in voluntary non-profit hospitals in Pennsylvania. The feasibility of using tax-free revenue bonds as an alternative method of capital financing was explored, using data from the literature and a questionnaire survey of voluntary non-profit general hospitals in Pennsylvania.
Hospital Abstract 08943 AC

Leuthauser, Terry A.
An Analysis of the Extent to Which Nonprofit, Voluntary, Acute Care Hospitals Utilize the Bank Term Loan
University of Iowa, Iowa City, Iowa, 1973,168 pp.
Available from University Microfilms

Study investigated the extent to which hospitals utilize bank term loans as a means of capital financing. Data were gathered from literature and a questionnaire survey of 497 nonprofit voluntary acute care hospitals in Region Six of the AHA's list of registered hospitals. There were 200 returns from hospitals having less than 100 beds and 152 returns from hospitals with more than 100 beds. Findings indicate 42.1 percent of large hospitals and 28.5 percent of smaller hospitals utilized some type of bank term loan. Ordinary term loan was the most prevalent form of bank term loan used and construction and working capital requirements were preponderant reasons for incurrence of this debt. The $100,000–$500,000 range was most popular range of borrowing at an interest rate of 6–8.99 percent. Analysis indicated bed size was significantly related to extent of bank term loan utilization, i.e., the large hospitals utilize bank loans more regularly and anticipate future use more often than small hospitals. Only a very small num-

ber of hospitals indicated they had been refused term lending by a commercial bank.
Hospital Abstract 14012 AC

McDougal, Tommy R.
Some Effects of Cost Reimbursement on Capital Requirements of Hospitals
University of Alabama, Birmingham, Ala., 1970, 45 pp.
Available from University Microfilms

Study of the development of third party financing of health care based on information gained by personal interviews, examination of accounting records of a large non-profit hospital in Alabama and a survey of literature. Topics covered are: hospital and capital requirements; impacts of cost-reimbursement, Blue Cross-Blue Shield of Alabama corporation, survey of the major capital fund sources, and public expectations. Author's conclusions are: formulas of third party payers fragment health care financing, create financial responsibility gaps, do not make allowance for inflation or technological improvements, do not provide for long-term debt retirement, have unrealistic depreciation schedules, perpetrate time lags in payment which create continuing deficits in operating funds, support a dual reimbursement system, and contain inadequate plus factors. Also that hospitals are receiving fewer donations, need increased amounts of capital, and must have adequate financing. Author's recommendations: third-party payers should reimburse on a more realistic cost basis; new contracts should be negotiated with hospitals and third party payers; Blue Cross of Alabama needs to be involved in pilot studies to determine a new agreement between the Blue Cross and hospitals "which would spread the cost of hospital care more equitably among all purchasers and also reduce the charges made by hospitals."
Hospital Abstract AC1–5938

MacLeod, Roderick K.
Program Budgeting Works in Nonprofit Institutions
Harvard Business Review, Sept.-Oct., 1971, pp. 46–56

An exposition of a program budgeting and accounting system for non-profit institutions, based on the three years' experience of the South Shore Mental Health Center, Quincy, Massachusetts. Organization, staffing, operation and potential problems of the system are explained. Results of the program, considered a success by those concerned, are discussed and some recommendations

made for administrators and trustees of other institutions interested in a cost accounting system and in the control of money and materials contributed by supporters.
Hospital Abstract 08573 AC

Magerlein, David B.; Davis, Rick J.; Hancock, Walton M.
The Prediction of Departmental Activity and Its Use in the Budgeting Process
Bureau of Hospital Administration, the University of Michigan, Ann Arbor 48109, 1976, 27 pp.

Paper outlines construction of a demand-based flexible operating budget. Emphasis is on describing the methodology used in predicting departmental activity, an essential element in developing such a budget. Predictions of hospital activity measures (admissions, patient days, outpatient visits, budget point) and time related variables (month, year) are used to predict each departmental activity through application of multiple linear regression. Data used were extracted from internal statistical reports of a 475-bed nonprofit, nongovernmental urban hospital for the 55 month period, January 1972 through July 1976. Statistical results for 13 hospital departments are presented and demonstrate the accuracy of models used. Paper also depicts the use of flexible budgeting to determine cost savings due to hospital resizing and includes an outline of an entire flexible budgeting system.
Hospital Abstract 17888 AC

Massachusetts Hospital Association
Follow-Up Analysis: Methods and Procedures for Minimizing Financial Loss Risk and Accounts Receivable
Division of Systems Engineering, the Association, Boston, Mass., 1969, 41 pp.
Available from University Microfilms

Description of a system designed to control the losses incurred through the granting of credit to hospital patients. Both the inpatient and outpatient applications of the system are described. Sample forms are also included.
Hospital Abstract AC3017

Massell, A. P.; Williams, A. P.
Comparing Costs of Inpatient Care in Teaching and Non-Teaching Hospitals: Methodology and Data
Rand Corporation, 1700 Main St., Santa Monica, CA 90406, 1977, 71 pp.

This publication identifies and evaluates options for analyzing the costs of inpatient care in teaching and non-teaching hospitals.

The report considers problems of research design, alternative analytic models, and data availability—and the relationship of each to health care reimbursement policy issues. A substantial component of the assessment is devoted to the availability of data that would permit analysis of both physician costs and hospital costs.
Hospital Abstract 19293 AC

Menzel, Helen L.
Health Maintenance Organization Budget Indicators: A Tool for Planning and Policy Analysis
University of Washington, Seattle, Wash., 1975, 127 pp.
Available from University Microfilms

The author describes HMOs and some major issues related to the planning, development, and operation of these organizations. After this introductory material is presented, she presents a set of budget indicators for use in planning and operating HMOs. The indicators include: sources of revenue; allocation of resources, including priorities of activities; and a determination of financial condition through the use of certain ratio formulas.
Hospital Abstract 14330 AC

Micah Corporation
The Micah System for Hospital Cost Analysis
The Micah Corporation, Ann Arbor, Mich., 1968, 30 pp.

Describes a computerized system employing matrix inversion for solving simultaneous equations to compute total departmental costs in a hospital cost finding procedure. The Micah system is said to simplify procedures because "accountants need only supply the direct costs of the departments of a hospital and one set of distributing statistics for each department that is distributed to others." Cost allocations are then automatically made by computer to as many as 250 calculating centers without need of any particular order of distribution and with the ability to distribute a single department's cost on several bases, if desired.
Hospital Abstract AC1032

Muenzberg, Michael W.
A Comparative Study of the Personnel Costs of Primary Care Nursing Stations and Modified Team Nursing Stations
University of Minnesota, Minneapolis, Minn., 1975, 63 pp.
Available from University Microfilms

Study assesses personnel and administrative costs per patient of primary nursing care units and modified team nursing units. Au-

thor collected data on number of hours worked for each category
of personnel per shift, classification for three primary and three
modified team nursing stations at the Miller Division of United
Hospitals Inc., St. Paul, Minnesota. No differences in personnel
costs or administrative costs per patient were found between primary care nursing stations and modified team nursing stations.
Hospital Abstract 14356 AC

Muller, Charlotte and Worthington, Paul
  Factors Entering Into Capital Decisions of Hospitals
Center for Social Research, City University of New York, New York, New
  York, c. 1967, 40 pp.

Paper reports a study conducted among 40 voluntary hospitals
in New York City to determine relationship between movement of
variables which reflect hospital services currently produced and
demanded and rate of investment. Data were taken from annual
reports to United Hospital Fund for period 1946–1965. Time series were developed for investment in plant and equipment, extensive and intensive aspects of services provided and extent of
teaching commitment and activity. Hospitals were classified in
four groups for analysis by teaching status—the highest class having a major medical school affiliation. It was hypothesized that the
teaching commitment of hospitals would be associated with
strength of demand for plant and equipment. Principal findings or
regression analyses were: when annual aggregates for 40 hospitals
are treated as variables, 68 percent of variance in annual real investment is explained by three factors: yearly changes in output
index; yearly changes in ratio of semi-private days to admissions;
and an allowance for a distributed lag in carrying out desired
investment projects. In cross-section analysis of means for each
variable, lags disappear and 56 percent of variance is explained by
mean annual admissions and extent of teaching commitment. Further research into effect of variation in supply of capital funds and
possible advantage to important teaching hospitals is planned.
Hospital Abstract ACO–5274

Nestman, Lawrence J.
  **Responsibility Accounting. A Tool to Better Planning and Cost Control
  in the Hospital**
Hospital Administration in Canada, Vol. 16, No. 2, Feb. 1974, pp. 45–48,
  50–52

Paper reviews basic concepts of responsibility accounting, and
discusses advantages and disadvantages of installing and operat-

ing a responsibility accounting system in the hospital. Responsibility accounting is defined as a system that recognizes responsibility and decision levels in a hospital typically indicated by the organization chart. It assigns costs to individuals who are responsible for the costs, so that they may be held accountable. A practical illustration of how responsibility accounting works in the budgeting process is presented. It is concluded that careful consideration should be made of both advantages and disadvantages before implementing the system.
Hospital Abstract 12217AC

Ofer, Aharon R.
Third Party Reimbursement and the Evaluation of Leasing Alternatives
Topics in Health Care Financing, 3:1, 1976, pp. 51–67.

Article discusses advantages and disadvantages involved in the leasing of hospital equipment and describes the various types of leasing arrangements and how third party payors classify them for reimbursement purposes. Distinction is made between true leases and financial leases; in the former case, the hospital has no ownership rights during or after the lease period and the lessor assumes the risk during or after the lease period and the lessor assumes the risk of obsolesence. In a financial lease, the lease period corresponds to the economic life of the equipment. Third parties recognize full lease payments as allowable cost only if the lease is a true lease. If the lease is a financial lease, the hospital is reimbursed only for imputed interest charges and depreciation. Guidelines for identification of a true lease are presented and evaluation is made of four alternatives for acquiring equipment in terms of comparative monetary cost and cash flow produced: outright purchase with cash; purchase using time-sales contract; acquisition with a financial lease; and acquisition with a true lease.
Hospital Abstract 17068 AC

Pavony, William H., et al.
Budgeting: A Traditional Tool Enters the 70s
Hospital Financial Management, Vol. 24, No. 12, December 1970, pp. 3–27.
Pavony, William H. and Gass, Anthony D.
"How Budgeting Can Help The Hospital Achieve Its Goals"

A demonstration of how the budget program can be woven into management by objectives.
Howe, Robert L.
"A Practical Approach to Budgeting"

A step-by-step guide to the development of a budgeting program.

Boer, Germaine B. and Parris, Walter K.
"Flexible Budgeting: A Cost Control Tool"
   An explanation of appropriate planning and control measures in cost analysis.
Anton, Chris J.
"The Six Month Budget: Key to Sounder Planning"
   The use of the six month budget as a part of effective long range planning is explained.
Conort, Frank E.
"Why Hospitals Needs Statistics"
   Several reasons for and uses of data on patients and utilization of facilities are explored.
Nash, Arthur
"How Detailed and Frequent Should Budget Reporting Be? Part I"
   This is the first of a seven part series on budgeting and deals with the frequency with which reports would be rendered, as well as the degree of sophistication they should possess.
   Hospital Abstract AC1–6796

Platou, Carl N. and Rice, James A.
   Multihospital Holding Companies
Harvard Business Review, Vol. 50, No. 3, May-June 1972.

   Article outlines application of the holding company concept to a group of medical care facilities, using information from the Fairview Hospitals, an affiliation of Minnesota hospitals developing a multihospital organization. Major benefits cited of the hospital holding company are: economies of scale resulting from superior management and centralization of certain specialized activities; broader range of services and facilities at the local level; and improved capital resources and operating efficiency that protect the solvency of each local unit. Data from the Fairview hospitals indicate they have achieved savings in a reduction of personnel, inventory, purchasing and payroll costs and have been able to generate additional revenue of $2.00 per patient day through the development of the multihospital holding company.
   Hospital Abstract 08756 AC

Robbins, Jennifer
   Uses of Population-Based Data for Rate Setting
Harvard Center for Community Health and Medical Care, 1976, 35 pp.

   The expansion of data bases for rate setting to include information about the population receiving services, the utilization of services, and service outcome is explored. Rationale for the popula-

tion-based approach to rate setting and examples of application of the population-based rate setting and examples of application of the population-based approach are reviewed. The kinds of problems in medical care delivery revealed through population-based data analysis are discussed, drawing from the experience of population-based data systems in (Maine, Vermont, and Rhode Island). The kinds of data such a system requires are outlined, and comments are offered concerning the availability and reliability of these data. It is suggested that reviews of hospital utilization and quality of patient care cannot be dealt with as processes separable from reviews of the manpower, facilities, equipment, and dollars used in delivering that care.
Hospital Abstract 17774 AC

Rowland, Diane
Transition to Uniform Accounting and Reporting for Hospitals: Some Perspectives From Participants
Harvard Center for Community Health Medical Care, 1976, 55 pp.

Problems encountered by hospitals in California and Washington in adapting to new systems of uniform accounting and reporting are discussed. Until 1975 the 750 hospitals in these two States used accounting and reporting practices designed solely to provide their managers with the information they needed for internal accountability and control and to meet the requirements of various reimbursing bodies. The systems subsequently introduced by the California Health Facilities Commission and the Washington Hospital Commission were designed to be compatible with individual management needs, but also to meet the external reviewers' needs for data to permit comparative analysis. The legal bases for the California and Washington systems are reviewed, and the time frame for implementation of the two systems is described. Brief descriptions are provided of both systems, and efforts to accommodate external need for uniformity to the hospitals' individual needs are discussed. Problems encountered by the hospitals as they implemented the new systems are reviewed, including those associated with timing, administrative burdens and implementation costs, computer problems, agreements with certified public accountant firms, and burdens on small hospitals. Potential benefits resulting from the transition are pointed out. Specific problems with units of measure and account classification are identified. Implications for future implementation efforts are discussed.
Hospital Abstract 17775 AC

Rumford, David M.
  An Analysis of the Financial Ramifications of Exchanging Inpatient Services
Xavier University, Cincinnati, Ohio, 1974, 55 pp.
Available from University Microfilms

This study results from a proposal to eliminate duplication of obstetric and pediatric services in a community served by two short-term acute care hospitals. The proposal calls for Hospital A to close its pediatric service and assume responsibility for all obstetric services, and Hospital B to close its obstetric service in exchange for all pediatric service responsibility. The total operational impact of the exchange on Hospital A is analyzed in four steps: 1) analysis of demand for obstetric services; 2) analysis of alternative plans to meet demand; 3) projection of financial statements for alternative plans; and 4) financial comparison of the alternatives and the status quo.

The study results in the recommendation that Hospital A not participate in the proposed exchange of services as to do so would place the hospital in an untenable and detrimental financial position. The study demonstrates a situation in which a plan to combine services to eliminate duplication by means of remodeling would be more costly than a plan calling for new construction. Hospital Abstract 13957 AC

Sahney, Vinod K.; Knappenberger, Allan H; Colter, Daniel; Chowdry, Vimal
  A Small Hospital Budgeting System
Wayne State University, Detroit, 1975, 20 pp., Available Center for Hospital Management Engineering, 840 North Lake Shore Drive, Chicago 60611.

Budgeting systems that could be used to provide management controls as well as meet the requirements of PL92-603 were developed for four small hospitals. The systems developed did not differ significantly from those used by larger hospitals, but their use required a substantially greater education effort due to the backgrounds of the managers and department heads. The budget document developed showed man-hours and other production-oriented figures as well as monetary figures. Monthly and quarterly reports were generated as well as the annual budget figures. Among the difficulties were the large effects created by changes in clinic practice patterns because of the small number of physicians per hospital. Hospital Abstract 18821 AC

Salkever, David S.; Bice, Thomas W.
The Impact of Certificate-of-Need Controls on Hospital Investment
Health and Society, 54:2, 1976, pp. 185–214.

Certificate-of-Need (CON) controls over hospital investment have been enacted by a number of states in recent years and the National Health Planning and Resources Development Act of 1974 provides strong incentives for adoption of CON in additional states. In this study, the questions that have been raised about the effectiveness of CON controls are reviewed and then quantitative estimates of the impact of CON on investment are developed. These estimates show that CON did not reduce the total dollar volume of investment but altered its composition, retarding expansion in bed supplies but increasing investment in new services and equipment. The authors suggest that this finding may be due to (1) the emphasis in CON laws and programs on controlling bed supplies and (2) a substitution of new services and equipment for additional beds in response to financial factors and organizational pressures for expansion. Finally, they caution against the conclusion that CON controls should be broadened and tightened, though the results might be so interpreted, because of the practical difficulties involved in reviewing and certifying large numbers of small investment projects.
Hospital Abstract 16984 AC

Sattler, Frederic L.
A Rational Look at the Hospital and Debt Financing
Hospital Topics, Vol. 53, No. 1, Jan.-Feb. 1975, pp. 16, 18, 20

Author discusses debt financing in the non-profit hospital.
Hospital Abstract 13739 AC

Shifman, Elliot L.
An Approach to Resource Allocation Decision Making; Development of Per Capita Service Unit Costs
The University of Michigan, Ann Arbor, Mich., 1972, 39 pp.
Available from University Microfilms

Paper outlines an approach for rational resource allocation using various types of data that are available or can be developed. Types of data analyzed are: health (index of degenerative morbidity, index of nondegenerative morbidity and mortality indices); utilization; population; and measures of cost. A per discharge unit cost is developed by applying the cost-revenue ratio to the average charge per discharge for a particular service or per outpatient treatment. A per capita service unit cost is developed by multiply-

ing total number of discharges of each type of patient times per unit discharge service unit cost and dividing this figure by relevance based population estimate for the hospital's service area. Per capita service unit costs allow for comparison of inter-hospital performance and intra-hospital evaluation of prospective marginal investment opportunities. An illustrative example of type of data which should be gathered and developed for this approach is presented in a case study of Annapolis Hospital in Wayne, Michigan.
Hospital Abstract 08792 AC

Shifman, Elliot; Walls, Edward
Guidelines for Consideration of Capital Financing and Alternative Debt Financing Methods
Metropolitan Health Planning Corporation, Cleveland, 1975, 19 pp.

Guidelines are presented for use by hospitals in determining the most appropriate and effective means for financing necessary capital improvements. The guidelines were developed by the Metropolitan Health Planning Corporation in Cleveland, Ohio. They are intended to assist in health care cost containment and in the development of an efficient health delivery system.
Hospital Abstract 17835 AC

Sister Marlene Fox
A Comparative Study of Educational and Occupational Backgrounds, Position, Role, and Duties of Financial Managers of Hospitals and Industrial Enterprises
George Washington University, Washington, D.C., 1970, 102 pp.
Available from University Microfilms

Study investigates how the educational and occupational background, position, role and duties of the hospital financial manager compare with those of the industrial financial manager. Related literature was reviewed to formulate the types of information gathered from interviews with the financial managers of ten hospitals and ten industrial firms which were similar in gross annual revenue and located within the New York City and Nassau County area. Study reveals that hospital financial managers tend to be slightly younger, have less tenure in the current organization, and receive lower annual salaries than their industrial counterparts. Hospital and industrial financial managers have comparable formal educational background, while difference is shown with regard to prior occupational experience. In the area of continuing education, namely, affiliations with professional organizations and attendance at educational meetings, hospital financial managers

tend to be more active than industrial financial managers. Relationship to the chief executive is similar for the two; however, industrial financial managers reveal considerable strength in relationship to the governing board. The scope of duties and responsibilities of industrial financial managers indicate they are generally recognized as members of the top management team, whereas hospital financial managers are not.
Hospital Abstract ACO–7355

Sister Mary Reginald Gawel
  Internal Control
Xavier University, Cincinnati, Ohio, 1970, 71 pp.
Available from University Microfilms

An analysis was made of the accounting function of internal control in four large teaching hospitals in the Twin City metropolitan area. Data were gathered from questionnaires and interviews with controllers and fiscal managers. Study found a great degree of difference in the internal control operation in the four hospitals, which was attributed to the type of hospital: federal, state, city-county or county hospital. Lack of internal control was found to be a significant problem in the city-county hospital. Generally, the controllers saw the necessity of internal control, but study concludes fiscal managers were indifferent to internal control systems because they received appropriations on an annual budget and did not have to meet expenses from revenue. Thesis also develops a manual for internal control which includes a definition of terms, organizational chart, forms and an outline of control procedures.
Hospital Abstract ACO–5820

Sister Mary Daniel Udelhofen
  Accounts Receivable: The Crisis Produced by Lack of Internal Control
Xavier University, Cincinnati, Ohio, 1974, 99 pp.
Available from University Microfilms

Research conducted during this study revealed numerous findings on the problems of disproportionately high accounts receivable. The findings centered primarily on four departments: admitting, billing, credit and collection, and medical records, which shared several problems while manifesting conditions that were uniquely problematic. The study also examines approaches that may be instrumental in problem reconciliation.
Hospital Abstract 13073 AC

Smith, Stephen W.
  Leasing: An Effective Source of Capital Asset Financing
Hospital Financial Management, Vol. iv, No. 9, Sept. 1974, pp. 36–41

Leasing, as a source of capital asset financing, is discussed in this article. A lease is defined as an agreement that gives the lessee the right to use the equipment for a specified period for a monthly payment without building up equity in the equipment; that has a term of at least two years less than the guideline life of the property; is written with a third party that has no other connection with the lessee; and that does not cover property which has an exceedingly high removal cost. Author then lists several advantages of leasing over other means of financing. Among these are: 1) it's a good hedge against inflation; 2) it reduces costs of replacing equipment before obsolescence; and 3) it provides a flexible instrument of long term financing. In the final section of the article, considerations involved with negotiating a lease are discussed. Included in this section are: the advantages of competitive bidding; specifications needed in renewal options; estimation of the physical life of the equipment; and methods of payment. Hospital Abstract 13531 AC

Spiegel, James E.
  Utilization of Tax Exempt Revenue Bonds for Financing Capital Expansion Requirements of Community Hospitals
University of Iowa, Iowa City, Iowa, 1974, 92 pp.
Available from University Microfilms

Thesis outlines major considerations of the borrower and lender concerning a long-term loan and specifically evaluates tax-exempt bonds as a long-term technique for financing capital expansion requirements of community hospitals. Analysis indicates two major factors a lender will consider are the need for the facility or project and sufficiency of cash flow to repay the loan. Some elements considered important to the borrower were: cost of debt; amount of debt; restriction on future borrowing; and prepayment provisions. Analysis of tax-exempt revenue bonds indicated they possess a significant cost advantage over other debt techniques, particularly for loans of more than $5 million, and much flexibility in the event future borrowing is required. Analysis also indicates they have stringent prepayment provisions, restrictions on use of income, acceptable construction financing requirements, and some marketability deficiencies which thesis concludes should be eliminated as their usage is increased. They also were found to have possible legal implications that might bar their utilization by

hospitals desirous of minimizing government control of their institutions. Thesis also outlines current status of tax-exempt bond legislation and describes procedural steps necessary to employ this technique with extensive reference to the Ohio Hoffman Act.
Hospital Abstract 14241 AC

Stambaugh, Jeffrey L.
A Study of the Sources of Capital Funds for Hospital Construction
Duke University, Durham, N.C., 1966, 64 pp.
Available from University Microfilms

In this study the author attempts to present an up-to-date data analysis of the source of capital funds for hospital construction. In addition to information obtained from the hospital literature, the author also sent out a questionnaire to 150 sample groups of hospitals engaged in construction projects, asking them to list their construction funds in the following source categories: Hill-Burton; Long-term Borrowing by Hospital; Bonded Indebtedness by a Taxing Agency; Private Contribution; Hospital Reserves; and Miscellaneous: 95.3% responded. A detailed presentation of data is given in several charts and tables.
Hospital Abstract AC0010

Talcott, Bruce E.
Comparative Analysis of Capital Equipment Budgeting Systems in Health Care Institutions
Available from National Technical Information Services, Springfield, Va.
Document No. AD-787 367/2GA, 1974, 126 pp.

The thesis presents a study of capital equipment investment budgeting procedures in the health care industry. It discusses capital equipment investment philosophy in general, and addresses a few of the contemporary problems and corresponding solutions contained in current health care literature. The thesis also describes the specific capital equipment budgeting systems of three segments of the health-care industry; Navy hospitals, Veterans Administration hospitals; and non-federal hospitals. Three case studies in capital equipment budgeting—Naval Regional Medical Center, Oakland; Veterans Administration Hospital, Martinez; and Fairmont General Hospital, Alemeda County—are presented to illustrate each of the three segments addressed.
Hospital Abstract 13456 AC

Tierney, Thomas M. and Sigmond, Robert M.
Could Capitation Ease Blue Cross Ills?
Modern Hospital, Vol. 105, No. 2, Aug. 1965, pp 103–106

Findings of a trial of direct payment of subscriber revenues to hospitals in Yuma County, Arizona. A drop in utilization of 7.5 percent was found in the first year, due to shorter average stays in county hospitals.
Hospital Abstract AC3002

Vraciu, Robert
Capital Investment Decisions for Hospitals: A Conjoint Measurement Approach
Cornell University, 1977, 231 pp. Available from University Microfilms Inc.

This study focused primarily on the use of managerial decision models for capital investment decisions in hospitals. Two categories of such models are identified: prescriptive and evaluative. The use of prescriptive models is criticized because of their reliance on an operationally defined organizational objective function which is likely to be misspecified for hospitals. The use of existing evaluation models is criticized for only partially synthesizing the characteristics of investments and relying upon decision makers to relate the synthesized and unsynthesized information to the organization's objective function. A hospital's objective function is viewed as an amalgamation (unspecified) of the objectives of some set of decision-influencing individuals. The proposed methodology first sought to partition this set of individuals into homogeneous groups (on the basis of preferences); second, sought to estimate an evaluation function for each group which represents the fully synthesized information about the investment characteristics (obtained from each respondent); and finally, sought to explicitly define conflicts within this set in terms of competing perspectives, leaving the synthesis of these perspectives to the decision makers. The model is applied to a realistic decision situation to illustrate its usefulness to decision makers. It is concluded that a conceptual approach which allows individuals (who are influential in hospital decisions) to fully synthesize investment characteristics and to define trade-offs explicitly in terms of competing perspectives, is an improvement over existing prescriptive and evaluative models.
Hospital Abstract 18915 AC

Wade, Charles M.
A Capital Equipment Budgeting System Applicable to Selected Midsouth Not-For-Profit Community Hospitals
University of Mississippi, 1977, 251 pp. Available University Microfilms Inc.

The primary objective of this study was to determine how not-for-profit community hospitals should make capital equipment in-

vestment decisions. Nine not-for-profit community hospitals with one hundred beds or more in the Midsouth were studied. Their capital equipment investment procedures and practices and their capital equipment expenditures for one year were examined. The study concluded that (1) the hospitals studied are profit motivated, (2) the not-for-profit hospital industry is characterized by oligopoly-price leadership, (3) the hospitals studied operate under conditions of rigid self-imposed capital rationing, and (4) they do not use accepted financial techniques in allocating resources to capital equipment investments. The result of the study was that a capital equipment investment system was recommended for the not-for-profit community hospitals studied. Their system is theoretically correct and incorporates analysis of incremental cash flows related to capital equipment investment proposals.
Hospital Abstract 18916 AC

Walls, Edward L.
Estimating Voluntary Hospital Debt Capacity
Harvard University Business School, Cambridge, Mass., 1970
Available from Harvard University Library in xerox or microfilm copies—
    prices on application to the library

This thesis proposes a framework for estimating debt capacity of voluntary nonprofit hospitals. More specifically it investigates debt capacity when a major share of revenue is received from cost-based reimbursement not including capital allowances. As a result it analyzes and describes the impact of cost-based reimbursement upon hospital capital financing.

The research was stimulated by the facts that hospitals need approximately ten billion dollars for renovation and new construction and that debt is increasingly used as a financing vehicle, but that industry opinions as to how much debt can safely be contracted by individual institutions vary from zero to 100 percent of the funds needed. A major goal was to develop useful guidelines for hospitals and lenders. The research was funded by an exploratory grant from the Department of Health, Education and Welfare.

The methodology was to 1) survey existing literature on hospital borrowing and financial management, 2) interview lenders and borrowers across the country to determine current debt practices and criteria, 3) analyze the financial environment to formulate a normative approach to measuring debt capacity, 4) test this normative approach by estimating the debt capacity of a typical hospital, 5) analyze the results, and 6) formulate general conclusions.

Interviews across the country and available literature indicated that external sources of capital are declining relative to need and the spread of cost-based reimbursement without capital allowances threatens hospital ability to generate capital internally. The focus of research then became the estimation of hospital debt capacity in the expected future environment, where most revenue will come from cost-based reimbursement. Massachusetts was chosen as the locale for case research because hospitals there receive as much as 80 percent of revenue from cost-based reimbursement formulas without capital allowances.

In this situation it was found that normative behavior is to attempt to break even on operations, thereby generating net cash flow available for debt servicing in amounts equal to annual depreciation expense. If this is achieved then debt capacity of a new hospital can approximate 60 percent of fixed asset value, but less than 50 percent of total asset value. Capacity is limited by 1) debt maturities shorter than the depreciable life of assets, 2) operating losses caused by unreimbursed bad debts and charity care and welfare reimbursement at less than cost, and 3) the necessity to divert net cash flow into working capital items. Factors which may increase debt capacity include 1) nonoperating income, 2) depreciation from assets already owned, and 3) use of accelerated depreciation.

The procedure recommended for estimating debt capacity consists of 1) a study of industrial trends, opportunities, and requisites for success, 2) non-financial analysis of the individual institution, and 3) financial analysis of net cash flows available for debt service. Where cost-based reimbursement without capital allowances is dominant normative net flows will approximate depreciation expense and analysis emphasizes the forecasting of depreciation flows. Where cost-based reimbursement does not dominate or includes capital allowances net income can add to net flows and analysis is similar to that of a commercial business.

The significance of the findings is that 1) spread of cost-based reimbursement without capital allowances will intensify the hospital capital shortage, thereby causing deterioration of current facilities and impeding development of a comprehensive health care delivery system, and 2) federal and state guaranty of loans and subsidization of interest will be ineffective because they ignore the main problem which is a lack of access to new capital, and 3) a logical solution is to link supply and demand by including capital allowances in reimbursement.

Hospital Abstract AC4–6779

Walters, James E.; Watson, Hugh J.
Building a Budget: Three Generations
Hospital Financial Management, 31:9, 1977, pp. 10–18.

This article illustrates the application of three levels of sophistication in constructing budgets for hospital financial management planning purposes: line item budgeting; deterministic mathematical models; and probabilistic estimates. It is pointed out that most hospitals practice line item budgeting with some movement toward deterministic mathematical models. Whether probabilistic estimation becomes prevalent depends on its perceived and actual usefulness.
Hospital Abstract 19045 AC

Young, Larry H.
An Analysis of the Utilization of Resources by Various Patient Groups to Establish a Set of Variable Inclusive Rates
Duke University, Durham, N.C., 1971, 72 pp.
Available from University Microfilms

Discusses a proposed rate structure for hospitals which uses weighted statistics to reflect differences in the complexity of various patient groups. Ten categories of patients who use hospital resources are defined and methods described for measuring the service or activity of departments. The feasibility of a variable-inclusive rate determination is analyzed. Some obstacles to implementation of such a rate structure are discussed, including the problem of physicians remuneration. Writer believes that advantages outweigh disadvantages, however. Numerous cost and resource utilization tables are included.
Hospital Abstract AC2–7715

Weinstein, Milton C.; Stason, William B.
Foundations of Cost-Effectiveness Analysis for Health and Medical Practices
New England Journal of Medicine, March 31, 1977, pp. 716–721.

Limits on health-care resources mandate that resource-allocation decisions be guided by considerations of cost in relation to expected benefits. In cost-effectiveness analysis, the ratio of net health-care costs to net health benefits provides an index by which priorities may be set. Quality-of-life concerns, including both adverse and beneficial effects of therapy, may be incorporated in the calculation of health benefits as adjustments to life expectancy. The timing of future benefits and costs may be ac-

counted for by the appropriate use of discounting. Current decisions must inevitably be based on imperfect information, but sensitivity analysis can increase the level of confidence in some decisions while suggesting areas where further research may be valuable in guiding others. Analyses should be adaptable to the needs of various health-care decisions makers, including planners, administrators and providers.
Hospital Abstract 19411 HC

Zaretsky, Henry W.
  The Effects of Patient Mix and Service Mix on Hospital Costs and Productivity
Topics in Health Care Financing, 4, 2, 1977, pp. 63–82.

The article describes a study which compared costs and productivity among 176 acute care California hospitals, using a cost function which takes into account differences in case mix and service mix. Data sources were the AHA 1971 Annual Survey, California Health Data Corporation, and PAS. Case mix, service mix, economic and short-run capacity utilization variables used in the cost model are described. The model was estimated through linear regression. Results indicate that when adjustments are made for service mix and case mix, size or volume does not greatly influence cost per case. The simple positive correlation between size and costliness was found to be due to the fact that larger hospitals in general treat more complex patients and provide more costly services than do smaller institutions. Results suggest fairly constant returns to scale when account is taken of service mix and case mix. When case mix is not controlled, the estimates suggest decreasing returns to scale. It is concluded that the findings have crucial implications for planning and economic regulation policies.
Hospital Abstract 19339 HC

ADMINISTRATION

Mankin, Douglas.; Glueck, William F.
  Strategic Planning
Hospital and Health Services Administration, 22, 2, 1977, pp. 6–22.

A study of 15 Missouri hospitals designed to find whether the hospitals used strategic planning, and if those that did were more successful in reaching their objectives. The study found that the hospitals did not formally plan their strategies in detail. The au-

thors predict that formalized strategic planning is essential and will be developed through continuing education and outside reading for administrators. The excuse that the hospital industry is too dynamic to formulate long-range plans is not accepted, and the point is made that long-range planning should replace a procedure of reacting to individual situations.
Hospital Abstract 19437 AB

HEALTH SERVICES

Averill, Richard F.; McMahon, Laurence F., Jr.
A Cost Benefit Analysis of Continued Stay Certification
Medical Care, XV:2, 1977, pp. 158–173.

A large portion of the resources of the Professional Standards Review Organization Program have been directed toward the review of inpatients to determine their need for continued hospitalization. The primary goal of this review process is the containment of hospital costs through the elimination of unnecessary patient hospitalization. A cost benefit analysis of this review process shows that the potential financial savings accrued are unlikely to offset the costs associated with the review procedure.
Hospital Abstract 18380 HE

Bellin, Lowell E.; Kavaler, Florence; Weitzner, Martin; Feldman, Louis; Hamlin, Robert
Hospital Cost and Use Control Via New York Health Department
Health Services Reports Vol. 88, No. 2, Feb. 1973, pp. 133–140

Authors discusses a six month feasibility study designed by the New York City Department of Health to change the department's regulatory powers into effective ways of screening and auditing hospital costs and of expanding service and productivity. Four hospitals were examined, one from each major type: voluntary teaching, voluntary nonteaching, municipal, and proprietary. Hospital size ranged from 150 to 1,000 beds; percentage of Medicaid patient days ranged from 32 to 86.

Using the field audit method, each hospital's data systems were reviewed for specifics that provided measures of hospital use, cost, and productivity. Authors proposed four interrelated methods to constrain costs of inpatient hospital care: 1) greater prudence, selflessness, and responsibility on the part of physicians; 2) provision of excellence in service and efficiency in operation by administrators; 3) cost constraints of hospital care by Blue Cross and

other insurance carriers; and 4) more active governmental participation in hospital cost control regulations.
Hospital Abstract 12602 HE

Clark, Bliss B.; Lamont, Gwynn X.
  Accurate Census Forecasting Leads to Cost Containment
Hospitals, 50:11, 1976, pp. 43–48.

The article presents a model that helped achieve accurate hospital census forecasts for eight medical-surgical units. Seven steps
used in developing the model included obtaining and evaluating
an historical data base, classification of discrete events affecting
the census, and projection of potential impact of future discrete
events on the census. The forecast was used in planning personnel and bed utilization, with resulting savings. Accuracy of the
forecast is illustrated.
Hospital Abstract 16786 HE

Cooper, Barbara S.; Worthington, Nancy L.; Piro, Paula A.
  National Health Expenditures: Calendar Years 1929–1972
Research and Statistics Note, No. 3, Feb. 6, 1974, 14 pp.

Report presents data on health spending in the United States for
1972. Tables include data on national health expenditures by
source and percentage of gross national product for selected years
1929–72; national health expenditures by type of expenditure and
source of funds 1970–72; expenditures for health services and supplies under public programs 1970–72; distribution of personal
health care expenditures for selected years 1950–72; aggregate
and per capita national health expenditures for selected years
1929–72; and the amount and percent of personal health care
expenditures met by third parties in 1972.
Hospital Abstract 12136 HE

Council of State Governments
  **Health Cost Containment: The Connecticut, Maryland, and New Jersey
  Responses**
The Council, Lexington, KY, 1976, 74 pp.

Report describes health cost containment program in Connecticut, Maryland and New Jersey, three states which have chosen to
intervene directly by regulating hospital rates. Their experiences
suggest they are making some progress in limiting the rise in
medical care costs. Report also outlines important considerations
in creating a health cost regulatory commission. Chief factors to be

considered include: structural characteristics of the existing system; State government's organization for health matters; manpower requirements; and State responses to federal legislation. It is concluded whether a regulatory commission will be successful in a particular State depends on the circumstances pertaining to these four factors.
Hospital Abstract 17720 HE

Davis, Karen
Relationship of Hospital Prices to Costs
Applied Economics, Vol. 4, 1971, pp. 115–125

The ratio of hospital prices to average costs of providing hospital care is studied. Empirical evidence presented in this paper contradicts the prevailing view that hospitals merely attempt to recover costs in their pricing policy. In addition, the view that the excess of price over average cost is merely an attempt on the part of the hospital to accumulate sufficient revenue to make needed investment is not substantiated. Instead, price-average cost ratios are found to be sensitive to certain demand and supply conditions.

Most importantly, price-average cost ratios are higher in states with higher per capita incomes, particularly in the earlier part of the 1960s. The importance of this factor has declined in recent years, perhaps because of the decline in the role of the private sector in financing hospital care. This evidence, however, provides some information on how market forces would work if the trend towards public financing of hospital care should be reversed.
Hospital Abstract 09128 HE

Davis, Karen
Rising Hospital Costs: Possible Causes and Cures
Bulletin of the New York Academy of Medicine, Nov. 1972.

This report discusses causes of hospital inflation, and their policy implications, among them: 1) shifts in demand, 2) labor cost, 3) wasteful capital expenditures, 4) cost reimbursement and hospital inefficiency, 5) changing medical technology, and 6) the expanded role of community hospitals. Various components of hospital costs are discussed in an effort to determine a correct view of hospital inflation. The author suggests policies to combat inflation could be: 1) movement toward direct controls, or 2) incentives to encourage better performance of private market.
Hospital Abstract 09131 HE

Denver, G. Alan
Guidelines for Health Status Measurement
Georgia Department of Human Resource, Atlanta, 1974, 74 pp.

An approach to measuring health status at the local level is
outlined in guidelines directed to health systems agencies (HSAs).
The HSA is urged first to develop policy statements reflecting a
holistic approach to changing disease patterns. Approaches to determining health goals and objectives are suggested. Criteria for
selecting a health status index are outlined, eight methods of calculating health indexes are described, and a conceptual model
suggesting the direction in which HSAs should move in developing measures of health status is cited. Categories of data and specific data sets required for health status measurement within the
context of the model, methods of evaluating health programs, and
appropriate applications of each type of evaluation are noted.
Strategies for effecting changes in health status and the inclusion
of the strategies in evaluation design are discussed. Application of
an epidemiological model to policy analysis is demonstrated.
Hospital Abstract 19148 HE

Elnicki, Richard A.
Effect of Phase II Price Controls on Hospital Services
Health Services Research, Vol. 7, No. 2, Summer 1972, pp. 106–117

Nonmaternity cost data from three Connecticut hospitals are
analyzed to determine the contribution to total costs per discharge
made by increases in cost per unit of service and by increases in
units of service per discharge between 1960 and 1969. The portion
of the percentage growth of total costs that is due to increased
units of service per discharge is compared with the percentage
growth in total costs allowable under the hospital price control
regulations of the Economic Stabilization Act, and the implicit
consequences for expansion of hospital services under the Act are
discussed.
Hospital Abstract 09220HE

Feldstein, Martin S.
The Rising Cost of Hospital Care
Information Resources Press, Washington, D.C., 1971, 88 pp.

The author makes the point that one factor which should be
considered as causing the rising costs of hospital care in addition
to sharply increased wages and other costs is the change in the
product, the hospital care itself. Rising income and more comprehensive insurance coverage have changed the patient's expecta-

tion of care; through present methods of financing care the hospital can provide more expensive care than the patient may need or want; and technical change in care may not necessarily be technical progress though costs can be increased per day of hospital care. And, almost as an afterthought: "The current approach to medical research may be based toward prcducing information that favors cost-increasing innovations."
Hospital Abstract 09092 HE

Feldstein, Martin; Taylor, Amy
   Rapid Rise in Hospital Costs
Harvard University, Boston, 1977, 76 pp.
Available National Technical Information Service HRP-0016527/4WW

An analysis of causes contributing to inflation in hospital costs is presented. It focuses on the cost of a day of inpatient care in short-term general hospitals, and makes use of statistics from the Bureau of Labor Statistics, Department of Labor, and from the American Hospital Association. The major conclusion is that the rapid, continuous increase in hospital costs results from the fundamental and continuously changing character of the service provided by the hospitals and that this change has been induced by a growth of insurance. The effect of prepaying for health care through insurance has been to encourage hospitals to provide a more expensive product than most consumers actually wish to purchase. The explanation of rising hospital costs lies not so much in changing wage rates or other input prices as in a changing product and the increased rate at which that product is consumed. The prices of various inputs that comprise total costs (e.g., wages, purchase of equipment) are not at the heart of hospital cost inflation. The problem is instead the overconsumption of the hospital's product, which is manifested in the growing number of hospital employees and the rapidly increasing volume of equipment purchases. The findings support earlier conclusions that persistent inflation in hospital cost is attributable to the basic structure of the hospital industry and not to a single, transient factor. Supporting data are included.
Hospital Abstract 18741 HE

Ferguson, Carl; Lee, Maw Lin; Wallace, Richard
   Effects of Medicare on Hospital Use: A Disease Specific Study
University of Missouri, Columbia, Mo., c. 1975, 20 pp.

Paper presents an analysis of the impact of Medicare on hospital use for 23 disease categories, using data from Missouri hospitals

for the period 1965–1971. Comparison of utilization data from the period 1965–66 (pre-Medicare) with data after Medicare was implemented indicated the proportion of patients age 65 and over has increased from 20 to 24 percent, number of total patient days for this group increased from 34 to 40 percent and length of stay increased from an average of 12 days to over 13 to 15 days. Analysis of utilization by age group shows impact of Medicare on hospital use was greater for 75 and over group than for the 65–74 age group. Analysis of disease categories shows largest increases in utilization occurred in disease categories where risk of dying and degree of severity of medical problem was relatively low. Paper points out these findings are consistent with Feldstein's suggestion that greatest impact of Medicare was on use of discretionary types of medical service. It is concluded, however, this requires further in-depth analysis because marginal benefit may decline as additional care is provided within each disease category and thus marginal benefits associated with increased days of care effected by Medicare may be the same in high risk and low risk disease categories.
Hospital Abstract 12144 HE

Fetter, Robert B.; Mills, Ronald E.; Riedel, Donald C.; Thompson, John D.
The Application of Diagnostic Specific Cost Profiles to Cost and Reimbursement Controls in Hospitals
Yale University Center for Study of Health Services, 77 Prospect St., New Haven, CT, 38 pp.

Paper describes a cost and reimbursement control system for hospitals which was developed to generate hospital budgets based on types of patients served. Classes of patients are categorized according to clinical attributes such as diagnoses and surgical procedures and for each class a profile of resources consumed is determined. The profiles are expressed as revenues generated by charging departments and as costs, direct and indirect, for all services. Using a forecast of patient load by class, budgets are computed from cost profiles and revenues determined from charging profiles. By means of variance analysis, the profiles can be used to determine effect of changes in case mix as well as in patient care processes. The effect on revenues of different reimbursement mechanisms can also be projected as a function of the case mix.
Hospital Abstract 17294 HE

Folsom, M.B.; Weaver, W.; Kernan, F.; Molony, J.P.; Park, R.H.; Straus, J.I.; Willis, W.
Governor's Committee on Hospital Costs: Summary of Findings and Recommendations
New York State Journal of Medicine, Aug. 1, 1965, pp. 2,030–2,044

A committee appointed by Governor Nelson Rockefeller and headed by Marion B. Folsom, former Secretary of Health, Education and Welfare, was commissioned to study the causes of rising costs of hospital care in New York and make recommendations for action. This article summarizes findings and conclusions. These included: more effective use of hospitals over weekends; pooling of maternity beds in multi-hospital communities; joint purchasing; and the elimination of duplication of highly specialized facilities. The use of pre-admission testing, of self care, home care, long-term care, and drug formularies were all recommended as means of reducing patients' bills. Medical review procedures and better hospital managment were called for to ensure better patient care and more efficient use of facilities. It was also suggested doctors could use the hospital for ambulatory diagnostic services and thus increase the institution's revenues.

In New York the committee believed more persons should be covered by hospital insurance. They therefore suggested a state law calling for employed persons and families to be covered by Blue Cross or insurance plans financed one-half each by employer and employee. Consolidation of New York Blue Cross plans was recommended, with control to be tripartite (divided between hospital-medical persons, subscribers, and general public). Other suggestions included: return to community rating by Blue Cross and with extension of benefits; allowing insurance carriers to experiment with pilot plans without being committed irrevocably to trial benefits; a uniform and better financial and statistical report system by hospitals; the assumption by the community of the additional costs incurred by teaching hositals for educational and internship programs; full payment to hospitals by government for care of the medically indigent; and realignment of the New York State organization of governmental health agencies.
Hospital Abstract HE0107

Foster, Richard W.; Phillip, P. Joseph; Hai, Abdul; Jeffers, James R.
The Nature of Hospital Costs: Three Studies
Hospital Research and Education Trust, 840 North Lake Shore Drive, Chicago, IL 60611, 1976, 268 pp.

These three papers commissioned by the AHA Board of Trustees concern various aspects of hospital costs: (1) "The Financial Structure of Community Hospitals: Impact of Medicare" by Richard W. Foster presents results from a study of financial statements of a stratified sample of 462 community hospitals certified as Medicare providers for the period 1962 to 1970. Various aspects of the hospital's financial position were analyzed—revenues, expense, assets, and liabilities. The major conclusion is that the overall financial position of hospitals deteriorated slightly following enactment of Medicare. Deterioration is seen in the rise of liabilities relative to assets despite a simultaneous increase in net income relative to total revenue. Paper concludes this reflects the failure of nondebt sources of funds other than patient revenue to expand as rapidly as hospital operations. Present methods of financing hospital care cannot be relied on in the future without altering the present trend of increasing quality, quantity and variety of services. (2). "Hospital Costs: An Investigation of Causality" by P. Joseph Phillip and Abdul Hai is a cross-sectional investigation of causal links between hospital cost behavior and external, product-type, and input-type factors. A synthesis of factor analysis and regression analysis developed to minimize problems of multicollinearity and interaction effects was used. The sample included all but 581 hospitals of the 5,789 community hospitals registered with the AHA in 1973. Dependent variables were Expenses per Day (EPD) and Expenses per Admission (EPA). Major findings were: a.) External factors, e.g. sociodemographic, demographic (uncontrollable), account for 20.49% of the differences in EPD and 23.6% of differences in EPA. A definite causal link was found between insurance and pre-admission cost; b.) Product-type factors (controllable in the long-run) accounted for 19.8% of difference in EPD and 34.4% of differences in EPA; c.) Input-type factors (controllable in the intermediate to long-run) account for 33.4% and 13.4% of differences in EPD and EPA respectively. Of these factors, staffing intensity of "other" personnel is most important cause of per diem and per admission cost increases. 3.) "Indexes of Factor Input Price, Service Intensity and Productivity for the Hospital Industry" by P. Joseph Phillip, James R. Jeffers and Abdul Hai. Review of the background, development and results from a study of the impact of changes in these three factors on changes in the cost of the Patient Day. The study used a model developed by Jeffers in 1972 which characterizes the hospital as a multi-service production unit that combines labor and nonlabor inputs into a set of services rendered to patients and which furnishes a means of decomposing inter-temporal changes in per unit costs into changes in factor prices and service intensity and offsetting or accentuating changes in productivity. Model was applied to data from a selected sample of 594 hospitals in the HAS program for years 1969–1974. Results show over a five year period adjusted cost per day increased 66.76% or 13.35% annually (compared to Price Index of 36.83% or 7.37% annually.) A major factor was service intensity which rose by 5.11% per year. Productivity registered a 2.3% annual increase. Model is also used to analyze changes in these indexes according to geographic region in the U.S.

Hospital Abstract 19796 HE

Ginsburg, Paul B.
Impact of Economic Stabilization Program on Hospitals and Hospital Care
Michigan State University, East Lansing, 1976, 119 pp.
Available National Technical Information Service PB263 341/0WW

The report involved an analysis of the effects of the economic stabilization program on hospitals. It includes discussion of the environment and development of the controls and analytical models, and presentation of econometric results, as well as a survey of hospital perceptions of the controls and their results. The study concludes that the regulations affecting hospitals were ill-suited to their objective of cost containment and that the program did not in fact reduce hospital inflation in any appreciable degree.

Hospital Abstract 17838 HE

Griffith, John R.; Hancock, Walton M.; Munson, Fred C.
Practical Ways to Contain Hospital Costs
Harvard Business Review, Nov.-Dec. 1973, pp. 131–139

The basis of this article stems from four years of close study in different cities of two medium-sized hospitals which have been unequally successful in tightening control over costs. Concentrating on what can be realistically expected, the authors focus on four areas: planning of facilities and services, scheduling of patients and patient services, medical control of facilities utilization and quality of service, and administrative control of manpower and expenditures. An essential ingredient of cost containment is measures by which trustees and administrators can gauge their performance according to norms and standards. Also essential, they maintain, is communitywide planning.

Hospital Abstract 12223 HE

Havighurst, Clark C., ed.; Mechanic, David; Lave, Judith R.; Lave, Lester B.; Kessel, Reuben; Roemer, Milton I.; Worthington, William; Silver, Laurens H.; Chapman, Carleton B.; Talmadge, John M.; Stevens, Rosemary; Stevens, John.
Health Care: Part I
Law and Contemporary Problems, Vol. 35, No. 2, Spring 1970, pp. 223–425

This symposium on health care presents papers which describe present health care system's deficiencies, suggest policy considerations and alternatives, discuss the need for maintaining high quality standards, and develop some of the political background involved in the formulation of a national health care program. Papers include:

"Problems in the Future Organization of Medical Practice" by David Mechanic. Discusses some of the major difficulties existing in present health care system and problems that proposals for national health insurance must confront.

"Medical Care and Its Delivery: An Economic Appraisal" by Judith R. Lave and Lester B. Lave. Paper discusses some aspects of the structure of medical care industry with special emphasis on important interrelationships that must be considered in formulating policy. Important issues enumerated: factors affecting individual's decision to seek medical care; extent of substitution that can be obtained in treating a patient; concept of the paramedic; mode of delivering medical care; and interrelationships between financing and costs.

"The AMA and The Supply of Physicians" by Reuben A. Kessel. Describes the role of AMA in determining the rate of output of physicians and in circumscribing the choice of contractual relationships between physicians and patients, with particular reference to the influence of the Flexner report.

"Controlling and Promoting Quality in Medical Care" by Milton I. Roemer. Paper focuses on nine social mechanisms of control to assure quality in the medical care system and discusses some of current issues in legislation on controlling the quality of medical care.

"Regulation of Quality of Care in Hospitals: The Need for Change" by William Worthington and Laurens H. Silver. Paper examines major agencies which regulate quality of care at state and federal level and how they are affected by federal health benefits legislation and evaluates the role of the federal government in maintaining minimum standards of care in hospitals.

"Historical and Political Background of Federal Health Care

Legislation" by Carleton B. Chapman and John M. Talmadge. Paper traces historical and political background of important federal health care legislation beginning with the first health laws passed during President Washington's administration.

"Medicaid: Anatomy of a Dilemma" by Rosemary Stevens and Robert Stevens. This analysis of the Medicaid program includes information on public health care prior to Medicaid, financial pressures on and from Medicaid and an evaluation of its administration. It is concluded the faults of Medicaid are epitomized by lax administration and unanticipated costs were inherent even in the legislation.

Hospital Abstract 08303 HE

Havighurst, Clark C.; Falk, I.S.; Wolkstein, Irwin; Phelan, Jerry; Erickson, Robert; Fleming, Scott; Steinwald, Bruce; Neuhauser, Duncan; Priest, A.J.G.; Carlson, Rick; Ludlum, James E.; Cantor, Norman L.
Health Care: Part II
Law and Contemporary Problems, Vol. 35, No. 4, Autumn 1970, 254 pp.

This issue examines various facets and legal implications of the problems of improving the delivery of health care to all the population. Included are:

"National Health Insurance: A Review of Policies and Proposals" by I.S. Falk. Discusses evolution of the social policy that medical care should be available to everyone and its implications for a national insurance plan. Details provisions of current legislative proposals now pending including: Catastrophic Illness Expense Plans; Medicredit; Healthcare; Ameriplan; Nixon Program; and Health Security Plan.

"Medicare 1971: Changing Attitudes and Changing Legislation" by Irwin Wolkstein. Discusses provisions of H.R.1., a proposed bill which would change provisions of Medicare, Medicaid, modify Social Security benefits and drastically revise the welfare programs.

"Health Maintenance Organizations and the Market for Health Services" by Clark C. Havighurst. Paper discusses policies needed to obtain best possible implementation of the Health Organization Maintenance concept.

"Group Practice Prepayment: An Approach to Delivering Organized Health Services" by Jerry Phelan, Robert Erickson and Scott Fleming. Paper identifies principal characteristics of group practice prepayment plans and describes six plans currently serving 50,000 members.

"The Role of the Proprietary Hospital" by Bruce Steinwald and

Duncan Neuhauser. Paper describes history of the proprietary hospital, its role in the hospital industry and summarizes main issues surrounding proprietary hospitals including professional ideology, proprietary chains, selective admissions and proprietary versus voluntary hospitals.

"Possible Adaptation of Public Utility Concepts in the Health Care Field" by A.J.G Priest. Discusses application of fixing public utility rates and practices by regulatory commissions to the regulation of medical care costs.

"Health Manpower Licensing and Emerging Institutional Responsibility for the Quality of Care" by Rick J. Carlson. Analyzes the current licensure system for health professionals and its effect on the quality of health care and presents a proposal for reform.

"Physician-Hospital Relations: The Role of Staff Privileges" by James E. Ludlam. Delineates current trends and cross currents in physician-hospital relationships and suggest patterns for the future.

"The Law and Poor People's Access to Health Care" by Norman L. Cantor. Paper contends low income is the primary causal factor in the failure of poor persons to obtain health care and analyzes potential legal channels for increasing the access of poverty populations to health care.

Hospital Abstract 08131 HE

Health Insurance Association of America
Survey of Hospital Semi-Private Room Charges as of January 1977
The Association, New York, 1977, 21 pp.

Statistical data on the cost of a hospital semi-private room as of January 1977 were obtained in a mail survey conducted by the Health Insurance Association of America. Questionnaires were sent to 3,943 nongovernmental short-term hospitals in the United States and Puerto Rico; responding were 2,787 hospitals, or 70.6 percent of the total sample. Questions in the survey applied only to medical-surgical semi-private accommodations and excluded pediatric, intensive care, cardiac care, extended care, self-care, psychiatric, and tuberculosis beds. Hospitals were requested to indicate how many semi-private beds they had and daily room and board rates for such beds, including three-bed and four-bed accommodations. Data on semiprivate room rates are tabulated and matched with the responses of a similar survey conducted in July 1976.

Hospital Abstract 19483 HC

Kashef, Morteza
Optimization of a Distributed System of Medical Care
Stanford University, Stanford, Calif., 1974, 311 pp.
Available from University Microfilms

Two essential components of a medical care delivery system are the providers of medical care services (facilities and manpower) and the consumers of the services (patients). In many cases, an administrative or decision-making body oversees and facilitates the interaction of the two components; when this third component is present, we term the system an integrated medical care delivery system (IMCDS).

This thesis discusses the general problem of determining feasible or optimal organizational alternatives for the IMCDS. A methodology is developed whereby the problem can be decomposed to evaluation of system organization alternatives and optimum copayment mechanisms. The methodology is general and can be applied to analysis and synthesis of a variety of medical care systems.

Part of this dissertation describes the application of the methodology to the IMCDS of San Mateo County, California, where the objective is to provide medical care services to a select group of the medically indigent. The problem involves the evaluation of and selection between centralized, county-operated IMCDS (the status quo) and a decentralized health care delivery system.

Other topics discussed in the dissertation include a critique of current methodology in health systems analysis. In addition, the potential application of the methodology to programs such as national health insurance, Medicaid, and prepaid health plans is discussed in some detail.
Hospital Abstract 13394 HE

Killian, Michael C.
Patients Are Paying the Bill For Government Regulation
Michigan Hospitals, 14, 2, 1978, pp. 2–5

The study was done to measure hospital costs directly attributable to meeting requirements of government regulations. The study, conducted in six Michigan hospitals, found that more than $24, on the average, was added to the patients' bills. The costs incurred by each of the hospitals are categorized in six government regulations considered: utilization review, plant codes, personnel management, medical arbitration, certificate of need, and reimbursement mechanics.
Hospital Abstract 19345 HC

Lave, Judith R.; Leinhardt, Samuel
An Evaluation of a Hospital Stay Regulatory Mechanism
American Journal of Public Health 66:10, 1976, pp. 959–967

The results of an evaluation of a predischarge utilization review program (PDUR) for Medicaid Patients are presented. A group of hospitals in Allegheny County, Pennsylvania, participated in this program on a voluntary basis prior to the program's being mandated statewide. All other hospitals in the county experienced retrospective review of Medicaid cases. The analysis incorporates both types of hospitals in a quasi-experimental design. It was found that during the period studied the length of stay of Medicaid patients fell proportionately more than that of the Blue Cross patients in both groups of hospitals; the relative decrease in the length of stay began to occur prior to the introduction of the PDUR program, but no differential effect of the PDUR review process could be demonstrated. The decline in the length of stay was, however, more continuous and smooth in those hospitals participating in the program.
Hospital Abstract 17745 HE

Lille, Kenneth; Danco, Walter
Organizing a Cost Containment Committee in the Hospital
American Hospital Association, 840 North Lake Shore Drive, Chicago, IL 60611, 1976, 47 pp.

A suggested approach for the organization of a hospital cost containment committee is designed to coordinate various methodologies used by hospitals to provide economical and high quality service. The recommendation is made that a cost containment committee must be fully integrated into the total administrative system of a hospital in order to be effective. Cost containment in the hospital industry is defined to encompass the use of human resources and physical assets in a manner that insures the economical delivery of high quality care. Considerations involved in the organization of such a committee are examined. Forms and tools to assist hospital administrators in planning and organizing the committee are included and resource materials for the committee members are reported. Information is presented on the structure of a cost containment committee, cost containment terminology, and processes by which a committee performs its work. Resources are listed in an appendix; a bibliography is provided.
Hospital Abstract 18583 HE

National Center for Health Services Research
Controlling the Cost of Health Care
The Center, 3700 East-West Highway, Hyattsville, MD, 20782, 1977, 22 pp.

This report summarizes some of the research findings that relate to the rising costs of health services. In particular, the report describes what is known about the consequences and effectiveness of various strategies intended to reduce or minimize increases in the costs of such services. The findings presented in this paper deal with only a limited part of the literature in this area. Particular emphasis is given to the results of studies supported by the National Center for Health Services Research.
Hospital Abstract 17813 HE

Newhouse, Joseph P.
Income and Medical Care Expenditure Across Countries
Rand Corporation, Santa Monica, CA 90406, 19 pp.

This paper examines the relationship between a country's medical care expenditures and its income. The study covers 13 so-called developed countries. The comparison shows that per capita income can explain much of the cross-national variation in expenditures. The amount of funds spent on medical care is directly proportional to gross domestic product per capita, but the proportion of income spent decreases.
Hospital Abstract 16962 HE

Rhode Island Health Services Research, Inc.
The Impact of Varying Economic Conditions on the Use of Community Hospitals in Rhode Island
The Corporation, 1977, 46 pp.

The report presents the results of an analysis of changes in hospital utilization which resulted from the economic conditions of 1974–75. The study analyzes three measures of hospital use (discharges, days, and lengths of stay) for all hospitals in Rhode Island for the years from 1970 to 1975 and characteristics of the population (age, socioeconomic status and source of payment). Despite the dramatic rise in unemployment in Rhode Island during the recession, the effects on hospital utilization and provider rationing were minimal. A significant shift in source of payment from private to public sources during the period was observed and there appeared to be a tendency to postpone elective surgery. Other-

wise, longer-term trends, particularly declines in lengths of stay, continued.
Hospital Abstract 19366 HF

Senate Subcommittee
Competition in the Health Services Market
Hearings before the Subcommittee on antitrust and monopoly of the Committee on the Judiciary United States Senate Ninety-third Congress, Second Session, Part I, 1974, 606 pp.
Available from Superintendent of Documents, U.S. Government Printing Office, Washington, D.C. 20402 for $4.95

Report presents the testimony given before the U.S. Senate Subcommittee on Antitrust and Monopoly on May 14 and 15, 1974 regarding the effectiveness of competition in keeping health care costs down and improving the quality of care delivered. The testimony given concerns the state of competition in four major areas of the health care industry: planning; organization; delivery; and financing. Important areas to be probed during the hearings were: unnecessary government restraints on trade; overly restrictive certificate-of-need and license laws; extent of government financing of health care; and restraints on trade coming from the American Medical Association and member associations—especially the impact on HMOs and alternatives to cost plus reimbursement.
Hospital Abstract 17981 HE

Surles, Kathryn B.; Johnson, Paul V.; Overby, Robert C.
Empirical Study of Alternative Health Indexes
North Carolina Department of Human Resources, Raleigh, 1976, 26 pp.

Four methods of arriving at an index of health-principal components, complete factor analysis, summed z-scores and summed rankings—are compared on the basis of their application to natality statistics for North Carolina for 1969 through 1973. The analysis proceeds on the assumption that an index should measure a precise functional area as opposed to the overall health or social well-being of a community. Thus, the four methods are used to develop indexes for a functional area called "conditions surrounding birth." The variables employed include nine identified as being discriminatory with respect to the outcome of pregnancy and four variables reflecting outcomes of pregnancy. Neither the summed z-scores nor the summed ranks method resulted in an acceptable index. Both principal components and complete factor analysis are demonstrated to be credible procedures, with principal components judged the most acceptable method. (Abstract

from *Government Reports Announcements and Index,* Jan. 20, 1978, adapted, p. 53)
Hospital Abstract 19152 HE

INSURANCE

American Association of Medical Clinics
An Administrative Information System for a Group Practice Developing a Prepaid Health Plan
The Association, Alexandria, Va., c. 1975, 45 pp.

Report describes an administrative information system (AIS) that was developed for prepaid health plans (HMOs). A manual version of the system was initially developed at St. Louis Park Medical Center in Minnesota. The AIS described in this report is a modified and improved version in which several processes are computerized. Following the introductory section of the paper, Section 2 of the report outlines the approach used in designing AIS which included: establishment of general design criteria; determination of HMO administrative functions; and development of information required to accomplish the administrative functions. Section 3 describes AIS. An overall flow chart summarizes relationship between the system's physical components (input forms, data files and output, and processing components) and manual procedures or computer programs required to process the data. Objectives, narrative description and flow chart of each of five processing components are included. In Section 4 each physical component is catalogued and described. The appendices include an overview description of an accounting system to support a prepaid health plan and a description of the role of AIS in evaluating financial success of a prepaid health plan.
Hospital Abstract 13162 IN

American Association of Medical Clinics
A Financial Evaluation System for a Group Practice Developing a Prepaid Health Plan
The Association, Alexandria, Va., 1973, 47 pp.

Purpose of this study is to present an approach to evaluating the financial success of a prepaid health plan; to offer an overview of how information generated by this financial evaluation system supports this approach; and to explain the methodology required for gathering and developing the necessary input data for group practices developing a prepaid health plan. In the first section, a clinic's participation in a prepaid health plan is examined in respect to the desirability of prepaid delivery relative to fee-for-service delivery, its ability to operate if it were not in a group practice, and the short term cash flow potential. A method for gathering information on: fee equivalents, fully allocated costs, clinical costs, nonclinical expenses, and health plan revenue are discussed in the second section. The third section is a detailed description of methodology and implementation procedures used in this evaluation system.

Hospital Abstract 13158 IN

American Association of Medical Clinics
Income Distribution: An Abstract and Analysis
The Association, Alexandria, Va., 1974, 146 pp.

Manual presents information on income distribution plans for group practices. Part I discusses 12 basic factors that should be considered in development of an income distribution plan by a medical group: equal distribution versus productivity; measurement of productivity; level of professional training; seniority; management duties of physicians; fringe benefits; disposition of income from laboratory, x-ray and other ancillary services; allocation of overhead costs; form of legal organization; objectives of an income distribution plan; flexibility; and intangible factors. Part II includes sample income distribution plans from 17 clinics which illustrate methods for determining phsyician income. Part III presents selected articles relevant to income distribution and a bibliography for additional references.

Hospital Abstract 13163 IN

American Hospital Association
Ameriplan: A Proposal for the Delivery and Financing of Health Services in the United States
The Association, Chicago, Ill., 1970, 99 pp.

Monograph describes Ameriplan, the proposal of the AHA's Special Committee on the Provision of Health Services to restructure and finance a delivery system of health care that is considered more accessible, comprehensive and relevant to the needs of the community. Ameriplan involves the formation of Health Care Corporations at the community level, composed of existing health care provider organizations. The Health Care Corporation would have a primary geographic assignment established by a State Health Commission; more than one Health Care Corporation may be assigned to the same area, however. Its primary responsibility is the provision of health care services to its registrants. It would

also act as a fiscal agency, receiving and disbursing money for the payment of health services. A National Health Commission would be the primary agency responsible for the continuing assessment of the effectiveness of Ameriplan. It would be responsible for adopting regulations to create uniform benefit packages and state scope, standards of quality, and comprehensiveness of health services. Federal and state legislation is needed to implement the proposal and create the State and National Health Commissions. The financing system recommended would utilize all existing sources of funds and be based on each citizen's ability to pay, except for the aged for whom coverage would be prepaid.
Hospital Abstract IN3–6696

Anderson, Odin W.
**National Health Insurance: Implications for the Management
of Hospitals**
American College of Hospital Administrators, Chicago, Ill., 1974, 90 pp.

Report presents findings and conclusions of the special Study Commission established by ACHA to define issues and make recommendations about basic administrative principles essential to success of any proposed national health insurance program. There are three major elements of consideration in the study: an evaluation of the background of current controversies and legislative proposals in the health care field; elucidation of the attitudes and experiences of hospital administrators with respect to problems of health care delivery and proposed solutions; and a detailed classification and analysis of the various legislative proposals for national health care insurance. This analysis is intended to furnish some criteria against which to measure feasibility of actions implicit and explicit in the legislation, adequacy of financial resources allocated for operating and capital expenditures, efficacy of controls on funding, volume of services, personnel and quality levels, and likelihood of achieving equality of access and cost sharing.
Hospital Abstract 14306 IN

Anderson, Odin W. and May, J. Joel
**The Federal Employees Health Benefits Program, 1961–1968: A Model
for National Health Insurance?**
Center for Health Administration Studies, University of Chicago, Chicago, Ill., 1971, 60 pp.

An evaluation of the Federal Employees' Health Benefits Program as a model for national health insurance in the U.S. Legislative history of the program, its scope and administration are discussed. Data collected by the Civil Service Commission on cost, use and enrollment are analyzed. The FEHB Program is described as one which was acceptable at the time of its adoption to all groups at interest (government, employees, providers and insurance agencies) and would be feasible as a national program. A two-class system of medical care could be avoided by allowing low-income individuals a choice of coverage through governmental subsidization.

Hospital Abstract IN4–7739

Barton, David M.
Alternative Institutional Arrangements for Medical Care Insurance
University of Virginia, Charlottesville, Va., 1974, 175 pp.
Available from University Microfilms

In situations where an insured individual has some control over the expected value of an insured loss, economic theory predicts that inefficiency will result since insured individuals will have reduced incentives for loss avoidance. Such a tendency on the part of insured individuals poses a problem of "moral hazard" for the insurer. As a result, the cost of insurance is higher and/or the amount of risk spreading is less than would be the case if the probability or size of the loss were unaffected by individual behavior.

This study deals with organizations which contract to both insure for medical expenses and supply medical services. In this study such organizations are termed "insurer-providers." This particular contractual arrangement is viewed as a device to eliminate the inefficiency resulting from moral hazard. Two implications concerning such insurance arrangements are derived and tested.

The expected utility position of an individual insured by an insurer-provider is compared with that achieved when insured by a conventional insurance firm.

Comparing the results of two maximization problems, it is shown that the expected utility position of the insured individual is greatest when insured by the insurer-provider. Furthermore, on the assumption that the price elasticity of demand for medical services is not greater than unity—it is shown that the quantity of medical services consumed when the insured is covered by the conventional insurance policy is greater than that consumed when covered by the insurer-provider. Two implications emerge from the analysis: 1) Insurer-provider type arrangements will be observed to offer insurance against some contingencies not insured, or insured less frequently, by conventional insurance firms. (2) Compared to conventional insurance firms, the expected value of

medical services consumed per insured individual will be less for populations insured for the same risk by insurer-providers. These two implications are tested using data on benefit structures and data on medical services utilization for populations insured by the two types of insurance arrangements.
Hospital Abstract 13685 IN

Bauer, Katharine G.
Containing Costs of Health Services Through Incentive Reimbursement
Cases in Health Services, Series No. 4, Dec. 1973, 293 pp.

Report presents 13 case studies of approaches taken by various third party sponsors including Medicare and Medicaid programs and Blue Cross plans to contain medical costs by control incentives linked to reimbursement. Each of the case reports describes the plan's sponsorship and stated purposes, types of performance sponsor seeks to encourage, methods for measuring performance, incentives offered and formulae for their calculations. Where available, results are also presented. Reports are organized in six sections, according to types of cost control approaches taken by third party sponsors: industrial engineering and cost monitoring; global performance strategy; prospective rate setting and target budgets; comprehensive approach to incentives; reaching practicing physician; and attempts to contain overall patient care costs. Most plans were initiated in response to some local manifestation of a crisis in health care costs and most were entered into as experiments, designed to test out new methods of reimbursement, and deal with a sizeable number of hospitals or physicians in a given geographic area.
Hospital Abstract 12135 IN

Berry, Ralph E., Jr.
Prospective Reimbursement in New York
Inquiry, 13, 4, 1976, pp. 288–301

The impact of the introduction of Medicare and Medicaid, national wage and price control, and New York's prospective reimbursement program are analyzed to determine if hospital cost inflation is of the "demand-pull" nature. Results indicated that is probably the case. Further analyses of New York's reimbursement program shows that the constraints imposed "worked"—net revenues decreased: however, constraints against excess capacity probably accounted for the increase in the average length of stay and occupancy rates, and deficits occurring in the hospital's operation

would be the basis for increases in reimbursement in following years.
Hospital Abstract 19124 IN

Blair, Roger D.; Ginsburg, Paul B.; Vogel, Ronald J.
  Blue Cross-Blue Shield Administration Costs: A Study of Non-Profit Health Insurers
Economic Inquiry 13:2, 1975, pp. 237–251

Administrative costs are examined for Blue Cross and Blue Shield for 1975. Two aspects of the Blue Cross and Blue Shield programs are examined in depth: (1) the costs incurred by each as an intermediary or a carrier for the Medicare program: and (2) the potential efficiencies of merging Blue Cross and Blue Shield when the two plans operate separately in a single area. Analysis of 1971 and 1972 cost data leads to the conclusion that the Blue Cross and Blue Shield programs evidence substantial managerial slack. Variance in costs is much smaller for those costs associated with Medicare administration than for those associated with the direct business of Blue Cross and Blue Shield. Although cost advantages can be demonstrated for a merged organizational form, this form is not prevalent. The evidence suggests that Blue Cross and Blue Shield have not taken advantage of potential economies of scale to reduce the cost of health insurance, but have instead dissipated the potential savings in increased administrative costs.
Hospital Abstract 17772 IN

Blue Cross Association and National Association of Blue Shield Plans
  The Effect of Deductibles, Coinsurance and Copayment on Utilization of Health Care Services: Opinions and Impressions from Blue Cross and Blue Shield Plans
The Associations, Chicago, Ill. c. 1972, 15 pp.

Report of a survey of 60 Blue Cross and Blue Shield Plans to determine the impact of deductibles, coinsurance and copayment provisions on health care utilization. Purpose of the study was to aid the national associations in deciding whether to continue their emphasis on first dollar coverage. Answers to survey questions indicated that personnel of many plans around the country believed that large deductibles, and coinsurance provisions curb utilization, but may also constitute a barrier to needed care. However, very little concrete evidence was produced to support this contention. Poll also indicated that the public will most often select comprehensive plans when given a choice. Included in the paper are a short summary of the background of deductibles, coin-

surance and copayment and tables showing survey results.
Hospital Abstract IN1–7704

Brian, Earl W. and Gibbens, Stephen F.
California's Medi-Cal Copayment Experiment
Medical Care, Vol. 12, No. 12, Dec. 1974, Supplement, 303 pp.

Report describes a study conducted to evaluate an experiment on copayment in the California Medi-Cal (Medicaid) program. About 30 percent of those eligible for Medi-Cal were required to pay $1.00 for each of their first two visits to providers each month and 50¢ for each of the first two prescriptions they had filled each month. Copayment was required only of those who had specific property or resources above a defined level. Data were gathered from: claims paid by the program to all providers for all services performed; household surveys of Medi-Cal beneficiaries before and after copayment requirements; mailed questionnaires sent to samples of Medi-Cal providers; and a household survey of average Californians. Findings indicate copayment reduced beneficiary utilization, but did not completely control it. Data indicated copayment did result in a decline in preventive care, but there was no instance found where a condition was classified as significant and the subject gave copayment as a reason for not going to the doctor. Data also indicate a lower use of drugs among copayers but little or no difference was found between copayers' and noncopayers' use of drugs judged to be most important for management or control of serious health care diseases. Findings for other services and a comparison of average Californian utilization with Medi-Cal population are also discussed.
Hospital Abstract 13433 IN

Chao, Cedric C.
Cost and Quality Control in the Medicare/Medicaid Program—Concurrent Review
Harvard Civil Right-Civil Liberties Law Review, 11, 3, 1976, pp. 664–700

The effectiveness of concurrent review as a means of preventing the improper utilization of medical resources under the Medicare and Medicaid programs is evaluated. Possible policy objections to concurrent review which must be addressed by persons seeking to reduce costs and improve the quality of health services are noted. Major problems faced by Medicare and Medicaid are identified as rising costs and uneven quality of care. The achievement of government objectives through concurrent review is assessed. It is concluded that statutory and constitutional objectives to concur-

rent review can be overcome, but that it may be difficult to determine the effectiveness of concurrent review in achieving its defined objectives. It is recommended that a flexible approach, to concurrent review and alternative utilization control techniques be adopted in order to meet the objective of high quality health care at a reasonable cost.
Hospital Abstract 19489 HF

Chawla, Marshall; Steinhardt, Bruce J.
Episode of Care Accounting Methodology For a Cost-Effectiveness Approach to Quality Assurance in a Health Maintenance Organization
Group Health Association, Inc., Washington, D.C., 1975, 323 pp.

A methodology is described for evaluating and promoting cost-effectiveness in health maintenance organizations (HMO's), using an episode of care accounting framework. Methods for reallocating constrained resources, based on an analysis of cost-effectiveness, are detailed. A technical description of a standard accounting and statistical information system, required for analyzing the quality of care provided by HMO's and their cost-effectiveness, is presented. Costs of constituent elements of an episode of care, particularly professional medical services, are identified. The results of time studies of two ambulatory health care settings are presented. It is concluded that a significant amount of variations in professional resources consumed by patients can be attributed to their different diagnoses or medical problems and may be predictable. The methodology is considered useful for internal HMO management, cross-HMO comparisons, and the implementation of uniform cost-reporting requirements. Appendixes contain narrative information and tabular data and HMO cost-effectiveness.
Hospital Abstract 18867 IN

Coombes, David H.
A Comparative Study of the Effects of Certain Selected Variables as Factors Influencing the Attitudes of Medical Staff Physicians Toward the Medicare Program
University of Minnesota, Minneapolis, Minn., 1969, 103 pp.
Available from University Microfilms

Physician attitudes toward the Medicare program were studied in a sample of 639 medical staff members of Baptist Hospital, Memphis, Tennessee. Study hospital was a large specialty private, church-related hospital. Questionnaires were mailed to 639 staff members with 345 usable responses. The relationship of age, political party affiliation, size of medical practice, level of graduate medical education, geographic region where educated, and method of payment for services rendered to attitudes toward four aspects of the Medicare Program was tested, using a chi-square test at .05 level of significance. The four questions studied were: degree of satisfaction with Medicare Program; its extension to all citizens; continued utilization of the Program; and financing of outpatient drug costs. The study found that a majority of the physicians sampled are dissatisfied with the present Medicare Program, but would continue to utilize its provisions. Physicians indicated strong opposition toward any extension of health insurance benefits to all citizens either under Medicare or via similar programs and to financing of outpatient prescription drug costs. The data showed a significant (negative) response between the south central region as location for education and attitudes toward Medicare and financing drug costs. The study also found a significant relationship between party affiliation and attitudes. A majority of Republicans were dissatisfied with Medicare and majority of Democrats favored it, but both groups were opposed to extending benefits to other age groups. Many physicians indicated objection to the procedure of direct billing. The study found that there is still a great deal of patient confusion over Medicare provisions and recommends a concentrated public relations program and re-examination of direct billing procedures by Social Security Administration.

Hospital Abstract IN4087

Cooper, Barbara S. and Worthington, Nancy L.
Comparison of Cost and Benefit Incidence of Government Medical Care Programs, Fiscal Years 1966 and 1969
Social Security Administration, Washington, D.C., Staff Paper No. 18, DHEW Pub. No. (SSA) 75–118–52, 93 pp.

Study is a cost-benefit comparison of 11 government medical care programs. Among these programs are Workmen's Compensation, Medicare, and Temporary Disability Insurance. Purpose of study is to determine how the cost incidence and benefit incidence of these medical care plans were distributed among the states; which people in the various states bore the heaviest tax burden and which people benefited the most; and if there has been a change in who pays and who receives Medicare and Medicaid benefits since their inceptions. Several conclusions of this study are that benefits were greatest in states where the targeted population was greatest; and federally financed programs are, on the whole, fiscally progressive while state and locally financed programs are fiscally regressive. Statistics pertaining to allocation of expenditures and costs by state are presented in an appendix. Hospital Abstract 13527 IN

Davidson, Stephen M. and Wacker, Ronald C.
Community Hospitals and Medicaid
Medical Care, Vol. xii, No. 2, Feb. 1974, pp. 115–130

The study examines Medicaid utilization patterns, determining the extent to which Medicaid recipients in a Chicago community use hospitals in their own communities. Data from the February 1970 Hospital Discharge Study show that substantial numbers of Medicaid patients bypass nearby community hospitals and receive care instead in more distant teaching hospitals. In addition to possible harmful medical consequences, this pattern turns out to be much more expensive to the state's Medicaid program than care in closer community hospitals would be. Possible reasons for these patterns are suggested, implications for planning are discussed, and questions for further research are identified.
Hospital Abstract 11937 IN

Davis, Karen
Medicaid Payments and Utilization of Medical Services by the Poor
Inquiry, 13, 2, 1976, pp. 122–135.

This paper summarizes the major benefits provided and persons served by Medicaid and assesses the impact of medical services and financial hardship inflicted on the poor by high medical bills. Analysis indicated that the rural, black and non-welfare poor have not received a proportionate share of medical benefits and that the Medicaid program overall has not reduced the percentage of their income the poor must spend on medical care.
Hospital Abstract 19125 IN

Davis, Karen
National Health Insurance: Benefits, Costs and Consequences
Brookings Institution, Washington, D.C., 1975, 194 pp.

Seven major national health insurance proposals introduced in Congress are analyzed. The approaches taken by the proposals to financing health care vary from tax subsidies for the purchase of private insurance, through a combination of private and public insurance, to coverage that is predominantly publicly financed. Each proposal is examined against a set of questions derived from the three basic goals which are: (1) to ensure that all Americans have access to adequate medical care; (2) to eliminate the finan-

cial hardship of large medical bills; and (3) to limit the rise in health care costs. The following questions are addressed: who should be covered; what services should be covered; what the roles of consumers, employers, insurance companies, and State and Federal government should be; how the plan should be paid. The costs of each plan and how they would be borne by patients and taxpayers of different levels are weighed against the plan's benefits and measured by how well it fulfills the stated goals. Although no one proposal is endorsed, a set of requirements are set forth for any plan that is to achieve the desired goals.
Hospital Abstract 17407 IN

Donabedian, Avedis
A Review of Some Experiences with Prepaid Group Practice
School of Public Health, The University of Michigan, Ann Arbor, Mich., 1965, 80 pp.

Analyzes available published information on expenditures, utilization, and quality of prepaid plans, together with surveys of subscriber attitudes. Two tables describe member physician attitudes. The author notes that "only those studies which permit fairly valid comparison" are included. References are described in an annotated bibliography and data are presented in detailed appendix tables.
Hospital Abstract HE0123

Donabedian, Avedis and Thorby, Jean A.
The Systematic Impact of Medicare
Medical Care Review, Vol. 26, No. 6, June 1969, pp. 567–585

Bibliography of 67 items and review article discussing the impact of Medicare on use, prices, voluntary health insurance and provider agencies, and individuals. There is brief reference to the degree of protection, quality of care, the impact on public welfare and civil rights aspects. Public health departments are included among the provider agencies discussed.
Hospital Abstract IN4084

Dowling William L.
Prospective Reimbursement of Hospitals
Inquiry, Vol. xi, No. 3, Sept. 1974, pp. 163–180

Paper develops a framework for examining different approaches to prospective reimbursement, identifies areas of hospital performance that might be affected by prospective reimbursement, suggests changes in hospital performance that might occur under different approaches to prospective reimbursement, and discusses alternative methods that can be used to set budgets or rates prospectively. Paper points out acceptability to hospitals of any rate-setting method, assuming participation is not mandated, probably depends more on expected payment level than on method used to determine rates. It is concluded for any rate-setting method to be acceptable to the AHA, it must meet financial requirements of hospitals as defined in the AHA statement, its rates must apply equally to all patients and third party payers, and rate-setting process must include provisions for full hearing of a hospital's budget justification, automatic approval of rate proposals not acted on within 90 days, planning agency approval of proposed capital projects, emergency adjustments of rates and appeal rights including judicial review.

Hospital Abstract 13263 IN

Dowling, William L.; House, Peter J.; Lehman, Jeffrey M.; Mead, Gary L.; Teague, Nancy; Trivedi, Vandan; Watts, Carolyn A.
Prospective Reimbursement in Downstate New York and Its Impact on Hospitals: A Summary
Center for Health Services Research, University of Washington, 1976, 93 pp.

Study evaluated the impact of New York Blue Cross and Medicaid prospective reimbursement systems (PR) begun in 1970 on hospital costs and operations in downstate New York (DNY). The PR system was developed under New York's Cost Control Act and was designed to keep hospital cost increases in line with inflation in the general economy. Cost containment impact of PR was examined by two methods: a comparison of DNY hospitals before and after PR and comparisons with a control group and nation as a whole; and by estimated cost functions for DNY and control hospitals that isolate cost trends for the pre-PR (1968–69) and post-PR (1969–74) periods and comparing rates of decline in cost increases for the two groups. Both methods produced consistent results and show PR substantially slowed the rate of cost increases in DNY hospitals for both adjusted cost per day and adjusted cost per case. Analysis of PR impact on DNY hospital operations compared to the control group shows these significant results: admissions increased faster; length of stay decreased more slowly; intensity of services increased more slowly; amenity level decreases; and efficiency decreased more slowly. Analysis also showed financial status of DNY hospitals deteriorated substantially during 1968–74 period. Blue Cross and Medicaid prospective rates consistently fell below their own definitions of cost as well as average cost for all patients. It is concluded PR contributed to financial problems of DNY hospitals, but there were other contributing factors such as ambulatory care losses, Economic Stabilization Program and general economic conditions. Final section of the report examines important issues regarding a PR system. Both sides of each issue are presented with any available evidence to support or refute them.

Hospital Abstract 17525 IN

Eilers, Robert D.
Postpayment Medical Expense Coverage: A Proposed Salvation for Insured and Insurer
Blue Cross Association, Chicago, Ill., 1969, 15 pp.

The author proposes postpayment medical expense coverage as the most realistic method of overcoming present inadequate insurance payments for a large portion of families' total health care expenditures. Postpayment provides credit for medical care. The carrier pays provider's total bill with provision for periodic repayment by the individual to the carrier of the noninsured portion. The author discusses services to be included, repayment time periods and interest rates. Governmental repayment might be arranged for the indigent. Despite unsettled aspects such as legal difficulties, risk and eligibility, the author believes the plan should be given exhaustive study for its many advantages to society.

Hospital Abstract IN1036

Elliott, William B.
An Investigation of Some Effects of the New York State Prospective Reimbursement Program on a Group of Upstate Hospitals
Cornell University, 1976, 326 pp. Available from University Microfilms.

This study examined some results of New York State regulations under a prospective reimbursement program. An analysis was made to determine if the controls worked to restrain cost increases. A second concern was the effects of regulatory pressure on hospitals and the populations they serve. The study was conducted on a population of twenty-two hospitals within a single region in upstate New York. A group of one hundred and forty-four hospitals from the Hospital Administrative Services data base was used as a control. Most data was drawn from financial reports. The results about the effectiveness of the regulations are somewhat ambiguous. The enactment of the regulation does coincide

with a significant decline in per diem revenue for the New York group. There is also a large but nonsignificant decline in the rate of growth of total expenses. Relative to the control group there was no notable change in the rate of increase in per diem expenses or total revenue. This pattern resulted in a marked decline in net income for the New York group. Wealthy hospitals appeared to be more successful in avoiding the effects of the regulations than poorer hospitals.
Hospital Abstract 18914 IN

Evans, Robert G.
Efficiency Incentives in Hospital Reimbursements
Harvard University Library, Cambridge, Mass., 1970

Thesis analyzed the effect of reimbursement plans on incentives for efficiency in the hospital industry. Study begins with the premise that hospitals produce too much care too expensively and the present means of payment of hospitals encourage waste. Data are presented to show rapid increase in resource utilization by hospitals in the last two decades is not related to any equivalent measurable increase in health and that health can be maintained with a much lower level of hospital activity input. An explicit model of hospital management is constructed to explain hospital technical and economic inefficiency. The model is then used to interpret various reimbursement plans as varying specifications of the relation between hospital size and growth variables and current cost levels. It is shown some plans provide opportunities for the hosital to subvert the plan by behavior aimed at changing the terms of the reimbursement function; others encourage expansion of output to earn bonuses for "efficiency"; and none provides a strong tradeoff between future growth and current slack. It is concluded some form of negotiated fixed price system is required and capitation provides maximum incentives for technical and economic efficiency, but feasibility considerations tend to favor fixed pricing of case types across hospitals. The impact of efficiency incentives on the quality of care is discussed and it is concluded the concept of quality is so diffuse and nebulous that an incentive plan should not be rejected unless it can be proved to reduce quality. Empirical data from the Ontario hospital system are then presented which indicate differences in diagnostic mix of patient load have a strong influence on costs per day and per case which argues further for use of fixed-price case-type schedules of payment.
Hospital Abstract INO–6252

Feldstein, Paul J.
An Analysis of Reimbursement Plans in *Reimbursements for Medical Care*
Office of Research and Statistics, Social Security Administration, Washington, D.C., 1968, pp. 23–54

A study of reimbursement plans in terms of lower cost incentives, greater efficiency in hospital procedures and accounting methods, and in terms of maintaining quality care. Various payment plans are discussed as to their Long and Short Term Marginal Costs, and as to their ability to strike a balance between efficiency, low-cost, and quality. Conclusions suggest: relative reimbursement, capitation, group prepayment, incentives aimed at results rather than means, reimbursement based on relative performance, effective use of a variety of health facilities all within a plan that counterchecks for levels of quality, should be elements of a reimbursement plan.
Hospital Abstract IN0012

Feldstein, Paul J.
Prepaid Group Practice: An Analysis and Review
Bureau of Hospital Administration, The University of Mich., June 1971, 147 pp.
Available from University Microfilms

Study presents a framework for analysis of prepaid group practices (PPGP) and a comparison of these with alternative delivery systems. The net effect on per unit costs of alternative delivery systems is determined by: standardizing for different outputs produced; standardizing different population groups being serviced and their differences in demand for medical services; and isolating differences in per unit cost of providing care that are a result of differences in the organization of delivery. Study then analyzes the effect of economies of scale in medical services to determine whether a change in the delivery system such as a PPGP must be of a certain size so as not to suffer from higher per unit costs of providing care. Study also investigates the effect of different methods of physician reimbursement on costs and utilization and reviews studies on physician and consumer satisfaction with PPGPs found in the literature. A review is also made of various studies and analyses which show differences in utilization and expenses of PPGP vs. a fee-for-service delivery system. These data are then applied to the Lansing, Michigan area to determine potential savings that might accrue under a PPGP that duplicated utilization rates and costs of a "typical" PPGP. Findings indicate for the total Lansing

population, the annual savings would be $10 million, due to reduced hospitalization rates for a PPGP. If only 30,000 of the population were enrolled, the annual savings for a family of three is calculated to be $165. It is concluded that PPGP does offer an immediate and long-run alternative for provision of health services and the most feasible method of organization is to have physician groups form into PPGPs, responsible for the entire package of medical care, and purchase from existing facilities and specialties those services they do not maintain themselves.
Hospital Abstracts IN2–6952

Feldstein, Paul J.
  A Proposal for Capitation Reimbursement to Medical Groups for Total Medical Care in *Reimbursement Incentives for Medical Care.*
Office of Research and Statistics, Social Security Administration, Washington, D.C., 1968, pp. 87–103

A proposal to develop a capitation reimbursement system under Medicare that pays organized groups of doctors who share facilities and expenses. Increased efficiency, decreased costs, and methods of implementation are discussed, as well as the maintenance of quality care and freedom of choice for patients.
Hospital Abstract IN0011

Feldstein, Paul J. and Waldman, Saul
  Financial Position of Hospitals in the Early Medicare Period
Social Security Bulletin, Oct. 1968

Data on prices, expenses, and utilization for community short term hospitals are presented and analyzed for the years from 1960 to 1967. Implementation of Medicare, expansion of Medicare and other government programs, an above-average rise in hospital charges, substantial increases in hospital expenses, and moderate increases in hospital utilization and occupancy rates are among the developments affecting hospitals in the period since June, 1966. Authors conclude that in the period following the start of Medicare, the financial situation of most hospitals improved.
Hospital Abstract IN4–6097

Feldstein, Paul J. and Waldman, Saul
  The Financial Position of Hospitals in the First Two Years of Medicare
Inquiry, Vol. vi, No. 1, March 1969, pp. 19–27.

Analysis of effect of Medicare on financial position of hospitals was made by examining revenue and expense data of community non-federal short-term hospitals from AHA before Medicare (1960–65 average) and two years later implementation, 1966–67.

These data show substantial rise in net revenues first year of Medicare, small and medium hospitals showing greatest gains. Net revenues fell second year of Medicare but exceeded pre-Medicare levels. Larger hospitals which serve fewer aged patients experienced less improvement after start of Medicare.
Hospital Abstract IN4080

Filerman, Gary L. and Shattuck, Frances M.
The Senate Rejects Health Insurance for the Aged.
The University of Minnesota, Minneapolis, Minn., c. 1967, 136 pp.
Available from University Microfilms

A detailed historical study of health insurance bills before Congress during the years 1952–1962. The authors chronologically trace the fate of the many bills and amendments which originated between the time the Murray-Dingell bill of 1952 was introduced to the defeat of the proposed Anderson-Javitz Amendment in the Senate in 1962. The Forand bill is followed to its defeat and the Kerr-Mills bill to its enactment. The attempts to bring about a health care bill linked to Social Security are followed through the Eisenhower administration and that of Kennedy to 1962. The power struggles involving the executive branch of the government, the American Medical Association, the UAW-CIO, the liberals vs. the conservatives, the party politics and the legislative maneuvering are all minutely described. The study ends with the description of the attempts to pass the King-Anderson bill and the Anderson-Javitz amendment in the 1962 Congress.
Hospital Abstract IN4003

Gartside, Foline E.
Causes of Increase in Medicaid Costs in California
Health Services Reports, Vol. 88, No. 3, March 1973, pp. 225–235

This study analyzes the fivefold increase in the costs of California public welfare medical care program over a six year period. Price increases, growth in the eligible population and increased use of services due to expanded benefits and per capita changes in utilization have all contributed to the rise in expenditures. Price increases account for approximately half of the net six-year increase of $640 million. Growth in the eligible population and greater use of services were almost equal in causing the remaining increased costs. Distribution of the cost increase factors among the major types of service show that their effects vary widely. The basic data from which the results were drawn are shown.
Hospital Abstract 12140 IN

Gartside, Foline E.; Hopkins, Carl E.; Roemer, Milton I.
Medicaid Services in California Under Different Organizational Modes
School of Public Health, University of California, Los Angeles, 1973, 99
pp.

This is a comparative study to determine if organizational mode
of delivery affects volume, costs, quality and outcomes of services
to Medicaid beneficiaries in California. Six organizational modes
were selected for the study: three open market (free choice, fee-
for-service) modes; and three organized delivery modes. Each set
of three included one prepaid or capitation health plan operating
as a demonstration pilot project of the Medi-Cal program and two
other modes without Medi-Cal capitation agreements and differing in objectives, controls and financing. Each mode served at
least 3,000 Medi-Cal beneficiaries. Report describes administrative structures and organizational methods of each of the six
modes and analyzes the patterns of use, costs, and certain indicators of the adequacy of their services. Data for the six modes were
obtained for years 1969 and 1970.

Major findings of the study are: Organizational differences were
found to be associated with measurable differences in nature of
services accessible to and received by Medi-Cal beneficiaries,
their volume and costs and, to the limited extent observable, in
their quality and outcomes. Structure of the modes determined
their flexibiltiy in locating facilities in areas of accessibility to the
poor, in scope of benefits provided and in control of quality. While
no mode was found to include all factors considered desirable in
delivery of health care services, it is concluded net potential of
organized modes for effective health service is somewhat greater
than that of open market modes.
Hospital Abstract 12141 IN

Hardwick, C.P.; Myers, Susan B.; Shlomo, Larry
The Effect of a Co-pay Agreement on Hospital Utilization
Blue Cross of Western Pennsylvania, Pittsburgh, Pa., 1971, 19 pp.

Study undertaken by Blue Cross of Western Pennsylvania, in
1971, to investigate whether a copayment insurance plan alters
hospital use. The report discusses 1969 inpatient claims for two
groups: Group A, having a full-service benefit contract; and Group
B, having the same benefits but with a copayment by the subscriber of five dollars per day. The design controls for differences
in age, sex, marital status and geographical residence. Effect of
copayment on hospital use was measured by the following five
indices: average length of stay; average benefits per admission;

average benefits per day; admissions per 1,000 members; and patient days per 1,000 members. The overall conclusion of the study is that a five dollar per day copayment has no significant effect on hospital use, as measured by the above indices.
Hospital Abstracts IN1–7455

Hardwick, C. Patrick; Myers, Susan B.; Woodruff, Linnis
Incentive Reimbursement: Prospects, Proposals, Plans and Programs
Blue Cross of Western Pennsylvania, Pittsburgh, Pa., 1969, 81 pp.

A collection of precis of recent articles and papers on incentive reimbursements grouped under the following headings: "Proposals and Programs of Blue Cross Plans," "Capitation Plans," "Other Suggested Plans," and "Health Manpower—Hospital Effectiveness."
Hospital Abstract IN3–5494

Hardwick, C.P. and Wolfe, Harvey
A Multifaceted Approach to Incentive Reimbursement
Medical Care, Vol. 8, No. 3, May-June 1970, pp. 173–188

This multifaceted approach to incentive reimbursement details three distinct experiments that are being tested in Western Pennsylvania. The departmentalized plans involve the placement of industrial engineers in three hospitals to work as an arm of the hospital's administrative team in seeking and analyzing potential cost-reduction situations and making recommendations to improve the existing system. Incentives are paid to hospitals on the basis of real savings made for each program that is implemented. The second approach described utilizes multivariate regression analysis in determining the coefficients which express the relationship between total cost and such independent variables as services, education, case-mix, medical staff composition, and location. Incentives are an integral part and will be paid on the difference between projected and actual costs. The other approach involves a negotiated budget-incentive in which an effort has been made to control hospital expenditures through accurate forecasting and agreement as to reasonableness of them. Evaluation of these alternatives should contribute significantly to the identification of those that are most feasible for general application. In addition, the effectiveness of each method in checking hospital costs will aid in the determination of which approach should be developed and refined further so that cost consciousness and efficiency become prime hospital objectives.
Hospital Abstract IN2–5615

Heaton, Harley L.; Johnson, Stephen P.; Fox, Kathryn E.; Koontz, Michael D.; Rhodes, John H.
Analysis of the New Jersey Hospital Prospective Reimbursement System: 1968–1973.

The analysis of the prospective reimbursement system utilized in 89 short term, general, acute care hospitals in New Jersey from 1968–1973 is discussed. A description and history of the New Jersey Prospective Reimbursement Program, best categorized as a budget review system, is presented. The evaluation addresses itself to the following hypotheses: (1) when under the prospective reimbursement program, hospitals will contain the rate of cost increases from year to year; (2) hospitals under the program will maximize productivity; (3) due to cost minimization, there will be a decrease in quality of care following entry into the program. No statistically significant relationships between prospective reimbursement as practiced in the State of New Jersey and hospital cost, productivity, or quality of care were demonstrated.
Hospital Abstract 18897 IN

Hedinger, Frederic R.
The Social Role of Blue Cross: Progress and Problems
Inquiry, Vol. v, No. 2, June 1968, pp. 3–12

This article traces the historical background and philosophical roots of Blue Cross and discusses the influence exerted by the entrance of the commercial insurance industry into the field of hospital care financing. Local control, community rating and full-service benefits are explored from the philosophical and competitive viewpoint. Author concludes that Blue Cross is closer to the commercial insurance than the social insurance model and suggests two points of view (1) that Blue Cross has fulfilled its original mission with the acceptance of a new field of service or (2) that Blue Cross is a failure because many of its social points of philosophy have been discarded or modified.
Hospital Abstract IN2019

Hill, Daniel B.
An Economic Analysis of Health Insurance with Special Reference to Blue Cross
Purdue University, Lafayette, Ind., 1971, 183 pp.
Available from University Microfilms

Study examines the role which health insurance plans occupy in the United States health sector economy. Using the Blue Cross system of health insurance, representing a midpoint between the

commercial health insurance companies and government health insurance programs, as a focus, an optimal health insurance plan is developed. This optimal plan takes into account standards of health in service benefit structures, alternative methods of financing personal health care expenses, methods of reimbursing providers of health care services, and associated activities which influence the quantity, distribution, and costs of health care services, and associated activities which influence the quantity, distribution, and costs of health care services. The Blue Cross example is introduced to study the feasibility of using the optimal plan concept as a blueprint for the operation of a private health insurance plan. The assumptions used in developing the optimal plan are summarized into six major assumptions, which were then tested within the constraints imposed by existing data. Data are drawn from Blue Cross sources, an experiment in which the author participated and various published sources. Results are discussed, and some broad policy implications are considered.
Hospital Abstract IN1–7670

Institute of Medicine
Medicare-Medicaid Reimbursement Policies
The Institute, National Academy of Medicine, Washington, D.C., 1976, 406 pp.

This is the final report on studies conducted by the Institute of Medicine concerning alternative equitable methods of reimbursing physicians under Medicare and Medicaid in hospitals which have teaching programs approved under the Social Security Act of 1973. Data were gathered from a national survey questionnaire sent to 1400 teaching hospitals in the U.S. and detailed field investigations of 96 teaching hospitals. Analysis indicated that house officers have more responsibility and less supervision by teaching physicians when they are taking care of non-private patients. The 20 hospitals in the sample with mostly non-private patients included 19 that were publically owned, 11 of which used cost-based or compensation related methods of payment for physicians' services. The nine others used fee-based methods. The study evaluated six alternative methods for Medicare reimbursement of physicians' services in teaching hospitals: present policy; conventional fee; proposed "fees" or "costs" under Section 227 of the 1973 Social Security Act; unified payment; and lump sum payment. Analysis indicated no one method would constitute appropriate and equitable compensation in all teaching hospital circum-

stances. In analyzing the effect of current reimbursement policies on specialty and geographic distribution of physicians and the training of foreign medical graduates (FMGs), the study found that primary care is generally undersupplied and surgery oversupplied. Data indicated that Medicaid and Medicare favored present patterns of the educational process and greater specialization more than the establishment of new training-ambulatory care. Data also show that prevailing changes and general pattern of physician fees tend to be higher in areas with high physician-to-population ratios. High Medicare fees were also associated with concentration of hospital beds and medical schools, high income areas, large metropolitan areas and West Coast counties. The study found that the more closely a hospital is affiliated with a medical school, the less likely it is to have an above average concentration of FMGs. Because of the decreasing number of positions likely to be available for FMGs, the study recommends elimination of existing incentives for physician immigration, including removal of Medicine as a shortage profession under Department of Labor's Schedule A.
Hospital Abstract 18619 IN

Lewis, Charles E. and Keairnes, Harold W.
  Controlling Costs of Medical Care by Expanding Insurance Coverage
  The New England Journal of Medicine, Vol. 282, No. 25, June 18, 1970, pp. 1,405–1,412

Special benefits were provided without additional charge to a randomly selected group of 5,000 subscribers of a Blue Cross plan. These benefits covered the costs of diagnostic and treatment services rendered outside hospitals. The experimental benefits did not affect hospitalization and patterns of care: no significant reductions were noted in admissions, days of stay and payments among the experimental and two control groups. Our observations support others indicating that coverage for ambulatory care does not reduce costs for hospital services as organized at present.

Despite an intensive informational campaign, few subscribers and physicians were aware of the change of benefits. The expected relation between income and frequency of physician contact was not evident among those receiving special benefits. Of all the special benefits paid, 18 percent were for psychiatric services to 0.7 percent of the subscribers; 8.7 percent of physicians in practice received 44 percent of all special-benefit dollars.
Hospital Abstract IN2–5864

Lynch, Catherine
  Reimbursement of Hospitals by Blue Cross: The Need for Subscriber Participation

Columbia Journal of Law and Social Problems, 11:2, 1975, pp. 189–230.

The reimbursement technique of Associated Hospital Services (AHS), A Blue Cross Plan in the New York City metropolitan area, is examined, and the internal review mechanism by which hospitals may appeal reimbursement rates is explored. AHS uses a complex formula to determine the rates at which it will reimburse member hospitals. Per diem reimbursable expense is the central concept of the reimbursement formula; it is computed for each hospital by dividing the number of patient days into the hospital's total reimbursable expense (both operating expense and capital costs). The per diem reimbursable expense for the base year is 2 years prior to the year for which rates are promulgated. The AHS reimbursement approach also considers capital improvement, community service costs, and research and educational programs. The rate review procedure is quasi-judicial and involves a hearing at which parties can be represented by counsel and post-hearing briefs. This mechanism has been successful in developing objective standards to be applied in determining whether a hospital is entitled to rate relief. An alternative to the adversary procedure is a settlement procedure. Governmental approval of reimbursement stems from the recognition that reimbursement rates determine premiums and that hospitals must receive third-party reimbursements to meet the health care needs of the community. A plan for subscriber participation in the ratemaking and approval process is proposed. (Author's abstract adapted)
Hospital Abstract 17834 IN

McCarthy, Carol
  Incentive Reimbursement as an Impetus to Cost Containment

Inquiry, 12, 4, 1975, pp. 320–329.

This paper describes and compares five experimental incentive reimbursement programs which utilize industrial engineering, budgetary or physician-expander approaches. It also outlines a number of methods for calculating incentive payments and presents recommendations to stimulate greater success through the incentive reimbursement approach.
Hospital Abstract 19127 IN

Markel, Gene A.
Pre-Case Reimbursement for Medical Care
Pennsylvania Blue Shield, Camp Hill, PA 17011, 1977, 62 pp.

An experimental program was established to test and evaluate the concept of reimbursing physicians for in-hospital medical care on a case basis, instead of the traditional disaggregated fee-for-service approach. Physician reimbursement amounts were based upon patient's discharge diagnoses, using a schedule of diagnosis categories based upon ICDA classifications. Primary research objectives were to test the effects of per case reimbursement upon inpatient hospital utilization, and to determine any associated changes in medical care costs. Comparisons with cross-sectional and longitudinal control groups indicate some modest favorable changes in average length-of-stay, with concomitant potential cost savings.
Hospital Abstract 17719 IN

Menchik, Mark D.
Hospital Use Under Medicaid In New York City
New York City Rand Institute, 1977, 244 pp.

Findings from an analysis of inpatient hospital utilization by New York City's (NYC) Medicaid population are presented. Data were taken from hospital claims approved for payment from May–December 1973. The study developed procedures for the regular production of two computerized client-oriented files to facilitate the analysis: Medicaid Admission File; and User History File. Analysis indicates that the blind and disabled have the highest rate of hospitalization in the welfare population, but all groups of welfare recipients studied have hospital use rates higher than corresponding persons in the total NYC population; heavy users constitute 8 percent of all users, but account for 48 percent of the hospital days for all Medicaid users and 45 percent of all Medicaid hospital costs, averaging $7302 in hospital costs compared with $450 for light users. It is suggested that explanation for the extensive hospitalization of the Medicaid population include: poor health status; disincentives to obtaining early ambulatory care; inadequacy of post-discharge care; and lack of incentives for hospitals to shorten stays. The study recommends focusing surveillance and utilization review procedures on heavy users and orienting medical counseling and comprehensive testing to heavy users.
Hospital Abstract 19291 HF

Michigan Blue Shield
Blue Shield of Michigan Family Health Expenditure Survey 1972–1973
Michigan Blue Shield, Detroit, Mich., 1975, 32 pp.

This study investigates how the Blue Cross-Blue Shield population compares with those having other types of coverage or no insurance at all, and reports on the amount that Blue Cross-Blue Shield subscribers were obliged to spend in utilizing services not covered by their insurance. The investigation was inaugurated in order to furnish this information by gathering demographic data and out-of-pocket health care disbursement information. Data were collected from families living within the city of Detroit first in September 1971-August 1972, then again in September 1972-August 1973. The second sample is compared to the first in order to observe if any particular trends exist in any of the variables analyzed.
Hospital Abstract 13271 IN

Morehead, Mildred A.; Zanes, Anne; Donaldson, Rose
Attitudes, Utilization, and Out-of-Pocket Costs for Health Services
School of Public Health and Administrative Medicine, Columbia University, New York, N.Y., 1967, 170 pp.
Available from University Microfilms

Report of household interviews of selected families participating in the Teamster Comprehensive Care Program (TCP). Study was designed to measure costs, attitudes, and utilization by participating families, and to focus on factors leading families to participate in TCP. Four principal groups were sampled: those who joined TCP when there was no charge for the program, and those who did not; and those who joined TCP who had previously agreed to pay $4.00 a week per family for health services and those who were not in the program. Findings show that those who did not join TCP reported higher utilization of health services, higher costs, and no difference in number or type of reported illness than those who did join, indicating that the apparent motivation to join TCP was more for the financial security of the plan than for actual medical necessity.
Hospital Abstract IN3019

Newhouse, Joseph P. and Taylor, Vincent
Medical Costs, Health Insurance, and Public Policy
Rand Corporation, Santa Monica, Calif., c. 1969, 27 pp.

The paper reports on health insurance in relation to excessive

medical costs and discusses a number of constructive steps that could be taken to modify the effects of insurance. A new type of hospital insurance, which has been termed variable cost insurance, is proposed. By greatly increasing consumer concern with hospital costs, variable cost insurance should slow the rise in these costs. It would also affect inequities in the present insurance system.
Hospital Abstract IN1–5532

O'Donnell, Paul J., Jr.
A Consideration of Third Party Cost Reimbursement and Its Influence on the Price of Patient Care in Hospitals
Xavier University, Cincinnati, Ohio, 1970, 27 pp.
Available from University Microfilms

Report of a study made of third-party reimbursement of hospital costs and of alternatives to current systems of payment. The history of cost reimbursement in the United States is traced to the present time; state and federal programs and the role of Blue Cross are discussed. The phenomenon of increased costs of health care resulting from a cost-based system of reimbursement is examined; other factors, such as increasing demands for service, inflation, higher wages and salaries and the cost of new technology are also considered. It is recommended that a capitation, or per capita, system of reimbursement to medical groups be instituted. Such a system is described and its advantages explained.
Hospital Abstract IN0–5854

Phelps, Charles E. and Newhouse, Joseph P.
Coinsurance and the Demand for Medical Services
Rand Corporation, Santa Monica, Calif., 1974, 63 pp.

Paper analyzes consumers' response to changes in the coinsurance rate for various medical services. Using a formal model of utility maximization, a model of demand for medical services is developed for when reimbursement insurance is present and when there are time costs involved in purchasing medical care. A number of data sources are used to estimate elasticities of demand for medical care services and these results are compared with results of three other studies. Results show services with a relatively high time price exhibit relatively low coinsurance or price elasticities. Services with relatively high money-price to time-price ratio show considerably higher own-price elasticities. Services with coinsurance rates near zero show low-price elasticities. In percentage terms, it is estimated eight to seventeen percent more services would be demanded at a zero coinsurance rate than at a 25 percent rate. A pattern of low elasticity for hospital services, larger one for office visits and largest for home visits is developed in the zero to 25 percent range of coverage. Paper concludes evidence indicates coinsurance is not irrelevant to choice; irrespective of who makes the decision, greater coinsurance implies less use of services and the amount of reduction varies by type of service.

Hospital Abstract 13674 IN

Rabin, David L.; Bice, Thomas W.; Starfield, Barbara
Use of Health Services by Baltimore Medicaid Recipients
Medical Care, Vol. 12, No. 7, July 1974, pp. 561–570

Medicaid legislation intended to remove financial barriers to health care for the poor. A household interview survey of the Metropolitan Baltimore area in 1968–69 shows that persons on Medicaid are the highest users of health services. More Medicaid recipients in Baltimore visited a physician in two weeks and one year; more were admitted one or more times to a hospital. The total number of days in a hospital per 100 persons was considerably greater for Medicaid adults.

Higher utilization of health services in Baltimore can be explained by the fact that Medicaid recipients are sicker than the rest of the population. Fewer Medicaid recipients are healthy; more are acutely, chronically, or acutely and chronically ill; more are chronically ill with impairment.

The higher rate of chronic illness accounts for higher hospital use for the working age population. When compared by morbidity categories, ill Medicaid recipients are using services at least at the same level as others, but healthy Medicaid recipients are using more services.

Hospital Abstract 12635 IN

Restuccia, Joseph D. and Chernow, Robert A.
Utilization and Cost of Mental and Health Benefits: A Comparison of Insurance Plans
School of Public Health, University of California, Berkeley, Calif., 1974, 23 pp.
Available from University Microfilms

This paper provides an insight into the problems surrounding the exclusion of mental illnesses in health insurance and prepayment plans, and describes the emerging public policies that foster benefits for mental illness. The paper is designed to help persons

planning or managing medical care programs to understand mental health benefits. The authors review and analyze comparative experience among health plans and insurers, and identify important factors affecting utilization and costs.
Hospital Abstract 13313 IN

Riedel, Donald C.; Walden, Daniel C.; Singsen, Antone G.; Meyers, Samuel; Krantz, Goldie; Henderson, Marie
Federal Employees Health Benefits Program Utilization Study
U.S. DHEW Pub. No. (HRA) 75–3125. Public Health Service, Rockville Md., 1975, 144 pp.

This report is a comparative utilization study of two alternate forms of health maintenance organization. The purpose of the study is to identify the factors that account for the observed lower rate of hospital admissions experienced by beneficiaries of a prepaid group health association, in contrast to subscribers of a traditional fee-for-service plan. The authors describe these two health plans presenting a comparison of premiums and benefits. Preliminary findings are reported in the following areas: (1) rates of hospital admissions for plan subscribers; (2) sex and age composition for each plan membership; (3) proportion of each subscriber group admitted to teaching hospitals; (4) attendance to plan subscribers by specialized physicians; (5) diagnostic-specific rates for subscribers to the two plans; (6) comparative admission rates; and (7) comparative lengths of hospital stay.
Hospital Abstract 14018 IN

Rosett, Richard N.
Role of Health Insurance in the Health Services Sector
National Bureau of Economic Research, Inc., New York, 10010, 1976, 548 pp.

Research papers on the market for health insurance, the effects of health insurance on the market for health services, and on national health insurance were organized for a conference sponsored by the Universities-National Bureau Committee for Economic Research. The subjects of examination include a welfare analysis of changes in health coinsurance rates, the joint demand for health insurance and preventive medicine, group health insurance as a local public good, and the demand for reimbursement insurance. The effects of insurance on the health services market are studied in relation to the demand for health care among the urban poor, the family provision of children's health, the price and income elasticities of medical care services, physician fee inflation as evidenced in the 1960's. Several aspects of national health insurance

are investigated: (1) mortality, disability, and the normative economics of Medicare; (2) the impact of Medicare and Medicaid on access to medical care; (3) the expenditure, utilization, and pricing of insured health care in Canada; and (4) the effect of national health on the price and quantity of medical care.
Hospital Abstract 17765 IN

Rowland, Diane
Data Rich and Information Poor; Medicare's Resources for Prospective Rate Setting
Harvard Center for Community Health and Medical Care, Boston, 1976, 171 pp.

Hospital and related Medicare data collected and used by the Social Security Administration are reviewed with a view toward their potential uses for hospital rate setting. An overview of the two separate but coordinated insurance coverages under Medicare—hospital insurance (Part A) and supplementary medical insurance (Part B)—is provided. The five computer tapes comprising the basic records for the Medicare program are then described: the master eligibility record, the provider of service record, the hospital insurance utilization record, the medical insurance payment record, and the bill summary record. The statistical analyses and reports derived from these basic records for administrative and evaluative use are discussed. A separate section is then devoted to the annual Medicare cost reports and other sources of hospital cost data, such as the Office of Research and Statistics hospital cost monitoring project. The strengths and limitations of the Medicare data base are then assessed in terms of the potential information requirements of prospective rate setting activities for Medicare. It is noted that, were rate setting mandated for the Medicare program, significant alterations would have to be made in the Medicare data base and its management.
Hospital Abstract 18047 IN

Saward, Ernest W.
The Relevance of Prepaid Group Practice to the Effective Delivery of Health Services
U.S. DHEW, Public Health Service, Health Services and Mental Health Administration, Office of Group Practice Development, Washington, D.C., 1969, 24 pp.

The paper discusses five major problems of administering medical services: 1) the rising cost of medical care; 2) absence of quality standards; 3) manpower shortage; 4) technology gap, and 5) expectation gap between patients' expectations and actual treat-

ment. Dr. Saward proposes the Kaiser Health Plan as an answer to some of these problems and outlines its six basic tenets: 1) prepayment; 2) group practice; 3) medical center facilities; 4) voluntary enrollment; 5) capitation payment; and 6) voluntary coverage. The effectiveness of the Kaiser system is summarized.
Hospital Abstract IN2–6599

Scitovsky, Anne A.; McCall, Nelda
Coinsurance and the Demand for Physician Services: Four Years Later
Social Security Bulletin, 40:5, 1977, pp. 19–27.

In 1971 a study was made of the effects of a 25-percent coinsurance provision on the demand for physician services under a comprehensive prepaid plan for medical care. Comparing physician utilization rates in 1966 (the year before coinsurance was introduced) and 1968 (the first calendar year after the change) showed that coinsurance led to a 24-percent decline in the per capita number of all physician visits that held true regardless of how the data were examined—whether by demographic characteristics of the study population, physician specialization, or place of visit. This effect of coinsurance could be temporary—a kind of shock effect that would wear off. Since there was no conclusive proof of this hypothesis, the authors conducted a followup study, comparing physician utilization rates in 1972 and 1968. They found no evidence of any upward trend in the use of physician services. The overall utilization rate was much the same in 1972 and in 1968, and the rates of the demographic subgroups and types of visits were either much the same or slightly lower. Equally important was the finding that the plan had become relatively unattractive for families in the lowest socioeconomic group who constituted a smaller proportion of the 1972 plan membership than of the pre-coinsurance membership.
Hospital Abstract 17936 IN

Sigmond, Robert M.
Capitation as a Method of Reimbursement to Hospitals in a Multihospital Area in *Reimbursement Incentives for Medical Care*
Office of Research and Statistics, Social Security Administration, Washington, D.C., 1968

A plan for reimbursing hospitals on a per capita basis, thus encouraging efficiency and discouraging overextended care. The Yuma County Blue Cross Plan is used as a successful example of the concept. Objections to the idea are also discussed briefly.
Hospital Abstract IN0013

Skinner, Douglas; Meltzer, Alfred
Analysis of Prospective Reimbursement Systems: Western Pennsylvania
Applied Management Science, Inc., Silver Spring, MD, 1975, 269 pp.

The major findings and recommendations of an experiment for assessing the impact of prospective reimbursement on the behavior of participating institutions in terms of changes in costs and quality of care and the applicability of such a prospective reimbursement system in other locations is discussed. The study evaluates the Blue Cross of Western Pennsylvania (BCWP) Prospective Reimbursement (PR) system which operated in 5 rural hospitals during FY 72–74. The system involved budget review and the application of formulas in the computation of the rate of reimbursement. Total and per diem cost increases were lower in the prospective reimbursement hospitals as compared with the control hospitals. The cost containment results were achieved mainly through the actions of administrators to increase volume and improve efficiency. Outpatient volume increased and the number of admissions increased in response to new services and efforts to recruit additional medical staff. Several findings concerning the behavioral characteristics of key participants in the rural community hospital sector were presented.
Hospital Abstract 18862 IN

Social Security Administration
Financing Mental Health Care Under Medicare and Medicaid
Office of Research and Statistics, Social Security Administration, Washington, D.C., Research Report No. 37, 1971

This report analyzes the use of and expenditures for psychiatric services for the aged under Medicare and Medicaid, especially as these relate to the limitations on mental illness coverage under these programs. Appended are a legislative history of federal financing of psychiatric services and an outline of optional coverage and exclusions in state Medicaid programs. For the years 1967–70 this report outlines the use of Medicare and Medicaid resources for psychiatric services on a state-by-state basis.
Hospital Abstract 12211 IN

Stuart, Bruce C.
Who Gains from Public Health Programs?
The Annals of the American Academy of Political and Social Science, Jan. 1972, pp. 145–150

Analysis of the economic impacts arising from the introduction of Medicare and Medicaid into federal and state budgets leads one to question the actual magnitude of gains which recipients can expect to obtain from new funding in the health area. A modified cost-benefit analysis of Medicare/Medicaid income effects on program recipients, non-recipients, and physicians from 1966 to 1968 shows that scarcely 56 percent of the $14.8 billion spent on the two programs represented gains to recipients. Over the same period, physicians received average net gains of between $5,400 and $7,400 over what would have been the case in the absence of both programs. The implications of these findings apply as much to the several proposals for national health insurance as they do to Medicaid and Medicare. It can be shown that the President's health insurance plan, among others, would result in a similar if not larger unintended allocation of public funds. This raises serious questions of equity in the development of national health policy. Hospital Abstract 08427 IN

Thompson, John L.
Third Party Involvement in Emergency Medical Services
Blue Shield of Massachusetts, Inc., Boston, 1975, 90 pp.

Third-party involvement in emergency medical services (EMS) need not be confined to the traditional role of reimbursement for covered services. Medicare, Blue Cross, Blue Shield, and commercial insurers can effectively, creatively, and positively impact the EMS delivery system. In this report data related to benefit coverages are briefly reviewed and innovative approaches to third-party involvement in legislation, training, and public education are identified. Based primarily on the experience of Blue Shield of Massachusetts, but also incorporating the activities of other third-parties, the report explores the interface between third-party payers and the public and private ambulance community. Further, the report describes the cooperative working arrangement that existed in Massachusetts between government and private industry in the planning, implementation, and evaluation of a statewide EMS system. The intent of this work is to provide a model for other communities to more fully utilize third-parties as an integral resource in the development of EMS systems throughout the country.
Hospital Abstract 18145 IN

Velthuis, Philip B.
The Hospital-Blue Cross Relationship Post-Medicare
Washington University, Saint Louis, Mo., 1968, 74 pp.
Available from University Microfilms

Study examined effect of Medicare legislation on relationship between Blue Cross and 72 nonfederal, general acute AHA affiliated hospitals in St. Louis area. All hospitals in sample had contracts with Blue Cross and were eligible to participate in Medicare. Questionnaires were mailed to the 72 hospital administrators with 46 usable responses. Two hypotheses were tested: 1.) since Medicare legislation, with Blue Cross acting as administrative intermediary for Medicare, friction between Blue Cross and hospitals has decreased; 2.) in cases where hospital contracts, in force prior to Medicare, contained unenforced controls and restrictions on hospitals similar to Medicare requirements, Blue Cross has used advent of Medicare to attempt stricter enforcement. Findings indicate a worsening of relations between Blue Cross and the hospitals but data were not sufficient to positively relate increased friction to advent of Blue Cross as administrative intermediary for Medicare. There was some indication of stricter Blue Cross contract enforcement but insufficient positive responses to apply this to any other Blue Cross plans. Shortcomings of questionnaire and limiting factors which may have affected study are discussed. Copy of questionnaire is in appendix.
Hospital Abstract IN2028

Waldman, Saul
Average Increase in Costs: An Incentive Reimbursement Formula for Hospitals in *Reimbursement Incentives for Medical Care*
Office of Research and Statistics, Social Security Administration, Washington, D.C., 1968, 15 pp.

A plan for an average increase in costs' reimbursement that defines a plan to emphasize hospital incentive and efficiency, while not encouraging overuse of facilities or extended length of stay, yet still maintaining high quality of care. Problems of the plan discussed are: treatment of extraordinary costs, methods for grouping hospitals to establish "averages," amelioration of financial loss, insuring highest quality of care, and implementation of the plan.
Hospital Abstract IN0014

Waldman, Saul
Tax Credits for Private Health Insurance: Cost Estimates for Alternative Proposals for 1970
Medical Care, Vol. viii, No. 5, Sept.-Oct. 1970, pp. 353–367

Among the recent proposals for a Federal program to finance the health care costs of the nation are plans to provide tax credits against the individual income tax to offset the cost of premiums for private health insurance. A cost analysis of four tax credit proposals is presented, including a plan limited to the poor, a proposal by Professor Rashi Fein of Harvard University, a bill (H.R. 9835) introduced by Representative Fulton of Tennessee, and the "Medicredit" plan of the American Medical Association. The methodology employed is to analyze the cost of the four plans on a comparable basis (assuming a $500 maximum tax credit) so that variations in the costs of the plans reflect differences in their eligibility and related provisions. On this basis, the gross costs of the four plans range from $6 billion to $21 billion. An analysis is provided concerning the effect of tax credit proposals on federal and state expenditures for the Medicaid program, and the gross costs are adjusted for the estimated reduction in these expenditures. A further adjustment is made for the projected reduction in the amount of deductions for medical expenses taken on income tax returns. After the two types of adjustments, the costs of the plans range from $5 billion to $17 billion.

Hospital Abstract IN1–6243

Wirick, Grover
Hospital Use and Characteristics of Michigan Blue Cross Subscribers: An Analytical Interview Survey
Bureau of Hospital Administration, The University of Michigan, Ann Arbor, Mich., 1972, 208 pp.

A two-stage probability sample of Michigan Blue Cross subscribers was interviewed in depth with the objective of determining whether demographic and social characteristics of subscribers and their families, and knowledge of, and attitudes toward hospital insurance and related health subjects influenced the amount of hospital care consumed. Interview data were augmented by Blue Cross records on enrollment and service rendered. The period studied was March 1, 1968 to May 31, 1969, and over 700 interviews were obtained. A small sample of physicians was also interviewed to determine how they saw their role in hospital utilization.

Two highly sophisticated statistical techniques were employed to analyze the results, a multiple classification analysis and a new computer program called automatic interaction detection (AID) III, both based on analysis of variance. The emphasis in model construction was on finding of interactions, i.e., situations where the relationship between the dependent variable and specific predictor variables is different among different subgroups of the population.

Findings failed to support the hypothesis that experience rating (setting insurance rates on the basis of recent experience for particular groups) tends to limit hospital use. A number of variables, including marital status, age, race, occupation, and income, were found to account systematically for a modest amont of hospital use, but numerous complex interactions limit the usefulness of these relationships. Limitations on the model and data gathering instruments were found to confuse the nature of the effect of subscriber opinions about hospitals and doctors on hospital use, and no effect of subscriber opinions about insurance and Blue Cross on hospital use could be found.

An interesting finding of the doctor survey was an apparent disinterest on the part of physicians in the prcblems of rapidly rising hospital costs, especially as these problems affect the hospitals and patients.

Hospital Abstract 09231 IN

Witkin, Erwin
The Impact of Medicare
Thomas Publishing Co., Springfield, Ill., 1971, 286 pp.

A history of the Medicare program and its present impact on health care delivery in this country, by the former Chief Medical Consultant to the Bureau of Health Insurance of the Social Security Administration.

Hospital Abstract 08572 IN

Wolkstein, Irwin
The Legislative History of Hospital Reimbursement in *Reimbursement Incentives for Medical Care*
Office of Research and Statistics, Social Security Administration, Washington, D.C., 1968, 21 pp.

A concise history of hospital cost reimbursement from 1920 to the present including explanations of: Blue Cross; Plans in Philadelphia, Cleveland, New York; The Forand Bill, King Anderson Bills, Medicare; and legislation before Cor.gress in 1968. Also discussed are the AHA's recommended principles for hospital reimbursement, and how reimbursement can be an incentive for economy and efficiency.

Hospital Abstract IN0003

MANPOWER

Ambrose, Donald M.
A Sensor and Monitor for a Manpower Control System
University of Michigan, Ann Arbor, Mich., 1973.
Available from University Microfilms.

This paper describes a manpower control system designed for a 287 bed community hospital. The control system is meant to monitor the use of manpower in an attempt to improve manpower allocation decisions. Specifically, the paper cites some of the relevant literature on the topic, and describes in detail the design of a four-level comparison Manpower Report and how it should be used. The author also discusses the mechanics of the generation of the report. The Report: details of hours used and dollars expended, comparing actual performance against a standard of expected performance; and flags problem areas based on preestablished control limits. The Report is designed to be generated by a computer, using payroll information as a data base for actual performance and the yearly budget as the standard of expected performance. The goal of the system is to improve the use of manpower and thus control the cost of the hospital's largest operating expenditure, personnel.
Hospital Abstract 10391 MP

UTILIZATION REVIEW

California Medical Association
Guidelines for Utilization Review
The Association, San Francisco, Calif., 1965, 31 pp.

Produced as a guide for medical staffs in developing utilization review plans. Outlines in detail four factors in medical staff utilization review function: 1. Various medical staff bylaw provisions that can be adopted; 2. Organization and composition of committee for utilization review; 3. Relationship to claims administration and review; 4. Methodology for procedures including sampling techniques, clarification of term "extended duration," methods of gathering information and transmitting to review committee and arrangements for committee reports and their dissemination. Appendices include samples of suggested forms, description of 2-phased stratified random sampling technique, a prototype utilization review plan for 200 bed hospital and current statements by national leaders about utilization review functions.
Hospital Abstract HE0135

List of Publishers and Sources

Abstracts of Health Care Management Studies
  M2240 School of Public Health
  The University of Michigan
  Ann Arbor, Mich 48109

The Accounting Review
  1507 Chicago Ave.
  Evanston, Ill. 60201

The University of Alabama
  Graduate Program in Hospital Administration
  Birmingham, Ala. 35233

American Association of Medical Clinics
  P.O. Box 949
  Alexandria, Va. 22313

American College of Hospital Administrators
  840 North Lake Shore Drive
  Chicago, Ill. 60611

American Hospital Association
  840 North Lake Shore Drive
  Chicago, Ill. 60611

American Institute of Industrial Engineering
  345 E. 47th St.
  New York, N.Y. 10017

American Journal of Public Health
  1015 Eighteenth St., N.W.
  Washington, D.C. 20036

American Management Association
  135 W. 50th St.
  New York, N.Y. 10020

Annals of the American Academy of Political and Social Sciences
  3937 Chestnut St.
  Philadelphia, Pa. 19104

Applied Economics
  Pergamon Press
  Maxwell House
  Fairview Park
  Elmsford, N.Y. 10523

Aspen Systems Corporation
20010 Century Boulevard
Germantown, Maryland 20767

Association of American Medical Colleges
2530 Ridge Ave.
Evanston, Ill. 60201

Ballinger Publishing Co.
17 Dunster St.
Harvard Square
Cambridge, Mass. 02138

Baylor University—Army
U.S. Army Medical Field Service School
Brooke Army Medical Center
Fort Sam Houston, Tex. 78234

Blue Cross Association
840 North Lake Shore Drive
Chicago, Ill. 60611

Blue Cross Reports
840 North Lake Shore Drive
Chicago, Ill. 60611

Blue Cross of Western Pennsylvania
One Smithfield St.
Pittsburgh, Pa. 15222

The Brookings Institution
1775 Massachusetts Ave., N.W.
Washington, D.C. 20036

Bulletin of the New York Academy of Medicine
2 East 103rd St.
New York, N.Y. 10029

Bulletin of the Operations Research Society of America
Mt. Royal and Guilford Ave.
Baltimore, Md. 21202

University of California—Los Angeles
Program in Hospital Administration
School of Public Health
Los Angeles, Calif. 90024

Catholic Hospital Association
1438 S. Grand Blvd.
Saint Louis, Mo. 63104

Cases in Health Services
Schering Library of Health Care
Harvard Center for Community Health and Medical Care
643 Huntington Ave.
Boston, Mass. 02115

University of Chicago
Graduate Program in Hospital Administration
5720 South Woodlawn Ave.
Chicago, Ill. 60637

The University of Chicago Press
5750 Ellis Ave.
Chicago, Ill. 60637

Citizens Research Council of Michigan
500 Guardian Building South
Detroit, Mich. 48226

City University of New York
Center for Social Research
33 W. 42nd St.
New York, N.Y. 10036

College and University Press
263 Chapel St.
New Haven, Conn. 06513

Columbia University
Graduate Program in Hospital Administration
600 West 168th St.
New York, N.Y. 10032

The Committee for National Health Insurance
806 15th St., N.W.
Washington, D.C. 20005

Community Systems Foundation
1130 Hill Street
Ann Arbor, Mich. 48104

Coopers and Lybrand
1900 Three Girard Plaza
Philadelphia, Pa. 19123

CSF, Ltd.
3001 S. State Street
Ann Arbor, Mich. 48104

Dell Publishing Company, Inc.
750 Third Ave.
New York, N.Y. 10017

Doubleday & Co., Inc. (Anchor Books)
501 Franklin Ave.
New York, N.Y. 11531

Duke University
Graduate Program in Hospital Administration
Box 3018
Durham, N.C. 27706

Financial Management
University of Akron
Akron, Ohio 44304

The George Washington University
Department of Health Care Administration
Washington, D.C. 20006

University of Georgia Press
Waddell Hall
Athens, Ga. 30602

Group Health Association of America, Inc.
  Suite 203
  1717 Massachusetts Ave., N.W.
  Washington, D.C. 20036
Halsted Press
  605 Third Ave.
  New York, N.Y. 10016
Harvard Business Review
  Soldiers Field
  Boston, Mass. 02163
Health Administration Press
  M2240 School of Public Health
  The University of Michigan
  Ann Arbor, Mich. 48109
Health Insurance Institute
  277 Park Ave.
  New York, N.Y. 10017
Health Insurance Statistics
  Social Security Administration
  Washington, D.C. 20201
Health Services Reports
  Superintendent of Documents
  Government Printing Office
  Washington, D.C. 20402
Health Services Research
  840 North Lake Shore Drive
  Chicago, Ill. 60611
D.C. Heath Co.
  Lexington, Mass. 02173
Holden-Day Publishing Co.,
  500 Sansome St.
  San Francisco, Calif. 94111
Holt, Rinehart and Winston, Inc.
  383 Madison Ave.
  New York, N.Y. 10017
Hospital Accounting
  see *Hospital Financial Management*
Hospital Administration
  840 North Lake Shore Drive
  Chicago, Ill. 60611
Hospital Administration in Canada
  1450 Don Mills Road
  Don Mills, Ontario, Canada
Hospital Financial Management
  666 North Lake Shore Drive, Suite 245
  Chicago, Ill. 60611
Hospital Forum
  4777 Sunset Blvd.
  Los Angeles, Calif. 90027

Hospital and Health Services Administration
    840 North Lake Shore Drive
    Chicago, Ill. 60611

Hospital Progress
    1438 S. Grand Blvd.
    Saint Louis, Mo. 63104

Hospital Research and Educational Trust
    840 North Lake Shore Drive
    Chicago, Ill. 60611

Hospitals
    840 North Lake Shore Drive
    Chicago, Ill. 60611

Hospital Topics
    4747 W. Peterson Ave.
    Chicago, Ill. 60646

Information Resources Press
    2100 M St., N.W., Suite 316
    Washington, D.C.

Inquiry
    840 North Lake Shore Drive
    Chicago, Ill. 60611

Institute of Gerontology
    The University of Michigan
    Ann Arbor, Mich. 48109

University of Iowa
    Graduate Program in Hospital and Health Administration
    S-517 Westlawn
    Iowa City, Iowa 52241

Richard D. Irwin, Inc.
    1818 Ridge Rd.
    Homewood, Ill. 60430

Journal of American Osteopathic Association
    212 E. Ohio St.
    Chicago, Ill. 60610

Kaiser Foundation
    300 Lakeside Drive
    Oakland, Calif. 94604

Law and Contemporary Problems
    Duke Station
    Durham, N.C.

McGraw-Hill Book Company, Inc.
    Princeton Rd.
    Hightstown, N.J. 08520

Management of Personnel Quarterly
    Graduate School of Business Administration
    The University of Michigan
    Ann Arbor, Mich. 48109

Manitoba Hospital Association
   377 Colony St.
   Winnipeg 2 Manitoba, Canada

Massachusetts Hospital Association
   5 New England Executive Park
   Burlington, Mass. 01803

Medical Care
   East Washington Square
   Philadelphia, Pa. 19105

Medical Care Review
   The School of Public Health
   The University of Michigan
   109 S. Observatory
   Ann Arbor, Mich. 48109

Medical College of Virginia
   Virginia Commonwealth University
   Department of Hospital and Health Administration
   MCV Station
   Richmond, Va. 23298

Medical Group Management
   956 Metropolitan Bldg.
   Denver, Colo. 80202

Mentor Books
   New American Library, Inc.
   1301 6th Ave.
   New York, N.Y. 10019

The Micah Corporation
   P.O. Box 152
   Ann Arbor, Mich. 48107

Michigan Blue Shield
   600 E. Layfayette
   Detroit, Mich. 48226

Michigan State Department of Social Services
   Lewis Cass Bldg.
   Lansing, Mich. 48913

Michigan State University
   East Lansing, Mich.

The University of Michigan
   Bureau of Health Economics
   The School of Public Health
   109 S. Observatory St.
   Ann Arbor, Mich. 48109

The University of Michigan
   Program and Bureau of Hospital Administration
   The School of Public Health II
   1420 Washington Heights, Third Floor
   Ann Arbor, Mich. 48109

The University of Michigan
   The School of Public Health
   109 S. Observatory
   Ann Arbor, Mich. 48109

Milbank Memorial Fund Quarterly
   40 Wall Street
   New York, N.Y. 10005

Mimir Publishers, Inc.
   1405 Monroe St.
   Madison, Wisc. 53711

University of Minnesota
   The Program in Hospital Administration
   Box 87
   Mayo Building
   Minneapolis, Minn. 55455

MIT Press
   28 Carleton St.
   Cambridge, Mass. 02142

The Modern Hospital
   1050 Merchandise Mart
   Chicago, Ill. 60654

C.V. Mosby Co.
   3207 Washington Blvd.
   St. Louis, Mo. 63103

National Center for Health Services Research
   U.S. Department of Health, Education and Welfare
   3700 East-West Highway
   Hyattsville, Maryland 20782

National Cooperative Services Center for
   Hospital Management Engineering
   840 North Lake Shore Drive
   Chicago, Ill. 60611

National Technical Information Services
   5285 Port Royal Rd.
   Springfield, Va. 22161

New England Journal of Medicine
   10 Shattuck St.
   Boston, Mass. 02115

New York State Journal of Medicine
   Medical Society of the State of New York
   750 Third Ave.
   New York, N.Y. 10017

Office of Research and Statistics
   Social Security Administration
   Washington, D.C. 20201

Physicians' Record Co.
   3000 S. Ridgeland Ave.
   Berwyn, Ill. 60402

University of Pittsburgh
  Health Law Center
  Pittsburgh, Pa. 15213
Frederick A. Praeger, Publishers
  111 Fourth Ave.
  New York, N.Y. 10003
Prentice-Hall, Inc.
  Englewood Cliffs, N.J. 07632
Pressler Publications
  Bloomington, Ind. 47401
Public Affairs Press
  419 New Jersey Ave.
  Washington, D.C. 20003
Public Health Reports
  Superintendent of Documents
  Washington, D.C. 20402
Quarterly Journal of Economics
  Harvard University Press
  79 Garden St.
  Cambridge, Mass. 02138
Rand Corporation
  1700 Main St.
  Santa Monica, Calif. 90406
Random House, Inc.
  457 Madison Ave.
  New York, N.Y. 10022
Reinhold Publishing Corporation
  430 Park Ave.
  New York, N.Y. 10022
Research and Statistic Notes
  Social Security Administration
  Washington, D.C. 20203
Rinehart, Winston
  see Holt, Reinhart and Winston
The Ronald Press Co.
  79 Madison Ave.
  New York, N.Y. 10016
W.B. Saunders Co.
  W. Washington Square
  Philadelphia, Pa. 19105
Social Security Bulletin
  Superintendent of Documents
  Washington, D.C. 20402
Spectrum Publications, Inc.
  Flushing, N.Y. 11352
Charles C. Thomas Publishing Co.
  301–377 E. Lawrence
  Springfield, Ill. 62705

Trinity University Press
  715 Stadium Drive
  San Antonio, Texas 78284

U.S. Department of Health, Education & Welfare
  330 Independence Ave. S.W.
  Washington, D.C. 20201

U.S. Government Printing Office
  Superintendent of Documents
  Washington, D.C. 20402

University Microfilms, Inc. (Division of Xerox Corp.)
  300 N. Zeeb Rd.
  Ann Arbor, Mich. 48106

Wadsworth Publishing Co., Inc.
  Belmont, Calif. 94002

John Wiley & Sons, Inc.
  605 Third Ave.
  New York, N.Y. 10015

Xavier University
  Graduate Program in Hospital Administration
  Victory Parkway
  Cincinnati, Ohio 45207

Yale University
  Program in Hospital Administration
  School of Medicine
  60 College St.
  New Haven, Conn. 06510

Index